Bisping/Amtsberg   Colour Atlas for the Diagnosis of Bacterial Pathogens in Animals
Farbatlas zur Diagnose bakterieller Infektionserreger der Tiere

Colour Atlas for the Diagnosis of Bacterial Pathogens in Animals

Professor Dr. Wolfgang Bisping
Institute for Microbiology and Infectious Diseases
of the Veterinary College Hanover

Professor Dr. Gunter Amtsberg
Institute for Microbiology and Infectious Diseases
of the Veterinary College Hanover

Translated into English by
Dr. Walter Siller · Edinburgh
Dr. James Phillips · Edinburgh

223 illustrations (180 in colour) and 96 tables

Paul Parey Scientific Publishers · Berlin and Hamburg

Farbatlas zur Diagnose bakterieller Infektionserreger der Tiere

Professor Dr. Wolfgang Bisping
Institut für Mikrobiologie und Tierseuchen
der Tierärztlichen Hochschule Hannover

Professor Dr. Gunter Amtsberg
Institut für Mikrobiologie und Tierseuchen
der Tierärztlichen Hochschule Hannover

Ins Englische übertragen von
Dr. Walter Siller · Edinburgh
Dr. James Phillips · Edinburgh

Mit 223 Abbildungen, davon 180 farbig, und 96 Tabellen

Verlag Paul Parey · Berlin und Hamburg

Authors' addresses:
Professor Dr. med. vet. Wolfgang Bisping/
Professor Dr. med. vet., Dr. med. vet. habil.
Gunter Amtsberg
Institut für Mikrobiologie und Tierseuchen
der Tierärztlichen Hochschule Hannover
Bischofsholer Damm 15
D-3000 Hannover 1

Translators' Addresses:
W. G. Siller, B. Sc., Dr. Med. Vet., M. R. C. V. S.,
Ph. D., F. R. C. Path., F. R. S. E.
13, Swanston Grove, Edinburgh EH10 7BN, Scotland
J. E. Phillips, B. Sc., D. V. M. & S., M. R. C. V. S.,
Department of Veterinary Pathology,
University of Edinburgh, Scotland

Anschrift der Verfasser:
Professor Dr. med. vet. Wolfgang Bisping/
Professor Dr. med. vet., Dr. med. vet. habil.
Gunter Amtsberg
Institut für Mikrobiologie und Tierseuchen
der Tierärztlichen Hochschule Hannover
Bischofsholer Damm 15
D-3000 Hannover 1

Anschrift der Übersetzer:
W. G. Siller, B. Sc., Dr. Med. Vet., M. R. C. V. S.,
Ph. D., F. R. C. Path., F. R. S. E.
13, Swanston Grove, Edinburgh EH10 7BN, Scotland
J. E. Phillips, B. Sc., D. V. M. & S., M. R. C. V. S.,
Department of Veterinary Pathology,
University of Edinburgh, Scotland

CIP-Titelaufnahme der Deutschen Bibliothek

Bisping, Wolfgang:
Colour atlas for the diagnosis of bacterial pathogens in animals / Wolfgang Bisping ; Gunter Amtsberg. Ins Engl. übertr. von Walter Siller ; James Phillips. – Berlin ; Hamburg : Parey, 1988
    Parallelsacht.: Farbatlas zur Diagnose bakterieller Infektionserreger der Tiere
    ISBN 3-489-50716-9
NE: Amtsberg, Gunter:

Cover design: Jan Buchholz und Reni Hinsch,
D-2000 Hamburg 73

© 1988 Paul Parey Scientific Publishers, Berlin and Hamburg. Addresses: Lindenstr. 44–47, D-1000 Berlin 61; Spitalerstr. 12, D-2000 Hamburg 1

ISBN 3-489-50716-9 · Printed in Germany

This work is subject to copyright. All rights are reserved, whether the whole or part of the material is concerned, specifically those rights of translation, reprinting, re-use of illustrations, recitation, broadcasting, reproduction on microfilms or in other ways, and storage in data banks. Duplication of this publication or parts thereof is only permitted under the provisions of the German Copyright Law of September 9, 1965, in its version of June 24, 1985, and a copyright fee must always be paid. Violations fall under the prosecution act of the German Copyright Law.

Typesetting and printing: Saladruck, Steinkopf & Sohn,
D-1000 Berlin 36
Lithography: O. R. T. OffsetReproTechnik
Kirchner + Graser, D-1000 Berlin 61
Binding: Lüderitz & Bauer Buchgewerbe,
D-1000 Berlin 61

Einband: Jan Buchholz und Reni Hinsch,
D-2000 Hamburg 73

© 1988 Verlag Paul Parey, Berlin und Hamburg.
Anschriften: Lindenstr. 44–47, D-1000 Berlin 61;
Spitalerstr. 12, D-2000 Hamburg 1

ISBN 3-489-50716-9 · Printed in Germany

Das Werk ist urheberrechtlich geschützt. Die dadurch begründeten Rechte, insbesondere die der Übersetzung, des Nachdrucks, des Vortrages, der Entnahme von Abbildungen, der Funksendung, der Mikroverfilmung oder der Vervielfältigung auf anderen Wegen und der Speicherung in Datenverarbeitungsanlagen, bleiben, auch bei nur auszugsweiser Verwertung, vorbehalten. Eine Vervielfältigung dieses Werkes oder von Teilen dieses Werkes ist auch im Einzelfall nur in den Grenzen der gesetzlichen Bestimmungen des Urheberrechtsgesetzes der Bundesrepublik Deutschland vom 9. September 1965 in der Fassung vom 24. Juni 1985 zulässig. Sie ist grundsätzlich vergütungspflichtig. Zuwiderhandlungen unterliegen den Strafbestimmungen des Urheberrechtsgesetzes.

Satz und Druck: Saladruck, Steinkopf & Sohn,
D-1000 Berlin 36
Schrift: Borgis Garamond (Satzsystem Linotype 202)
Lithographie: O. R. T. OffsetReproTechnik
Kirchner + Graser, D-1000 Berlin 61
Bindung: Lüderitz und Bauer Buchgewerbe,
D-1000 Berlin 61

Preface

Numerous and often complex bacteriological diagnostic techniques may be necessary for a rapid and reliable detection and subsequent identification of the great variety of bacterial pathogens that can affect animals.

A compromise may sometimes have to be reached in the demonstration of bacteria of veterinary importance, especially in their identification. This is because a balance has to be struck between the practitioner's reasonable requirements for a rapid, economical and clinically useful diagnosis and the bacteriologist's aim at obtaining a definitive identification of the pathogen. This is a fundamental problem of clinical bacteriology which has not yet been wholly solved.

It is hoped, however, that this book may throw light on this problem and that it may also give an indication of how some of these difficulties may be overcome by the application of suitable investigative methods. Thus it was envisaged as a manual for the diagnosis of bacterial pathogens. The bacteria of veterinary importance and their significance to animals and man are discussed; the appearance of these organisms, their properties and methods of identification are presented in pictorial and tabular form. Therefore, this book provides the practising veterinarian, the laboratory worker and the student with an easy and quick means of orientation. In selecting the test procedures preference has been given to those methods which could be performed with relative ease in routine laboratories. Similarly, the literature references were chosen from readily accessible sources wherever possible. An appendix of recipes for media was intentionally omitted, since the manufacturers of culture media provide extensive literature on this subject. If special culture media have been recommended then their composition is always given in the text.

We thank Drs. Walter Siller and James Phillips for their proficient translation of the manuscript into English and for their many critical comments. Finally we wish to express our gratitude to Drs.

Vorwort

Für die erfolgreiche Durchführung der bakteriologischen Diagnostik, die eine möglichst schnelle und exakte Diagnose bakterieller Infektionserreger zum Ziel hat, bedarf es des Einsatzes zahlreicher Nachweisverfahren und vielfältiger Identifizierungsmethoden, um die Fülle der bei Tieren vorkommenden Erregerarten zuverlässig erfassen zu können.
Der Nachweis und insbesondere die Identifizierung der veterinärmedizinisch bedeutsamen Bakterien muß oft ein Kompromiß sein zwischen den berechtigten Erwartungen des praktizierenden Tierarztes nach einer klinisch verwertbaren, schnellen und kostengünstigen Diagnose und dem Verlangen des Bakteriologen, sein Ergebnis möglichst genau abzusichern. Dies ist das Kernproblem jeder klinischen Bakteriologie, das aber leider in vielen Fällen noch immer nicht optimal gelöst ist.
Das Buch möchte zur Verdeutlichung dieses Problems beitragen und gleichzeitig Möglichkeiten aufzeigen, wie durch den gezielten Einsatz geeigneter Untersuchungstechniken dieser Problematik entgegen gewirkt werden kann. Es wurde deshalb als Leitfaden für die Diagnose bakterieller Infektionserreger konzipiert. Die Zusammenstellung der veterinärmedizinisch wichtigsten Bakterien mit einleitenden Hinweisen auf ihre Bedeutung für Tier und Mensch sowie die Darstellung ihrer Erscheinungsformen, Eigenschaften und Nachweisverfahren in Abbildungen und Tabellen sollen dem Tierarzt in Labor und Praxis, den technischen Mitarbeitern und den Studenten eine möglichst leichte und schnelle Orientierung ermöglichen. Bei der Auswahl der Untersuchungsmethoden sind insbesondere solche Verfahren bevorzugt worden, die im Routinelabor relativ leicht durchführbar sind. Auch bei der Aufführung der weiterführenden Literatur sind leicht zugängliche Arbeiten besonders berücksichtigt worden. Auf einen Anhang mit Nährbodenrezepturen wurde bewußt verzichtet, da die Nährbodenhersteller hierzu umfangreiches Informationsmaterial bereitstellen. Soweit besondere Nährmedien empfohlen werden, erfolgen entsprechende

h. c. Friedrich Georgi and his staff for the excellent and considerate manner in which they have looked after the production of this book.

Wolfgang Bisping Hannover,
Gunter Amtsberg Spring 1988

Hinweise auf deren Zusammensetzung im Text. Den Herren Dr. Walter Siller und Dr. James Phillips danken wir für die sachkundige Übersetzung des Manuskriptes in die englische Sprache sowie für die vielen kritischen Anregungen, die dabei entstanden sind, nicht zuletzt sei dem Verlag Paul Parey, Herrn Dr. h. c. mult. Friedrich Georgi und seinen Mitarbeitern für die ausgezeichnete und verständnisvolle verlegerische Betreuung gedankt, die dieses Buch erst möglich gemacht hat.

Wolfgang Bisping Hannover,
Gunter Amtsberg im Frühjahr 1988

Contents / Inhalt

Gram-positive cocci 15
Grampositive Kokken 15

1	Family: Micrococcaceae	15	1	Familie: Micrococcaceae	15
1.1	Species: Staphylococcus (St.)	16	1.1	Gattung: Staphylococcus (St.)	16
1.1.1	Staphylococcus aureus	16	1.1.1	Staphylococcus aureus	16
1.1.2	Staphylococcus hyicus	23	1.1.2	Staphylococcus hyicus	23
1.1.2.1	Staphylococcus hyicus subsp. hyicus	23	1.1.2.1	Staphylococcus hyicus subsp. hyicus	23
1.1.2.2	Staphylococcus hyicus subsp. chromogenes	25	1.1.2.2	Staphylococcus hyicus subsp. chromogenes	25
1.1.3	Coagulase negative Staphylococci	26	1.1.3	Koagulasenegative Staphylokokken	26
1.1.3.1	Staphylococcus epidermis	26	1.1.3.1	Staphylococcus epidermis	26
1.1.3.2	Staphylococcus saprophyticus	26	1.1.3.2	Staphylococcus saprophyticus	26
1.2	Genus: Micrococcus (M.)	26	1.2	Gattung: Micrococcus (M.)	26
	Bibliography	27		*Literatur*	27
2	Family: Streptococcaceae	28	2	Familie: Streptococcaceae	28
2.1	Genus: Streptococcus (Sc.)	28	2.1	Gattung: Streptococcus (Sc.)	28
2.1.1	Streptococci of cattle	33	2.1.1	Streptokokken des Rindes	33
2.1.1.1	Streptococcus agalactiae	33	2.1.1.1	Streptococcus agalactiae	33
2.1.1.2	Streptococcus dysgalactiae	34	2.1.1.2	Streptococcus dysgalactiae	34
2.1.1.3	Streptococcus uberis	34	2.1.1.3	Streptococcus uberis	34
2.1.1.4	Other streptococci	35	2.1.1.4	Andere Streptokokken	35
2.1.2	Streptococci of the horse	35	2.1.2	Streptokokken des Pferdes	35
2.1.2.1	Streptococcus zooepidemicus	35	2.1.2.1	Streptococcus zooepidemicus	35
2.1.2.2	Streptococci equi	35	2.1.2.2	Streptococcus equi	35
2.1.3	Streptococci of the pig	36	2.1.3	Streptokokken des Schweines	36
2.1.3.1	Streptococci of group E	37	2.1.3.1	Streptokokken der Gruppe E	37
2.1.3.2	Streptococci of group L	37	2.1.3.2	Streptokokken der Gruppe L	37
2.1.3.3	Streptococci of group P	37	2.1.3.3	Streptokokken der Gruppe P	37
2.1.3.4	Streptococci of groups R, S and T	37	2.1.3.4	Streptokokken der Gruppen R, S und T	37
2.1.3.5	Group U streptococci	38	2.1.3.5	Streptokokken der Gruppe U	38
2.1.3.6	Group V streptococci	38	2.1.3.6	Streptokokken der Gruppe V	38
2.1.3.7	Streptococcus equisimilis	38	2.1.3.7	Streptococcus equisimilis	38
2.1.4	Enterococci	39	2.1.4	Enterokokken	39
2.1.5	Streptococcus pneumoniae	40	2.1.5	Streptococcus pneumoniae	40
	Bibliography	42		*Literatur*	42
3	Family: Peptococcaceae	44	3	Familie: Peptococcaceae	44
	Bibliography	44		*Literatur*	44

Gram-positive, non-spore-forming rods 45
Grampositive, sporenlose Stäbchen 45

1	**Genus: Corynebacterium**	45	1	**Gattung: Corynebacterium**	45
1.1	Corynebacterium (Actinomyces) pyogenes	45	1.1	Corynebacterium (Actinomyces) pyogenes	45
1.2	Corynebacterium renale	48	1.2	Corynebacterium renale	48
1.3	Corynebacterium pseudotuberculosis	50	1.3	Corynebacterium pseudotuberculosis	50
1.4	Corynebacterium (Rhodococcus) equi	51	1.4	Corynebacterium (Rhodococcus) equi	51
1.5	Corynebacterium (Eubacterium) suis	53	1.5	Corynebacterium (Eubacterium) suis	53
1.6	Other Corynebacteria	54	1.6	Weitere Corynebakterien	54
	Bibliography	55		*Literatur*	55
2	**Genus: Listeria (L.)**	56	2	**Gattung: Listeria (L.)**	56
2.1	Listeria monocytogenes	56	2.1	Listeria monocytogenes	56
	Bibliography	62		*Literatur*	62
3	**Genus: Erysipelothrix (E.)**	63	3	**Gattung: Erysipelothrix (E.)**	63
3.1	Erysipelothrix rhusiopathiae	63	3.1	Erysipelothrix rhusiopathiae	63
	Bibliography	68		*Literatur*	68
4	**Genus: Lactobacillus (L.)**	69	4	**Gattung: Lactobacillus (L.)**	69
	Bibliography			*Literatur*	
5	**Renibacterium salmoninarum**	71	5	**Renibacterium salmoninarum**	71
	Bibliography	71		*Literatur*	71

Gram-positive spore-forming organisms 72
Grampositive Sporenbildner 72

1	**Genus: Bacillus (Bac.)**	72	1	**Gattung: Bacillus (Bac.)**	72
1.1	Bacillus anthracis	72	1.1	Bacillus anthracis	72
1.2	Bacillus cereus	76	1.2	Bacillus cereus	76
1.3	Bacillus larvae	77	1.3	Bacillus larvae	77
1.4	Bacillus alvei	77	1.4	Bacillus alvei	77
1.5	Group of Gram-positive, non-pathogenic, aerobic, spore-forming bacilli	77	1.5	Gruppe der grampositiven, apathogenen, aeroben Sporenbildner	77
	Bibliography	79		*Literatur*	79
2	**Genus: Clostridium (Cl.)**	79	2	**Gattung: Clostridium (Cl.)**	79
2.1	Clostridia as cause of blackleg and wound clostridiosis	82	2.1	Clostridien als Erreger des Rauschbrandes und von Wundclostridiosen	82
2.1.1	Clostridium chauvoei	82	2.1.1	Clostridium chauvoei	82
2.1.2	Clostridia as causes of wound infections	82	2.1.2	Clostridien als Erreger von Wundclostridiosen	82
2.2	Clostridium septicum, cause of braxy	88	2.2	Clostridium septicum als Ursache des Labmagenpararauschbrandes	88
2.3	Clostridium novyi type B, cause of infectious necrotic hepatitis	88	2.3	Clostridium novyi Typ B als Ursache der nekrotischen Hepatitis	88
2.4	Clostridium novyi type D (Cl. haemolyticum) cause of bacillary haemoglobinuria	88	2.4	Clostridium novyi Typ D (Cl. haemolyticum) als Erreger der »bazillären Hämoglobinurie«	88
2.5	Clostridium novyi type C, cause of an osteomyelitis	88	2.5	Clostridium novyi Typ C als Erreger einer Osteomyelitis	88

2.6	Clostridium perfringens cause of enterotoxaemias, food poisoning and some other diseases	89	2.6	Clostridium perfringens als Ursache von Enterotoxämien, Lebensmittelvergiftungen und einigen anderen Erkrankungen	89
2.7	Clostridium sordellii, cause of enteritis and toxaemia	93	2.7	Clostridium sordellii als Ursache von Darmerkrankungen und Toxämien	93
2.8	Clostridium difficile, cause of intestinal disorders	93	2.8	Clostridium difficile als Ursache von Darmerkrankungen	93
2.9	Clostridium spiroforme infections	94	2.9	Clostridium spiroforme-Infektionen	94
2.10	Clostridium tetani	94	2.10	Clostridium tetani	94
2.11	Clostridium botulinum	95	2.11	Clostridium botulinum	95
	Bibliography	98		Literatur	98

Actinomyces, Dermatophilus, Nocardia 101
Actinomyces, Dermatophilus, Nocardia 101

1	Actinomyces (Ac.)	101	1	Actinomyces (Ac.)	101
2	Nocardia (N.)	103	2	Nocardia (N.)	103
3	Dermatophilus (D.)	105	3	Dermatopilus (D.)	105
	Bibliography	106		Literatur	106

Mycobacteria 108
Mykobakterien 108

1	Tubercle bacilli and atypical mycobacteria	108	1	Tuberkelbakterien und atypische Mykobakterien	108
	Bibliography	118		Literatur	118
2	Mycobacterium paratuberculosis	119	2	Mycobacterium paratuberculosis	119
	Bibliography	120		Literatur	120

Gram-negative, aerobic or micro-aerophilic or facultatively anaerobic rods, with simple cultural requirements 121
Gramnegative, aerob oder mikroaerophil oder fakultativ anaerob wachsende, in der Kultur anspruchslose Stäbchen 121

1	Oxidase-positive and fermentative bacteria	123	1	Oxidasepositive und fermentative Bakterien	123
1.1	Genus: Pasteurella (P.)	123	1.1	Gattung: Pasteurella (P.)	123
1.1.1	Pasteurella multocida	126	1.1.1	Pasteurella multocida	126
1.1.2	Pasteurella haemolytica	130	1.1.2	Pasteurella haemolytica	130
1.1.3	Pasteurella pneumotropica	133	1.1.3	Pasteurella pneumotropica	133
1.1.4	Pasteurella ureae	133	1.1.4	Pasteurella ureae	133
1.1.5	Pasteurella gallinarum	133	1.1.5	Pasteurella gallinarum	133
1.1.6	Pasteurella aerogenes	133	1.1.6	Pasteurella aerogenes	133
1.1.7	Pasteurella anatipestifer	133	1.1.7	Pasteurella anatipestifer	133
	Bibliography	134		Literatur	134
1.2	Genus: Actinobacillus (Act.)	135	1.2	Gattung: Actinobacillus (Act.)	135
1.2.1	Actinobacillus lignieresii	137	1.2.1	Actinobacillus lignieresii	137
1.2.2	Actinobacillus equuli	137	1.2.2	Actinobacillus equuli	137
1.2.3	Actinobacillus suis	138	1.2.3	Actinobacillus suis	138
	Bibliography	138		Literatur	138
1.3	Family Vibrionaceae	139	1.3	Familie: Vibrionaceae	139
1.3.1	Genus: Vibrio (V.)	139	1.3.1	Gattung: Vibrio	139

1.3.1.1	Vibrio metschnikovi	139		1.3.1.1	Vibrio metschnikovi	139
1.3.1.2	Vibrio anguillarum	139		1.3.1.2	Vibrio anguillarum	139
1.3.1.3	Vibrio parahaemolyticus	140		1.3.1.3	Vibrio parahaemolyticus	140
1.3.2	Genus: Aeromonas (A.)	140		1.3.2	Gattung: Aeromonas	140
1.3.2.1	Aeromonas hydrophila, A. caviae and A. sobria (motile aeromonads)	141		1.3.2.1	Aeromonas hydrophila, A. caviae und A. sobria (bewegliche Aeromonaden)	141
1.3.2.2	Aeromonas salmonicida (non-motile aeromonads)	143		1.3.2.2	Aeromonas salmonicida (unbewegliche Aeromonaden)	143
	Bibliography	145			Literatur	145

2	**Oxidase-positive and oxidative bacteria**	**146**		**2**	**Oxidasepositive und oxidative Bakterien**	**146**
2.1	Genus: Pseudomonas (Ps.)	146		2.1	Gattung: Pseudomonas (Ps.)	146
2.1.1	Pseudomonas aeruginosa	146		2.1.1	Pseudomonas aeruginosa	146
2.1.2	Other pseudomonas species	149		2.1.2	Weitere Pseudomonas-Arten	149
2.1.3	Pseudomonas mallei	149		2.1.3	Pseudomonas mallei	149
2.1.4	Pseudomonas pseudomallei	151		2.1.4	Pseudomonas pseudomallei	151
	Bibliography	151			Literatur	151
2.2	Flavobacterium	152		2.2	Flavobacterium	152

3	**Oxidase-positive glucose-inactive bacteria**	**153**		**3**	**Oxidasepositive und glucoseinaktive Bakterien**	**153**
3.1	Genus: Alcaligenes (A.)	153		3.1	Gattung: Alcaligenes (A.)	153
	Bibliography	153			Literatur	153
3.2	Genus: Bordetella (B.)	153		3.2	Gattung: Bordetella (B.)	153
3.2.1	Bordetella bronchiseptica	153		3.2.1	Bordetella bronchiseptica	153
3.2.2	Bordetella avium	156		3.2.2	Bordetella avium	156
	Bibliography	156			Literatur	156
3.3	Genus: Neisseria (N.)	157		3.3	Gattung: Neisseria (N.)	157
	Bibliography	158			Literatur	158
3.4	Genus: Moraxella (M.)	158		3.4	Gattung: Moraxella (M.)	158
3.4.1	Subgenus: Moraxella	158		3.4.1	Subgenus: Moraxella	158
3.4.1.1	Moraxella bovis	158		3.4.1.1	Moraxella bovis	158
3.4.2	Subgenus Branhamella	159		3.4.2	Subgenus: Branhamella	159
3.4.2.1	Moraxella (Branhamella) ovis	159		3.4.2.1	Moraxella (Branhamella) ovis	159
3.4.2.2	Moraxella (Branhamella) cuniculi	159		3.4.2.2	Moraxella (Branhamella) cuniculi	159
3.4.2.3	Moraxella (Branhamella) caviae	159		3.4.2.3	Moraxella (Branhamella) caviae	159
3.4.2.4	Moraxella (Branhamella) catarrhalis	160		3.4.2.4	Moraxella (Branhamella) catarrhalis	160
	Bibliography	160			Literatur	160

4	**Oxidase-negative and fermentative bacteria**	**160**		**4**	**Oxidasenegative und fermentative Bakterien**	**160**
4.1	Enterobacteriaceae	160		4.1	Enterobacteriaceae	160
4.1.1	Genus: Escherichia (E.)	160		4.1.1	Gattung: Escherichia (E.)	160
4.1.1.1	Escherichia coli	160		4.1.1.1	Escherichia coli	160
	Bibliography	168			Literatur	168
4.1.2	Genus: Citrobacter (C.)	169		4.1.2	Gattung: Citrobacter (C.)	169
	Bibliography	170			Literatur	170
4.1.3	Genus: Salmonella (S.)	171		4.1.3	Gattung: Salmonella (S.)	171
	Bibliography	182			Literatur	182
4.1.4	Genus: Shigella (Sh.)	182		4.1.4	Gattung: Shigella (Sh.)	182
	Bibliography	183			Literatur	183
4.1.5	Genus: Edwardsiella (Ed.)	184		4.1.5	Gattung: Edwardsiella (Ed.)	184
4.1.5.1	Edwardsiella tarda	184		4.1.5.1	Edwardsiella tarda	184
4.1.5.2	Edwardsiella ictaluri	185		4.1.5.2	Edwardsiella ictaluri	185
	Bibliography	185			Literatur	185
4.1.6	Genus: Klebsiella (K.)	186		4.1.6	Gattung: Klebsiella (K.)	186
4.1.6.1	Klebsiella pneumoniae subsp. pneumoniae	187		4.1.6.1	Klebsiella pneumoniae subsp. pneumoniae	187

4.1.6.2	Klebsiella oxytoca	188	4.1.6.2	Klebsiella oxytoca	188
	Bibliography	188		*Literatur*	188
4.1.7	Genus: Enterobacter (Eb.)	189	4.1.7	Gattung: Enterobacter (Eb.)	189
	Bibliography	191		*Literatur*	191
4.1.8	Genus: Hafnia (H.)	191	4.1.8	Gattung: Hafnia (H.)	191
	Bibliography	192		*Literatur*	192
4.1.9	Genus: Serratia (Sr.)	192	4.1.9	Gattung: Serratia (Sr.)	192
	Bibliography	193		*Literatur*	193
4.1.10	Genus: Proteus, Providencia, Morganella	195	4.1.10	Gattungen: Proteus, Providencia, Morganella	195
4.1.10.1	Genus: Proteus (Pr.)	195	4.1.10.1	Gattung: Proteus (Pr.)	195
4.1.10.2	Genus: Providencia (Prov.)	196	4.1.10.2	Gattung: Providencia (Prov.)	196
4.1.10.3	Genus: Morganella (Mg.)	197	4.1.10.3	Gattung: Morganella (Mg.)	197
	Bibliography	197		*Literatur*	197
4.1.11	Genus: Erwinia	197	4.1.11	Gattung: Erwinia	197
	Bibliography	199		*Literatur*	199
4.1.12	Genus: Yersinia (Y.)	200	4.1.12	Gattung: Yersinia (Y.)	200
4.1.12.1	Yersinia pseudotuberculosis	200	4.1.12.1	Yersinia pseudotuberculosis	200
4.1.12.2	Yersinia enterocolitica	203	4.1.12.2	Yersinia enterocolitica	203
4.1.12.3	Yersinia frederiksenii, Y. intermedia, Y. kristensenii	206	4.1.12.3	Yersinia frederiksenii, Y. intermedia, Y. kristensenii	206
4.1.12.4	Yersinia ruckeri	207	4.1.12.4	Yersinia ruckeri	207
	Bibliography	208		*Literatur*	208
5	**Oxidase-negative and oxidative or glucose-inactive bacteria**	209	5	**Oxidasenegative und oxidative oder glucoseinaktive Bakterien**	209
	Genus: Acinetobacter (A.)	209		Gattung: Acinetobacter (A.)	209
5.1	*Bibliography*	211	5.1	*Literatur*	211
6	**Further Gram-negative, oxidase-negative and rarely encountered bacteria**	212	6	**Weitere gramnegative, oxidasenegative und selten vorkommende Bakterien**	212
6.1	Genus: Francisella (Fr.)	212	6.1	Gattung: Francisella (Fr.)	212
6.1.1	Francisella tularensis	212	6.1.1	Francisella tularensis	212
6.1.2	Francisella novicida	213	6.1.2	Francisella novicida	213
	Bibliography	213		*Literatur*	213
6.2	Genus: Streptobacillus	213	6.2	Gattung: Streptobacillus	213
	Bibliography	214		*Literatur*	214

Gram-negative, comma-shaped or spiral bacteria (Family: Spirillaceae) 215
Gramnegative, komma- bis spiralförmige Bakterien (Familie: Spirillaceae) 215

1	**Genus: Spirillum**	215	1	**Gattung: Spirillum**	215
2	**Genus: Campylobacter (C.)**	215	2	**Gattung: Campylobacter (C.)**	215
2.1	Campylobacter infections of the reproductive organs	217	2.1	Campylobacter-Infektionen der Geschlechtsorgane	217
2.1.1	Campylobacter fetus subsp. venerealis	217	2.1.1	Campylobacter fetus subsp. venerealis	217
2.1.2	Campylobacter fetus subsp. fetus	217	2.1.2	Campylobacter fetus subsp. fetus	217
2.1.3	Campylobacter sputorum subsp. bubulus	218	2.1.3	Campylobacter sputorum subsp. bubulus	218
2.1.4	Diagnosis of the genital Campylobacter infections	219	2.1.4	Diagnose der genitalen Campylobacter-Infektion	219
2.1.4.1	Identification of causal agent	219	2.1.4.1	Erregernachweis	219

2.1.4.2	Biochemical differentiation	220	2.1.4.2	Kulturell-biochemische Identifizierung	220
2.1.4.3	Serological identification	223	2.1.4.3	Serologische Identifizierung	223
2.1.5	Aerotolerant Campylobacter (Campylobacter cryaerophilia)	223	2.1.5	Aerotolerante Campylobacter (Campylobacter cryaerophilia)	223
2.2	Campylobacter infections of the gut	224	2.2	Campylobacter-Infektionen des Darmes	224
2.2.1	Campylobacter jejuni	224	2.2.1	Campylobacter jejuni	224
2.2.2	Campylobacter coli	226	2.2.2	Campylobacter coli	226
2.2.3	Campylobacter laridis	226	2.2.3	Campylobacter laridis	226
2.2.4	Diagnosis of infections by C. jejuni and C. coli	227	2.2.4	Diagnose der Campylobacter jejuni- und Campylobacter coli-Infektion	227
2.2.5	Campylobacter sputorum subsp. mucosalis	228	2.2.5	Campylobacter sputorum subsp. mucosalis	228
2.2.6	Campylobacter hyointestinalis	228	2.2.6	Campylobacter hyointestinalis	228
2.2.7	Campylobacter fecalis	228	2.2.7	Campylobacter fecalis	228
	Bibliography	229		*Literatur*	229

Haemophilic bacteria 232
Hämophile Bakterien 232

1	**Genus: Haemophilus (H.)**	232	1	**Gattung: Haemophilus (H.)**	232
1.1	Haemophilus infections in pigs	236	1.1	Haemophilus-Infektionen beim Schwein	236
1.1.1	Haemophilus suis	236	1.1.1	Haemophilus suis	236
1.1.2	Haemophilus parasuis	236	1.1.2	Haemophilus parasuis	236
1.1.3	Haemophilus pleuropneumoniae	236	1.1.3	Haemophilus pleuropneumoniae	236
1.2	Haemophilus infections in poultry	238	1.2	Haemophilus-Infektionen beim Geflügel	238
1.2.1	Haemophilus paragallinarum	238	1.2.1	Haemophilus paragallinarum	238
1.2.2	Haemophilus avium	238	1.2.2	Haemophilus avium	238
1.3	Haemophilus haemoglobinophilus	239	1.3	Haemophilus haemoglobinophilus	239
1.4	Haemophilus somnus	239	1.4	Haemophilus somnus	239
1.5	Haemophilus (Taylorella) equigenitalis	241	1.5	Haemophilus (Taylorella) equigenitalis	241
2	**Genus: Histophilus**	242	2	**Gattung: Histophilus**	242
2.1	Histophilus ovis	242	2.1	Histophilus ovis	242
	Bibliography	243		*Literatur*	243

Brucellae 246
Brucellen 246

1	**Brucella (Br.) melitensis, Br. abortus and Br. suis**	247	1	**Brucella (Br.) melitensis, Br. abortus und Br. suis**	247
1.1	Properties, demonstration and identification	247	1.1	Eigenschaften, Nachweis und Bestimmung	247
1.2	Serological diagnosis	252	1.2	Serologische Diagnose	252
2	**Brucella ovis**	257	2	**Brucella ovis**	257
3	**Brucella canis**	258	3	**Brucella canis**	258
	Bibliography	259		*Literatur*	259

Gram-negative anaerobic rods ... 263
Gramnegative, anaerobe Stäbchen ... 263

1	**Family: Bacteroideaceae** ... 263
1.1	Genus: Bacteroides (Ba.) ... 263
1.2	Genus: Fusobacterium (F.) ... 271
1.2.1	Fusobacterium necrophorum ... 272
1.2.2	Other types of Fusobacterium ... 274
	Bibliography ... 275

1	**Familie: Bacteroideaceae** ... 263
1.1	Gattung: Bacteroides (Ba.) ... 263
1.2	Gattung: Fusobacterium (F.) ... 271
1.2.1	Fusobacterium necrophorum ... 272
1.2.2	Weitere Fusobacterium-Arten ... 274
	Literatur ... 275

Spirochaetes (Family: Spirochaetaceae) ... 277
Spirochäten (Familie: Spirochaetaceae) ... 277

1	**Genus: Leptospira (L.)** ... 277
1.1	Properties of leptospires ... 279
1.2	Diagnostic demonstration of causal organism ... 281
1.3	Serological diagnosis ... 283
	Bibliography ... 285
2	**Genus: Treponema (T.)** ... 286
2.1	Treponema hyodysenteriae ... 286
2.2	Treponema innocens ... 291
	Bibliography ... 292

1	**Gattung: Leptospira (L.)** ... 277
1.1	Eigenschaften der Leptospiren ... 279
1.2	Diagnostischer Erregernachweis ... 281
1.3	Serologische Diagnose ... 283
	Literatur ... 285
2	**Gattung: Treponema (T.)** ... 286
2.1	Treponema hyodysenteriae ... 286
2.2	Treponema innocens ... 291
	Literatur ... 292

Rickettsiae and Chlamydias ... 294
Rickettsien und Chlamydien ... 294

1	**Rickettsiae** ... 294
1.1	Coxiella (C.) burnetii ... 294
	Bibliography ... 298
1.2	Ehrlichia (E.) ... 299
1.3	Cowdria, Anaplasma, Aegyptianella ... 299
1.4	Haemobartonella (H.) ... 299
1.5	Eperythrozoon (Ep.) ... 300
	Bibliography ... 300
2	**Chlamydia (Chl.)** ... 301
2.1	Chlamydia psittaci ... 302
	Bibliography ... 304

1	**Rickettsien** ... 294
1.1	Coxiella (C.) burnetii ... 294
	Literatur ... 298
1.2	Ehrlichia (E.) ... 299
1.3	Cowdria, Anaplasma, Aegyptianella ... 299
1.4	Haemobartonella (H.) ... 299
1.5	Eperythrozoon (Ep.) ... 300
	Literatur ... 300
2	**Chlamydia (Chl.)** ... 301
2.1	Chlamydia psittaci ... 302
	Literatur ... 304

Mycoplasms ... 306
Mykoplasmen ... 306

1	**Genus: Mycoplasma (M.)** ... 306
2	**Genus: Ureaplasma** ... 311
3	**Genus: Acholeplasma (A.)** ... 312
4	**Diagnosis of mycoplasma infections** ... 312
4.1	Morphology and staining methods ... 312

1	**Gattung: Mycoplasma (M.)** ... 306
2	**Gattung: Ureaplasma** ... 311
3	**Gattung: Acholeplasma (A.)** ... 312
4	**Diagnose der Mykoplasmeninfektion** ... 312
4.1	Morphologie und färberische Darstellung ... 312

4.2	Cultural isolation of mycoplasms	313	4.2	Kulturelle Isolierung der Mykoplasmen	313
	Identification of mycoplasms	315	4.3	Identifizierung der Mykoplasmen	315
4.3	Serological diagnosis of mycoplasmosis	319	4.4	Serologische Diagnose von Mykoplasmen	319
4.4	Bibliography	320		Literatur	320

Appendix 324
Anhang 324

1	Abbreviations	324	1	Abkürzungen	324
2	Taxonomy and nomenclature of bacteria of veterinary importance	326	2	Systematik und Nomenklatur der veterinärmedizinisch bedeutsamen Bakterien	326
3	Bacteriological stains	333	3	Bakterienfärbungen	333
3.1	Dyes and staining solutions	333	3.1	Farbstoffe und Farbstofflösungen	333
3.2	Staining methods	334	3.2	Färbemethoden	334
4	Index	338	4	Sachverzeichnis	338

Gram-positive Cocci

1 Family: Micrococcaceae

This family includes spherical bacteria with an average diameter of 1 µm. Cell division takes place in more than one plane and this results in either irregular clusters or an orderly arrangement in the form of packets of four. They are catalase positive.

The family is comprised of the species Staphylococcus, Micrococcus and Planococcus (mobile cocci). Their differentiation is given in table 1.

The oxidation-fermentation test, whereby glucose is broken down anaerobically *(Staphylococcus)*, aerobically *(Micrococcus)* or not at all, has been used to differentiate the species. However, because of its wide margin of error this test often gives rise to wrong diagnoses. The reaction to lysostaphin and lysozyme, as well as the ability to form acid from glycerol in the presence of 0.4 µg erythromycin per ml, have been established as the criteria for species identification. It is also possible to differentiate between staphylococci and micrococci by virtue of the difference in their resistance to furazolidone.

Table 1: Differentiation between *Staphylococcus* and *Micrococcus* (28, 30)

Properties	*Staphylococcus*	*Micrococcus*
Gram positive, spherical cells	+	+
Grouping: irregular clusters	+	+
packets of four	−	+
Fermentation of glucose	+	v$^-$
Resistance to lysostaphin[1] (200 µg/ml)	−	+
Resistance to lysozyme (25 µg/ml)	−	v
Aerobic acid formation on glycerol-erythromycin medium	+	−
Growth on furazolidone-containing media, Furazolidone (20 µg/ml) — peptone agar	−	+

[1] Lysostaphin is a metabolite of *St. staphylolyticus*; it has a lytic action on *St. aureus*

1.1 Species: Staphylococcus (St.)

This species encompasses non-motile cocci, measuring between 0.5 and 1.5 µm, which form into irregular clusters. They are facultative anaerobes but grow best under aerobic conditions and have no special nutritive requirements. The optimum temperature lies between 30 °C and 40 °C. Other properties of the species are listed in table 1.

1.1.1 Staphylococcus aureus

■ **Occurrence and veterinary significance**
St. aureus occurs in man and practically all species of animals. Apart from a clinically latent infection of the skin and mucous membranes, it causes acute to chronic purulent inflammations of all organ systems, including wound infections, purulent catarrh of mucous membranes, abscesses, boils, pyodermias, osteomyelitis, mastitis and it can lead to septicaemia. Botryomycosis is a chronic purulent, indurating infectious disease of horses, in which *St. aureus* is sequestrated in the typical granulomatous lesion.

The diagnostic procedure for identifying the organism is illustrated in figure 5 (p. 18).

■ **Morphology**
The Gram stain is best for the microscopic detection. In smears prepared from animal materials the cocci are usually extracellular, although a small proportion may have been phagocytosed. The extracellular cocci lie in irregular clusters, singly or more rarely in pairs (fig. 1).

■ **Culture**
St. aureus has no special nutrient requirements, so that it is possible to grow it even on simple media. It will grow within 12 to 24 hours in a simple broth, causing turbidity and sediment. On solid media (nutrient or blood agar) it will form medium-sized, smooth, irregular, golden-yellow colonies (fig. 2). The various forms of haemolysis become manifest on blood agar (fig. 2).
▷ Selective media: Various solid and liquid selective media have been developed for the isolation of staphylococci *(St. aureus* and *St. epidermidis)* from contaminated material. These are especially useful for the bacteriological examination of human foods. Potassium tellurite, lithium chloride, sodium azide, neomycin or polymyxin are added to these media by themselves or with sodium chloride in order to suppress the contaminating flora.

Such selective media are usually available commercially as poured plates; some examples are: Mannitol-salt-phenol red agar (fig. 4).

1.1 Gattung: Staphylococcus (St.)

Die Gattung umfaßt 0,5 bis 1,5 µm große, unbewegliche, in unregelmäßigen Haufen gelagerte Kokken. Sie sind fakultativ anaerob, wachsen jedoch am besten unter aeroben Bedingungen und stellen keine besonderen Nährbodenanforderungen. Das Temperaturoptimum liegt zwischen 30 °C und 40 °C. Weitere Gattungseigenschaften siehe Tab. 1.

1.1.1 Staphylococcus aureus

■ **Vorkommen und medizinische Bedeutung**
St. aureus kommt beim Menschen und bei praktisch allen Tierarten vor. Neben einer klinisch latenten Besiedlung der Haut und der Schleimhäute verursacht er akut bis chronisch verlaufende, eitrige Entzündungen in allen Organsystemen, z. B. Wundinfektionen, eitrige Schleimhautkatarrhe, Abszesse, Furunkel, Pyodermien, Osteomyelitis, Mastitis und kann zu einer Sepsis führen. Eine chronisch-eitrige, indurierende Infektionskrankheit des Pferdes, bei der *St. aureus* in drusenähnliche Herde eingeschlossen ist, wird als Botryomykose bezeichnet.

Der diagnostische Weg zum Erregernachweis ist in der Abb. 5 (S. 18) dargestellt.

■ **Morphologie**
Die mikroskopische Darstellung erfolgt am besten mit der Gram-Färbung. In Ausstrichen von tierischen Untersuchungsstoffen liegen die meisten Kokken extrazellulär, ein geringer Teil kann auch phagozytiert sein. Die extrazellulären Kokken liegen in unregelmäßigen Haufen, einzeln oder seltener paarweise (Abb. 1).

■ **Kultur**
St. aureus stellt keine besonderen Nährbodenansprüche, so daß seine Anzüchtung auch auf einfachen Nährböden gelingt. Innerhalb von 12 bis 24 h wächst er in einer einfachen Bouillon unter Trübung und Bodensatzbildung. Auf festen Nährböden (Nähr-, Blutagar) bilden sich mittelgroße, glatte, unregelmäßig goldgelbe Kolonien (Abb. 2). Auf Blutagar werden die verschiedenen Hämolyseformen ausgebildet (Abb. 2).
▷ Selektivnährböden: Für die Isolierung von Staphylokokken *(St. aureus* und *St. epidermidis)* aus einem kontaminierten Material sind verschiedene feste und flüssige Selektivnährböden entwickelt worden, die besonders in der Lebensmittelbakteriologie Anwendung finden. Zur Unterdrückung der Begleitflora sind diesen Nährböden einzeln oder in Kombination Kochsalz, Kaliumtellurit, Lithiumchlorid, Natriumacid, Neomycin oder Polymyxin zugesetzt.

Beispiele für derartige Selektivmedien, die mei-

Family: Micrococcaceae

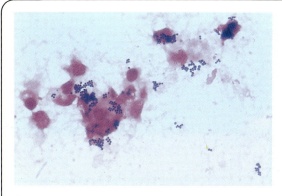
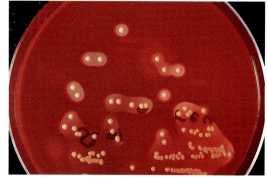
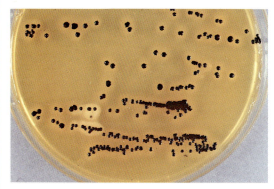
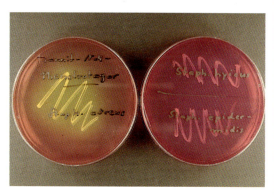

▲ Fig. 1: *Staphylococcus aureus*, mastitis milk smear, Gram stain. The cocci are arranged in irregular clusters. Magnification x 1000
▼ Fig. 3: *Staphylococcus aureus*, pure culture on Baird-Parker agar, colonies are black due to the reduction of tellurite. Halo-formation due to proteolysis and lipolysis. 72 h, 37 °C. Magnification x 0.4

▲ Abb. 1: *Staphylococcus aureus*, Ausstrich einer Mastitismilch, Gramfärbung, Lagerung der Kokken in unregelmäßigen Haufen, Abb.-M. 1000 : 1
▼ Abb. 3: *Staphylococcus aureus*, Reinkultur auf Baird-Parker-Agar, schwarze Kolonien durch Telluritreduktion, Ringbildung durch Proteo- und Lipolyse, 72 h, 37 °C, Abb.-M. 1 : 2,5

▲ Fig. 2: *Staphylococcus aureus*, pure culture on blood agar, haemolysis, 48 h. 37 °C. Magnification x 0.4
▼ Fig. 4: *Staphylococcus aureus* and *Staphylococcus epidermidis* culture on mannitol-salt-phenol red agar. *St. aureus*: yellow due to the fermentation of mannitol; *St. epidermidis* no fermentation of mannitol, therefore no colour change, 24 h, 37 °C. Magnification x 0.25

▲ Abb. 2: *Staphylococcus aureus*, Reinkultur auf Blutagar, Hämolyse, 48 h, 37 °C, Abb.-M. 1 : 2,5
▼ Abb. 4: *Staphylococcus aureus* und *Staphylococcus epidermidis*, Kultur auf Mannit-Kochsalz-Phenolrot-Agar, *St. aureus*: Gelbfärbung durch Mannitabbau, *St. epidermidis*: kein Mannitabbau und daher keine Verfärbung, 24 h, 37 °C, Abb.-M. 1 : 4

Yolk-tellurite-glycine-pyruvate agar after Baird-Parker; this medium contains lithium chloride and tellurite to inhibit contaminating flora and a suspension of yolk to demonstrate the presence of lipases, especially the yolk factor. *St. aureus* forms black (reduction of the tellurite), shiny colonies which are surrounded by clear areas, 2–5 mm wide. The colonies of *St. epidermidis* are appreciably smaller and irregular in shape (fig. 3).
Columbia-CNA agar which contains nalidixic acid and colistin sulphate for the selective culture of staphylococci and streptococci.

stens als Fertignährböden im Handel erhältlich sind, sind u. a.:
Mannit-Kochsalz-Phenolrot-Agar (Abb. 4).
Eigelb-Tellurit-Glycin-Pyruvat-Agar nach Baird-Parker, der Nährboden enthält Lithiumchlorid und Tellurit zur Hemmung der Begleitflora und Eigelbsuspension zum Nachweis von Lipasen, insbesondere des Eigelbfaktors. *St. aureus* bildet schwarze (Reduktion des Tellurits), glänzende Kolonien, umgeben von klaren, 2 bis 5 mm breiten Höfen. Die Kolonien von *St. epidermidis* sind wesentlich kleiner und von unregelmäßiger Form (Abb. 3).

Specimens
Organ samples, pus, milk, swabs from skin and mucosa etc.

Microscopic identification of pathogens
Gram stain, Gram-positive cocci lying singly or in irregular clusters

Cultural identification of pathogens
1. Enrichment in fluid media, nutrient broth or fluid selective medium, incubation for 24 h at 37 °C, subsequent isolation on solid media: blood agar or selective medium. 2. Solid nutrient media for direct culture or isolation from enrichment media, Blood agar: Characteristic, relatively large, white to yellow colonies with haemolysis (fig. 2).

Identification of St. aureus in pure culture
1. Microscopic examination: Gram-positive cocci. 2. Appearance of colonies: relatively large, white to yellow colonies with haemolysis. 3. a) Cultural and biochemical examination: Rapid identification of St. aureus on the basis of selected properties observed during routine tests: Haemolysis +, demonstration of the clumping factor with the slide method using rabbit plasma, commercial systems, e. g. the Staphy slide test (bio-Merieux), API STAPH System (4, 11, 22, 27). 3. b) Demonstration of other properties.

Reaction	St. aureus	St. hyicus subsp. hyicus	St. hyicus subsp. chromogenes	St. intermedius	St. epidermidis
Haemolysis — bovine RBC	+	−	−	+	−
— sheep RBC	+	v⁻	v⁻	+	v⁻
Mannitol aerobic	+	−	−	+	−
fermentation anaerobic	+	−	v⁻	−	−
Clumping factor (rabbit plasma)	+	v⁻	−	v⁺	−
Coagulase — rabbit plasma	+	v	−	+	−
— pig plasma	+	v⁺	−	−	−
Thermonuclease	+	+	−	+	−
Hyaluronidase	+	+	−	−	−
Yolk reaction	+	v⁺	−	−	−
Protein A	+	+	−	v	−
Tellurite reaction	+	v⁺	−	−	−
Pigment formation	+	−	+	−	−

Fig. 5: Detection and identification of coagulase-positive staphylococci

Abb. 5: Nachweis und Bestimmung koagulasepositiver Staphylokokken

Potassium rhodanid-actidione-sodium azide-yolk-pyruvate agar is used mainly in the examination of human foods (32).

Columbia-CNA-Agar, der Nalidixinsäure und Colistinsulfat zur selektiven Herauszüchtung von Staphylo- und Streptokokken enthält.
Kaliumrhodanid-Aktidion-Natriumacid-Eigelb-Pyruvat-Agar, der besonders in der Lebensmittelbakteriologie Anwendung findet (32).

■ Biochemical properties

St. aureus exhibits great metabolic selectivity, which permits its differentiation from other staphylococci. Many of the metabolic functions are recognized as features of pathogenicity (5, 6, 9). The most impor-

■ Kulturell-biochemische Eigenschaften

St. aureus zeigt eine große Stoffwechselaktivität, die seine Abgrenzung von anderen Staphylokokken erlaubt. Viele der Stoffwechselleistungen werden zugleich als Pathogenitätsmerkmale angesehen (5, 6,

Table 2: Haemolytic action on blood agar plates with various erythrocytes (5). This is complete haemolysis and includes »hot-cold-lysis« after 18 h at 37 °C and 1 h at 4 °C

Haemolysins	Erythrocytes of		
	Man	Rabbit	Sheep
α	−	+	+
β	−(+)	−	+
δ	+	+	+
αβ	−(+)	+	+
αβδ	+	+	+
βδ	+	+	+
	+	+	+

tant metabolic products are:

▷ Haemolysins: Most strains of *St. aureus* form haemolysins which may damage erythrocytes and other cell types. The α-, β- and δ-haemolysins are of medical and diagnostic importance and they are produced by a strain of staphylococci either singly or in various combinations (see table 2).

The α-haemolysin is found primarily in staphylococcal strains of human origin and produces a wide zone of complete haemolysis. The β-haemolysin occurs mainly in strains of animal origin and especially bovine. With incubation at 37 °C it produces an incomplete haemolysis, which develops into a complete haemolysis when held at 4 °C (»hot-cold lysis«).

δ-lysin produces a narrow, sharply defined zone of complete haemolysis and it is formed by strains of both human and animal origin. The types of erythrocytes suitable for demonstrating haemolysis are listed in table 3.

▷ Coagulases: These are enzyme-like substances which, in the presence of a plasma factor, convert fibrinogen into fibrin; they are characteristic for *St. aureus*.

The test is carried out with blood plasma obtained from citrated blood (1 volume of 4 % sodium citrate solution to 9 volumes of whole blood). Rabbit plasma is suitable for this test, also pig plasma, especially for strains of animal origin. For the investigation of staphylococcal strains derived from cattle one may use bovine plasma and, similarly,

Table 3: Suitability of erythrocytes of various animal species for the demonstration of staphylococcal haemolysins (Tube test) (5)

Haemolysins	Erythrocyte donor[1]
α	Rabbit (sheep)
β[2]	Sheep (ox, man)
γ	Rabbit (man)
δ	Man (rabbit, sheep, horse)

[1] The erythrocytes of animals in brackets are less suitable
[2] hot-cold-lysis

canine plasma for strains from dogs.

Tube method: 0.2 ml of a 24 hour broth culture is added to 0.5 ml of plasma that has been diluted 1 : 5. The reaction takes place within 3–4 hours at 37 °C, and ranges from loose clots to the formation of one complete clot.

▷ Clumping factor (CF): Almost all coagulase positive staphylococci form CF, so that this test can be used as a substitute for the coagulase method. The clumping factor reacts directly with the fibrinogen, without participation of a plasma factor, and leads to clumping of the staphylococci. The slide test is used in this method whereby the staphylococcal colonies are picked off the solid media and mixed with undiluted citrate plasma. In a positive test clumping occurs within a few minutes, but a control test should be carried out with physiological saline in order to eliminate false spontaneous reactions.

▷ Nucleases and Thermonucleases: The test is carried out on solid, DNase-containing media. DNase positive colonies hydrolyse the surrounding DNA. Therefore, after incubation the medium is acidified with 1N HCl, so that the DNA precipitates and causes tubidity, leaving clear zones around the DNase positive colonies. On media which contain not only DNA but also toluidine blue or methylene green, a positive colony is surrounded by a pink halo on the otherwise blue background or a clear halo on the green medium. (This is without the addition of HCl.) Nucleases are consistently produced by *St. aureus* and usually by *St. epidermidis*.

Heat resistant nucleases (thermonucleases) are always produced by *St. aureus* and *St. hyicus subsp. hyicus*, and they are therefore very typical for these species. The presence of thermonucleases is demonstrated in the agar diffusion test using the abovementioned media. The staphylococcal cultures or their supernatant are first heated to 100 °C for 15 minutes in a waterbath, in order to destroy the thermolabile nucleases. They are then placed into the wells of the medium. In food materials infected with *St. aureus* it is still possible to demonstrate thermostable nucleases, even after heat treatment when it is no longer possible to culture live staphylococci.

▷ Hyaluronidase: The presence of hyaluronidase can be demonstrated in the decapsulation test of MURRAY & PEARCE (23) which makes use of a capsule-forming strain of *Streptococcus equi*. The bacteria to be tested for the production of hyaluronidase and the streptococci are spread on the plate at right angles to one another. At the intersection of the streaks the streptococci will grow without mucus production if the test strain produces hyaluronidase (fig. 8).

▷ Protein A: This is a protein substance that is produced by most of the strains of *St. aureus* and *St. hyicus subsp. hyicus*. It is bound to the surface of the cell membrane and it reacts with the Fc fragment

Herkunft besonders Schweineplasma. Für die Untersuchung von Rinderstämmen kann bovines und von Hundestämmen canines Plasma benutzt werden.

Röhrchenmethode: 0,5 ml 1 : 5 verdünntes Plasma wird mit 0,2 ml einer 24stündigen Bouillonkultur versetzt. Die Reaktion tritt innerhalb von 3–4 h bei 37 °C ein, sie zeigt sich in der Bildung von lockeren Gerinnseln bis zur vollständigen Verklumpung des Inhalts.

▷ Clumping factor (CF): Fast alle koagulasepositiven Staphylokokken bilden CF, so daß dieser Test stellvertretend für den Koagulasenachweis geführt werden kann. Der CF reagiert direkt mit Fibrinogen ohne Vermittlung eines Plasmafaktors und führt zur Verklumpung von Staphylokokken. Der Nachweis geschieht im Objektträgertest, indem Staphylokokkenkolonien von festen Nährböden unverdünntem Citratplasma eingerieben werden, bei positivem Ausfall kommt es innerhalb weniger Minuten zu einer Verklumpung. Eine Kontrolle mit physiologischer Kochsalzlösung zur Ausscheidung von Spontanreaktionen ist erforderlich.

▷ Nukleasen und Thermonukleasen: Der Nachweis wird auf DNase-haltigen festen Nährböden geführt. DNase-positive Kolonien hydrolysieren in ihrer Umgebung DNS. Deswegen wird nach der Bebrütung der Nährböden mit 1 N HCl angesäuert, dadurch fällt die DNS aus (Trübung) und es entstehen um die DNase-positiven Kolonien Aufhellungshöfe. Auf Nährböden, die neben DNS Toluidinblau oder Methylgrün enthalten, bilden sich um die positiven Kolonien rosarote Höfe im sonst blauen oder helle Höfe im sonst grünen Nährboden (ohne Zugabe von HCl). Nukleasen werden regelmäßig von *St. aureus* und meistens auch von *St. epidermidis* gebildet.

Hitzeresistente Nukleasen (Thermonukleasen) werden regelmäßig von *St. aureus, St. hyicus subsp. hyicus* gebildet und sind somit für diese Arten besonders charakteristisch. Ihr Nachweis geschieht im Agardiffusionstest mit Hilfe der o. g. Nährböden. Die Staphylokokkenkulturen bzw. deren Überstände werden zur Zerstörung der thermolabilen Nukleasen vorher in einem Wasserbad 15 Minuten auf 100 °C erhitzt und dann in die Stanzlöcher des Nährbodens gegeben. Thermoresistente Nukleasen können auch in hitzebehandelten Lebensmitteln nachweisbar sein, die vorher mit *St. aureus* kontaminiert waren und in denen nach der Behandlung lebende Staphylokokken nicht mehr nachweisbar sind.

▷ Hyaluronidase: Der Nachweis kann im Dekapsulationstest nach MURRAY & PEARCE (23) unter Verwendung eines kapselbildenden *Streptococcus equi*-Stammes geführt werden. Die Impfstriche mit Streptokokken und dem auf Hyaluronidasebildung zu prüfenden Bakterienstamm werden senkrecht zueinander angelegt, im Berührungsbereich wachsen die Streptokokken schleimlos, wenn der geprüf-

of IgG. Its presence can be demonstrated with the slide test of Winblad & Erikson (39), which uses antibody-sensitized sheep erythrocytes. A loopful of staphylococcal culture is mixed on a slide with a suspension of erythrocytes. The slide is tilted back and forth and agglutination will take place, if the staphylococci contain protein A.

▷ Reduction of tellurite: This test relies on the reduction of tellurite salts to black metallic tellurium.

Test substrate: solid media containing potassium tellurite.

Potassium tellurite is contained in Vogel-Johnson's selective medium for staphylococci, which becomes selective for coagulase- and mannitol-positive staphylococci by the addition of lithium chloride (0.5 %). The medium also contains mannitol, glycerol and phenol red as indicator. Coagulase-positive staphylococci grow as black colonies with a yellow halo.

The characteristic features enumerated above can be present in various combinations in the different strains of staphylococcus. However, in routine diagnosis it is usually sufficient for an identification of *St. aureus* to demonstrate one to three of the typical and rapidly identifiable characteristics such as haemolysis, CF or protein A (fig. 5).

Because of the great variability in the metabolic reactions of *St. aureus* it is not always possible to classify certain strains satisfactorily. Numerous attempts have therefore been made to establish new types. Thus for example, haemolytic, CF-positive or negative, mannitol-negative staphylococci, which grow as white colonies, have been classified as *St. intermedius* (fig. 5) (9). They have been found in various animal species, especially in the dog and

te Stamm Hyaluronidase bildet (Abb. 8).

▷ Protein A: Es handelt sich um eine Eiweißsubstanz, die von den meisten *St. aureus-* und *St. hyicus* subsp. *hyicus-*Stämmen gebildet wird und an der Oberfläche der Zellwand gebunden ist. Protein A reagiert mit dem Fc-Fragment von IgG im Normalserum. Der Nachweis kann mit der Objektträgermethode nach Winblad & Erikson (39) unter Verwendung von mit Amboseptor sensibilisierten Schaferythrozyten geführt werden. Nach Einreiben einer Öse Staphylokokkenkultur in die Erythrozytensuspension tritt nach Schwenken des Objektträgers, und sofern die Staphylokokken Protein A besitzen, eine Agglutination auf.

▷ Tellurtreduktion: Es wird die Reduktion von Tellursalzen zu schwarzem metallischen Tellur nachgewiesen.

Testsubstrat: K-Tellurit-haltige feste Nährböden.

K-Tellurit als Zusatz zum Staphylokokken-Selektivagar nach Vogel-Johnson, dessen selektive Wirkung für koagulase- (mannit-)positive Staphylokokken durch den Zusatz von Lithiumchlorid (0,5 %) erreicht wird. Der Nährboden enthält ferner Mannit, Glycerin und Phenolrot als Farbindikator. Koagulasepositive Staphylokokken wachsen in schwarzen Kolonien mit gelbem Hof.

Bei den einzelnen Staphylokokkenstämmen kann jedoch das oben erläuterte Merkmalsschema unterschiedlich zusammengesetzt sein. Für die Identifizierung von *St. aureus* in der Routinediagnostik genügt es im allgemeinen, ein bis drei kennzeichnende und methodisch schnell erfaßbare Merkmale nachzuweisen, wie z. B. Hämolyse, CF oder Protein A (Abb. 5).

Die große Stoffwechselplastizität von *St. aureus*

Table 4: Enlarged system for the classification of staphylococci occurring in the bovine udder (16)

Tabelle 4: Erweitertes Schema zur Einteilung von Staphylokokken, die im Rindereuter vorkommen (16)

	St. aureus	St. intermedius	St. hyicus subsp. hyicus	St. hyicus subsp. chromogenes	St. epidermidis	St. capitis	St. hominis	St. haemolyticus	St. cohnii	St. warneri	St. saprophyticus
Coagulase	+	+	v	−	−	−	−	−	−	−	−
Catalase	+	+	+	+	+	+	+	+	+	+	+
Glucose fermentation	+	+	+	+	+	+	+	+	+	+	+
Thermolabile nuclease	+	+	+	(+)	−	−	−	−	−	−	−
Haemolysis	+	v	−	−	−	−	−	−	−	−	−
Acetoin	+	−	−	−	+	v	v	+	v	+	+
Saccharose fermentation	+	+	+	+	+	+	+	+	−	+	+
Trehalose fermentation	+	+	+	+	+	−	+	+	+	+	+
Mannitol fermentation	+	(+)	−	−	−	+	−	v	+	v	+
Phosphatase	+	+	+	+	+	−	−	−	−	−	−
Novobiocin inhibition (1.6 μg/ml)	−	−	−	−	−	−	−	−	−	+	+
Erythromycin inhibition (0.4 μg/ml)	+	+	+	+	+	+	+	+	+	+	+
Lysostaphin	+	+	−	−	−	−	−	−	−	−	−

in bovine mastitis (16). Table 4 contains an example of such a classification.

Furthermore *St. aureus* strains of man and a range of animals have host specific variants (e. g. *hominis, bovis, canis, gallinae*), which differ in their biochemical properties. Variable characteristics are, for example, the coagulase action on the plasma of various animal species (fig. 5), the fibrinolysin effect and the types of lysis and haemolysis (13, 14, 18, 24, 25). The host variant in the dog *(St. aureus var. canis)* which takes up an intermediate position between *St. aureus* and *St. epidermidis*, has more recently been classified as a separate species under the designation of *St. intermedius* (20). The majority of coagulase positive staphylococci isolated from dogs have been shown by their cultural and biochemical properties to be of this type (17).

In summary, therefore, it can be stated that the taxonomic classification of the genus *Staphylococcus* is not definitive and other types may yet be added.

■ Enterotoxins

These are extracellular, heat resistant toxins which are produced in food materials by some strains of *St. aureus* and cause food poisoning in man. At least five enterotoxins (A, B, C, D, E) are recognized and toxin C has two variants C_1 and C_2. Chemically they are proteins.

More of the strains that are isolated from man than from cattle produce enterotoxins. More than 50 % of the human strains from clinical material may produce enterotoxins.

Identification of staphylococci and enterotoxins in food materials

The demonstration of staphylococci by means of culture, best carried out on selective media (see p. 16), will only provide a partial answer to the possible presence of enterotoxins in the food because:

▷ not all strains of staphylococcus produce enterotoxins,
▷ even potential enterotoxin producers do not always form toxins,
▷ enterotoxins can be expected to be present only when bacterial counts have reached between 10^5 and 10^6 per g,

▷ enterotoxins are considerably more stable than the staphylococci and thus the absence of enterotoxins cannot be assumed even when only a few or no staphylococci are present (36).

In food materials which have been heated and in which staphylococci can no longer be cultured, the identification of thermonuclease can be used as an indicator of contamination (see p. 20).

Proof that an intoxication has occurred or that human beings are in real danger of intoxication can only be provided by the demonstration of enterotoxins in the food. But this is very costly and is usually restricted to specialized laboratories. An indication with strong probability is given when illness has occurred, the suspect food contains more than 10^5 staphylococci per gram and the isolated strain is one that is capable of producing enterotoxins.

To demonstrate their ability to produce enterotoxins, the staphylococci are grown on suitable media (e.g. brain-heart infusion broth) and the supernatant is used directly for the serological test. It is more difficult to demonstrate the toxins in food, because they have to be extracted and concentrated first. Various methods have been described for demonstrating toxins; these are listed by UNTERMANN (36). The micro-agar-gel diffusion test of WADSWORTH (38) adapted by CASMAN et al. (8) and modified by UNTERMANN (37) has been found very effective for the diagnosis of enterotoxins. FEY et al. (12) have reported on the use of the ELISA technique.

1.1.2 Staphylococcus hyicus
1.1.2.1 Staphylococcus hyicus subsp. hyicus

■ **Incidence and veterinary significance**
The causal agent of the weeping eczema (exudative epidermitis, seborrhoeic eczema) of pigs (3, 7, 31), which must be interpreted as a generalized disease because the kidneys, liver, central nervous system, joints etc. are also affected apart from the skin lesions. The bacterium is rarely encountered in cattle and poultry.
  Pemphigoid of piglets which is accompanied by pulmonary lesions (26) is caused by *St. aureus*.

■ **Morphology** (fig. 6)
The microscopic appearance is similar to that of *St. aureus*.

■ **Culture** (fig. 7)
On bovine blood agar *St. hyicus* grows as white,

kokken sind, so daß auch dann, wenn Staphylokokken nicht oder nur in geringen Keimzahlen vorhanden sind, die Abwesenheit des Enterotoxins nicht sicher angenommen werden kann (36).

In Lebensmitteln, die erhitzt worden sind und aus denen Staphylokokken kulturell nicht mehr nachweisbar sind, kann als Indikator der Kontamination die Thermonuklease nachgewiesen werden (s. S. 20).

Der alleinige Beweis einer stattgehabten Intoxikation oder einer konkreten Gefährdung des Menschen kann nur über den Enterotoxinnachweis aus dem Lebensmittel geführt werden. Dieser ist jedoch sehr aufwendig und meistens spezialisierten Laboratorien vorbehalten. Eine hohe Wahrscheinlichkeitsdiagnose ist jedoch nach Erkrankungen erlaubt, wenn in dem betreffenden Lebensmittel Staphylokokkenzahlen von mehr als $10^5/g$ festgestellt werden und der isolierte Staphylokokkenstamm Enterotoxin bilden kann.

Für den Enterotoxinnachweis von Staphylokokkenstämmen werden diese in geeigneten Nährböden (z. B. brain-heart-infusion-Bouillon) gezüchtet, und der Überstand kann unmittelbar für den serologischen Toxinnachweis benutzt werden. Schwieriger ist der Nachweis aus Lebensmitteln, da das Toxin vorher extrahiert und konzentriert werden muß. Für den Enterotoxinnachweis sind verschiedene Methoden beschrieben worden (Zusammenstellung bei UNTERMANN, 36), besonders bewährt hat sich der Mikro-Agargel-Diffusionstest nach WADSWORTH (38), der von CASMAN et al. (8) für die Enterotoxindiagnostik beschrieben wurde und von UNTERMANN (37) modifiziert wurde. Über die Anwendung der ELISA Technik haben FEY et al. (12) berichtet.

1.1.2 Staphylococcus hyicus
1.1.2.1 Staphylococcus hyicus subsp. hyicus

■ **Vorkommen und medizinische Bedeutung**
Erreger des nässenden Ekzems (exsudative Epidermitis, seborrhoisches Ekzem, Ferkelruß) des Schweines (3, 7, 31), das als eine Allgemeinerkrankung des Schweines aufzufassen ist, an der neben der äußeren Haut u. a. auch Niere, Leber, ZNS und Gelenke beteiligt sind. Selten kommt das Bakterium auch beim Rind und beim Geflügel vor.
  Das beim Saugferkel zusammen mit Lungenalterationen vorkommende Pemphigoid (26) wird durch *St. aureus* verursacht.

■ **Morphologie** (Abb. 6)
Das mikroskopische Bild entspricht *St. aureus*.

■ **Kultur** (Abb. 7)
St. hyicus wächst auf Rinderblutagar in weißen, an-

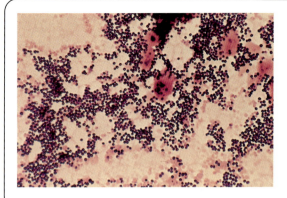
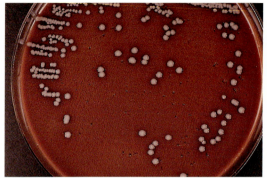
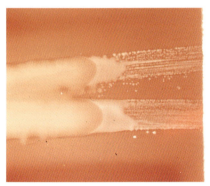
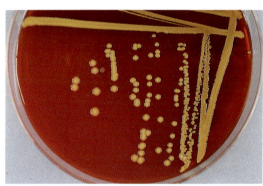

▲ Fig. 6: *Staphylococcus hyicus subsp. hyicus*, smear from skin lesion, Gram stain, irregularly distributed cocci. Magnification x 1000
▼ Fig. 8: Demonstration of hyaluronidase in *Staphylococcus hyicus* (right vertical inoculation streak). In the region of this streak there is no mucoid growth on *Streptococcus equi* (horizontal streak). Blood agar, 48 h, 37 °C. Magnification x 2

▲ Fig. 7: *Staphylococcus hyicus subsp. hyicus* pure culture on chocolate agar, white colonies surrounded by a dark rim. 24 h, 37 °C. Magnification x 0.4
▼ Fig. 9: *Micrococcus sp.*, pure culture on blood agar, yellow non-haemolytic colonies, 48 h, 37 °C. Magnification x 0.4

▲ Abb. 6: *Staphylococcus hyicus subsp. hyicus*, Ausstrich aus Hautveränderungen, Gram-Färbung, unregelmäßig gelagerte Kokken, Abb.-M. 1000 : 1
▼ Abb. 8: Hyaluronidasenachweis bei *Staphylococcus hyicus* (rechter senkrechter Impfstrich), im Bereich dieses Impfstriches unterbleibt das schleimige Wachstum von *Streptococcus equi* (waagerechte Impfstriche), Blutagar, 48 h, 37 °C, Abb.-M. 2 : 1

▲ Abb. 7: *Staphylococcus hyicus subsp. hyicus*, Reinkultur auf Kochblutplatte, weiße, von einem dunklen Rand umgebene Kolonien, 24 h, 37 °C, Abb.-M. 1 : 2,5
▼ Abb. 9: *Micrococcus sp.*, Reinkultur auf Blutagar, gelbe anhämolytische Kolonien, 48 h, 37 °C, Abb.-M. 1 : 2,5

non-haemolytic colonies. On chocolate agar after 20 hours incubation, a characteristic dark brown border, 1–2 mm in diameter, develops which intensifies after 24 to 48 hours to a 1 mm wide zone of lysis at the periphery of the colonies.

■ **Cultural and biochemical properties**
See figure 5 (1, 3, 10).

hämolysierenden Kolonien. Auf Kochblutagar bildet sich nach 20stündiger Bebrütung ein charaktistischer, ca. 1–2 mm breiter dunkelbrauner Hof, der sich nach 24–48 h an der Kolonieperipherie zu einer 1 mm breiten Lysiszone verstärkt.

■ **Kulturell-biochemische Eigenschaften**
Siehe Abb. 5 (1, 3, 10).

Family: Micrococcaceae

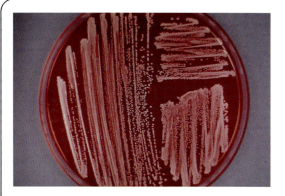
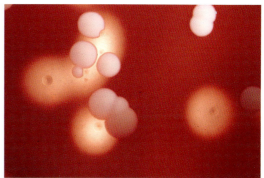
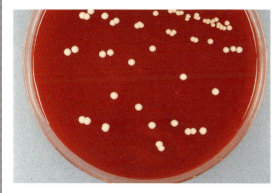
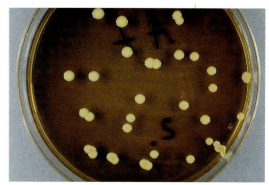

▲ Fig. 10: *Staphylococcus epidermidis*, pure culture on blood agar, white colonies without haemolysis, 24 h, 37 °C. Magnification x 0.4
▼ Fig. 12: Yeasts in pure culture on blood agar. The colonies of yeasts and *St. epidermidis* are so similar that they may be confused. Microscopic examination will provide the differentiation. 48 h, 37 °C. Magnification x 0.33

▲ Fig. 11: Mixed culture of *Staphylococcus epidermidis* and β-haemolytic streptococci on blood agar, 24 h, 37 °C. Magnification x 0.33
▼ Fig. 13: Yeasts in pure culture on Gassner agar. Differential diagnosis for *St. epidermidis* which is inhibited or at least retarded on Gassner medium. 48 h, 37 °C. Magnification x 0.33

▲ Abb. 10: *Staphylococcus epidermidis*, Reinkultur auf Blutagar, weiße Kolonien ohne Hämolyse, 24 h, 37 °C, Abb.-M. 1 : 2,5
▼ Abb. 12: Hefen, Reinkultur auf Blutagar, Hefen können nach dem Koloniebild mit *St. epidermidis* verwechselt werden, Differentialdiagnose durch mikroskopische Untersuchung, 48 h, 37 °C, Abb.-M. 1 : 3

▲ Abb. 11: Mischkultur mit *Staphylococcus epidermidis* und β-hämolysierenden Streptokokken auf Blutagar, 24 h, 37 °C, Abb.-M. 2 : 1
▼ Abb. 13: Hefen, Reinkultur auf Gaßner-Agar, Differentialdiagnose zu *St. epidermidis*, der auf der Gaßner-Platte nicht oder nur sehr verzögert wächst, 48 h, 37 °C, Abb.-M. 1 : 3

1.1.2.2 Staphylococcus hyicus subsp. chromogenes

This subspecies is of interest in differential diagnosis, since it occurs on the skin of pigs. The cultural and biochemical properties are given in table 4.

1.1.2.2 Staphylococcus hyicus subsp. chromogenes

Die Unterart ist von differentialdiagnostischem Interesse, da sie auf der Haut von Schweinen vorkommt. Kulturell-biochemische Eigenschaften erläutert Tab. 4.

1.1.3 Coagulase negative Staphylococci
1.1.3.1 Staphylococcus epidermidis

■ **Incidence and veterinary significance**

St. epidermidis is similar in distribution to St. aureus. It occurs on the skin and mucous membranes of man and animals and is often encountered in samples from these tissues. It is distinctly less pathogenic than St. aureus, but under favourable conditions it can also cause purulent lesions.

■ **Morphology**

In microscopic appearance and the arrangement of the cocci to one another are similar in St. epidermidis and St. aureus.

■ **Culture** (fig. 11)

St. epidermidis grows on the usual media without any special requirements as white, very rarely yellow to orange, lightly granular colonies. Initially broth becomes uniformly cloudy, this later clears as a sediment is formed. Selective media which also serve to identify St. epidermidis are listed on p. 16.

■ **Biochemical properties**

Typical strains of St. epidermidis are metabolically not very active when compared with St. aureus (fig. 5).

1.1.3.2 Staphylococcus saprophyticus

This is considered to be a non-pathogen but it is occasionally encountered in samples of animal origin. It also occurs in the air, soil, dust, milk products and the like.

These are spherical cells with a diameter between 0.5 and 1.5 µm, which are usually in irregular groups, sometimes in tetrads and packets.

On solid media they form smooth convex colonies, generally white occasionally yellow to orange. Metabolism is respiratory, a weak glucose fermentation can occur. Acid is formed from glucose, glycerol, lactose and saccharose.

1.2 Genus: Micrococcus (M.)

Spherical cells, 0.5 to 3.5 µm in diameter. The cocci occur in irregular groups clusters, in groups of four or in packets.

1.1.3 Koagulasenegative Staphylokokken
1.1.3.1 Staphylococcus epidermidis

■ **Vorkommen und medizinische Bedeutung**

St. epidermidis kommt in ähnlicher Verbreitung wie St. aureus auf der Haut und auf den Schleimhäuten von Mensch und Tier vor und wird oft in entsprechenden Untersuchungsmaterialien nachgewiesen. Im Vergleich zu St. aureus ist er deutlich weniger pathogen, kann jedoch unter günstigen Bedingungen ebenfalls eitrige Prozesse verursachen.

■ **Morphologie**

In seinem mikroskopischen Bild und in der Lagerung der Kokken zueinander gleicht St. epidermidis St. aureus.

■ **Kultur** (Abb. 11)

St. epidermidis wächst ohne besondere Ansprüche auf den üblichen Nährböden in weißen, sehr selten gelb bis orange pigmentierten, leicht granulierten Kolonien. Die Bouillon wird zunächst gleichmäßig getrübt, später bildet sich bei gleichzeitiger Klärung Bodensatz. Selektivmedien, die auch den Nachweis von St. epidermidis ermöglichen, sind auf S. 16 angeführt.

■ **Kulturell-biochemische Eigenschaften**

Im Vergleich zu St. aureus sind typische Stämme von St. epidermidis weitgehend stoffwechselinaktiv (Abb. 5).

1.1.3.2 Staphylococcus saprophyticus

Das Bakterium gilt als apathogen, wird jedoch zufällig aus tierischen Untersuchungsstoffen isoliert. Das weitere Vorkommen betrifft Luft, Erde, Staub, Milchprodukte u. ä.

Es handelt sich um kugelige Zellen mit einem Durchmesser von 0,5 bis 1,5 µm, die meistens in unregelmäßigen Haufen liegen und gelegentlich Tetraden und Pakete bilden können.

In der Kultur bilden sich glatte, konvexe Kolonien, die für gewöhnlich weiß aussehen, manchmal gelb bis orange gefärbt sein können.

Der Stoffwechsel ist respiratorisch, eine schwache Glucosefermentation ist möglich. Aus Glucose, Glycerin, Lactose und Saccharose wird Säure gebildet.

1.2 Gattung: Micrococcus (M.)

Kugelige Zellen mit einem Durchmesser von 0,5 bis 3,5 µm. Die Kokken sind in unregelmäßigen Haufen, als Viererkokken oder Paketkokken gelagert.

Family: Micrococcaceae

Micrococcus luteus, M. roseus, M. varians

■ **Incidence and veterinary significance**

The micrococci are widely distributed, they occur in soil, water, on the skin and mucous membrane of animals and they are therefore frequently encountered as contaminants; they are non-pathogenic.

■ **Culture** (fig. 9)

The micrococci grow aerobically and best at temperatures between 25 and 30 °C and they will tolerate up to 5 % salt in the medium. On solid media they form medium-sized, smooth, yellow *(M. luteus, M. varians)* or red *(M. roseus)* colonies.

■ **Biochemical properties**

The metabolism is strictly respiratory. They are very inactive in the breakdown of sugars; glucose is utilized oxidatively or not at all. They are catalase positive. The differentiation between micrococcus and staphylococcus spp. is shown in table 1.

Micrococcus luteus, M. roseus, M. varians

■ **Vorkommen und medizinische Bedeutung**

Die Mikrokokken kommen im Erdboden, Wasser, auf der Haut und den Schleimhäuten der Tiere weit verbreitet vor. Sie werden deswegen in den verschiedenen Untersuchungsmaterialien als Kontaminanten oft gefunden, sind jedoch nicht pathogen.

■ **Kultur** (Abb. 9)

Die Mikrokokken wachsen aerob und am besten bei einer Temperatur zwischen 25 und 30 °C, sie tolerieren bis zu 5 % Kochsalz im Nährmedium. Auf festen Nährböden wachsen sie in mittelgroßen, glatten, gelb *(M. luteus, M. varians)* oder rot *(M. roseus)* pigmentierten Kolonien.

■ **Kulturell-biochemische Eigenschaften**

Der Stoffwechsel ist streng respiratorisch. Hinsichtlich des Zuckerabbaues verhalten sie sich sehr inaktiv, Glucose wird oxydativ oder überhaupt nicht verwertet. Katalasepositiv. Die Abtrennung der Gattung *Micrococcus* von den Staphylokokken gibt Tab. 1 wieder.

Bibliography / Literatur

1. AMTSBERG, G. (1979): Vergleichende biochemische und serologische Untersuchungen an Staphylokokken von Schweinen und Rindern unter besonderer Berücksichtigung von Staphylococcus hyicus bzw. Staphylococcus epidermidis Biotyp 2. Zbl. Vet. Med. B, **26** 137–152.
2. AMTSBERG, G., & S. HAZEM (1978): Vergleichende experimentelle Untersuchungen zum Nachweis der Pathogenität von Staphylococcus hyicus des Schweines bzw. Staphylococcus epidermidis Biotyp 2 des Rindes an gnotobiotischen Ferkeln und Kaninchen. Berl. Münch. tierärztl. Wschr. **91**, 299–301.
3. AMTSBERG, G., W. BOLLWAHN, S. HAZEM, B. JORDAN & U. SCHMIDT (1973): Bakteriologische, serologische und tierexperimentelle Untersuchungen zur ätiologischen Bedeutung von Staphylococcus hyicus beim Nässenden Ekzem der Schweine. Dtsch. tierärztl. Wschr. **80**, 496–499, 521–523.
4. BIBERSTEIN, E. L., S. S. JANG & D. HIRSCH (1984): Species distribution of coagulase-positive staphylococci in animals. J. clin. Microbiol. **19**, 610–615.
5. BLOBEL, H., & J. BRÜCKLER (1980): Staphylokokken. In: H. BLOBEL & TH. SCHLIESSER (Hrsg.): Handbuch der bakteriellen Infektionen bei Tieren. S. 21–130. Jena: VEB Gustav Fischer.
6. BLOBEL, H., J. BRÜCKLER, D. KITZROW & W. SCHAEG (1977): Zur Pathogenität von Staphylokokken. Tierärztl. Umschau **32**, 350–353.
7. BOLLWAHN, W., K. H. BÄHR, A. S. HAZEM, G. AMTSBERG & U. SCHMIDT (1970): Experimentelle Untersuchungen zur Ätiologie des nässenden Ekzems der Schweine. Dtsch. tierärztl. Wschr. **77**, 601–603.
8. CASMAN, E. P., R. W. BENNETT, A. E. DORSEY & J. E. STONE (1969): The micro-slide gel double diffusion test for the detection and assay of staphylococcal enterotoxine. Hlth. Lab. Sci. **6**, 185–198.
9. DEVRIESE, L. A., & V. HAJEK (1980): Identification of pathogenic staphylococci isolated from animals and foods derived from animals. J. appl. Bact. **49**, 1–11.
10. DEVRIESE, L. A., V. HAJEK, P. OEDING, S. A. MEYER & K. H. SCHLEIFER (1978): Staphylococcus hyicus (Sompolinski 1953) comb. nov. and Staphylococcus hyicus subsp. chromogenes subsp. nov. Int. J. System. Bact. **28**, 482–490.
11. ESSERS, L., & W. BECKER (1985): Identifizierung koagulasenegativer Staphylokokken — Ein Methodenvergleich zwischen einem konventionellen Verfahren und einem kommerziellen Mikroidentifizierungssystem. Lab. med. **9**, 79–81.
12. FEY, H., G. STIFFLER-ROSENBERG, G. WARTENWEILER-BURKHARD, CHR. MÜLLER & O. RÜEGG (1982): Der Nachweis von Staphylokokken-Enterotoxinen (SST). Schweiz. Arch. Tierhk. **124**, 297–306.
13. GRÜN, L. (1968): Zur Bestimmung von Standortvarianten der Staphylokokken humaner und boviner Herkunft. Milchwissensch. **23**, 604–608.
14. HÁJEK, V., & E. MARSÁLEK (1969): Untersuchungen mit Staphylokokken bovinen Ursprungs (Staphylococcus aureus var. bovis). Zbl. Bakt. I. Orig. **209**, 154–168.
15. HIGGINS, R., & P. CHARTIER (1984): Contribution à l'identification des staphylocoques coagulase positive d'origine animale. Méd. Vét. du Québec **14**, 61–65.
16. HODGES, R. T., Y. S. JONES & J. T. S. HOLLAND (1984): Characterisation of staphylococci associated with clinical and subclinical bovine mastitis. N.Z. vet. J. **32**, 141–145.
17. HUMMEL, R. (1984): Epizootology of staphylococci, and some other remarks on the pathogenesis of staphylococcal infections in animals. In: W. MEYER (Hrsg.): Staphylokokken und Staphylokokken-Erkrankungen. S. 485–499. Jena: VEB Gustav Fischer.
18. HUMMEL, R., W. WITTE & W. WITTIG (1982): Vorkommen von Staphylococcus-aureus-Stämmen, die nicht einzuordnen sind in die hier bekannten Standortvarietäten, in pathologischen Prozessen von Haustieren. Arch. exp. Vet. med. **36**, 679–689.
19. KLOOS, W. E., & K. H. SCHLEIFER (1975): Simplified scheme for routine identification of human Staphylococcus species. J. clin. Microbiol. **1**, 82–86.
20. KOCUR, M. (1984): Taxonomy of the genus Staphylococcus. In: W. MEYER (Hrsg.): Staphylokokken und Staphylokokken-Erkrankungen. S. 17–27. Jena: VEB Gustav Fischer.

21. Lachica, R. V. F., C. Genigeorgis & P. D. Hoeprich (1971): Metachromatic agar-diffusion methods for detecting staphylococcal activity. Appl. Microbiol. 21, 585–587.
22. Langlois, B. E., R. J. Harmon & K. Akers (1983): Identification of Staphylococcus species of bovine origin with the API Staph-Ident System. J. clin. Microbiol. 18, 1212–1219.
23. Murray, R. G. EF., & R. H. Pearce (1949): The detection and assay of hyaluronidase by means of mucoid streptococci. Canad. J. Res. Sect. E 27, 254–264.
24. Pulverer, G. (1966): Vergleich pathogener Staphylokokken von Mensch und Tier. Zbl. Bakt. I. Orig. 201, 27–41.
25. Meyer, W. (1966): Differenzierungsschema für Standortvarianten von Staphylococcus aureus. Zbl. Bakt. I. Orig. 201, 465–481.
26. Matschullat, G., M. Rosenbruch & J. Woicke (1984): Eine durch Pemphigoid und Lungenalterationen gekennzeichnete Staphylokokkeninfektion bei Saugferkeln. Prakt. Tierarzt 65, 844–847.
27. Radebold, K., & L. Essers (1980): Zur Beurteilung des API-Staph-Systems für die routinemäßige Identifizierung von Staphylokokken. Ärztl. Lab. 26, 236–238.
28. Rheinbaben, K. E. v., & R. M. Hadlok (1981): Rapid distinction between micrococci and staphylococci with furazolidone agars. Antonie van Leeuwenhoek 47, 41–51.
29. Rheinbaben, K. E. v., & R. M. Hadlok (1980): Differenzierung von in Fleischerzeugnissen vorkommenden Mikroorganismen der Familie Micrococcaceae. schlachten u. vermarkten, 80, 333–364.
30. Schleifer, K. H., & W. E. Kloss (1975): A simple test system for the separation of staphylococci from micrococci. J. clin. Microbiol. 1, 337–338.
31. Schulz, W. (1970): Die Exsudative Epidermitis der Ferkel (Ferkelruß) — Untersuchungen zur Ätiologie und Pathogenese unter besonderer Berücksichtigung des Staphylococcus hyicus. Mh. Vet. Med. 25, 428–435.
32. Sinell, H.-J., & J. Baumgart (1967): Selektivnährböden mit Eigelb zur Isolierung von pathogenen Staphylokokken aus Lebensmitteln. Zbl. Bakt. I. Orig. 204, 248–264.
33. Terplan, G., H. Becker & K.-J. Zaadhof (1981): Eignung gebräuchlicher und neuer Medien zum Nachweis von St. aureus in Lebensmitteln und Möglichkeiten ihrer Qualitätskontrolle. Arch. Lebensmittelhyg. 32, 126–130.
34. Terplan, G., & K.-J. Zaadhof (1978): Nachweisverfahren für S. aureus in Lebensmitteln. Arch. Lebensmittelhyg. 29, 132–135.
35. Trolldenier, H. (1977): Antibiotika in der Veterinärmedizin. Jena: VEB Gustav Fischer.
36. Untermann, F. (1980): Staphylokokken-Enterotoxine. In: H. Blobel u. Th. Schliesser (Hrsg.): Handbuch der bakteriellen Infektionen bei Tieren. Bd. II. Jena: VEB Gustav Fischer.
37. Untermann, F. (1974): A modified microslide gel double diffusion test. Zbl. Bakt. I. Orig. A 229, 51–54.
38. Wadsworth, C. (1957): A slide microtechnique for the analysis of immune precipitates in gel. Int. Arch. Allergy 10, 355–360.
39. Winblad, S., & C. Erikson (1973): Sensitized sheep red cells as a reactant for Staphylococcus aureus protein A. Act. Path. Scand. 81, 150–156.

2 Family: Streptococcaceae

2.1 Genus: Streptococcus (Sc.)

This genus encompasses almost 40 species which either give rise to usually purulent inflammation or form part of the physiological flora of the body. Thus we differentiate:

Pathogenic streptococci. The individual species have become specially adapted to either man or certain animals, which have thus become the primary hosts (tab. 5), although there is no true host specificity.

Enterococci. These belong to the serological group D and their normal habitat is the gut of warm-

Table 5: Principal occurrence of the most important pathogenic streptococci of man and animals

Man	Horse	Ox	Pig
Sc. pyogenes	Sc. equi	Sc. agalactiae	Sc. group E
Sc. equisimilis	Sc. zooepidemicus	Sc. dysgalactiae	Sc. equisimilis
Sc. anginosus		Sc. uberis	Sc. group L
Sc. group G			Sc. group R
Sc. pneumoniae			Sc. group S
			Sc. group T
			Sc. group U
			Sc. group V

blooded animals. They are frequently encountered in food materials (see p. 39).

Oral streptococci are present in the oral cavities of man and animals. They include the serological groups H and K, and the unclassified species *Sc. sanguis*, *Sc. mutans*, *Sc. salivarius*, *Sc. viridans*, *Sc. milleri* and *Sc. MG*.

Lactis streptococci are non-pathogenic and do not occur in the animal body, except coincidentally. They include *Sc. lactis*, *Sc. cremoris* and *Sc. diacetylactis*. They are found in milk and milk products and are used as starter cultures in the production of fermented milk products.

The diagnostic procedure to demonstrate streptococcal infections is shown in figure 14.

■ Morphology
These are Gram-positive, round or ovoid cocci which, after division, lie in only one plane, either in pairs or in chains of various lengths. The diameter of the individual cocci is between 0.6 and 1.2 µm (figs. 15, 19 and 20).

■ Culture
▷ Fluid media: streptococci produce diffuse turbidity of the medium and/or sediment and develop

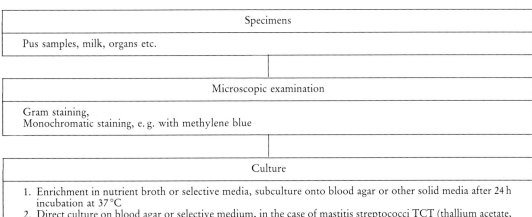

Specimens
Pus samples, milk, organs etc.

Microscopic examination
Gram staining, Monochromatic staining, e.g. with methylene blue

Culture
1. Enrichment in nutrient broth or selective media, subculture onto blood agar or other solid media after 24 h incubation at 37 °C 2. Direct culture on blood agar or selective medium, in the case of mastitis streptococci TCT (thallium acetate, crystal violet, toxin) medium or Edwards medium. 3. Culture for demonstrating anaerobic streptococci.

Biochemical reactions of pure cultures
Type of haemolysis, Metabolic performance, e.g. fermentation of carbohydrates, Determination of serological group CAMP test for the identification of Sc. agalactiae (fig. 17), The bacitracin test is used for the identification of group A streptococci, and group E streptococci may also be sensitive to bacitracin. Incubation at 45 °C in nutrient broth to identify enterococci, Sensitivity to optochin for the recognition of Sc. pneumoniae (fig. 26), Bile solubility test to identify Sc. pneumoniae.

Fig. 14: Examination sequence to demonstrate and identify streptococci

the typical chains.

Broth is used for enrichment in diagnosis, and selective substances may be added which will inhibit the contaminating flora. Such substances can be: sodium azide, crystal violet, kanamycin. An example is »Streptosel broth« which contains sodium azide, crystal violet and possibly kanamycin.

▷ Solid media: media containing blood are best suited for the isolation of these bacteria. Selective agents can be added to these as well and they might include nalidixic acid, polymyxin B sulphate, neomycin sulphate.

Such selective media can be obtained commercially or the selective substances may be purchased as supplements.

The special elements in the identification of mastitis streptococci are given on p. 33.

■ Biochemical properties

Streptococci are facultative anaerobes, their metabolism is homofermentative and the main endproduct of the glucose metabolism is dextro-rotary lactic acid. Their temperature optimum is 37 °C but some species can grow at 10 °C and 45 °C. In particular the pathogenic streptococci produce a series of extracellular substances known as toxins or aggressive enzymes and these are interpreted as evidence of pathogenicity. These include: streptolysins (haemolysins), streptokinase, streptodornase (deoxyribonuclease) and hyaluronidase.

Incubation in a CO_2-enriched atmosphere (5–10 %) will improve the growth on solid media (capnophilic behaviour).

■ Biochemical differentiation

Besides the serological grouping, the following cultural and biochemical characteristics are used in the identification of streptococci.

▷ Haemolysis. There are several forms of haemolysis:

α-haemolysis (fig. 23): incomplete haemolysis, immediately around the colony there are remains of erythrocytes and often a green colouration (breakdown of haemoglobin to the intermediate stage methaemoglobin), this is surrounded by a narrow second zone of complete haemolysis;

β-haemolysis (Figs. 21 and 22): complete haemolysis which consists of a relatively broad, sharply defined zone of complete lysis of both erythrocytes and haemoglobin;

γ-haemolysis: no alteration of either erythrocytes or haemoglobin.

▷ CAMP test. The CAMP test is used for the identification of *Sc. agalactiae* and of streptococci of groups E, P, K and U (see p. 33 and fig. 17).

▷ Bacitracin test. This test serves the recognition of

Bodensatzbildung und Ausbildung typischer Ketten.

In der Diagnostik wird die Bouillon zur Anreicherung benutzt, ihr können selektive Substanzen zugesetzt werden, die die Begleitflora hemmen, z. B.: Natriumsulfit, Natriumacid, Kristallviolett, Kanamycin. Ein Beispiel ist die »Streptosel-Broth«, die Natriumacid, Kristallviolett und eventuell Kanamycin enthält.

▷ Feste Nährböden: Für die Isolierung eignen sich am besten bluthaltige Nährböden, auch ihnen können selektiv wirkende Stoffe zugegeben werden, z. B. Nalidixinsäure, Polymyxin-B-Sulfat, Neomycinsulfat.

Derartige Selektivmedien werden als Fertignährböden oder die selektiven Substanzen als Supplemente im Handel angeboten.

Besonderheiten beim Nachweis von Mastitisstreptokokken siehe S. 33.

■ Kulturell-biochemische Eigenschaften

Streptokokken sind fakultative Anaerobier; ihr Stoffwechsel ist homofermentativ, hauptsächliches Endprodukt des Glucosestoffwechsels ist rechtsdrehende Milchsäure. Ihr Temperaturoptimum liegt bei 37 °C, einige Arten können bei 10 °C und 45 °C wachsen. Insbesondere die pathogenen Streptokokken bilden eine Reihe extrazellulärer Substanzen, die als Toxine oder aggressive Fermente anzusehen sind und als Pathogenitätsmerkmale gewertet werden, z. B. Streptolysine (Hämolysine), Streptokinase, Streptodornase (Desoxyribonuklease) und Hyaluronidase.

Die Wachstumsintensität auf festen Nährböden kann durch Bebrütung in einer CO_2-angereicherten Atmosphäre (5 bis 10 %) erhöht werden (kapnophiles Verhalten).

■ Kulturell-biochemische Differenzierung

Für die Bestimmung der Streptokokken werden neben der serologischen Gruppendiagnose folgende kulturelle und biochemische Merkmale benutzt.

▷ Hämolysine. Nach den Hämolyseformen kann man unterscheiden:

α-**Hämolyse** (Abb. 23): unvollständige Hämolyse, unmittelbar um die Kolonie findet man Erythrozytenreste und oft eine Vergrünung (Abbau des Blutfarbstoffes zur Zwischenstufe Methämoglobin), es folgt eine schmale zweite Zone mit totaler Hämolyse;

β-**Hämolyse** (Abb. 21 u. 22): vollständige Hämolyse, die aus einer relativ breiten, scharf begrenzten Zone mit vollständiger Lysis der Erythrozyten und des Blutfarbstoffes besteht;

γ-**Hämolyse**: keine Veränderung der Erythrozyten und des Blutfarbstoffes.

▷ CAMP-Test. Der CAMP-Test wird zur Identifizierung von *Sc. agalactiae* sowie von Streptokokken der Gruppen E, P, K und U eingesetzt (s. S. 33 u. Abb. 17).

β-haemolytic streptococci of group A, 95% of strains are inhibited by the antibiotic (disc test 0.1–0.2 units).

▷ Growth at a higher incubation temperature (45 °C) and in media containing 6% salt, 0.1% methylene blue or 40% bile: These methods are used mainly for the differentiation of enterococci (group D streptococci), which assume a special position from the biochemical viewpoint. In contrast to most of the other streptococci they will grow

a) at 45 °C,
b) in/on media containing 6% NaCl,
c) in sterile milk containing 0.1% methylene blue,
d) on media containing 40% ox bile (bile blood agar, SEELEMANN, 34).

▷ Fermentation of carbohydrates. These reactions are tested in the usual manner.

▷ Growth in litmus milk. The following reactions may be observed:
Blue colouration due to alkalinity (protein breakdown)
Red colour due to acidification (fermentation of lactose)
Clotting and separation of whey from the other milk constituents,
Loss of colour due to reduction of the indicator.

▷ Hippurate hydrolysis. A tube, containing 1 ml 1% sodium hippurate solution is heavily inoculated and incubated for 2 h at 37 °C in a waterbath. 0.2 ml of ninhydrin reagent is then added (3.5 g ninhydrin in 100 ml acetone and butanol 1 : 1). A positive reaction: purple colouration.

▷ Aesculin hydrolysis. Some streptococci are able to split the glycoside aesculin into δ-glucose and aesculetin. The test: culture in 0.1% aesculin broth and after incubation for 3 to 4 days, 1 ml of a 7% $FeCl_2$ solution is added (37). Positive result: greenish-black precipitate.

■ **Antigenic structure**

Steptococci have several antigens that are of practical importance for their classification and identification.

C-substance: This is a carbohydrate fraction of the cell membrane which usually contains rhamnose, glucose and galactose and forms the basis of the group classification of Lancefield.

Protein antigens (M-substance, T-substance) are of special significance for group A streptococci and serve for their type classification.

Serological test for group identification (precipitation): The C-polysaccharide antigen can be extracted from the cell membrane with, for example, hydrochloric acid, formamide, streptomyces albus enzyme or by autoclaving. The autoclave extract has proved adequate for practical purposes.

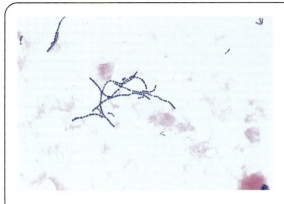
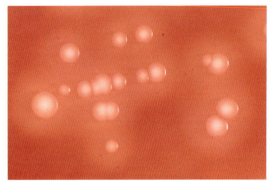
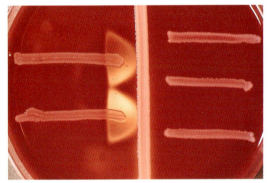
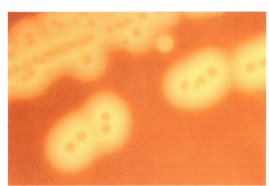

▲ Fig. 15: *Streptococcus agalactiae*, milk smear from mastitis, Gram stain, Gram-positive, long chains of cocci. Magnification x 1000
▼ Fig. 17: CAMP test for confirmation of *Streptococcus agalactiae*, vertical streak: *St. aureus*, left horizontal inoculation streaks: *Sc. agalactiae* with cup-shaped haemolysis, right horizontal streaks: *Sc. lactis* without haemolysis, 48 h, 37 °C. Magnification x 2

▲ Fig. 16: *Streptococcus agalactiae*, pure culture on blood agar, weak haemolysis, 48 h, 37 °C. Magnification x 4
▼ Fig. 18: *Streptococcus agalactiae*, pure culture on TCT medium with strong haemolysis, 48 h, 37 °C. Magnification x 2, transmitted light

▲ Abb. 15: *Streptococcus agalactiae*, Ausstrich von einer Mastitismilch, Gram-Färbung, grampositive, lange Kokkenketten, Abb.-M. 1000 : 1
▼ Abb. 17: CAMP-Test zur Bestimmung von *Streptococcus agalactiae*, senkrechter Impfstrich: *Staphylococcus aureus*, waagerechte linke Impfstriche: *Streptococcus agalactiae* mit schalenförmiger Hämolyse, waagerechte rechte Impfstriche: *Streptococcus lactis* ohne Hämolyse, 48 h, 37 °C, Abb.-M. 2 : 1

▲ Abb. 16: *Streptococcus agalactiae*, Reinkultur auf Blutagar mit einer schwachen Hämolyse, 48 h, 37 °C, Abb.-M. 4 : 1
▼ Abb. 18: *Streptococcus agalactiae*, Reinkultur auf TKT-Medium mit kräftiger Hämolyse, 48 h, 37 °C, Abb.-M. 2 : 1, Durchlichtaufnahme

Preparation of antigen (11)
1. Grow the bacterial strain in 40 ml glucose broth for 24 h
2. Centrifuge cells and suspended in 0.5 ml pyhsiological saline,
3. Add 1 drop of phenol red, neutralize with $^n/_{10}$ NaOH,
4. Autoclave at 120 °C (20 minutes)
5. Cool, re-neutralize, if necessary, remove cells by centrifugation

Antigenherstellung (11)
1. Stamm in 40 ml Glucosebouillon 24 h züchten,
2. Zellen abzentrifugieren und in 0,5 ml physiol. Kochsalzlösung suspendieren,
3. Zugabe eines Tropfens Phenolrot und Neutralisation mit $^n/_{10}$ NaOH,
4. autoklavieren bei 120 °C (20 min),
5. abkühlen lassen, evtl. nachneutralisieren und abzentrifugieren der Zellen,

6. The clear supernatant is used for the precipitation test.

The precipitation test is best carried out as a microcapillary test (12). Capillary tubes, about 4 cm long and internal diameter of 2–3 mm, are dipped into the serum, allowing a column of about 0.5 cm to rise. This is then placed, with the serum downwards, into a plasticine stand. Using a fine capillary pipette, the antigen is layered from above onto the serum. A precipitate will develop in 10 to 15 minutes at the interface.

The serological precipitation test can be simplified by using one of several test systems that have now been commercially developed, such as co-agglutination and latex agglutination. Co-agglutination uses group-specific antibodies, which are bound to the protein A of staphylococci. In latex agglutination the antibodies are bound to latex particles. The antigen is obtained from the cell wall of the streptococci by means of enzymic extraction with pronase B. The results obtained with these methods are in close agreement with those of the classical precipitation test (10, 22, 23).

2.1.1 Streptococci of cattle
2.1.1.1 Streptococcus agalactiae

Sc. agalactiae (see table 6. Figs. 15 to 18) is not only a widespread cause of bovine mastitis, but it also occurs with increasing frequency in man and in particular in certain disease processes of infants such as general infections and meningitis, and it is isolated from the urogenital tract and oro-pharyngeal region. Group B streptococci are rarely found in other animals (such as horses, pigs and sheep).

■ **Culture**

Broth: growth in chains of variable length and clouding of the medium with mucoid, flocculent sediment.
  Blood agar: α-, β- or γ-haemolysis.
▷ Cultural confirmation: Direct smear onto blood agar plates or a selective medium such as Edwards or TCT medium which contain thallium sulphate or acetate and crystal violet as inhibitor. The recognition of Sc. agalactiae is aided by the absence of aesculin hydrolysis or, in TCT agar, by the CAMP phenomenon elicited by the addition of St. aureus β-toxin (fig. 18).
  Enrichment in »streptosel« broth which contains sodium azide, crystal violet and kanamycin.
  The CAMP test: The positive outcome of the CAMP test (fig. 17) agrees to more than 90 % with the serological group determination. Even streptococci of groups E, P, K, U and V can give positive reactions with the CAMP test (37). A positive CAMP test is also possible between C. pseudotuber-

Table 6: The most important streptococci causing bovine mastitis

Properties	Sc. agalactiae	Sc. dysgalactiae	Sc. uberis
Morphology in infected material	Long chains with cocci in pairs palisade form	Chains of medium length, ovoid cocci	Ovoid cells in diploid form, chains up to medium length
Broth	Sediment, long chains	uniform turbidity, chains of medium length	uniform turbidity, small ovoid cocci, short to medium chains, diploid form
Haemolysis on blood agar	α, β, γ	α, β	α, γ, vir[3]
CAMP test	+	−	v⁻
Aesculin	−	−	+[2]
Hippurate hydrolysis	+	−	+
Mannitol fermentation	−	−	+
Sero-grouping	B	C	−[1]

[1] between 15 and 50 % of strains react with E serum;
[2] blackish colonies on TCT agar with added aesculin;
[3] viridans reaction

culosis and group B streptococci; the reaction is negative with group E streptococci (31).

■ **Antigenic structure**

Sc. agalactiae has the group B antigen. 7 type antigens are known. WIESNER (43) and SCHÜTZ et al. (33) have described the serological identification of group B streptococcal antigen in milk. In this test the sediment from 10 ml milk is incubated in broth for 24 h. The B-antigen is extracted with pronase E from the enriched streptococci and the antigen is then confirmed by means of immuno-electrophoresis.

2.1.1.2 Streptococcus dysgalactiae

Apart from cattle, *Sc. dysgalactiae* (table 6) occurs also in sheep (mastitis, metritis), but it is very rarely isolated from other animals.

The metabolic functions used to identify this streptococcus are not very characteristic, so that the determination of the group antigen is of greatest significance.

2.1.1.3 Streptococcus uberis

Although *Sc. uberis* (table 6) causes mastitis it is also found on the outer skin, the muzzle, the skin of the udder and the genital mucosa (41).

■ **Antigenic structure**

There is no group antigen, but between 15 and 50 % of strains react with group E serum.

2.1.1.4 Other streptococci

Besides the types mentioned above one can occasionally encounter other streptococci in individual cattle and especially in mastitis. Examples are *Sc. pyogenes*, streptococci of groups G, L, P (8, 39, 40).

2.1.2 Streptococci of the horse
2.1.2.1 Streptococcus zooepidemicus

Sc. zooepidemicus (tab. 7, figs. 19 and 21) is a pyogenic organism that affects the widest range of animals, but it is most common in equidae.

2.1.2.2 Sc. equi

Compare table 7, figures 20 and 21.

Table 7: The group C pyogenic streptococci of the horse

Feature	*Sc. zooepidemicus*	*Sc. equi*
Clinical picture	Purulent wound infections inflammation of the reproductive organs (sterility in the mare), pneumonia, arthritis, mastitis, septicaemia, paralysis of older foals, latent infection of the mucous membranes	Strangles, less commonly infections of the reproductive organs (sterility in the mare 14, 15), generalized infections of foals
Morphology in native material	ovoid cells, short to medium long chains	ovoid to spherical cells, chains of variable lengths, palisade form
Blood agar	β-haemolysis	β-haemolysis, mucoid growth because of capsule formation (fig. 22)
Broth	flocculent slimy sediment, short to medium length chains	flocculent slimy sediment, particularly long chains (fig. 20)
CAMP test	−	−
Aesculin	v	−
Mannitol	v	−
Lactose	+	−
Sorbitol	+	−
Trehalose	−	−

Table 8: Characteristic reactions in the identification of β-haemolytic streptococci of group C

Species	Sorbitol	Trehalose
Sc. equisimilis	−	+
Sc. zooepidemicus	+	−
Sc. equi	−	−

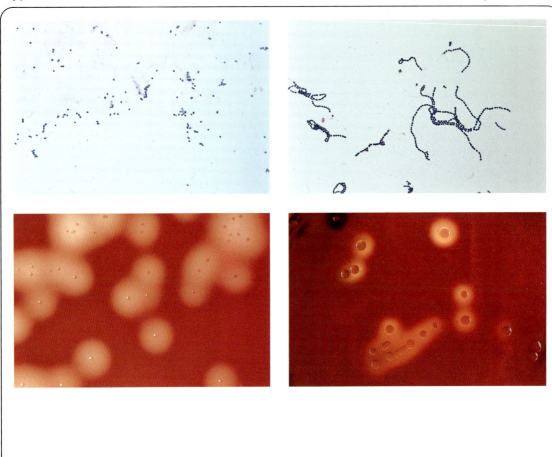

▲ Fig. 19: *Streptococcus zooepidemicus*, smear from a blood agar culture, Gram stain, ther are no distinct streptococcal chains. Magnification x 1000
▼ Fig. 21: *Streptococcus zooepidemicus*, pure culture with β-haemolysis on blood agar, 24 h, 37 °C. Magnification x 2

▲ Fig. 20: *Streptococcus equi*, smear from a broth culture, Gram stain, note the long streptococcal chains. Magnification x 1000
▼ Fig. 22: *Streptoccocus equi*, pure culture with β-haemolysis on DST blood agar, moist mucoid colonies, 24 h, 37 °C. Magnification x 2

▲ Abb. 19: *Streptoccocus zooepidemicus*, Ausstrich von einer Blutagarkultur, Gram-Färbung, es fehlt die Ausbildung deutlicher Streptokokkenketten, Abb.-M. 1000 : 1
▼ Abb. 21: *Streptococcus zooepidemicus*, Reinkultur mit β-Hämolyse auf Blutagar, 24 h, 37 °C, Abb.-M. 2 : 1

▲ Abb. 20: *Streptococcus equi*, Ausstrich von einer Bouillonkultur, Gram-Färbung, Ausbildung langer Streptokokkenketten, Abb.-M. 1000 : 1
▼ Abb. 22: *Streptococcus equi*, Reinkultur mit β-Hämolyse auf DST-Blutagar, schleimig-feuchte Kolonien, 24 h, 37 °C, Abb.-M. 2 : 1

2.1.3 Streptococci of the pig

Members of many serological groups have been isolated from pigs in recent years. It is often difficult to relate them aetiologically with certain clinical signs, their isolation may only be an indication of a latent infection. The following types and groups are mainly involved:

2.1.3 Streptokokken des Schweines

Beim Schwein sind in den letzten Jahren Vertreter vieler Serogruppen isoliert worden. Die ätiologische Zuordnung zu bestimmten Krankheitsbildern ist oft schwierig, oft ist ihr Nachweis nur Ausdruck einer latenten Infektion. Hauptsächlich handelt es sich um folgende Arten und Gruppen:

2.1.3.1 Streptococci of group E

These streptococci (tab. 9) are recognized as the cause of neck and cheek abscesses found particularly commonly in the USA. In the Federal Republic of Germany, this streptococcus can also frequently be isolated from pigs (e.g. from lymph nodes, but the typical clinical picture is hardly ever encountered [42]).

2.1.3.2 Streptococci of group L

Streptococci of this group (tab. 9) are among the most common to be isolated from pigs (3). They lead to latent infections (being located in the tonsils, lymph nodes and vaginal discharge), or they cause a variety of clinical conditions such as arthritis, meningoencephalitis, endocarditis, septicaemia (18, 42).

2.1.3.3 Streptococci of group P

Group P streptococci (tab. 9) were first isolated by MOBERG & THAL (25) from pigs with purulent pneumonia, polyarthritis and pericarditis.

2.1.3.4 Streptococci of groups R, S and T

Members of this group (tab. 9) have, so far, been isolated only from pigs. Groups R and S, and later group T, were drawn up by DE MOOR (6).

ELLIOT (7) named the group R streptococci *Sc. suis* type I and the group S streptococci *Sc. suis* type II. Both these were originally classified under the serological group D. The serological group S occurs only in piglets up to the 8th week of age and group R is seen mainly in older animals (9, 21, 32). Streptococci of group T are very rare. In such infections, however, the picture is dominated by the clinical signs of septicaemia and meningo-encephalitis; arthritis, pneumonia and endocarditis are more rare. Latent infections can occur, especially in the tonsils (4, 5, 19, 28). Group R streptococci can also occur in man, causing meningitis and other symptoms.

Blood agar: β-haemolysis, but also α- or γ-haemolysis. In group R streptococci the type of haemolysis depends on the species from which the blood was obtained. In horse, pig and rabbit blood agar β-haemolysis is observed while α-haemolysis occurs on blood agar made with bovine or ovine blood.

■ Biochemical properties
The action spectrum of streptococci from groups

R, S and T is largely uniform, but raffinose is fermented only by groups R and T. For further details see table 9.

Table 9: Differentiation of the most important β-haemolytic streptococci of the pig (11, 42)

Character	Sc. equisimilis	E	P	R	S	T	U	V
				Streptococci of groups				
Haemolysis	β	β	β or γ	β, α, γ	β, α, γ	β, α, γ	β	β
Broth	long chains flocculent sediment	medium long chains sediment	short-medium length chains uniform turbidity or flocculence	small cocci lying singly or on diploid form, uniform turbidity				
CAMP test	−	+	+	−	−	−	+	+
Growth in 40 % bile	−	−	−	−	−	+	+	−
Aes	v	+	+	+	+	+	+	−
Hip	−	−	+	−	−	−	−	−
Inu	−	−	−	+	+	+	−	−
Man	−	+	+	−	−	−	+	+
Raf	−	−	−	+	−	+	v⁻	+
Sor	−	+	v	−	−	−	+	v⁺
Tre	+	v⁺	+	+	+	+	+	v⁺
VPR	−	+	−	−	−	−	−	−

2.1.3.5 Group U streptococci

Streptococci of group U (tab. 9) are relatively rare organisms that probably occur only in pigs; they have been isolated from tonsils or pathological lesions.

Blood agar: β-haemolysis may develop only under anaerobic conditions. All strains are sensitive to bacitracin (20, 37, 38). They grow on 4 % NaCl agar.

2.1.3.6 Group V streptococci

Streptococci of this group (tab. 9) were isolated from abnormal lymph nodes by JELINKOVÁ & KUBIN (16).

2.1.3.7 Streptococcus equisimilis

Although man is the primary host of Sc. equisimilis (tab. 9), it does occur with relative frequency also in pigs in the form of latent infections (mucous membranes, lymph nodes) or as the cause of generalized infections, polyarthritis, pneumonia and the like.

Family: Streptococcaceae

2.1.4 Enterococci
(group D streptococci)

Opinions vary about the taxonomic definition of enterococci. According to the classification used here the enterococci are equated with group D streptococci.

■ **Incidence and veterinary significance**

Enterococci are ubiquitous in the faeces of man and animals, in sewage, on plants, in animal and human food and in milk. Their physiological habitat is the gut of man and animals. They are of subordinate importance as pathogens in animals, although isolated cases have been described in cattle, sheep, pigs, horses, poultry and other animals as causes of mastitis, pneumonia, vaginitis, endocarditis, septicaemia etc. In the pig- and especially in the poultry-industries epidemic outbreaks have been reported with mortality from 1% to 26%. Among the causal organisms isolated were *Sc. bovis*, *Sc. faecalis* and *Sc. faecium*. It is possible that there are particularly virulent strains among the enterococci (for a literature review see HAHN, 11). *Sc. equinus* is found primarily in the gut of the horse, *Sc. bovis* in the intestinal tract of ruminants.

The following belong to the group of enterococci:

Sc. faecalis var. faecalis
Sc. faecalis var. liquefaciens
Sc. faecalis var. zymogenes
Sc. faecium
Sc. durans
Sc. equinus
Sc. bovis

Sc. durans is considered a variant but Bergey's Manual lists it as synonymous with *Sc. faecium*.

■ **Morphology**

Spherical to ovoid cells with a diameter of 0.5 to 1 µm. The cells of *Sc. faecalis* and *Sc. faecium* are elongated in the direction of the chain. The cocci lie in pairs or chains of varying length, which may sometimes be very short.

■ **Culture**

Broth: They usually grow in short to medium long chains and cause pronounced turbidity of the medium. Blood agar: various forms of haemolysis see table 10.

■ **Biochemical properties**

The enterococci are distinctly different in their biological properties from all other streptococci. A particularly characteristic feature is their ability to grow in or on media containing 6.5% NaCl (excep-

2.1.4 Enterokokken
(Streptokokken der serologischen Gruppe D)

Hinsichtlich der taxonomischen Abgrenzung der Enterokokken bestehen unterschiedliche Ansichten. In der hier gewählten Einteilung werden die Enterokokken mit der Gruppe der D-Streptokokken gleichgesetzt.

■ **Vorkommen und medizinische Bedeutung**

Die Enterokokken kommen ubiquitär in Fäces von Mensch und Tier, in Abwässern, an Pflanzen, in Futter- und Lebensmitteln und in Milch vor. Ihr physiologischer Standort ist der Darm von Mensch und Tier. Als Krankheitserreger des Tieres sind sie von untergeordneter Bedeutung, in Einzelfällen sind sie beim Rind, Schaf, Schwein, Pferd, Geflügel und bei einigen anderen Tierarten als Ursache von Mastitis, Pneumonie, Vaginitis, Endokarditis, Sepsis u. ä. beschrieben worden. In der Ferkel- und vor allem in der Geflügelhaltung sind seuchenartige Verlaufsformen mit einer Mortalität von 1 bis 26 % beschrieben worden, als Erreger wurden dabei u. a. *Sc. bovis*, *Sc. faecalis* und *Sc. faecium* gefunden. Möglicherweise gibt es unter den Enterokokkenarten besonders virulente Stämme (Literaturzusammenstellung bei HAHN, 11). *Sc. equinus* kommt besonders häufig im Darm des Pferdes, *Sc. bovis* im Darm der Wiederkäuer vor.

Zu den Enterokokken gehören:

Sc. faecalis var. faecalis
Sc. faecalis var. liquefaciens
Sc. faecalis var. zymogenes
Sc. faecium
Sc. durans
Sc. equinus
Sc. bovis

Sc. durans wird als eine Variante und nach Bergey's Manual als ein Synonym von *Sc. faecium* angesehen.

■ **Morphologie**

Sphärische bis ovoide Zellen mit einem Durchmesser von 0,5 bis 1 µm. Bei *Sc. faecalis* und *Sc. faecium* sind die Zellen in Kettenrichtung verlängert. Die Kokken liegen in Paaren oder unterschiedlich langen Ketten, oft in kurzen Ketten.

■ **Kultur**

Bouillon: Wachstum meist in kurzen bis mittellangen Ketten unter starker Trübung der Bouillon. Blutagar: Verschiedene Hämolyseformen zeigt Tab. 10.

■ **Kulturell-biochemische Eigenschaften**

Die Enterokokken weichen in ihren biologischen Eigenschaften von den übrigen Streptokokken deutlich ab. Für sie besonders charakteristische Eigenschaften sind das Wachstum in oder auf Nähr-

Table 10: Characteristic biochemical properties of enterococci (11)

Tabelle 10: Charakteristische kulturell-biochemische Eigenschaften der Enterokokken (11)

	Sc. faecalis var. faecalis	*Sc. faecalis var. liquefaciens*	*Sc. faecalis var. zymogenes*	*Sc. faecium*	*Sc. durans*	*Sc. equinus*	*Sc. bovis*
Haemolysis	γ	γ	β	α, vir	α, β, vir	α, γ	α, γ
Growth at 45 °C	+	+	+	+	+	+	+
Growth in 40 % bile	+	+	+	+	+	+	+
Growth in 0.1 % methylene blue	+	+	+	+	+	−	v
Growth in Litmus milk	AcC	AcCw	AcC	AcC	AcC		AcC
Reduction of K-tellurite	+	+	+	−	−	−	−
Fermentation of arginine	+	+	+	+	+	−	−
Fermentation of mannitol	+	+	−	+	−	−	−
Fermentation of lactose	+	+	+	+	+	−	+
Fermentation of glycerine (anaerobic)	+.	+	+	−	−	−	−
Fermentation of gelatine	−	+	−	−	−	−	−
Fermentation of starch	−	−	+	−	−	−	+

Ac = acid production, C = clotting, w — whey production

Ac = Rötung, C = Gerinnung, w — Molkebildung

tion *Sc. equinus*), 40 % bile or 0.1 % methylene blue. (*Sc. bovis* is variable and *Sc. equinus* exhibits no growth). All enterococci will grow at 45 °C. For further biochemical details see table 10.

böden mit 6,5 % NaCl (Ausnahme *Sc. equinus*), 40 % Galle oder 0,1 % Methylenblau (*Sc. bovis* unterschiedliches Verhalten, *Sc. equinus* kein Wachstum). Alle Enterokokken wachsen bei 45 °C. Weitere biochemische Eigenschaften siehe Tabelle 10.

■ **Antigenic structure**
Group antigen D.

■ **Antigenstruktur**
Gruppenantigen D.

2.1.5 Streptococcus pneumoniae
(Syn.: *Diplococcus pneumoniae*, Pneumococcus)

2.1.5 Streptococcus pneumoniae
(Syn.: *Diplococcus pneumoniae*, Pneumokokken)

■ **Incidence and veterinary significance**
Sc. pneumoniae is primarily a human pathogen (pneumonia with a high incidence of bacteraemic forms). In calves it can cause a septic bronchopneumonia. Furthermore, it has been identified in bovine mastitis, in bronchopneumonia and metritis of sheep and in generalized infections of monkeys and laboratory animals (mice, rats, guinea pigs, rabbits). Man is frequently the source of the infection (anthropozoonosis) (13).

■ **Vorkommen und medizinische Bedeutung**
Sc. pneumoniae ist in erster Linie ein Krankheitserreger des Menschen (Pneumonie mit hohem Anteil bakteriämischer Verlaufsformen). Beim Kalb kann eine septische Bronchopneumonie auftreten. Ferner werden beim Rind Mastitiden, beim Schaf Bronchopneumonien und Metritiden, bei Affen und bei Labortieren (Maus, Ratte, Meerschweinchen, Kaninchen) Allgemeininfektionen beobachtet. Infektionsquelle ist oft der Mensch (Anthropozoonose) (13).

■ **Morphology**
These are oval diplococci, 0.5 to 1.25 μm in diameter. Short chains do sometimes occur. The cocci may have a lancet-like appearance and the flat sides of the pair are apposed, so that the pointed surfaces are free (fig. 25). Capsules are formed in animal material and in young cultures. These are recog-

■ **Morphologie**
Es handelt sich um ovale Diplokokken (Durchmesser 0,5 bis 1,25 μm), gelegentlich kommen auch kurze Ketten vor. Die Kokken können lanzettähnlich aussehen, wobei die Kokken eines Paares mit abgeflachter Seite aneinanderliegen und die Gegenseiten zugespitzt sind (Abb. 25). In tierischem Ma-

Family: Streptococcaceae

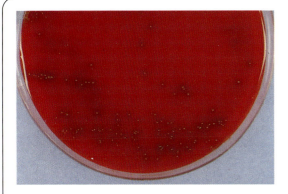
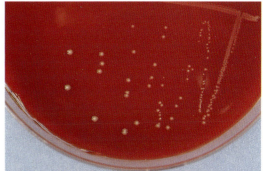
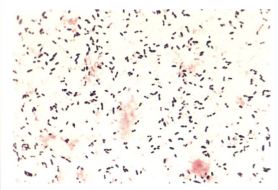
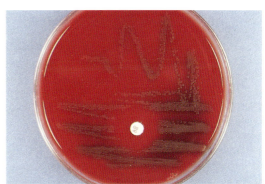

▲ Fig. 23: Streptococcal colonies turning green, blood agar, 48 h, 37 °C. Magnification x 0.4
▼ Fig. 25: *Streptococcus pneumoniae (Diplococcus pneumoniae)*, culture smear, characteristic diplococcal arrangement, Gram stain. Magnification x 1000

▲ Fig. 24: *Peptococcus indolicus*, anaerobic incubation, blood agar, 48 h, 37 °C. Magnification x 0.4
▼ Fig. 26: *Streptococcus pneumoniae*, optochin test: growth inhibition in the region of the diffusion zone, blood agar, colonies turning partially green, 24 h, 37 °C. Magnification x 0.33

▲ Abb. 23: Vergrünend wachsende Streptokokken, Blutagar, 48 h, 37 °C, Abb.-M. 1 : 2,5
▼ Abb. 25: *Streptococcus pneumoniae (Diplococcus pneumoniae)*, Kulturausstrich, charakteristische Diplokokkenlagerung, Gram-Färbung, Abb.-M. 1000 : 1

▲ Abb. 24: *Peptococcus indolicus*, anaerobe Bebrütung, Blutagar, 48 h, 37 °C, Abb.-M. 1 : 2,5
▼ Abb. 26: *Streptococcus pneumoniae*, Optochintest: Wachstumshemmung im Bereich der Diffusionszone, Blutagar, teilweise vergrünendes Wachstum, 24 h, 37 °C, Abb.-M. 1 : 3

nized in methylene blue staining, whereby the blue diplococci are surrounded by a transparent zone (unstained capsules).

■ Culture
The pneumococci grow on blood agar as flat colonies with smooth borders. They measure 1 to 2 mm and the centres show a ring-like depression below the level of the periphery. α-haemolysis with

terial und jungen Kulturen werden Kapseln gebildet, die nach Methylenblaufärbung erkennbar sind, indem die blau gefärbten Diplokokken von einem durchsichtigen Hof (ungefärbte Kapsel) umgeben sind.

■ Kultur
Die Pneumokokken wachsen auf Blutagar in flachen, glattrandigen, 1 bis 2 mm großen Kolonien, deren Zentren gegenüber dem ringförmig erhöhten Rand eingedellt sind. Es tritt eine α-Hämolyse mit

green colouration appears (fig. 26). Type III *(Sc. mucosus)* shows mucoid growth which is increased in an atmosphere of 10 % CO_2.

■ Biochemical properties

Bile solubility and optochin sensitivity are particularly important for the identification of pneumococci.

Bile solubility: This is based on the triggering of an autolytic amidase. The test is carried out by adding to broth culture or a suspension of bacteria in physiological saline, an equal quantity of a 10 % solution of sodium taurocholate. Within 10 to 15 minutes the pneumococci are dissolved and the liquid becomes clear.

Optochin sensitivity: The test is based on the growth inhibition of optochin on pneumococci. This is still effective in dilutions of 1 : 500,000. The test is most easily performed as a diffusion test whereby the appropriate discs are laid onto the inoculated medium (fig. 26).

■ Antigenic structure

More than 80 pneumococcal serotypes have been identified. The capsular polysaccharide antigens form the basis of the test, but the nomenclature of these antigens is not uniform. Neufeld identified types I, II, III and X, where X is a collective group which contains all further types. Other classification make use of arabic figures and letters, but the identification of the serotypes is less important for practical purposes of diagnosis. More than 80 % of all human pneumococcal infections are caused by 14 serotypes, particularly types 1–9. In animals types 4–47 are most prominent and in particular 6, 8, 18 and 19. The identification of the capsule type is achieved with the capsular swelling reaction. If pneumococci in natural material (e. g. peritoneal exudate from inoculated mice) are mixed with antigen on a slide, then in a positive case, the capsule swells.

■ Animal experiment

Mice will die 24 hours after intraperitoneal injection and the pneumococci can be demonstrated microscopically and on culture in the heart blood and organs.

■ Kulturell-biochemische Eigenschaften

Für die Bestimmung der Pneumokokken sind die Gallelöslichkeit und die Optochinempfindlichkeit besonders wichtig.

Gallelöslichkeit: Sie beruht auf der Aktivierung einer autolytischen Amidase. Der Nachweis geschieht, indem einer 24stündigen Bouillon oder einer Keimsuspension in physiol. Kochsalzlösung die gleiche Menge einer 10%igen Na-Taurocholatlösung zugesetzt wird. Pneumokokken werden innerhalb von 10 bis 15 Minuten gelöst und die Flüssigkeit klärt sich.

Optochinempfindlichkeit: Der Test beruht auf der Wachstumshemmung der Pneumokokken durch Optochin, das noch in Verdünnungen von 1 : 500 000 wirksam ist. Der Nachweis geschieht am leichtesten im Diffusionstest, indem dem beimpften Nährboden entsprechende Blättchen aufgelegt werden (Abb. 26).

■ Antigenstruktur

Von den Pneumokokken sind über 80 Serotypen bekannt. Grundlage dieser Einteilung sind die Polysaccharidantigene der Kapselsubstanz. Die Bezeichnung der Antigene ist unterschiedlich. Von NEUFELD wurden die Typen I, II, III und X unterschieden, wobei X eine Sammelgruppe darstellt, die alle weiteren Typen enthält. In anderen Einteilungen werden arabische Zahlen und Buchstaben benutzt. Für die praktische Diagnostik ist die Feststellung des Serotyps von untergeordneter Bedeutung. Beim Menschen verursachen 14 Serotypen, insbesondere die Typen 1–9, über 80 % aller Erkrankungen. Beim Tier überwiegen die Typen 4–47, besonders 6, 8, 18 und 19. Der Nachweis des Kapseltyps erfolgt mit der Quellungsreaktion. Wenn Pneumokokken in nativem Material (z. B. Peritonealexsudat aus Mäuseversuch) auf dem Objektträger mit Antiserum vermischt werden, kommt es zu einer Anschwellung der Kapsel.

■ Tierversuch

Nach ip. Infektion sterben Mäuse innerhalb 24 h, und aus dem Herzblut und den Organen können die Pneumokokken mikroskopisch und kulturell nachgewiesen werden.

Bibliography / Literatur

1. BLOM, E., & O. RØMER (1961 a): On the occurrence of β-hemolytic streptococci in bull semen. Proc. IV. Intern. Congr. Anim. Reprod.
2. BLOM, E., & O. RØMER (1961 b): Om forekomsten af β-haemolytiske streptokokker i tyresperma. Medlemsbl. for danske Drylaegeforening **44**, 741–748.
3. BOCKLISCH, H., & V. ZEPEZAUER (1979): Zur Streptokokkeninfektion des Schweines. Mh. Vet. Med. **34**, 841–846.
4. CLAUSEN, H. M. (1980): Kulturelle und tierexperimentelle Untersuchungen zum Vorkommen und zur Bedeutung von Streptokokken der Serogruppe R beim Schwein. Vet. Med. Diss. Hannover.

5. CLIFTON-HADLEY, F. A., J. L. ALEXANDER, I. UPTON & W. P. H. DUFFUS (1984): Further studies on the subclinical carrier state of Streptococcus suis type 2 in pigs. Vet. Rec. 114, 513–518.
6. DE MOOR, C. E. (1957): Een nieuwe streptococcus haemolyticus (Lancefield groep R). Berichten Rijks Institut Volksgezondheit 174–177.
7. ELLIOT, S. D. (1966): Streptococcal infection in young pigs. J. Hyg. Camb. 64, 205–212.
8. ENGEBRETSEN, I. (1970): Group P-streptococci. Occurrence and characteristics of strains isolated from bovine mastitis and from the environment. Nord. Ved. Med. 22, 510–516.
9. FIELD, H. J., D. BUNTAIN & J. T. DONE (1954): Studies on piglet mortality. I. Streptococcal meningitis and arthritis. Vet. Rec. 66, 453–455.
10. HAHN, G. (1980): Identifizierung von Streptokokken verschiedener serologischer Gruppen unter Verwendung der Latex-Agglutination. Lab. med. 4, 102–106.
11. HAHN, G. (1980): Streptokokken. In: H. BLOBEL & TH. SCHLIESSER (Hrsg.): Handbuch der bakteriellen Infektionen bei Tieren. Bd. II, S. 161–278. Stuttgart: Gustav Fischer.
12. HAHN, G., W. HEESCHEN & A. TOLLE (1970): Streptococcus. Eine Studie zur Struktur, Biochemie, Kultur und Klassifizierung. Kieler Milchwiss. Forschungber. 22, 333–546.
13. HAMMER, D. (1961): Die Immunisierung trächtiger Rinder gegen Pneumokokken-Polysaccharide und die biologische Bedeutung der im Kolostrum ausgeschiedenen spezifischen Antikörper. Zbl. Vet. med. 8, 369–402, 405–450.
14. HAWARI, A. D., & B. SONNENSCHEIN (1981): Untersuchungen zur Differenzierung von aus Geschlechtsorganen sowie Feten isolierten β-hämolysierenden Streptokokken. Berl. Münch. tierärztl. Wschr. 94, 101–103.
15. HENSEL, L. (1962): Differenzierung der von den Genitalschleimhäuten des Pferdes isolierten β-hämolysierenden Streptokokken. Zuchthyg. 6, 285–293.
16. JELINKOVÁ, J., & V. KUBIN (1974): Proposal of a new serological group V of haemolytic streptococci isolated from swine lymph nodes. Int. J. System. Bact. 24, 434–437.
17. JONES, J. E. T. (1976): The serological classification of streptococci isolated from diseased pigs. Brit. Vet. J. 132, 471–478.
18. JONES, J. E. T. (1976): The carriage of beta-hemolytic streptococci by healthy pigs. Brit. Vet. J. 132, 276–283.
19. KOEHNE, G., R. L. MADDUX & W. D. CORNELL (1979): Lancefield group R streptococci associated with pneumonia in swine. Am. J. Vet. Res. 40, 1640–1641.
20. KUNTER, E. (1982): Bericht des Streptokokken-Referenzzentrums über die 1968–1980 vom Schwein isolierten Streptokokken. 1. Mitt.: Serologische Gruppenzugehörigkeit und pathogene Bedeutung. 2. Mitt.: Chemotherapeutikaempfindlichkeit. Arch. exp. Vet. med. 36, 279–296, 785–799.
21. KUNTER, E., & W. WITTIG (1976): R- und S-Streptokokkeninfektionen beim Schwein. Arch. exp. Vet. med. 30, 211–216.
22. LÖGERING, H. J. (1981): Vergleichende Untersuchung fünf verschiedener Methoden zur Gruppenbestimmung von β-hämolysierenden Streptokokken. Zbl. Bakt. I. Orig. A 248, 437–445.
23. MARX, M. (1985): Zur Differenzierung β- bzw. δ/(β)-hämolysierender Streptokokken unter besonderer Berücksichtigung serologischer »Schnellverfahren«. Berl. Münch. tierärztl. Wschr. 98, 208–216.
24. MANTOVANI, A., R. ESTANI, D. SCIARRA & P. SIMONELLA (1961): Streptococcus L infection in the dog. J. small anim. Pract. 2, 185–194.
25. MOBERG, K., & E. THAL (1954): β-hämolytische Streptokokken einer neuen Lancefield-Gruppe. Nord. Vet. Med. 6, 69–72.
26. OHLSEN, S. H. (1956): Weitere Untersuchungen mit Streptokokken der Gruppe L beim Rind. Nord. Vet. Med. 8, 777.
27. OHLSEN, S. J. (1959): Group L-streptococci as a cause of mastitis. Int. Dairy Congr. 1, 92–98.
28. POWER, S. B. (1978): Streptococcus suis type 2 infection in pigs. Vet. Rec. 102, 215–216.
29. RICKERT, J., H. M. CLAUSEN, G. AMTSBERG, C. MEIER & G. HAHN (1982): Bakteriologische Untersuchungen zum Vorkommen von Streptokokken der serologischen Gruppe R bei klinisch gesunden Schweinen. Prakt. Tierarzt 63, 1054–1058.
30. SADATSUNE, T., & G. MORENO (1975): Contribution to the study of hemolytic streptococci isolated from dogs. Arq. Inst. Biol., São Paulo, 42, 257–264.
31. SKALKA, B., J. SMOLA & J. PILLICH (1979): Diagnostical availability of the hemolytically active exosubstance of Corynebacterium pseudotuberculosis for isolation and identification of Streptococcus agalactiae and its comparison with the beta toxin of Staphylococcus aureus. Zbl. Vet. Med. B 26, 679–687.
32. SCHOON, H. A., G. SCHAIBLE, G. AMTSBERG, M. ROSENBRUCH & G. HAHN (1980): Zum Vorkommen einer Leptomeningitis beim Schwein, hervorgerufen durch Streptokokken der Serogruppe R. Prakt. Tierarzt 61, 1035–1044.
33. SCHÜTZ, M., H. LAUTH & H. U. WIESNER (1984): Optimierung des serologischen Suchtestes mit der Counter-Immun-Elektrophorese sowie des kulturellen Nachweises von Streptococcus agalactiae in Milchproben. Arch. Lebensmittelhyg. 35, 58–60.
34. SEELEMANN, M. (1954): Biologie der Streptokokken. 2. Aufl. Nürnberg: Hans Carl.
35. SKOVGAARD, N. (1967): Untersuchungen über den Ursprung der Gruppe L Streptokokken und Staphylokokken in Lebensmitteln. Nord. Vet. Med. 19, 240–248.
36. THAL, E., & K. MOBERG (1953): Serologische Gruppenbestimmung der bei Tieren vorkommenden β-hämolytischen Streptokokken. Nord. Vet. Med. 5, 835–846.
37. THAL, E., & G. OBIGER (1969): Das CAMP-Phänomen der Sc. agalactiae und der neuen serologischen Streptokokkengruppe »U« sowie weiterer Bakterienarten. Berliner Münchener tierärztl. Wschr. 82, 126–130.
38. THAL, E., & O. SÖDERLIND (1966): Ny serologisk grupp U av beta-hämolserande streptoccer isolerade fran svin. Statens Veterinärmed. Anstalt 50, 1–4.
39. WATTS, J. L., S. C. NICKERSON & J. W. PANKEY (1984): A case study of Streptococcus group G infection in a dairy herd. Vet. Microbiol. 9, 571–579.
40. WEIGT, U., & E. GRUNERT (1964): Durch seltene Streptokokkengruppen verursachte Mastitiden und deren klinisches Bild. Dtsch. tierärztl. Wschr. 71, 1–5.
41. WEISSER, W. (1981): Ein Beitrag zu Klassifizierung der wichtigsten vergrünenden Streptokokken des weiblichen bovinen Genitaltraktes. Zbl. Vet. Med. B 28, 59–68.
42. WEISSER, W., & J. KÖHLER (1982): Kulturelle Untersuchung von Schlachtschweine-Lymphknoten auf das Vorkommen von β-hämolysierenden Streptokokken. Tierärztl. Umschau 37, 338–344.
43. WIESNER, H.-U. (1979): Serologischer Nachweis von B-Streptokokken-Antigen in Herdensammelmilch. Arch. Lebensmittelhyg. 30, 46–48.

3 Family: Peptococcaceae

In this family are grouped anaerobic Gram-positive cocci, which reside normally in the intestinal canal of man and animals.

Some have been isolated in human disease, but so far there is no information about their pathogenic importance in animals. The following genera are differentiated in this family:

Peptococcus whose species lie singly, in pairs, tetrads or in irregular clusters, but not cube-shaped packets and only rarely do they form short chains;

Peptostreptococcus and *Ruminococcus*, form pairs, or chains of various lengths. The genus Ruminococcus is found commonly in the rumen;

Sarcina forms three-dimensional packets, consisting of 8 or more cocci.

Peptococcus indolicus (*Micrococcus indolicus*, CHRISTIANSEN, 2), is not mentioned in the 8th edition of Bergey's manual (1974), but it is claimed to be of importance in the development of bovine mastitis due to *C. pyogenes*, *P. indolicus* has often been isolated, together with the latter from cases of pyogenes mastitis (4, 5). It has also been found in cattle with healthy udders (6, 7). CHIRINO-TREJO & PRESCOTT (1) have discovered *P. indolicus* in pneumonic lungs of cattle where again it was associated with *C. pyogenes*. For the cultural properties consult figure 24.

3 Familie: Peptococcaceae

In dieser Familie werden anaerobe, grampositive Kokken zusammengefaßt, die normalerweise im Darmkanal von Mensch und Tier vorkommen.

Sie sind gelegentlich beim Menschen aus Krankheitsprozessen isoliert worden, über ihre Bedeutung als Krankheitserreger bei Tieren liegen noch keine gesicherten Kenntnisse vor. Innerhalb der Familie werden folgende Gattungen unterschieden:

Peptococcus, deren Arten einzeln, in Paaren, Tetraden oder unregelmäßigen Haufen liegen und keine kubischen Pakete und sehr selten kurze Ketten bilden;

Peptostreptococcus und *Ruminococcus* bilden Paare oder kurze bis lange Ketten, die Gattung *Ruminococcus* kommt besonders im Pansen vor;

Sarcina bildet dreidimensionale Pakete, die aus 8 oder mehr Kokken bestehen.

Peptococcus indolicus (*Micrococcus indolicus*, CHRISTIANSEN, 2), in der 8. Aufl. von Bergey's manual (1974) nicht aufgeführt, soll eine Bedeutung für die Entstehung der durch *C. pyogenes* verursachten Mastitis des Rindes haben. Diese Keimart wurde häufig bei der Pyogenes-Mastitis zusammen mit *C. pyogenes* isoliert (4, 5), sie konnte auch bei eutergesunden Rindern nachgewiesen werden (6, 7). *P. indolicus* wurde von CHIRINO-TREJO & PRESCOTT (1) in Lungen von Rindern mit Pneumonien gefunden, auch hier vergesellschaftet mit *C. pyogenes*. Kulturelles Wachstum siehe Abb. 24.

Bibliography / Literatur

1. CHIRINO-TREJO, J. M., & J. F. PRESCOTT (1983): The identification and antimicrobial susceptibility of anaerobic bacteria from pneumonic cattle lungs. Can. J. Comp. Med. **47**, 270–276.
2. CHRISTIANSEN, M. (1934): An anaerobic, gas-producing, indol-positive Micrococcus. Acta path. microbiol. scand. Supp. XVIII, 42–63.
3. HOI SÖRENSEN, G. (1976): Studies on the occurrence of Peptococcus indolicus and Corynebacterium pyogenes in apparently healthy cattle. Acta vet. scand. **17**, 15–24.
4. HOI SÖRENSEN, G. (1974): Studies on aetiology and transmission of summermastitis. Nord. Vet. Med. **26**, 122–136.
5. STUART, P., D. BUNTAIN & R. G. LANGRIDGE (1951): Bacteriological examinations of secretions from cases of summermastitis and experimental infection of nonlactating udders. Vet. Rec. **63**, 451–453.
6. TOLLE, A., V. FRANKE & J. REICHMUTH (1983): Zur C. pyogenes-Mastitis — Bakteriologische Aspekte. Dtsch. tierärztl. Wschr. **90**, 256–260.
7. WEBER, A., TH. SCHLIESSER & G. STEINER (1977): Zum kulturellen Nachweis von anaeroben Kokken, insbesondere von Micrococcus indolicus in Milchsekretproben von Rindern mit sogenannter Sommermastitis. Dtsch. tierärztl. Wschr. **84**, 165–167.

Gram-positive, non-spore-forming rods
Grampositive, sporenlose Stäbchen

1 Genus: Corynebacterium

This genus contains pleomorphic, non-acid fast, Gram-positive rods which do not form spores. The polymorphism is expressed in the irregular shape and staining. Occasionally these rods have a slightly curved, comma-like appearance (*C. renale*) and club-shaped thickening.

The genus contains numerous species of which only a few are pathogenic to animals or man. The animal pathogens are non-motile and their biochemical properties are in part variable. It may, in fact, not be possible to identify strains which deviate in their properties (45).

1.1 Corynebacterium (Actinomyces) pyogenes

C. pyogenes differs considerably from the type species of the genus *Corynebacterium* (*C. diphtheriae*) and for this reason it has been recommended that it be transferred to the genus *Actinomyces* (8, 37).

■ **Incidence and veterinary significance**

C. pyogenes causes purulent inflammatory processes, especially in ruminants and pigs (abscesses, mastitis, pneumonia, endometritis, endocarditis, arthritis and the like). Latent infections often occur in healthy animals e.g. in the genital tract of cattle (26, 32).

■ **Morphology**

The best method for identification is the Gram stain. In pus smears the rods, 0.5–2 µm in length and 0.2–0.3 µm in thickness, are scattered irregularly through the field. The bacteria lie in no particular arrangement (figs. 27 and 28). Coccoid forms are

1 Gattung: Corynebacterium

Die Gattung enthält pleomorphe, nichtsäurefeste, grampositive Stäbchen, die keine Sporen bilden. Der Polymorphismus zeigt sich in der unregelmäßigen Gestalt und Färbung, die Stäbchen sind gelegentlich leicht kommaförmig gebogen (*C. renale*) und keulenförmig verdickt.

Die Gattung enthält zahlreiche Arten, von denen nur einige tier- oder menschenpathogen sind. Die tierpathogenen Arten sind unbeweglich, ihre kulturell-biochemischen Eigenschaften sind teilweise inkonstant. In ihren Eigenschaften abweichende Stämme sind oft nicht endgültig zu bestimmen (45).

1.1 Corynebacterium (Actinomyces) pyogenes

C. pyogenes unterscheidet sich in seinen Eigenschaften von der Typspezies der Gattung *Corynebacterium* (*C. diphtheriae*) wesentlich, es ist deswegen empfohlen worden, es in die Gattung *Actinomyces* zu überführen (8, 37).

■ **Vorkommen und medizinische Bedeutung**

C. pyogenes verursacht eitrige Entzündungsprozesse, insbesondere bei den Wiederkäuern und beim Schwein (Abszesse, Mastitis, Pneumonien, Endometritis, Endokarditis, Arthritis u. ä.). Bei gesunden Tieren bestehen oft latente Schleimhautinfektionen, so z. B. im Genitaltrakt der Rinder (26, 32).

■ **Morphologie**

Zum Nachweis eignet sich am besten die Gram-Färbung. In Ausstrichpräparaten aus Eiterungsprozessen findet man das 0,2 bis 0,3 µm dicke und 0,5 bis 2 µm lange Stäbchen unregelmäßig über das Gesichtsfeld verteilt, die Bakterien weisen keine

Fig. 27–30 see page 48.

Abb. 27–30 siehe Seite 48.

encountered especially in chronic conditions. The majority of bacteria are found extracellularly, although isolated ones are phagocytosed.

■ Culture
Media containing blood are most suited for the cultural identification, because a narrow β-haemolytic zone is formed. The colonies are small, about the size of a pin point, and transparent (fig. 29). The growth is much more rapid and profuse under anaerobic conditions and on glucose blood agar or on chocolate agar in a 10 % CO_2 atmosphere (figs. 32 and 33).

■ Biochemical properties
Serum plate of Loeffler: serum liquefaction (fig. 30), Litmus milk: turns red, clots and becomes peptonized. After 4 to 5 days, the contracted milk clot lies at the bottom of the tube under the whey, like a blood clot separates in serum (39). The following

besondere Zuordnung zueinander auf (Abb. 27 u. 28). Besonders in chronischen Prozessen treten kokkoide Formen auf. Die Bakterien liegen überwiegend extrazellulär, vereinzelt sind sie phagozytiert.

■ Kultur
Der kulturelle Nachweis geschieht am besten auf bluthaltigen Nährböden, dabei bildet sich nach 48 h eine schmale β-hämolytische Zone. Die Kolonien sind klein, etwa stecknadelstichgroß und durchsichtig (Abb. 29). Schneller und üppiger ist das Wachstum bei anaerober Bebrütung und unter Verwendung von Glucoseblutagar oder in 10%iger CO_2-Atmosphäre auf Kochblutagar (Abb. 32 u. 33).

■ Kulturell-biochemische Eigenschaften
Serumplatte nach Loeffler: Serolyse (Abb. 30), Lackmusmilch: Rötung, Gerinnung, Peptonisierung, nach 4 bis 5 Tagen liegt das zusammengepreßte Milchgerinnsel auf dem Boden des Röhrchens unter der Molke wie ein Blutkuchen im abgeschie-

Specimens
Pus, milk, secretions, mucosal swabs etc.

Microscopic examination
Gram stain: small, pleomorphic, Gram-positive rods, some of which may be curved

Cultural examination
1. Enrichment in fluid media, after 24 h subculture on blood agar. 2. Direct culture on blood agar, aerobic incubation at 37 °C. The growth of C. pyogenes will be substantially augmented on a Zeissler plate under anaerobic incubation (fig. 33) or on chocolate agar in an atmosphere of 10 % CO_2 (fig. 32).

Biochemical properties of pure culture					
Reaction	C. pyogenes	C. pyogenes atypical	C. renale	C. pseudo-tuberculosis	C. (Rhodococcus) equi
β-Haemolysis	+ (fig. 29)	+	–	(+)	–
Haemolysis inhibition	–	–	–	+ (fig. 39)	–
CAMP test	–	–	–	–	+ (fig. 42)
Gelatinase	+	v⁻	–	–	–
Serum liquefaction	+ (fig. 30)	v⁻	–	–	–
Litmus milk	RCP	RC(P)	A	unchanged	decolour.
Urea production	–	–	+	+	+
Nitrate reduction	–	–	–	–	+
Aesculin hydrolysis	–	–	–	–	–
Catalase production	–	–	+	+	+

Fig. 31: Isolation and identification of corynebacteria pathogenic to animals

Abb. 31: Nachweis und Bestimmung aerober tierpathogener Corynebakterien

sugars are fermented with acid formation: glucose, lactose, saccharose, maltose, galactose, xylose, adonitol, raffinose and salicin.

In the carbohydrate fermentation tests one can add bovine serum to the tubes in order to augment growth (24, 42) or the JAYNE-WILLIAMS basic medium (21) may be used.

The results of the carbohydrate fermentation are often inconstant and therefore the following properties are considered to be particularly characteristic: β-haemolysis, proteolysis or gelatinolysis, absence of urease production, the reduction of nitrate and the reddening, clotting and peptonization of litmus milk (fig. 31) (25, 45).

■ Toxin
C. pyogenes produces a filterable, thermolabile, haemolytic toxin (β-haemolysin), which is lethal to mice on intraperitoneal or intravenous injection. It is antigenic and can be neutralized by antibodies (15). It will produce inflammation and necrosis when injected intradermally into rabbits or guinea pigs.

■ Antigen structure
Serological tests, such as agar-gel precipitation, have been used to differentiate *C. pyogenes* from other corynebacteria (25). Strains from cattle, sheep and pigs react similarly.

■ Animal experiment
The pathogenicity of *C. pyogenes* for small laboratory animals is slight and variable. Abscesses develop after subcutaneous injection and the intraperitoneal or intravenous administration can lead to fatal general infections. In rabbits the intravenous injection results in abscess formation in the organs and the skeletal musculature and arthritis (12).

■ Atypical variants of C. pyogenes
Bacteria have been isolated from man and cattle, which resemble *C. pyogenes*, but deviate from them to some extent in certain properties. Their final classification is therefore unresolved. Usually these are haemolytic strains, which liquefy gelatine slowly or not at all, and differ in their ability to coagulate milk. These atypical strains behave biochemically very like those that have been isolated from purulent processes and pharyngeal smears of man (15, 16, 34).

denen Serum (39); Kohlenhydratfermentierung (Säurebildung) ist positiv bei Glu, Lact, Sac, Mal, Gal, Xyl, Ado, Raf und Sal.

Bei der Prüfung der Kohlenhydratspaltung kann den Röhrchen zur Wachstumsförderung Rinderserum zugesetzt werden (24, 42) oder es kann das Basalmedium nach JAYNE-WILLIAMS (21) verwendet werden.

Die Ergebnisse der Kohlenhydratspaltung sind oft nicht konstant, deswegen gelten folgende Eigenschaften als besonders charakteristisch: β-Hämolyse, Serolyse bzw. Gelatinolyse, fehlende Harnstoffspaltung und Nitratreduktion sowie Rötung, Gerinnung und Peptonisierung der Lackmusmilch (Abb. 31) (25, 45).

■ Toxin
C. pyogenes produziert ein filtrierbares, thermolabiles, hämolysierendes Toxin (β-Hämolysin), das bei Mäusen nach ip. oder iv. Injektion letal wirkt. Es wirkt antigen und kann durch Antikörper neutralisiert werden (15). Bei intradermaler Injektion an Kaninchen oder Meerschweinchen entstehen Entzündungen und Nekrosen.

■ Antigenstruktur
Zur serologischen Abgrenzung von *C. pyogens* von anderen Corynebakterien sind serologische Methoden benutzt worden, u. a. die Agargelpräzipitation (25), dabei reagieren Stämme von Rindern, Schafen und Schweinen übereinstimmend.

■ Tierversuch
Die Pathogenität von *C. pyogenes* für kleine Versuchstiere ist gering und unterschiedlich. Nach sbk. Injektion entstehen Abszesse und nach ip. oder iv. Injektion kann es zu einer tödlichen Allgemeininfektion kommen. Beim Kaninchen führt die iv. Infektion zu Abszessen in den Organen und in der Skelettmuskulatur sowie zu eitrigen Arthritiden (12).

■ Atypische Variante von C. pyogenes
Beim Menschen und beim Rind sind Bakterien isoliert worden, die *C. pyogenes* gleichen, aber in einigen Eigenschaften mehr oder weniger abweichen. Ihre endgültige Zuordnung ist noch offen. Es handelt sich meistens um hämolysierende Stämme, die Gelatine nicht oder verzögert verflüssigen und Abweichungen in der Milchgerinnung zeigen. Diese atypischen Stämme zeigen mit beim Menschen aus Eiterungsprozessen und Rachenabstrichen isolierten Stämmen biochemisch weitgehende Übereinstimmungen (15, 16, 34).

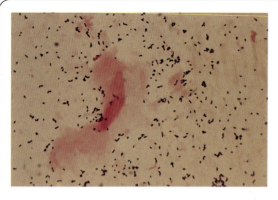
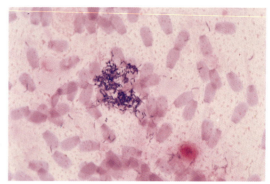
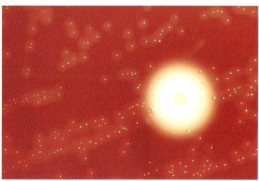
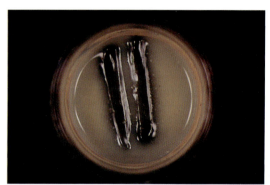

▲ Fig. 27: *Corynebacterium (Actinomyces) pyogenes*, Culture smear, Gram stain, pleomorphic, Gram-positive rods. Magnification x 1000
▼ Fig. 29: Mixed culture of *Corynebacterium (Actinomyces) pyogenes* and *Streptococcus zooepidemicus* on blood agar, aerobic incubation. *C. pyogenes* grows in small colonies with weak haemolysis, 24 h, 37 °C. Magnification x 4

▲ Fig. 28: *Corynebacterium (Actinomyces) pyogenes*, smear from purulent orchitis in a bull, Gram stain. Magnification x 1000
▼ Fig. 30: *Corynebacterium (Actinomyces) pyogenes*, pure culture on Loeffler serum, serum liquefaction, 48 h, 37 °C. Magnification x 0.25

▲ Abb. 27: *Corynebacterium (Actinomyces) pyogenes*, Kulturausstrich, Gram-Färbung, polymorphe, grampositive Stäbchen, Abb.-M. 1000 : 1
▼ Abb. 29: Mischkultur mit *Corynebacterium (Actinomyces) pyogenes* und *Streptococcus zooepidemicus* auf Blutagar, aerobe Bebrütung. *C. pyogenes* wächst in kleinen Kolonien mit einer schwachen Hämolyse, 24 h, 37 °C, Abb.-M. 4 : 1

▲ Abb. 28: *Corynebacterium (Actinomyces) pyogenes*, Ausstrich aus einer eitrigen Hodenentzündung eines Rindes, Gram-Färbung, Abb.-M. 1000 : 1
▼ Abb. 30: *Corynebacterium (Actinomyces) pyogenes*, Reinkultur auf der Serumplatte nach Loeffler, Serolyse, 48 h, 37 °C, Abb.-M. 1 : 4

1.2 Corynebacterium renale

■ Incidence and veterinary significance

C. renale is recognized as the organism causing a purulent pyelonephritis in cattle, but rarely in other animals. A latent colonization of the bovine genital tract and the prepuce in particular, is much more common. Therefore, this bacterium is consistently found in the semen of healthy bulls, without caus-

1.2 Corynebacterium renale

■ Vorkommen und medizinische Bedeutung

C. renale gilt als Erreger einer eitrigen Pyelonephritis des Rindes und sehr selten bei anderen Tierarten. Sehr viel häufiger ist eine latente Besiedlung der Genitalschleimhäute des Rindes, insbesondere des Präputiums. Dementsprechend wird das Bakterium regelmäßig im Sperma gesunder Bullen gefun-

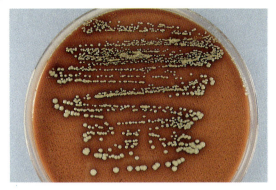
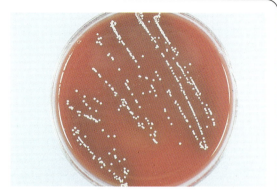
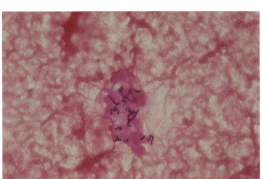
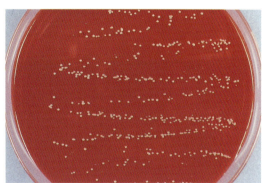

▲ Fig. 32: *Corynebacterium (Actinomyces) pyogenes*, pure culture on chocolate agar, incubation in an atmosphere of 10% CO_2; a distinct enhancement of growth in comparison with the aerobic incubation, 48 h, 37°C. Magnification x 0.25
▼ Fig. 34: *Corynebacterium renale*, urine smear from a pyelonephritic ox. Gram stain. Magnification x 1000

▲ Fig. 33: *Corynebacterium (Actinomyces) pyogenes*, pure culture on a Zeissler plate. Anaerobic incubation produced a distinctly heavier growth than under aerobic incubation, 48 h, 37°C. Magnification x 0.25
▼ Fig. 35: *Corynebacterium renale*, pure culture on blood agar, small white, dry colonies, slightly adherent to the medium, 72 h, 37°C. Magnification x 0.4

▲ Abb. 32: *Corynebacterium (Actinomyces) pyogenes*, Reinkultur auf Kochblutagar, Bebrütung in 10%iger CO_2-Atmosphäre, deutlich verstärktes Wachstum im Vergleich zu der aeroben Bebrütung, 48 h, 37°C, Abb.-M. 1 : 4
▼ Abb. 34: *Corynebacterium renale*, Harnausstrich von einem Rind mit Pyelonephritis, Gram-Färbung, Abb.-M. 1000 : 1

▲ Abb. 33: *Corynebacterium (Actinomyces) pyogenes*, Reinkultur auf Zeißler-Platte. Anaerobe Bebrütung, deutlich verstärktes Wachstum im Vergleich zur aeroben Bebrütung, 48 h, 37°C, Abb.-M. 1 : 4
▼ Abb. 35: *Corynebacterium renale*, Reinkultur auf Blutagar, weiße, kleine trockene, dem Nährboden leicht anhaftende Kolonien, 72 h, 37°C, Abb.-M. 1 : 2,5

ing any demonstrable damage to the semen (6, 26).

Within this species there are at least three types (I, II, III) which can be identified serologically and biochemically (17, 19, 46, 48). They all cause pyelonephritis, but they differ in virulence. *C. cystitidis* (type III) is the most virulent and type II (*C. pilosum*) the least (18).

den, ohne daß eine spermienschädigende Wirkung nachweisbar ist (6, 26).

Innerhalb der Spezies lassen sich serologisch und biochemisch mindestens drei Typen unterscheiden (I–III) (17, 19, 46, 48). Diese Typen sollen hinsichtlich der Auslösung der Pyelonephritis eine unterschiedliche Virulenz besitzen, die beim Typ III (*C. cystitidis*) am stärksten und beim Typ II (*C. pilosum*) am schwächsten ist (18).

■ Morphology
This is a pleomorphic rod, measuring 0.7 to 3.0 µm (fig. 34).

■ Culture
C. renale grows best on media containing blood. After 48 hours incubation it forms white colonies, about pin head size, which adhere lightly to the medium (fig. 35). No haemolysis is produced.

■ Biochemical properties
See figure 31.

■ Antigenic structure
C. renale has a specific antigenic structure and it can therefore be differentiated from other corynebacteria of the bovine genital tract by agar-gel precipitation (25) and immunofluorescence (1).

1.3 Corynebacterium pseudotuberculosis
Syn.: *C. pseudotuberculosis ovis*, Preisz-Nocard bacillus)

■ Incidence and veterinary significance
The cause of pseudotuberculosis of sheep and goats, which in rare cases may also affect cattle and other animals and induce ulcerative lymphangitis in solipeds (4).
Infections are rare in other animals.

■ Morphology
A short, pleomorphic rod, ranging from 0.5 to 1–3 µm.

■ Culture
C. pseudotuberculosis grows on simple media as aerobe or facultative anaerobe. Growth can be increased by the addition of blood or an atmosphere of CO_2.
The colonies are white, dry and with sharp borders. A narrow haemolytic zone often develops on blood agar (fig. 38). The action of the haemolysin is augmented in the CAMP test by *C. equi* (11). On the other hand, *C. pseudotuberculosis* inhibits the action of the β-haemolysin of *St. aureus*, when it is streaked on a blood agar plate across the staphylococcal inoculation, in the CAMP test (fig. 39) (13, 14).

■ Biochemical properties
See figure 31. Further fermentation reactions are: arabinose –, glucose +, dulcitol –, saccharose v, galactose +, trehalose –, lactose v, maltose +, mannitol v⁻, raffinose v and xylose v.

Fig. 36–39 see page 52.

■ **Toxins**

It is likely that toxins are produced. Broth filtrates are dermo-necrotic and lethal to mice.

■ **Animal experiments**

Mice are variably susceptible. The intravenous infection takes in 90.7 % of animals, and the subcutaneous route is successful in 21.2 % of mice. An orchitis is induced when guinea pigs are injected intraperitoneally (12).

1.4 Corynebacterium (Rhodococcus) equi

Its inclusion in the genus *Corynebacterium* is debateable, for this bacterium is also classed under the genus *Rhodococcus* along with other cocci, coccoid or coryneform rods which produce red colonies (5).

■ **Incidence and veterinary significance**

This bacterium has been found in several animal species. It is most important as the cause of a purulent pneumonia in foals, but it does infect other organs of horses, such as the genital tract and kidneys. In isolated cases it can induce pneumonias and other diseases in none-equine species (cattle, pigs, sheep, cats etc.). Furthermore, *C. equi* has been isolated from tuberculosis-like lesions in the lymph nodes especially the mesenteric lymph nodes of cattle and pigs. It can also be isolated from faecal samples of cattle and pigs (3, 10, 28). Infections of man are very rare (5).

■ **Morphology**

In animal tissues *C. equi* is usually coccoid to ovoid in shape (fig. 40), but in broth the rods tend to be longer.

■ **Culture**

C. equi is an aerobe or facultative anaerobe. It forms moist, mucoid colonies, which are white at first (fig. 41), but may later become reddish. There is no haemolysis on blood agar. In the CAMP test *C. equi* gives a positive reaction to the haemolysin of *St. aureus* (fig. 42), as it does with *C. pseudotuberculosis*. The basis of this reaction is a substance, known as the »equi factor«, which is formed by all strains of *C. equi* and which is antigenically active (11, 35, 40).

Media containing nalidixic acid, novobiocin, cycloheximide and potassium tellurite are used for selective primary culture from animal tissues (28).

■ **Toxine**

Mit dem Vorhandensein von Toxinen muß gerechnet werden. Bouillonkulturfiltrate wirken dermonekrotisch und mäuseletal.

■ **Tierversuch**

Mäuse sind unterschiedlich empfänglich. Die iv. Infektion haftet bei 90,7 %, die sbk. bei 21,2 % der Tiere. Die ip. Infektion von Meerschweinchen führt zur Orchitis (12).

1.4 Corynebacterium (Rhodococcus) equi

Die Zugehörigkeit zur Gattung *Corynebacterium* ist offen, das Bakterium wird auch mit anderen rot wachsenden Kokken oder kokkoiden bis coryneformen Stäbchen zur Gattung *Rhodococcus* gezählt (5).

■ **Vorkommen und medizinische Bedeutung**

Das Bakterium kommt bei verschiedenen Tierarten vor. Am wichtigsten ist es als Ursache von eitrigen Pneumonien bei Fohlen, es kommt beim Pferd aber auch in anderen Organen vor (Genitaltrakt, Niere). In Einzelfällen kann es Pneumonien oder andere Erkrankungen auch bei anderen Tieren hervorrufen (Rind, Schwein, Schaf, Katze u.a.). Ferner wurde *C. equi* aus tuberkuloseähnlichen Prozessen in Lymphknoten von Rind und Schwein isoliert, insbesondere aus den Mesenteriallymphknoten. Es kann ferner aus Kotproben von Rindern und Schweinen isoliert werden (3, 10, 28). Sehr selten kommen Infektionen beim Menschen vor (5).

■ **Morphologie**

In tierischen Untersuchungsstoffen besitzt *C. equi* meitens eine kokkoide bis ovoide Gestalt (Abb. 40), längere Stäbchenformen finden sich in Bouillonkulturen.

■ **Kultur**

C. equi wächst aerob und fakultativ anaerob. Es bilden sich feuchte, schleimige, zunächst weiße Kolonien (Abb. 41), die sich später rötlich färben können. Auf Blutagar kommt es zu keiner Hämolyse. Im CAMP-Test mit dem β-Hämolysin von *St. aureus* reagiert *C. equi* positiv (Abb. 42), ebenso mit *C. pseudotuberculosis*. Grundlage der Reaktion ist eine Exosubstanz (»Equi-Faktor«), die von allen *C. equi*-Stämmen gebildet wird und antigen wirksam ist (11, 35, 40).

Zur selektiven Herauszüchtung aus einem Untersuchungsmaterial sind Nährböden mit Zusatz von Nalidixinsäure, Novobiocin, Cycloheximid und Kaliumtellurit benutzt worden (28).

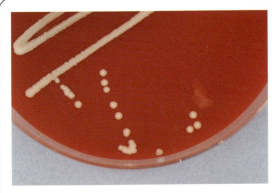
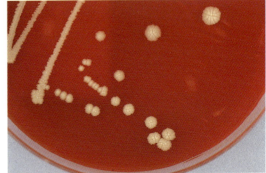
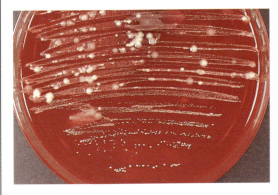
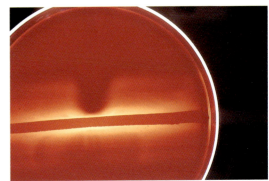

▲ Fig. 36: *Corynebacterium bovis*, pure culture on blood agar, smooth edged white colonies, 48 h, 37 °C. Magnification x 0.4
▼ Fig. 38: *Corynebacterium pseudotuberculosis (ovis)*, direct culture from the purulent lesion in a ram's testis. The larger colonies are contaminants, blood agar, 24 h, 37 °C. Magnification x 0.4

▲ Fig. 37: *Corynebacterium xerosis*, pure culture on blood agar, dry, greyish-white, wrinkled colonies, 48 h, 37 °C. Magnification x 0.4
▼ Fig. 39: *Corynebacterium pseudotuberculosis (ovis)* (upper vertical streak), inhibits the action of β-haemolysins from *Staphylococcus aureus*, (horizontal streak), blood agar, 48 h, 37 °C. Magnification x 0.4, transmitted light

■ Biochemical properties
The biochemical properties are not very distinctive. *C. equi* ferments glucose, reduces nitrates and is catalase- and urease-positive (28) (fig. 31).

■ Antigenic structure
At least 7 types of capsular antigens can be differentiated. But there appears to be no relationship between the origin of the strains and their antigenic structure (28).

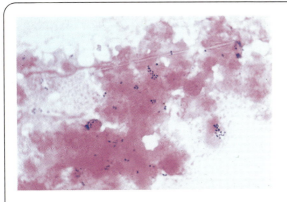
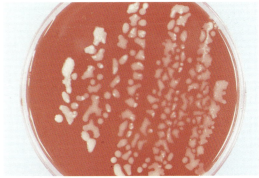
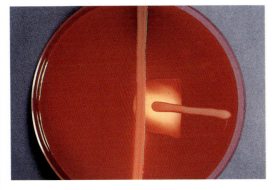
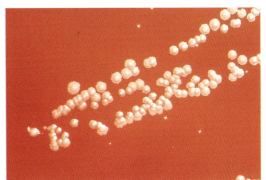

▲ Fig. 40: *Corynebacterium equi*, lung smear of a foal, Gram stain, Gram-positive coccobacilli. Magnification x 1000
▼ Fig. 42: *Corynebacterium equi*, positive CAMP test, horizontal streak: *C. equi*, vertical inoculation streak: *St. aureus*, 24 h, 37 °C. Magnification x 0.4

▲ Fig. 41: *Corynebacterium equi*, pure culture on blood agar, mucoid growth in confluent greyish-white colonies, 24 h, 37 °C. Magnification x 0.4
▼ Fig. 43: *Corynebacterium suis*, pure culture on Zeissler agar after anaerobic incubation, greyish-white colonies with textured surface and irregular border, 5 d, 37 °C. Magnification x 2.6

▲ Abb. 40: *Corynebacterium equi*, Ausstrich aus der Lunge eines Fohlens, Gram-Färbung, grampositive, kokkoide Stäbchen, Abb.-M. 1000 : 1
▼ Abb. 42: *Corynebacterium equi*, positiver CAMP-Test, waagerechter Impfstrich: *C. equi*, senkrechter Impfstrich: *Staphylococcus aureus*, Blutagar, 24 h, 37 °C, Abb.-M. 1 : 2,5

▲ Abb. 41: *Corynebacterium equi*, Reinkultur auf Blutagar, schleimiges Wachstum in zusammenfließenden, grauweißen Kolonie, 24 h, 37 °C, Abb.-M. 1 : 2,5
▼ Abb. 43: *Corynebacterium suis*, Reinkultur auf Zeißler-Agar nach anaerober Bebrütung, weißgraue, trockene, undurchsichtige Kolonien mit strukturierter Oberfläche und unregelmäßigem Rand, 5 d, 37 °C, Abb.-M. 2,6 : 1

1.5 Corynebacterium (Eubacterium) suis

■ **Incidence and veterinary significance**
C. suis is recognized as the cause of purulent cystitis, ureteritis and pyelonephritis of the pig. Breeding sows are most frequently affected. But the bacterium also occurs on the preputial mucosa of boars (22, 23, 30, 43, 44).

1.5 Corynebacterium (Eubacterium) suis

■ **Vorkommen und medizinische Bedeutung**
C. suis gilt als Erreger einer eitrigen Zystitis, Ureteritis und Pyelonephritis beim Schwein. Zuchtsauen sind am häufigsten erkrankt. Das Bakterium kommt ferner häufig auf der Präputialschleimhaut von Schweinen vor (22, 23, 30, 43, 44).

The bacteriological detection and identification of the bacterium are compiled in figure 44.

Der bakteriologische Nachweis und die Bestimmung des Bakteriums sind in der Abb. 44 zusammengestellt.

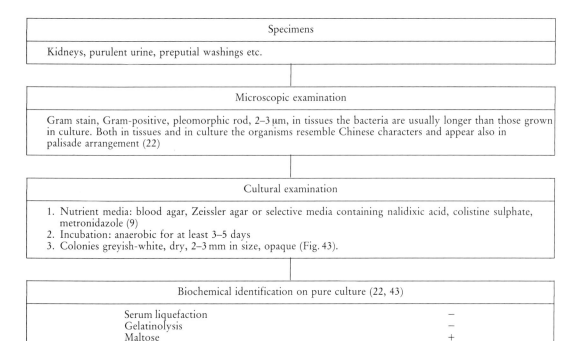

Fig. 44: Detection and identification of *Corynebacterium suis*

Abb. 44: Nachweis und Bestimmung von *Corynebacterium suis*

1.6 Other Corynebacteria

Apart from the above-mentioned corynebacteria which are known animal pathogens and whose bacteriological characters are sufficiently defined, there are still others occurring in animals, test for whose identification often produce rather unsatisfactory results, but the following types can be differentiated:

C. bovis is a saprophyte found in the teat canal of cows and has been isolated in cases of mastitis (20, 38). MÜNKER & KLEIKAMP (26) have found this bacterium in bovine semen. It will grow on the usual media, forming colonies after 48 hours that are about the size of a pin head, with a rough surface and serrated border (fig. 36). *C. bovis* is biochemically not very active, but this activity can be stimulated by the addition to the medium of calf serum or Tween 80. Glucose, maltose and galactose are fermented, nitrate reduction is negative and urease is not formed.

C. kutscheri, which occurs mainly in mice, less

1.6 Weitere Corynebakterien

Neben den erwähnten Corynebakterien, die eine bekannte Tierpathogenität besitzen und bakteriologisch ausreichend definiert sind, kommen beim Tier noch weitere Corynebakterien vor. Untersuchungen zu ihrer Bestimmung bringen oft kein befriedigendes Ergebnis, jedoch werden mindestens noch folgende Arten unterschieden:

C. bovis, ein Saprophyt, der im Zitzenkanal des Rindes angetroffen wird, es wurde auch im Zusammenhang mit Mastitiden isoliert (20, 38). MÜNKER & KLEIKAMP (26) fanden das Bakterium in Rindersperma. Es wächst auf den üblichen Nährböden und bildet nach 48 h etwa stecknadelkopfgroße Kolonien mit einer rauhen Oberfläche und einem zerklüfteten Rand (Abb. 36). *C. bovis* ist biochemisch wenig aktiv, die Aktivität kann jedoch durch Zugabe von Kälberserum oder Tween 80 zum Medium gesteigert werden. Vergoren werden Glucose, Maltose und Galactose, die Nitratreduktion ist negativ, Urease wird nicht gebildet.

frequently in rats and guinea pigs, leads to the formation of abscesses in various organs.

C. xerosis is a commensal on the mucosa, mainly of man. It may also be encountered as a contaminant in animal materials. It grows on blood agar (fig. 37) as smooth or rough, greyish-white colonies that may even be slightly yellow or brown.

C. kutscheri, das besonders bei Mäusen und seltener bei Ratten und Meerschweinchen vorkommt und zu einer multiplen Abszeßbildung in verschiedenen Organen führt.

C. xerosis, Kommensale auf der Schleimhaut hauptsächlich des Menschen. Kann als Kontaminant auch in tierischen Untersuchungsstoffen vorkommen. Es wächst auf Blutagar in glatten bis rauhen (Abb. 37), grauweißen Kolonien, die leicht gelb bis bräunlich gefärbt sein können.

Bibliography / Literatur

1. ADDO, P. B., & I. E. COOK (1979): Specific immunofluorescence of Corynebacterium renale. Brit. Vet. J. 135, 50–54.
2. ARTHUR, S. H. (1949): Some observations on pyelonephritis and its treatment with penicillin. Vet. Rec. 61, 257–259.
3. BARTON, M. D., & K. L. HUGHES (1980): Corynebacterium equi: a review. Vet. Bull. 50, 65–80.
4. BAUMANN, R. (1957): Die geschwürige Lymphgefäßentzündung der Einhufer (Lymphangitis ulcerosa). Wiener tierärztl. Mschr. 44, 292–296.
5. BÜRGER, H., & H. E. MÜLLER (1982): Rhodococcus isoliert aus Glutäalabszeß. Infection 10, 343–346.
6. BRATKE, E. (1952): Vorkommen und Bedeutung von Corynebacterium renale und pyogenes bei der künstlichen Besamung des Rindes. Berl. Münch. tierärztl. Wschr. 65, 247–250.
7. BULLING, E. (1954): Über die Wirkung einiger Antibiotika auf Corynebacterium pyogenes. Berl. Münch. tierärztl. Wschr. 67, 381–384.
8. COLLINS, M. D., & D. JONES (1982): Reclassification of Corynebacterium pyogenes (Glage) in the genus Actinomyces as Actinomyces pyogenes comb. nov. J. Gen. Microbiol. 128, 901–903.
9. DAGNALL, G. J. R., & J. C. T. JONES (1982): A selective medium for the isolation of Corynebacterium suis. Res. Vet. Sci. 32, 389–390.
10. ELLIOT, G., H. K. LAWSON & C. P. MACKENZIE (1986): Rhodococcus equi infection in cats. Vet. Rec. 118, 693–694.
11. FJØLSTAD, M. (1970): The CAMP phenomenon of Corynebacterium equi and its application on the isolation of this bacterium. Proc. 11th Nordic Vet. Congr., Bergen, S. 286.
12. HARTWIGK, H. (1966): Das Tierexperiment mit tierpathogenen Corynebakterien. In: Handbuch der exp. Pharmakologie. Bd. 16/10, S. 39–77. Berlin: Springer.
13. HARTWIGK, H. (1963): Antihämolysinbildung beim Tier vorkommender β-hämolytischer Corynebakterien. Zbl. Bakt. I. Orig. 191, 274–280.
14. HARTWIGK, H. (1963): Antihämolysinbildung bei Corynebacterium pseudotuberculosis ovis. Berl. Münch. tierärztl. Wschr. 76, 222–224.
15. HARTWIGK, H. (1961): Atypische Merkmale von Corynebacterium pyogenes beim Rind. Dtsch. tierärztl. Wschr. 68, 38–41.
16. HARTWIGK, H., & S. GRUND (1960): Atypische Corynebakterien beim Rind. Zbl. Bakt. I. Orig. 179, 499–508.
17. HIRAI, K., & R. YANAGAWA (1967): Nutritional requirements of Corynebacterium renale. Jap. J. Vet. Res. 15, 121–134.
18. HIRAMUNE, T., S. INUI, N. MURASE & R. YANAGAWA (1971): Virulence of three types of Corynebacterium renale in cows. Am. J. Vet. Res. 32, 237–242.
19. HIRAMUNE, T., N. MURASE & R. YANAGAWA (1970): Distribution of the types of Corynebacterium renale in cows of Japan. Jap. J. Vet. Sci. 32, 235–242.
20. HOUKANEN-BUZALSKI, T., T. K. GRIFFIN & F. H. DODD (1984): Natural infection of the bovine mammary gland with Corynebacterium bovis. J. Dairy Res. 51, 371–374.
21. JAYNE-WILLIAMS, D. J., & T. M. SKERMAN (1966): Comparative studies on coryneform bacteria from milk and dairy sources. J. appl. Bact. 29, 72–92.
22. JONES, J. E. T. (1980): Zystitis und Pyelonephritis bei Sauen. Dtsch. tierärztl. Wschr. 87, 443–445.
23. JONES, J. E. T., E. FARRIES & D. SMIDT (1982): Untersuchungen zum Vorkommen von Corynebacterium suis bei Wild- und Hausschweinen in der Bundesrepublik Deutschland. Dtsch. tierärztl. Wschr. 89, 110–112.
24. KIELSTEIN, P., & W. KÖTSCHE (1966): Untersuchungen zur biochemischen und serologischen Abgrenzung von Corynebakterien tierischer und menschlicher Herkunft. Mh. Vet. Med. 21, 20–26.
25. KIELSTEIN, P., & W. KÖTSCHE (1963): Zur Differenzierung der aus tierischem Untersuchungsmaterial stammenden Corynebakterien. Arch. exp. Vet. med. 17, 449–460.
26. MÜNKER, W., & I. KLEIKAMP (1960): Untersuchungen über die Corynebakterien im Bullensperma. Berl. Münch. tierärztl. Wschr. 73, 151–153.
27. MUTIMER, M. D., & J. B. WOOLCOCK (1981): Some problems associated with the identification of Corynebacterium equi. Vet. Microbiol. 6, 331–338.
28. MUTIMER, M. D., & J. B. WOOLCOCK (1980): Corynebacterium equi in cattle and pigs. Vet. Quarterly 2, 25–27.
29. MUTIMER, M. D., J. F. PRESCOTT & J. B. WOOLCOCK (1982): Capsular serotypes of Rhodococcus equi. Aust. Vet. J. 58, 67–69.
30. NARUCKA, U., & J. F. WESTENDORP (1972): Corynebacterium suis bij het varken II. Tijdschr. Diergeneesk. 97, 642–652.
31. NARUCKA, U., & J. F. WESTENDORP (1971): Corynebacterium suis bij het varken. Tijdschr. Diergeneesk. 96, 399–404.
32. NATTERMANN, H., & F. HORSCH (1977): Zur Pathogenese der Corynebacterium-pyogenes-Mastitis des Rindes. Mh. Vet. Med. 32, 342–345.
33. NATTERMANN, H., & F. HORSCH (1976): Chemotherapeutikaresistenz bei Corynebacterium pyogenes. Mh. Vet. Med. 31, 441–446.
34. PATOCKA, M. F. (1958): Durch atypische Corynebakterien verursachte Infektionen. Anthropoozoonosy, Prag, Kongreßbericht, 375.
35. PRESCOTT, J. F., M. LASTRA & L. BARKSDALE (1982): Equi factors in the identification of Corynebacterium equi Magnusson. J. clin. Microbiol. 16, 988–990.
36. PURDON, M. R., A. SEAMAN & M. WOODBINE (1958): The bacteriology and antibiotic sensitivity of Corynebacterium pyogenes. Vet. Rev. Annot. 4, 55–91.
37. REDDY, C. A., C. P. CORNELL & A. M. FRAGA (1982): Transfer of Corynebacterium pyogenes (Glage) Eberson to the genus Actinomyces as Actinomyces pyogenes (Glage) comb. nov. Intern. J. System. Bact. 32, 419–429.

38. Rizk, G., & P. Janetschke (1972): Über die Rolle von Corynebacterium bovis im Mastitisgeschehen und Untersuchungen zu seiner biochemischen Aktivität. Mh. Vet. Med. **27**, 470–471.
39. Rolle, M. (1929): Biologie des Bacterium pyogenes. Diss. Hannover.
40. Skalka, B., & A. Svastová (1985): Serodiagnostics of Corynebacterium (Rhodococcus) equi. Zbl. Vet. Med. B **32**, 137–142.
41. Schällibaum, M., H. Häni & J. Nicolet (1976): Infektion des Harntraktes beim Schwein mit Corynebacterium suis: Diagnose mit Immunfluoreszenz. Schweiz. Arch. Tierheilkd. **118**, 329–334.
42. Sørensen, G. H. (1974): Corynebacterium pyogenes. A biochemical and serological study. Acta vet. scand. **15**, 544–554.
43. Soltys, M. A. (1961): Corynebacterium suis associated with a specific cystitis and pyelonephritis in pigs. J. Path. Bact. **81**, 441–446.
44. Soltys, M. A., & F. R. Spratling (1957): Infectious cystitis and pyelonephritis of pigs. Vet. Rec. **69**, 500.
45. Stoll, L. (1960): Atypische Corynebakterien in der Milch. Berliner Münchener tierärztl. Wschr. **73**, 270–272.
46. Tinelli, R., A. Vallée, C. J. Guillon & A. Le Priol (1972): Étude serologique par diffusion en gel, de vingt-huit souches de Corynebacterium renale. Recl. Méd. vét. **148**, 1363–1368.
47. Yanagawa, R., & E. Honda (1978): Corynebacterium pilosum and Corynebacterium cystitidis two new species from cows. Intern. J. System. Bact. **28**, 209–216.
48. Yanagawa, R., R. Basri & K. Otsuki (1967): Three types of Corynebacterium renale classified by precipitin reaction in gels. Jap. J. Vet. Res. **15**, 111–119.
49. Zaki, M. M. (1965): Relation between staphylococcal β-lysin and different corynebacteria. Vet. Rec. **77**, 941.

2 Genus: Listeria (L.)

2.1 Listeria monocytogenes

■ **Incidence and veterinary significance**

L. monocytogenes is the causal organism of listeriosis, a ubiquitous sporadic infectious disease of man and animals.

Listerias occur in the soil and on plants; they are geophilic, facultative pathogens. In both man and animals the disease is often without clinical signs. Factors that reduce resistance, such as pregnancy, nutritional changes, virus infections and parasitic diseases tend to increase the likelihood of clinical manifestations in infections with *L. monocytogenes*. Listeriosis can occur in all domestic mammals, in wild and captive animals and in poultry, but sheep and cattle are most often affected. Various clinical forms have been observed in animals.
▷ Cerebral form: Meningo-encephalitis is the predominant form in sheep;
▷ Metrogenic form: Abortions, premature births or the foetus, although week, may be carried to term, septic metritis;
▷ A generalized infection, a granulomatosis with lesions in various organs, is seen especially in young animals, poultry and rodents;
▷ Mastitis;
▷ Latent infections.

Silage, and in particular poor quality (pH > 5.5) maize and grass silage wherein the organism can multiply, is the most important source of infection for ruminants, the species most commonly affected by listeriosis.

■ **Morphology**

In the S-form *L. monocytogenes* appears as a Gram-positive, motile, coccoid rod of 0.6 to 2 μm in

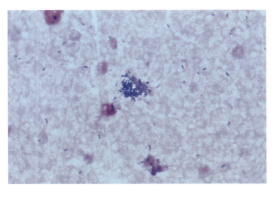
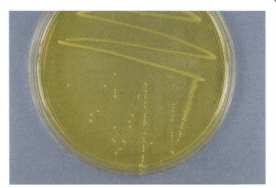
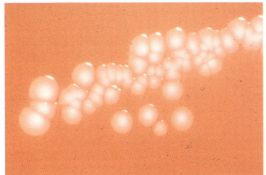
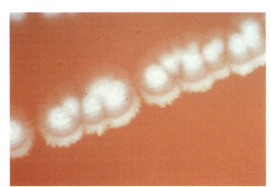

▲ Fig. 45: *Listeria monocytogenes*, smear from the heart of an experimentally infected mouse, Gram stain, Gram-positive rods. Magnification x 1000
▼ Fig. 47: *Listeria monocytogenes*, pure culture on blood agar, transparent borders with smooth borders, S-form, 48 h, 37 °C. Magnification x 5

▲ Fig. 46: *Listeria monocytogenes*, pure culture on selective medium (tryptose-nalidixic acid-trypaflavin agar), 72 h, 37 °C. Magnification x 0.4
▼ Fig. 48: *Listeria monocytogenes*, pure culture on blood agar, granular opaque colonies, R-form, 48 h, 37 °C. Magnification x 2

▲ Abb. 45: *Listeria monocytogenes*, Ausstrich vom Herzen einer experimentell infizierten Maus, Gram-Färbung, grampositive Stäbchen, Abb.-M. 1000 : 1
▼ Abb. 47: *Listeria monocytogenes*, Reinkultur auf Blutagar, glattrandige, durchscheinende Kolonien, S-Form, 48 h, 37 °C, Abb.-M. 5 : 1

▲ Abb. 46: *Listeria monocytogenes*, Reinkultur auf Selektivmedium (Tryptose-Naladixinsäure-Trypa-flavin-Agar,), 72 h, 37 °C, Abb.-M. 1 : 2,5
▼ Abb. 48: *Listeria monocytogenes*, Reinkultur auf Blutagar, granulierte, undurchsichtige Kolonien, R-Form, 48 h, 37 °C, Abb.-M. 2 : 1

length (fig. 45). In culture smears it is more common to find palisade, V- and Y-forms but his arrangement cannot be regarded as characteristic. R-forms can appear under favourable cultural conditions, and they develop long filamentous forms that can attain lengths of 50 and 100 µm.

At incubation temperatures of between 20 °C and 25 °C *L. monocytogenes* will produce 4 peritrichous flagella; the number decreases above 30 °C. When testing for motility in the hanging drop preparation

langes Stäbchen (Abb. 45). In Kulturausstrichen sind zwar häufiger Palisaden-, V- und Y-Formen zu sehen, dennoch kann die Anordnung der Kurzstäbchen zueinander nicht als besonders charakteristisch bezeichnet werden. Unter künstlichen Züchtungsbedingungen können R-Formen auftreten, deren Fäden eine Länge zwischen 50 und 100 µm erreichen.

Bei Züchtungstemperaturen von 20 bis 25 °C bildet *L. monocytogenes* 4 peritrich angeordnete Gei-

or on migration agar, it is necessary to incubate at 20 °C.

■ Culture

L. monocytogenes will grow on simple solid or fluid media. The addition of blood, serum or dextrose will augment growth. The bacteria will grow in a temperature range of 3 °C to 45 °C, with the optimum between 30 °C and 37 °C. Listeria thrives in a pH range of 5.6 to 9.6, and neutral or slightly alkaline media are preferred for primary culture. Incubation may be aerobic, but an atmosphere of 5–10 % CO_2 will improve growth.

Blood agar is well suited for the primary culture and after 24 h at 37 °C very small transparent colonies with smooth borders develop. After 48 h they measure between 0.5 and 2 mm, are greyish-white and surrounded by a narrow zone of haemolysis (fig. 47) (22).

There are also non-haemolytic listerias, which SEELIGER (23) classed as one of the non-pathogenic *L. innocua*. They are frequently isolated from human faecal samples, from plant remains and from soil samples.

If one suspects having grown colonies of *L. monocytogenes* on a transparent solid medium (nutrient or tryptose agar) the plate should be inspected under oblique transmitted light (11). Since colonies of the S-form will thereby take on a distinctive bluish-green to bluish-grey colour and a delicately textured surface, they can be rapidly identified in mixed cultures (8, 13, 16).

While freshly isolated strains occur almost exclusively in the smooth form, on artificial culture rough forms may also develop. Such colonies are of crumbly consistency and there is only a weak suggestion of haemolysis (fig. 48). In physiological saline the R-forms have a tendency towards spontaneous agglutination.

The S-form will cause slight turbidity in broth cultures within 24 to 48 hours. The intensity of this, which is dependent on the dose inoculated, can be considerably increased by the addition of glucose. In broth culture the R-form produces a granular, crumbly sediment.

■ The isolation of listeria from natural materials

If it is suspected that the material contains only a few listeria, then some form of enrichment is necessary. In the case of heavy contamination inhibitors, such as nalidixic acid, potassium thiocyanate and acridine dyes, can be added to the selective medium. The available media and the culture methods are summarized in figure 49.

■ Kultur

L. monocytogenes wächst auf einfachen festen und in flüssigen Nährmedien. Zusätze von Blut, Serum oder Traubenzucker wirken wachstumsfördernd. Das Wachstum erfolgt in einem Temperaturbereich von 3 bis 45 °C, das Optimum liegt zwischen 30 und 37 °C. Listerien gedeihen in einem pH-Bereich von 5,6 bis 9,6. Zur Anzüchtung werden neutrale oder schwach alkalische Nährmedien bevorzugt. Die Kultivierung wird unter aeroben Bedingungen vorgenommen, durch eine 5- bis 10%ige CO_2-Atmosphäre läßt sich das Wachstum verbessern.

Auf Blutagar, der zur Anzüchtung gut geeignet ist, bilden sich nach 24 h bei 37 °C sehr kleine, durchscheinende, glattrandige Kolonien, die nach 48 h eine grauweiße Farbe annehmen, etwa 0,5 bis 2 mm groß sind und von einem schmalen hämolytischen Hof (Abb. 47) umgeben werden (22).

Daneben gibt es anhämolysierend wachsende Listerien, die SEELIGER (23) der apathogenen Art *L. innocua* zuordnete. Sie werden häufig in Stuhlproben von Menschen, in Pflanzenresten und in Bodenproben nachgewiesen.

Für die Beurteilung der auf durchsichtigen Nährmedien (Nähragar, Tryptoseagar) gewachsenen *L. monocytogenes*-verdächtigen Kolonien wird die Schrägdurchleuchtung der Plattenkulturen empfohlen (11). Da die Kolonien der S-Form hierbei eine charakteristische blaugrüne bis blaugraue Farbe und eine zart gewebte Oberfläche (Textur) aufweisen, sind sie in Mischkulturen schnell zu identifizieren (8, 13, 16).

Während frisch isolierte Stämme fast ausschließlich in der Glattform erscheinen, können unter dem Einfluß von künstlichen Züchtungsbedingungen auch Rauhformen entstehen. Die Konsistenz dieser Kolonien ist bröckelig, die Hämolyse nur schwach angedeutet (Abb. 48). Die R-Formen neigen zu kräftiger Spontanagglutination in physiologischer Kochsalzlösung.

Die S-Form bildet in Nährbouillon innerhalb von 24 bis 48 h eine schwache Trübung aus, deren Intensität durch die Einsaatmenge sowie durch Zusatz von Glucose wesentlich gesteigert werden kann. Die R-Form zeigt in Nährbouillon einen körnig-krümeligen Bodensatz.

■ Isolierung von Listerien aus einem natürlichen Untersuchungsmaterial

Ist in dem Untersuchungsmaterial nur mit dem Vorkommen weniger Listerien zu rechnen, so muß zunächst eine Anreicherung durchgeführt werden. Bei Vorhandensein einer starken Begleitflora können den Anreicherungsmedien selektive Hemmsubstanzen zugesetzt werden, als solche haben sich

Solid selective media are available for direct culture and for subculture from enrichment media (fig. 49).

■ **Biochemical properties**

The biochemical reactions necessary for identification are presented in figure 49. Serotype 5 of L. monocytogenes shows deviations from the

Nalidixinsäure, Kaliumthiocyanat und Akridinfarbstoffe bewährt. Die in Frage kommenden Medien sowie das Kulturverfahren sind in der Abb. 49 zusammengestellt.

Für die Direktkultur sowie für die Abimpfungen aus den Anreicherungsmedien stehen feste Selektivnährböden zur Verfügung (Abb. 49).

■ **Kulturell-biochemische Eigenschaften**

Die zur Identifizierung erforderlichen biochemischen Reaktionen sind in der Abb. 49 dargestellt. Abweichungen vom charakteristischen biochemi-

Specimens
Cerebral form: brain stem, several sites of medulla oblongata Metrogenic form: placenta, amniotic fluid, content of foetal abomasum General infection: liver, lung, kidney, spleen Mastitis: milk Soil, silage, food material etc.

Cultural Isolation
1. Selective enrichment: Cold enrichment at 4 °C, tryptose broth or heart-brain infusion broth. Incubation time: 4 weeks to maximally 6 months. Subculture to solid (selective) medium weekly, later monthly. Enrichment at 22 °C: 3.75 % Potassium thiocyanate broth; Stuart medium with 40 µg/ml nalidixic acid and acridine dyes (e. g. trypaflavin). Incubation time 5 to 8 days. 2. Selective plates: Tryptose agar with added nalidixic acid (40 µg/ml) or potassium thiocyanate (to 3.75 %) in combination with acridine dyes (e. g. trypaflavin). Incubation time 1–2 days at 37 °C (fig. 46).

Identification of listeria in pure culture
1. Microscopic examination: Gram-positive rods
2. Appearance of colonies, under oblique transillumation of Henry, if necessary
3. Biochemical examination (after 24–48 hours incubation)[1]

Glu	+	Lact	v	Rha	v	Mal	+
Sac	v	Mnn	−	Sal	+	Ara	−
Xyl	−	Aes	+	H_2S	−	Gel	−
VPR	+	MR	+	Cat	+	Nit	−
Ure	−	Ind	−	Cit	−	Oxi	−
LDC	−	ODC	−	Mot (20 °C)	+	Hae	+

Biochemical differentiation of various Listeria species				
Species	CAMP test		Acid production from	
	St. aureus	C. (Rhodococcus) equi	D-xylose	L-rhamnose	methyl-D-mannoside
L. monocytogenes	+	−	−	+	+
L. ivanovii	−	+	+	−	−
L. innocua	−	−	−	+	+
L. welshimeri	−	−	+	v	+
L. seeligeri	+	−	+	−	−

[1] after SEELIGER (22, 23); GRAY & KILLINGER (9).
Fig. 49: Demonstration and identification of *Listeria spp.*

[1] nach SEELIGER (22, 23); GRAY & KILLINGER (9).
Abb. 49: Nachweis und Bestimmung von Listerien

characteristic biochemical reaction spectrum. These strains do not acidify trehalose, maltose, xylose, dextrin and salicin, nor do they hydrolyse aesculin (6, 12). The name *L. ivanovii* has been suggested for these strains (24).

Besides *L. innocua* other non-pathogenic listerias have been isolated from soil samples, plants and sheep faeces, these are: *L. welshimeri* and *L. seeligeri* (19, 20). In figure 49 it is shown how to distinguish between these new species and *L. monocytogenes*.

■ Toxins

L. monocytogenes produces a trypsin-sensitive and antigenic haemolysin, that lyses erythrocytes of various animal species and is lethal to mice. Its virulence in experimental animals is closely linked to its haemolytic capacity (29, 32, 34).

L. monocytogenes subjected to phenol-water extraction has rendered an endotoxin-like substance which is positive in the limulus test, pyrogenic in rabbits and lethal to chick embryos (30, 35).

There is also a monocytosis-producing agent (MPA) which causes the blood monocyte count of rabbits to rise. MPA is non-toxic and non-antigenic and it consists of various lipid components (31).

■ Antigenic structure

The various O- and H-antigens occur in diverse combinations in *L. monocytogenes*. A system, based on antigenic structure, was devised which would determine the serotype and enable the classification of all strains of *L. monocytogenes* to be established (6, 17, 22). Non-haemolytic strains of listeria *(L. innocua)* are classed mainly in O-group 6 (21).

The antigen identification is carried out either by means of tube agglutination or precipitation (22, 23, 25).

In the Federal Republic of Germany serotypes 1/2a and 4b are encountered almost exclusively. Serotype 1/2a is more common in Eastern Europe.

Serotyping is of subordinate importance in aetiological diagnosis, but in certain cases it can be of interest from an epidemiological viewpoint.

■ Animal experiment

The organism can be detected in the test material without the use of experimental animals, because the culture method invariably provides better results (22). But experimental animals are of importance for testing the virulence of already isolated

schen Reaktionsspektrum sind beim Serotyp 5 von *L. monocytogenes* festzustellen. Diese Stämme bilden aus Trehalose, Maltose, Xylose, Dextrin und Salizin keine Säure, außerdem wird Äskulin nicht hydrolysiert (6, 12). Für sie wurde die Artbezeichnung *L. ivanovii* vorgeschlagen (24).

Neben *L. innocua* wurden aus Bodenproben, Pflanzen, aber auch aus Kotproben von Schafen noch die apathogenen Listerienarten *L. welshimeri* und *L. seeligeri* isoliert (19, 20). Die Abgrenzung dieser neu beschriebenen Arten von *L. monocytogenes* ist aus Abb. 49 ersichtlich.

■ Toxine

L. monocytogenes produziert ein trypsinempfindliches und antigenwirkendes Hämolysin, das die Erythrozyten verschiedener Tierarten lysiert und für Mäuse eine letale Wirkung hat. Die Virulenz für Versuchstiere ist eng mit dem Hämolysevermögen gekoppelt (29, 32, 34).

Durch die Phenol-Wasser-Extraktion wurden von *L. monocytogenes* endotoxinähnliche Substanzen isoliert, die einen positiven Limulustest erbrachten, bei Kaninchen pyrogen und auf Hühnerembryonen toxisch wirkten (30, 35).

Außerdem wird ein monozytoseproduzierendes Agens (MPA) gebildet, das bei Kaninchen einen Anstieg der Monozyten im Blut hervorruft. Das MPA ist nicht toxisch und wirkt nicht antigen, es besteht aus verschiedenen Lipoidkomponenten (31).

■ Antigenstruktur

Die verschiedenen O- und H-Antigene treten bei *L. monocytogenes* in unterschiedlichen Kombinationen auf. Zur Bestimmung der Serotypen (Serovarietäten, Serovare) auf der Grundlage ihrer Antigenstruktur wurde ein Antigenschema erarbeitet (6, 17, 22), das eine serologische Einordnung aller *L. monocytogenes*-Stämme ermöglicht (Tab. 11). Anhämolysierende Listerienstämme *(L. innocua)* werden vorwiegen der O-Gruppe 6 zugeordnet (21).

Die Antigenbestimmung wird mit Hilfe der Röhrchenagglutination oder der Präzipitation durchgeführt (22, 23, 25).

In der Bundesrepublik Deutschland werden fast ausschließlich die Serotypen 1/2a und 4b gefunden. In Osteuropa ist der Serotyp 1/2a häufiger anzutreffen.

Die Serotypisierung ist für die ätiologische Diagnose von untergeordneter Bedeutung, sie kann in bestimmten Fällen aus epidemiologischer Sicht von Interesse sein.

■ Tierversuch

Für den Nachweis des Erregers im Untersuchungsmaterial ist der Tierversuch entbehrlich, da die kulturellen Anzüchtungsverfahren durchweg bessere Ergebnisse erbringen (22). Dagegen hat der Tierversuch für die Virulenzprüfung isolierter Stämme ne-

Table 11: Antigenic structure of listeria and serological examination methods for the diagnosis of listeriosis

Tabelle 11: Antigenstruktur der Listerien und serologischen Untersuchungsmethoden zur Diagnose der Listeriose

I. Antigenic structure of listeria species

Serotypes (18)		O-antigens (6, 22)													H-antigens			
		I	II	(III)	IV	(V)	VI	VII	VIII	IX	X	XI	XII	XIII	XV	A	B	C	D
1	1/2a	I	II	(III)												A	B		
	1/2b	I	II	(III)												A	B	C	
2	1/2c	I	II	(III)													B		D
3	3a		II	(III)												A	B		
	3b		II	(III)	IV											A	B	C	
	3c		II	(III)	IV												B		D
4	4a			(III)		(V)		VII		IX						A	B	C	
	4ab			(III)		V	VI	VII		IX						A	B	C	
	4b			(III)		V	VI									A	B	C	
	4c			(III)		V		VII								A	B	C	
	4d			(III)		(V)	VI		VIII							A	B	C	
	4e			(III)		V	VI		(VIII)	(IX)						A	B	C	
	5			(III)		(V)	VI		VIII		X					A	B	C	
	7?			(III)									XII	XIII		A	B	C	
List. spec.	6a (4f)			(III)		V	VI	VII		IX					XV	A	B	C	
	6b (4g)			(III)		V	VI	VII		IX	X	XI				A	B	C	

II. Serological diagnosis of listeriosis (1, 2)

Test method	Titre range suspicious	Titre range positive
Tube agglutination	1 : 160 + + to 1 : 320 + (Horse from 1 : 320)	1 : 320 + + (Horse from 1 : 640?)
Agglutination-growth test	1 : 200 to 1 : 400	1 : 400
Complement fixation test	1 : 5	1 : 10

strains along with the determination of the haemolytic potential. In mouse tests the LD$_{50}$ lies between 10^2 and 10^7 bacteria (3, 7). If the yolk sacs of 10-day old chick embryos are injected with 0.1 ml of a suspension containing 10^2 bacteria/ml, they will die within 2 to 5 days.

To differentiate virulent listeria strains from avirulent or from erysipelas bacteria Anton's eye test can be used in rabbits or guinea pigs (14, 23). A purulent conjunctivitis develops within 24 to 48 hours of instilling the bacteria into the conjunctival sac.

Non-haemolytic strains of *L. innocua* do not cause a fatal infection in mice, nor do they induce a conjunctivitis in rabbits or guinea pigs.

ben der Beurteilung des Hämolysevermögens Bedeutung. Hämolysierende Stämme sind virulent für Mäuse und Hühnerembryonen. Bei ip. Infektion der Maus liegt die LD$_{50}$ zwischen 10^2 und 10^7 Keimen (3, 7). Hühnerembryonen sterben innerhalb von 2–5 Tagen post infectionem ab, wenn die Eier nach 10tägiger Bebrütung durch Dottersackbeimpfung mit 0,1 ml Erregersuspension (10^2 Keime/ml) infiziert wurden.

Zur Abgrenzung virulenter Listerienstämme von avirulenten bzw. von Rotlaufbakterien kann der Antonsche Augenversuch an Kaninchen oder Meerschweinchen herangezogen werden (14, 23). Nach dem Einbringen der Erreger in den Konjunktivalsack entwickelt sich innerhalb von 24–48 h eine eitrige Konjunktivitis.

The transition from the S- to the R-form may be associated with a loss in virulence.

■ **Serological diagnosis**

The demonstration of antibodies in the patient's serum can be used for the diagnosis of listeriosis during life. In many cases however, the interpretation of the results causes difficulty, because antibodies have also been found in healthy animals and negative or only insignificant titres have been recorded in bacteriologically confirmed cases of listeriosis (14, 27). Serology is therefore to be looked upon merely as a diagnostic aid because it cannot provide the desired proof in clinically doubtful cases. The recommended serological methods are the tube agglutination test, complement fixation test and the agglutination growth test (literature in 2). The assessment follows the titre limits stated in table 11.

Anhämolysierende Stämme von *L. innocua* verursachen bei Mäusen keine tödlich verlaufende Infektion, sie sind auch nicht in der Lage, am Kaninchen- oder Meerschweinchenauge eine Konjunktivitis hervorzurufen.

Der Übergang von der S-Form in die R-Form kann mit einem Virulenzverlust einhergehen.

■ **Serologische Diagnose**

Der Antikörpernachweis im Patientenserum kann zur intravitalen Diagnose der Listeriose herangezogen werden. Die Befundinterpretation bereitet in vielen Fällen jedoch Schwierigkeiten, da auch bei gesunden Tieren häufig Antikörpertiter feststellbar sind und bei bakteriologisch gesicherten Listeriosen vielfach nur niedrige oder keine Titer gefunden werden (14, 27). Die Serologie kann deshalb nur als diagnostisches Hilfsmittel verstanden werden, da sie nicht in jedem Fall eine Objektivierung der klinischen Verdachtsdiagnose erbringt.

Als serologische Verfahren werden die Langsamagglutination, die Komplementbindungsreaktion und die Agglutinations-Wachstumsprobe empfohlen (Lit. bei 2). Die Beurteilung erfolgt nach dem in Tab. 11 aufgeführten Grenztitern.

Bibliography / Literatur

1. AMTSBERG, G. (1979): Epidemiologie und Diagnostik der Listeriose. Dtsch. tierärztl. Wschr. **86**, 253–257, 295–299.
2. AMTSBERG, G. (1980): Listerien. In: H. BLOBEL & T. SCHLIESSER (Hrsg.): Handbuch der bakteriellen Infektionen bei Tieren. Bd. II, S. 345–438. Jena: VEB Gustav Fischer.
3. BERGER, U. (1975): Einige Eigenschaften der Keimträgerstämme von Listeria monocytogenes. Med. Microbiol. Immunol. **161**, 215–229.
4. BOCKEMÜHL, J., E. FEINDT, E. HÖHNE & H. P. SEELIGER (1974): Acridinfarbstoffe in Selektivnährböden zur Isolierung von Listeria monocytogenes. II. Modifiziertes Stuart-Medium: ein neues Listeria-Transport-Anreicherungsmedium. Zschr. Med. Microbiol. Immunol. **159**, 289–299.
5. BRZIN, B., & H. P. SEELIGER (1975): A brief note on the CAMP phenomenon in Listeria. Proc. 6th Intern. Symp. on Listeriosis, Nottingham 1974, Leicester University Press, S. 34–38.
6. DONKER-VOET, J. (1966): A serological study on some strains of Listeria monocytogenes. Proc. 3rd Intern. Sympos. on Listeriosis, Bilthoven, S. 133–137.
7. EMÖDY, L., & B. RALOVICH (1975): Listeria infection in mice. Proc. 6th Intern. Sympos. on Listeriosis, Nottingham 1974, Leicester University Press, S. 131–139.
8. GRAY, M. L. (1967): A rapid method for the detection of colonies of Listeria monocytogenes. Zbl. Bakt. I. Orig. A, **169**, 373–377.
9. GRAY, M. L., & H. KILLINGER (1966): Listeria monocytogenes and listeric infections. Bacteriol. Rev. **30**, 309–382.
10. GROVES, R. D., & H. J. WELSHIMER (1977): Separation of pathogenic from apathogenic Listeria monocytogenes by three vitro reactions. J. clin. Microbiol. **5**, 559–563.
11. HENRY, B. S. (1933): Dissociation in the genus Brucella. J. Infect. Dis. **52**, 374–402.
12. IVANOV, I. (1975): Establishment of non-motile strains of Listeria monocytogenes type 5. Proc. 6th Intern. Sympos. on Listeriosis, Nottingham, 1974, Leicester University Press, S. 18–26.
13. JENTZSCH, K. D. (1962): Die Schrägdurchleuchtung von Plattenkulturen mit konstanten Bedingungen, eine wertvolle Untersuchungsanordnung für den Listeriennachweis bei der bakteriologischen Fleischuntersuchung. Fleischwirtschaft **14**, 523–525.
14. LEHNERT, CH. (1964): Bakteriologische, serologische und tierexperimentelle Untersuchungen zur Pathogenese, Epizootiologie und Prophylaxe der Listeriose. Arch. exp. Vet. med. **18**, 981–1027, 1247–1302.
15. LEHNERT, CH. (1965): Zur Züchtung von Listeria monocytogenes aus keimhaltigem Material. Zschr. ges. Hyg. **11**, 633–636.
16. OBIGER, G., & A. SCHÖNBERG (1973): Vergleichende Untersuchungen mit verschiedenen Nährmedien zur bakteriologischen Diagnose der Listeriose. Fleischwirtschaft **53**, 1452–1456.
17. PATERSON, J. S. (1939): Flagellar antigens of organisms of the Listerella. J. Path. Bact. **48**, 25–32.
18. PATERSON, J. S. (1940): The antigenic structure of organisms of the genus Listerella. J. Path. Bact. **51**, 427–436.
19. ROCOURT, J., & P. A. D. GRIMONT (1983): Listeria welshimeri sp. nov. und Listeria seeligeri sp. nov. Int. J. System. Bact. **33**, 866–869.
20. ROCOURT, J., & H. P. R. SEELIGER (1985): Distribution des espèces du genre Listeria. Zbl. Bakt. I. Orig. A, **259**, 317–330.
21. SCHOOFS, M. (1978): Kulturelle, biochemische und serologische Untersuchung an nicht-hämolysierenden Listeria-Stämmen. Med. Diss., Würzburg.
22. SEELIGER, H. P. (1958): Listeriose. Leipzig: J. A. Barth.
23. SEELIGER, H. P. (1961): Listeriosis. Basel, New York: S. Karger.
24. SEELIGER, H. P. R., J. ROCOURT, A. SCHRETTENBRUNNER, P. A. D. GRIMONT & D. JONES (1984): Listeria ivanovii sp. nov. Int. J. System. Bact. **34**, 336–337.

25. SEELIGER, H. P., & H. FINGER (1969): Analytical serology of Listeria. In: KWAPINSKI: Analytical serology of micro-organisms. Vol. 2. New York: J. Wiley & sons.
26. SEELIGER, H. P., & M. SCHOOFS (1977): Serological analysis of non hemolyzing strains of Listeria species. VII. Intern. Sympos. on the Problems of Listeriosis, Varna (Bulgaria), 3–4.
27. SEELIGER, H. P., H. FINGER & A. DIGOH (1969): Zur Epidemiologie der Listeriose. Listeria-Titerverteilung bei verschiedenen Bevölkerungsgruppen. Münch. Med. Wschr., 111, 2077–2081.
28. SEELIGER, H. P., F. SANDER & J. BOCKEMÜHL (1970): Zum kulturellen Nachweis von Listeria monocytogenes. Zschr. Med. Mikrobiol. Immunol., 155, 352–368.
29. SIDDIQUE, I. H., I. F. LIN & R. A. CHUNG (1974): Purification and characterization of hemolysin produced by Listeria monocytogenes. Am. J. Vet. Res., 35, 289–296.
30. SINGH, S. P., B. L. MOORE & I. H. SIDDIGEN (1981): Purification and further characterization of phenol extract from Listeria monocytogenes. Am. J. Vet. Res., 42, 1266–1268.
31. STANLEY, N. F. (1949): Studies on Listeria monocytogenes. I. Isolation of a monocytosis producing agent (MPA). Aust. J. Exp. Biol. Med. Sci., 27, 123–131.
32. SWORD, C. P., & G. C. KINGDON (1971): Listeria monocytogenes toxin. In: S. KADIS, T. C. MONTIE & S. J. AJE: Microbiol. toxins. Vol. II. A, Bacterial protein toxins. New York, London: Academic Press.
33. WEIS, J. (1975): The incidence of Listeria monocytogenes on plants and in soil. Proc. 6th Int. Symp. on Listeriosis, Nottingham 1974, Leicester University Press, 61–66.
34. WELSHIMER, H. J. (1968): Isolation of Listeria monocytogenes from vegetation. J. Bact., 95, 300–303.
35. WEXLER, H., & J. D. OPPENHEIM (1979): Isolation, characterization, and biological properties of an endotoxin-like material from the Gram-positive organism Listeria monocytogenes. Infect. Immun. 23, 845–857.

3 Genus: Erysipelothrix (E.)

3.1 Erysipelothrix rhusiopathiae
(Syn.: *Erysipelothrix insidiosa*)

■ **Incidence and veterinary significance**

E. rhusiopathiae cause erysipelas, a disease of world-wide distribution, which affects primarily the pig. In this species it is encountered mainly during the summer months and there are various forms:
▷ Acute erysipelas, a generalized infection, a bacteraemia, is characterized by the typical skin diamonds.
▷ Chronic erysipelas, on the other hand, causes arthritis, endocarditis, discospondylitis and skin necrosis.

The causal organism is excreted by affected animals in the faeces and urine. Infection is by the oral route. One may occasionally find erysipelas bacteria in the tonsils and faeces of healthy pigs. They have also been isolated from the soil, from sewage and fish and they participate in the process of putrefaction of organic material. Sheep up to 6 months of age can become infected with *E. rhusiopathiae* and they develop a chronic polyarthritis or septicaemia.

Infections are occasionally encountered in dogs, mice, dolphins and other animals and, among birds, the condition is important in turkeys and geese.

Erysipeloid can develop in man after wound infection. As a rule the infection remains localized, but in rare instances it spreads, leading to the development of arthritis, meningitis or endocarditis. Certain professions are exposed to special risk such as slaughtermen, veterinarians, agricultural workers, animal attendants, workers in the fish industry, all of whom may come in contact with infected material in the course of their daily work (3, 6).

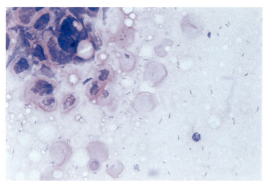
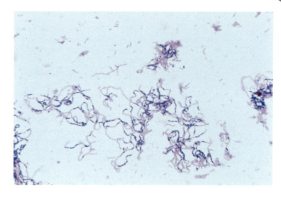
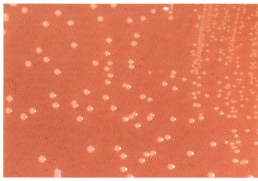
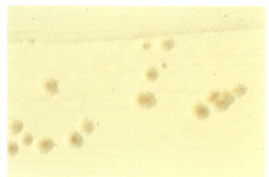

▲ Fig. 50: *Erysipelothrix rhusiopathiae*, smear from the spleen of an experimentally infected mouse, Gram stain, slender, Gram-positive rods, S-form. Magnification x 1000
▼ Fig. 52: *Erysipelothrix rhusiopathiae*, pure culture on blood agar, small, dew-drop colonies with smooth borders, S-form, 24 h, 37 °C. Magnification x 3.2

▲ Fig. 51: *Erysipelothrix rhusiopathiae*, smear from culture, Gram stain, Gram-positive bacterial filaments, R-form. Magnification x 1000
▼ Fig. 53: *Erysipelothrix rhusiopathiae*, pure culture on nutrient agar, granulated, opaque colonies with irregular borders, R-form. 48 h, 37 °C. Magnification x 3.2

▲ Abb. 50: *Erysipelothrix rhusiopathiae*, Milzausstrich von einer experimentell infizierten Maus, Gram-Färbung, grampositive, schlanke Stäbchen, S-Form, Abb.-M. 1000 : 1
▼ Abb. 52: *Erysipelothrix rhusiopathiae*, Reinkultur auf Blutagar, kleine, glattrandige, tautropfenförmige Kolonien, S-Form, 24 h, 37 °C, Abb.-M. 3,2 : 1

▲ Abb. 51: *Erysipelothrix rhusiopathiae*, Kulturausstrich, Gram-Färbung, grampositive Bakterienfäden, R-Form, Abb.-M. 1000 : 1
▼ Abb. 53: *Erysipelothrix rhusiopathiae*, Reinkultur auf Nähragar, granulierte, undurchsichtige Kolonien mit unregelmäßigem Rand, R-Form, 48 h, 37 °C, Abb.-M. 3,2 : 1

aufgrund ihrer Tätigkeit mit infiziertem Tiermaterial in Berührung kommen (3, 6).

■ Morphology

Erysipelothrix rhusiopathiae is a slim, Gram-positive, non-motile rod, that is generally straight, though sometimes curved. It measures 0.8 to 2.5 µm in length. In the S-form these rods lie singly, but in the R-form they form twisted filaments which may be more than 60 µm in length (figs. 50, 51).

The bacteria can readily become decolourized

■ Morphologie

Rotlaufbakterien sind grampositive, gerade, schlanke, seltener leicht gebogene, unbewegliche Stäbchen mit einer Länge von 0,8 bis 2,5 µm. Während die Stäbchen der S-Form einzeln liegen, bilden die der R-Form lange gewundene Fäden, die eine Länge von 60 µm und mehr erreichen können (Abb. 50 u. 51).

with the Gram stain, so that they appear as Gram-negative.

■ Culture

E. rhusiopathiae is a facultative anaerobe, which grows under aerobic conditions at 37 °C. It will multiply in a temperature range of 16 °C to 41 °C and a pH from 6.7 to 9.2. However, it prefers a pH of between 7.4 and 8.0. Growth can be improved by the addition of 5–10 % CO_2.

▷ Growth on solid media: Nutrient agar is used to differentiate between the two forms and on this medium the colonies of the smooth form are small and transparent with smooth edges and a diameter of about 1 mm. The R-form, on the other hand, produces colonies with irregular borders, a granular, flat-grey surface and the diameter can be more than 2 mm (fig. 53) (3, 6, 15).

Erysipelas bacteria grown on blood agar for 24 to 48 hours at 37 °C produce small greyish-white colonies with a diameter of 0.5 to 1.0 mm (fig. 52). The colonies are often surrounded by a narrow darker or greenish zone, so that these colonies resemble those of α-haemolytic streptococci. On dextrose blood agar (Zeissler plate), these characteristic colonies are clearly recognized within 24 h. The R-form will also grow on blood agar, producing larger colonies with rough surface and irregular outline.

Selective media, containing sodium azide, crystal violet, phenol and/or kanamycin as inhibitors, can be used for the detection of erysipelas bacteria in contaminated material (1, 3, 5, 6, 7).

▷ Growth in fluid media: The S-form produces a uniform turbidity in nutrient broth, the R-form a floccular, granular sediment.

Growth can be improved both in nutrient broth and on nutrient agar by the addition of serum (5 %) or glucose (1–2 %). Repeated subcultures on unsuitable media can change the S-form into the R-form.

Fluid media containing inhibitors can be used for selective enrichment.

The diagnostic use of cultures is summarized in figure 54.

■ Biochemical properties

The biochemical activity is not very pronounced in *E. rhusiopathiae* (fig. 54). 1 % peptone water containing 5 % horse serum is recommended for testing

■ Kultur

E. rhusiopathiae gehört zu den fakultativen Anaerobiern, die unter aeroben Bedingungen bei 37 °C angezüchtet werden. Sie vermehren sich in einem Temperaturbereich von 16 bis 41 °C und einem pH-Bereich von 6,7 bis 9,2, bevorzugt werden pH-Werte zwischen 7,4 und 8,0. Durch ein 5- bis 10%iges CO_2-Milieu läßt sich das Wachstum verbessern.

▷ Wachstum auf festen Nährböden: Auf Nähragar, der zur Unterscheidung der beiden Wuchsformen verwendet wird, wächst die Glattform in kleinen, glattrandigen, transparenten Kolonien mit einem Durchmesser bis zu 1 mm. Die R-Form bildet dagegen Kolonien mit unregelmäßigen Rändern und körniger, mattgrauer Oberfläche, der Koloniedurchmesser kann über 2 mm erreichen (Abb. 53) (3, 6, 15).

Auf Blutagar wachsen die Rotlaufbakterien innerhalb von 24 bis 48 h bei einer Bebrütung bei 37 °C in kleinen, grauweißen Kolonien, die einen Durchmesser von 0,5 bis 1,0 mm erreichen (Abb. 52). Häufig kommt es um die Kolonien zum Auftreten schmaler dunkler oder grünlicher Höfe, so daß diese Koloniemorphologie der der α-hämolysierenden Streptokokken sehr ähnlich ist. Auf dem Traubenzuckerblutagar (Zeißler-Platte) ist die beschriebene Koloniemorphologie innerhalb von 24 h deutlicher zu erkennen. Die R-Form wächst auf dem Blutagar in größeren Kolonien mit rauher Oberfläche und unregelmäßigem Rand.

Zum Nachweis von Rotlaufbakterien aus kontaminiertem Untersuchungsmaterial können Selektivmedien eingesetzt werden, die als Hemmittel Natriumacid, Kristallviolett, Phenol und (oder) Kanamycin enthalten (1, 3, 5, 6, 7).

▷ Wachstum in flüssigen Nährböden: In Nährbouillon bewirkt die S-Form eine gleichmäßige Trübung, die R-Form einen flockig-körnigen Bodensatz.

Das Wachstum läßt sich in der Nährbouillon oder im Nähragar durch den Zusatz von Serum (5 %) oder Glukose (1–2 %) verbessern. Die R-Form kann sich durch häufige Kulturpassagen auf ungünstigen Nährmedien aus der S-Form entwickeln.

Flüssige Nährmedien können ferner für die selektive Anreicherung unter Zusatz von Hemmstoffen eingesetzt werden.

Die diagnostische Verwendung der Kultur ist in der Abb. 54 zusammengestellt.

■ Kulturell-biochemische Eigenschaften

Die biochemische Aktivität ist bei *E. rhusiopathiae* nicht sehr ausgeprägt (Abb. 54). Zur Prüfung der Kohlenhydratspaltung wird 1%iges Peptonwasser

for carbohydrate fermentation. The use of yeast autolysate is also advised, because otherwise the results can be unclear and ambiguous (15).

The recommendations of the German Society for Hygiene and Microbiology (Deutsche Gesellschaft für Hygiene und Mikrobiologie) for the microbiological diagnosis of *Erysipelothrix* state that rabbit serum (1 ml rabbit serum to 4 ml medium) should be added to the usual biochemical media for the fermentation tests.

The triple sugar iron agar of Kligler is used for testing for hydrogen sulphide production.

Stab culture of erysipelas bacteria into nutrient gelatine causes the characteristic development of small lateral outgrowth which are reminiscent of a bottle brush.

mit Zusatz von 5 % Pferdeserum empfohlen. Außerdem wird der Zusatz von Hefeautolysat angeraten, da die Ergebnisse sonst undeutlich und widersprüchlich ausfallen können (15).

In den Richtlinien der Deutschen Gesellschaft für Hygiene und Mikrobiologie für die mikrobiologische Diagnostik von *Erysipelothrix* (1982) werden für die Fermentationsprüfung die üblichen biochemischen Medien mit Zusatz von Kaninchenserum (1 ml Kaninchenserum auf 4 ml Medium) vorgeschlagen.

Für die Schwefelwasserstoffbildung findet der Eisen-Dreizucker-Agar nach Kligler Verwendung.

Die Stichkultur von Nährgelatine mit Rotlaufbakterien führt nach einigen Tagen zum Auftreten von Ausläufern um den Stichkanal, dieses charakteristische Wachstum erinnert an die Form einer Gläserbürste.

Specimens
Organs, tonsils, joints etc.

Microscopic detection of organism in direct smears
Gram staining
Acute erysipelas: slender, Gram-positive rods, lying singly (S-form, fig. 50)
Chronic erysipelas: slender, Gram-positive rods (S-form) or filaments (R-form, fig. 51)

Examination by culture
1. Selective enrichment is necessary if a small number of bacteria are suspected in contaminated material, crystal violet-sodium azide-phenol-kanamycin broth, incubation 4 to 5 days at 37 °C, isolation by daily subculture onto solid media (see 2 below) (1, 3)
2. Solid media for direct culture or the isolation from enrichment broth,
blood agar: After 24 to 48 hours small, dew drop-like colonies without haemolysis (fig. 52), selective medium: Sodium azide-phenol-kanamycin-saccharose agar. The saccharose serves as indicator to exclude saccharose-positive streptococci (1, 3)
Incubation 24 to 72 h,
Erysipelas bacteria grow as colourless colonies.

Identification of E. rhusiopathiae in pure culture

1. Microscopic examination: Gram-positive rods, lying singly or in filaments (S- or R-form)

2. Assessment of colony morphology (S- or R-form)

3. Culture-biochemical examination

Glu (no gas)	+	Gal	+	Fru	+	Lac	+
Rha	−	Xyl	v	Man	−	Sac	−
Ind	−	Sal	−	Tre	−	Aes	−
Ure	−	H$_2$S	+	VPR	−	MR	−
Litmus milk	−	Nit	−	Cat	−	Gel	−[1]
				Serum liquefaction	−	Mot	−

[1] Growth in bottle-brush form

Fig. 54: Detection and identification of *Erysipelothrix rhusiopathiae*

[1] Wachstum in Form einer Gläserbürste

Abb. 54: Nachweis und Bestimmung von *Erysipelothrix rhusiopathiae*

■ Enzymes and toxins

Erysipelas bacteria form hyaluronidase and neuraminidase (9, 12) which are of importance as virulence factors, but these enzymes are not used for identifying the organism.

The presence of a thermolabile toxin is suspected on the basis of experiments with phenol-water extracts (3).

■ Antigenic structure

Serotypes A to O have been identified on the basis of various polysaccharide antigens (8, 10, 11, 16). Serotype A is generally responsible for the acute and peracute forms of erysipelas. Type B occurs mainly, though not exclusively, in the chronic forms (3, 4). Both types can be divided into further subgroups (10, 11) and the remaining types are found mainly in fish (C, D and E), in the tonsils of healthy pigs (G and H) and cattle (C and D) (6). However, the tonsils of healthy pigs also carry serotypes A and B (2). Erysipelas bacteria which lack type-specific antigens are classed in group N. N strains are not very virulent in pigs (6). Dissociation causes an alteration of the antigenic properties. The agar precipitation test with heat-stable or acid-soluble antigen (8, 10) is used for typing and to divide it into further subgroups (10, 11).

■ Animal experiments

Mice and pigs are used for testing the virulence of erysipelas bacteria. It must be borne in mind, of course, that the virulence assessed in mice is not immediately applicable to pigs. Pigs are infected by the cutaneous, oral or intravenous routes, while intraperitoneal injection is preferred for mice. Mice will die within 2 to 5 days and in pigs all the forms of acute erysipelas can develop. For virulence testing in pigs the method of choice is scarification (2), in which several strains can be tested in the same animal simultaneously. The severity of the inflammation that develops along the scarification lines and perhaps the transition into a generalized infection permits the virulence to be assessed quantitatively.

Dissociation usually causes a loss of virulence, but the results of virulence tests on dissociated cultures are very variable, because they still contain a proportion of non-dissociated organisms, which are selected in the experimental animal and produce full virulence.

In the majority of cases the diagnostic demonstration of the bacteria does not require animal inoculation, because culture and subsequent biochemical tests provide unequivocal results.

■ Enzyme und Toxine

Rotlaufbakterien bilden Hyaluronidase und Neuraminidase (9, 12), die als Virulenzfaktoren von Bedeutung sind. Zur Differenzierung der Erreger werden diese Enzyme nicht herangezogen.

Vermutet wird das Vorkommen eines thermostabilen Toxins, Hinweise hierfür ergaben Versuche mit Phenol-Wasser-Extrakten (3).

■ Antigenstruktur

Serologisch werden bei den Rotlaufbakterien aufgrund von verschiedenen Polysaccharidantigenen die Serotypen A bis O unterschieden (8, 10, 11, 16). Der Serotyp A verursacht in der Regel die akuten bis perakuten Verlaufsformen, der Typ B kommt überwiegend, aber nicht ausschließlich, bei den chronischen Formen vor (3, 4). Beide Typen lassen sich in weitere Subtypen unterteilen (10, 11), die übrigen Typen werden vorwiegend bei Fischen (C, D und E) oder in Tonsillen von gesunden Schweinen (G und H) und Rindern (C und D) gefunden (6). Daneben kommen in den Tonsillen gesunder Schweine auch die Serotypen A und B vor (2). Rotlaufbakterienstämmen, denen ein typspezifisches Antigen fehlt, werden der Gruppe N zugeordnet. N-Stämme besitzen für das Schwein eine geringe Virulenz (6). Die Dissoziation führt bei den Rotlaufbakterien zu einer Veränderung der antigenen Eigenschaften. Für die Typisierung wird die Agargelpräzipitation unter Verwendung von Kochantigenen oder säurelöslichen Antigenen (8, 10) benutzt.

■ Tierversuch

Für Virulenzprüfungen von Rotlaufbakterien werden Mäuse und Schweine verwendet. Hierbei muß berücksichtigt werden, daß die an Mäusen festgestellte Virulenz nicht ohne weiteres auf das Schwein übertragen werden kann. Schweine werden kutan, oral oder iv. infiziert, bei Mäusen wird die ip. Infektion bevorzugt. Die Mäuse sterben meistens innerhalb von 2 bis 5 d, bei den Schweinen können sich alle Formen des akuten Rotlaufs entwickeln. Bevorzugt für die Virulenztestung am Schwein wird die Skarifikationsmethode (2), bei der gleichzeitig mehrere Stämme an einem Tier geprüft werden können. Die Schwere der entzündlichen Veränderungen entlang dem Skarifikationsstrich sowie ein eventueller Übergang in eine Allgemeininfektion können quantitative Hinweise zum Virulenzgrad erlauben.

Eine Dissoziation bewirkt meistens einen Virulenzverlust. Die Ergebnisse von Virulenzprüfungen dissoziierter Kulturen sind sehr schwankend, da diese oft noch einen Anteil nicht dissoziierter Keime enthalten, der im Versuchstier selektiert wird und seine volle Virulenz entfalten kann.

Für den diagnostischen Erregernachweis ist der Tierversuch in der Mehrzahl der Fälle entbehrlich, da der kulturelle Nachweis und die nachfolgende

Table 12: Serological diagnosis of chronic erysipelas (3)

Tabelle 12: Serologische Diagnostik des chronischen Rotlaufs (3)

Reaction		Non-specific titre range	Specific titre range		
			low titre	moderate titre	high titre
Growth test	Main value	≥ 40 %	20 % 10 %	7 % 5 % 1 %	≤ 0.5 %
	value in parenthesis	≥ 5 %	1 % 0.5 %	0.25 % 0.125 % 0.0625 %	≤ 0.03125 %
Agglutination		1 : ≤ 80	160 320	620 1280 2560	≥ 5120

■ **Serological diagnosis**

Serological procedures have not gained any significance in the diagnosis of acute erysipelas, but in the chronic disease they can offer useful indications. Two methods are employed, tube agglutination using killed antigen and the agglutination growth test for which live antigen is required (3). The interpretation of the antibody titre is illustrated in table 12. According to this, non-specific and low titres indicate the absence of chronic erysipelas, moderately high specific titres suggest that the presence of disease is probable and with high specific titres the diagnosis is considered to be confirmed.

■ **Serologische Diagnose**

Zur Diagnose des akuten Rotlaufs haben serologische Verfahren keine Bedeutung erlangt, dagegen können sie in der Diagnostik chronischer Verlaufsformen brauchbare Hinweise erbringen. Zum Einsatz kommen die Langsamagglutination unter Verwendung von totem Antigen und die Agglutinations-Wachstumsprobe, bei der lebendes Antigen benötigt wird (3). Die Beurteilung der Antikörpertiter ist aus Tabelle 12 zu ersehen. Danach sprechen unspezifische und niedrige Titer gegen das Vorliegen von chronischem Rotlauf, bei mittleren spezifischen Titern ist das Vorliegen wahrscheinlich und bei hohen spezifischen Titern gilt die Diagnose als erwiesen.

Es sollte noch darauf hingewiesen werden, daß nur die kulturell-biochemische Differenzierung eindeutige Ergebnisse liefern.

Bibliography / Literatur

1. BÖHM, K. H. (1971): Neue Selektivnährböden für Rotlaufbakterien. Zbl. Bakt. I. Orig. A., 218, 330–334.
2. BÖHM, K. H. (1972): Vorkommen und mögliche Bedeutung von Rotlaufbakterien bei rotlaufunverdächtigen Schlachtschweinen. Schlacht-Viehhofztg. 72, 316–322.
3. BÖHM, K. H., W. BOLLWAHN & G. TRAUTWEIN (1980): Erysipelothrix. In: H. BLOBEL & T. SCHLIESSER (Hrsg.): Handbuch der bakteriellen Infektionen bei Tieren. Bd. II, S. 439–553. Jena: VEB Gustav Fischer.
4. BISPING, W. (1979): Kompendium der veterinärmedizinischen Mikrobiologie. Teil II: Spezielle Mikrobiologie und Mykologie. 3. Aufl. Hannover: M. & H. Schaper.
5. BRATBERG, A. M. (1981): Observations on the utilization of a selective medium for the isolation of Erysipelothrix rhusiopathiae. Acta vet. scand. 22, 55–59.
6. EISSNER, G., & F. W. EWALD (1973): Rotlauf. Jena: VEB Gustav Fischer.
7. EWALD, F. W. (1960): Differentialdiagnostische Gesichtspunkte bei der Diagnose des Schweinerotlaufs unter besonderer Berücksichtigung des Vorkommens von Streptokokken. Arch. Lebensmittelhyg. 11, 97–102.
8. EWALD, F. W. (1962): Typendifferenzierung von Erysipelothrix rhusiopathiae im Agargel. Berl. Münch. tierärztl. Wschr. 75, 71–73.
9. FRANKE, F., & C. SANNING (1971): Zur Hyaluronidasebildung bei Rotlaufbakterien. Berl. Münch. tierärztl. Wschr. 84, 28–30.
10. HEUNER, F. (1958): Über serologische Untersuchungen an Rotlaufstämmen. Arch. exp. Vet. med. 12, 40–61.
11. KUCSERA, G. (1962): Die Untersuchung von Schweinerotlaufbakterienstämmen mit der Präzipitationsprobe unter Anwendung verschiedener Antigenextraktionsmethoden. Acta vet. hung. 12, 43–51.
12. MÜLLER, H. E., & K. H. BÖHM (1973): Untersuchungen in vitro über die Neuraminidase bei Erysipelothrix insidiosa. Zbl. Bakt. I. Orig. A, 223, 220–227.
13. NØRRUNG, V. (1979): Two new serotypes of Erysipelothrix rhusiopathiae. Nord. Vet. Med. 31, 462–465.
14. Richtlinien für die mikrobiologische Diagnostik der Deutschen Gesellschaft für Hygiene und Mikrobiologie (1982): Isolierung und Identifizierung von Corynebakterium, Listeria und Erysipelothrix. Zbl. Bakt. I. Orig. A, 253, 43–60.
15. SEELIGER, H. P. R. (1975): Genus Erysipelothrix. In: R. E. BUCHANAN & N. E. GIBBONS, Bergey's manual of determinative bacteriology. 8th ed., S. 597. Baltimore: Williams & Wilkins.
16. TRUSZCZYNSKI, M. (1963): Investigations on the antigenic structure of the new Erysipelothrix insidiosa serotype. Bull. Vet. Inst. Pulawy 7, 85–92.

4 Genus: Lactobacillus (L.)

Lactobacilli are widely distributed in nature. They are found frequently in milk, meat and fish products and they are important in making silage, sauerkraut, yoghurt, cheese and other milk products. In man and animals they normally inhabit the mucosa of the digestive and genital tracts (5, 6). Since they produce metabolites of antibacterial potency, they have an antagonistic effect on other bacterial species. Preparations containing lactobacilli are available today which are used in the treatment of diarrhoea of young animals (2, 3, 4). Lactobacilli are of no pathogenic importance. They are of differential diagnostic interest in medical bacteriology and therefore their most important properties will be mentioned here.

■ Morphology
Lactobacilli are Gram-positive non-sporulating bacteria, which occur in long slender rods (fig. 55) or in short coccoid forms. They lie singly or in chains and they are usually non-motile. Their size generally varies between 1.5 and 6 µm (7).

■ Culture
Although lactobacilli are classed only as facultative anaerobes, they grow more rapidly and profusely under anaerobic than aerobic conditions. Some species flourish on solid media only in the presence of oxygen. They can multiply in a temperature range of 5 °C to 53 °C, but the optimum temperature lies between 30 °C and 40 °C. A pH range of 5.0 to 6.0 is preferred (7).

Lactobacilli grow on dextrose blood agar as small greyish-white colonies which often show the viridans effect (fig. 56). Rogosa agar (7) or tomato juice agar are recommended for specific primary culture (fig. 57). They can grow as either S- or R-forms. As fluid media one can use liver broth or nutrient broth containing 0.5 % glacial acetic acid (for its selective effect) or peptone yeast broth (1).

■ Biochemical properties
We differentiate between homo- and heterofermentative lactobacilli, depending on the metabolites that develop during carbohydrate breakdown. The homofermentative ones, which include, for example, *L. acidophilus*, *L. plantarum* and *L. casei* produce lactic acid as the main product. The heterofermentative species produce not only lactic acid but also acetic acid and CO_2.

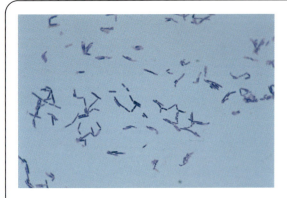
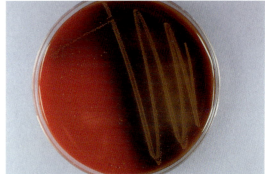
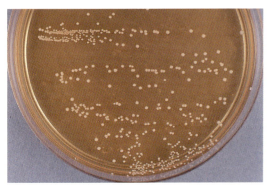
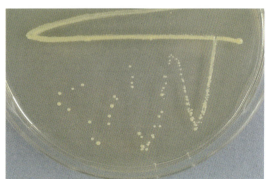

▲ Fig. 55: *Lactobacillus acidophilus*, culture smear, Gram stain, slender, Gram-positive rods. Magnification x 1000
▼ Fig. 57: *Lactobacillus acidophilus*, pure culture on Rogosa agar, greyish-white, shiny colonies with smooth borders, S-form, 48 h, 37 °C. Magnification x 0.4

▲ Fig. 56: *Lactobacillus acidophilus*, pure culture on blood agar, greenish growth, 48 h, 37 °C. Magnification x 0.25
▼ Fig. 58: *Renibacterium salmoninarum*, pure culture on selective agar, small, shiny, creamy-white colonies, 30 d, 17 °C. Magnification x 0.4

▲ Abb. 55: *Lactobacillus acidophilus*, Kulturausstrich, Gram-Färbung, grampositive, schlanke Stäbchen, Abb.-M. 1000 : 1
▼ Abb. 57: *Lactobacillus acidophilus*, Reinkultur auf Rogosa-Agar, grauweiße, glattrandige, glänzende Kolonien, S-Form, 48 h, 37 °C, Abb.-M. 1 : 2,5

▲ Abb. 56: *Lactobacillus acidophilus*, Reinkultur auf Blutagar, vergrünendes Wachstum, 48 h, 37 °C, Abb.-M. 1 : 4
▼ Abb. 58: *Renibacterium salmoninarum* Reinkultur auf Selektivagar, kleine, weiß-cremig glänzende Kolonien, 30 d, 17 °C, Abb.-M. 1 : 2,5

More than 20 species of lactobacilli are known and their differentiation is carried out by means of numerous biochemical reactions (7). Commercial kits are available for this purpose, e.g. API 50. Gas chromatographic test can also be helpful.

The diagnostic differentiation between lactobacilli and morphologically similar pathogens is presented in table 13.

L. buchneri, entstehen beim Abbau neben Milchsäure auch Essigsäure und CO_2.

Die Differenzierung der mehr als 20 bekannten Lactobacillus-Arten erfolgt mit zahlreichen biochemischen Reaktionen (7), hierfür gibt es auch handelsübliche Reaktionsreihen (z. B. API 50 CHL). Daneben können gaschromatographische Untersuchungen hilfreich sein.

Die differentialdiagnostische Abgrenzung der Gattung *Lactobacillus* von anderen morphologisch ähnlichen pathogenen Bakterien zeigt Tab. 13.

Table 13: The important differentiating properties of various Gram-positive bacteria

Properties	Lactobacillus spp.	Listeria monocytogenes	Erysipelothrix rhusiopathiae	Streptococcus spp.
Morphology	rods	rods	rods	cocci
Size in µm	1.5–6	0.5–2	0.8–2.5	1
Oxidation-fermentation test/glucose	F	F	F	F
Oxidase formation	–	–	–	–
Catalase formation	–	+	–	–
Nitrate reduction	–	–	–	–
H_2S production	–	–	+	–
Motility	–	+	–	–
β-haemolysis	–	+	–	+/–

Bibliography / Literatur

1. HOLDEMAN, L. V., E. P. CATO & W. E. C. MOORE (1977): Anaerobe laboratory manual. 4th ed. Anaerobe Laboratory Virginia Polytechnic Institute and State University, Blacksburg, Virginia.
2. JAHREIS, G., A. HENNING, H. BOCHER & K. GRUHN (1981): Zur Anwendung von Laktobazillen bei monogastrischen Nutztieren anstelle konventioneller Antibiotika. Mh. Vet.-Med. 36, 820–826.
3. MULLING, M., & W. GROSS (1980): Therapie des Kälberdurchfalls mit ferment- und milchsäurebakterienhaltigen Präparaten (Fermatolad, CTB Chemotherapia, Lactofermente, Selectavet). Tierärztl. Umschau 35, 379–382.
4. MULARIDHARA, K. S., G. G. SHEGGEGY, P. R. ELLIKER, D. C. ENGLAND & W. E. SANDIM (1977): Effect of feeding Lactobacilli on coliform and Lactobacillus flora of intestinal tissue and feces from piglets. J. Food Protect, 40, 288–295.
5. REUTER, G. (1965): Das Vorkommen von Laktobazillen in Lebensmitteln und ihr Verhalten im menschlichen Intestinaltrakt. Zbl. Bakt., I. Orig. 197, 468–487.
6. REUTER, G. (1972): Untersuchungen zur antagonistischen Wirkung der Milchsäurebakterien auf andere Keimgruppen der Lebensmittelflora. Zbl. Vet. Med. B 19, 320–334.
7. ROGOSA, M. (1974): Genus I. Lactobacillus Beijerinck 1901. In: R. E. BUCHANAN & N. E. GIBBONS (ed.): Bergey's Manual of Determinative Bacteriology. 8th ed., S. 576–593. Baltimore: Williams & Wilkins.

5 Renibacterium salmoninarum

The Gram-positive, non-sporulating bacterium is the cause of bacterial kidney disease of salmonid fish. It was first classed as a corynebacterium but, because of divergent bacteriological characteristics it is now assigned to its own genus.

In Germany the disease was first observed in 1984 (3). The small, coryneform bacterium can be demonstrated in culture and by immunofluorescence (4). Selective media have been described (1, 2), which contain cycloserine, polymyxin-B sulphate and oxolinic acid. These are incubated for 8–30 days at 18 °C (4).

Bibliography / Literatur

1. AUSTIN, B., T. M. EMBLEY & M. GOODFELLOW (1983): Selective isolation of Renibacterium salmoninarum. FEMS Microbiol. Letters 17, 11–14.
2. EVELYN, T. P. T. (1977): An improved growth medium for the kidney disease bacterium and some notes on using the medium. Bull. Off. Int. Epiz. 87, 511–513.
3. HOFFMANN, R., W. POPP & S. VAN DE GRAAFF (1984): Atypical BKD predominantly causing ocular and skin lesions. Bull. Europ. Ass. Fish Path. 4, 7–9.
4. PFEIL-PUTZIEN, C., R. HOFFMANN, W. POPP & M. SCHAUNER (1985): Zur Verbreitung der bacterial kidney disease (BKD) der Salmoniden in der Bundesrepublik Deutschland. Zbl. Vet. Med. B 32, 541–547.
5. SANDERS, J. E., & J. L. FRYER (1980): Renibacterium salmoninarum gen. nov. sp. nov. the causative agent of bacterial kidney disease in salmonid fishes. Int. J. System. Bact. 30, 496–502.
6. HOFFMANN, R., & C. PFEIL-PUTZIEN (1986): Bacterial kidney disease. Tierärztl. Prax. 14, 283–289.

Gram-positive spore-forming organisms
Grampositive Sporenbildner

1 Genus: Bacillus (Bac.)

Gram-positive, rarely Gram-variable, rods that are usually motile, form endogenous spores and grow aerobically.

1.1 Bacillus anthracis

■ **Incidence and veterinary significance**

Bac. anthracis is the organism causing anthrax in both man and animals. The animals most commonly to become affected by the disease under natural conditions are cattle, sheep, goats, buffalo, horses, camels, reindeer, elephant and mink. Birds, with the exception of the ostrich, are distinctly less susceptible, and only very occasionally do they succumb to the spontaneous disease (20). A subacute or chronic form is common in the pig and associated with a primary infection in the pharyngeal region (15). KAUKER (11) and KAUKER & ZETTEL (12) discuss the world-wide distribution of anthrax.

■ **Morphology**

Bac. anthracis is an aerobic sporulating organism. It is a non-motile, Gram-positive, cylindrical rod, 1 µm thick and 3–5 µm in length. Inside the host's body it forms a capsule which can be demonstrated by special stains (e.g. the one of Foth, page 336). In organ smears the bacilli lie either singly or in short chains of between 2 and 5 cells. Their ends appear sharply defined in stained preparations; they are convex where they meet another individual. This causes the threads to assume the so-called bamboo-stick form (fig. 59). Long chains of bacilli without capsules are formed in culture. Spores develop only in the presence of oxygen at temperatures above 12 °C.

■ **Culture**

Anthrax bacilli will grow on ordinary solid media

1 Gattung: Bacillus (Bac.)

Grampositive, selten gramlabile bis gramnegative, meistens bewegliche Stäbchen mit endogener Sporenbildung und aerobem Wachstum.

1.1 Bacillus anthracis

■ **Vorkommen und medizinische Bedeutung**

Bac. anthracis ist der Milzbranderreger bei Mensch und Tier. Unter den Tieren erkranken unter natürlichen Verhältnissen am häufigsten Rind, Schaf, Ziege, Büffel, Pferd, Kamel, Rentier, Elefant und Nerz. Eine deutlich geringere Empfindlichkeit weisen Vögel (Ausnahme: Strauß) auf, die nur ganz vereinzelt erkranken (20). Beim Schwein ist ein subakuter bis chronischer Verlauf mit einer primären Infektion im Rachenbereich häufig (16). Über die weltweite Verbreitung des Milzbrandes siehe KAUKER (11) und KAUKER & ZETTEL (12).

■ **Morphologie**

Bac. anthracis ist ein aerober Sporenbildner. Es handelt sich um ein unbewegliches, grampositives, zylindrisches, 1 µm dickes, 3–5 µm langes Stäbchen. Im Organismus wird eine Kapsel gebildet, die mit Spezialfärbungen (z. B. nach Foth, s. S. 336) darstellbar ist. Im Organausstrich liegen die Bazillen entweder einzeln oder in kurzen Verbänden von 2 bis 5 Bakterienzellen. Im gefärbten Präparat sind die Enden der Stäbchen scharf gekantet, die sich gegenüberliegenden Seiten tellerförmig eingebuchtet, was den in Fäden liegenden Bazillen die sog. »Bambusstabform« verleiht (Abb. 59). In der Kultur werden lange Fäden aus unbekapselten Bazillen gebildet. Sporen entstehen nur bei Anwesenheit von Sauerstoff und einer Temperatur von über 12 °C.

■ **Kultur**

Die Milzbrandbazillen wachsen auf den gebräuchli-

(agar, serum agar, blood agar) and, after 48 hours at 37 °C they form dull surface colonies of moderate size and greyish-white appearance (figs. 61 and 64). Under low magnification the colonies are seen to have curved, twisted processes radiating from their borders, which resemble locks of hair or plaits, and give the appearance of a medusa head or a woman's curly hair. No haemolysis is produced on blood agar (fig. 64). In broth, after 24 hour incubation, there is a floccular, cotton wool-like sediment while the supernatant liquid usually remains clear. Gelatine stab cultures present the slowly progressive »bottle brush« type of liquefaction, with the side-shoots radiating from the stab line.

■ **Biochemical properties** (fig. 63)
These are of subordinate importance for the identification of *Bac. anthracis*. Acid is formed from glucose, laevulose, maltose, saccharose, trehalose and dextrin. The Voges-Proskauer reaction is positive and nitrates are reduced to nitrites.
▷ Yolk reaction: This is in effect a demonstration of the presence of lecithinase which is positive in *Bac. anthracis* and *Bac. cereus* but negative in the others.
▷ Pearl-string test: When *Bac. anthracis* is grown for a few hours on solid media containing 0.5 I.U. penicillin/ml, the bacilli become spherical in appearance, resembling a string of pearls. This test is an adjunct to the rapid recognition of anthrax bacilli.
For further characteristics useful in the differential diagnosis see GIBSON & GORDON (5), SEIDL (18) and KRIEG (13).

■ **Serological detection of anthrax antigens**
If, because of advanced autolysis, for example, the anthrax bacilli are no longer demonstrable in the tissues, the thermoprecipitation test of ASCOLI can be applied (1). It may also be used for identifying strains of anthrax. The method is based on the demonstration of the anthrax antigens by precipitation. The procedure is as follows: 2 to 3 g of chopped organ material are briefly boiled and filtered through filter paper. Using a capillary pipette, precipitating anthrax serum is first placed into small precipitation tubes and then the clear extract is layered on top of the serum. In positive cases a ring of precipitation develops within a few minutes at the interface. This reaction can also be carried out as an OUCHTERLONY agar precipitation test (16). This thermoprecipitation test is not suitable for the examination of food materials and bone meal (10).

chen festen Nährböden (Nähragar-, Serumagar-, Blutagarplatten) und bilden nach 24 h aerober Bebrütung bei 37 °C oberflächliche, mittelgroße, matte Kolonien von grauweißlichem Aussehen (Abb. 61 u. 64). Bei schwacher Vergrößerung sind diese an ihren Rändern von ausstrahlenden, bogenförmig gewundenen, lockigen oder zopfartigen Ausläufern (Bazillenfäden) umgeben, die den Kolonien das Aussehen eines »Medusenhauptes« oder »gelockten Frauenhaares« verleihen. Auf Blutagar wird keine Hämolyse gebildet (Abb. 64). In der Bouillonkultur erscheint nach 24stündiger Bebrütung ein flockiger, watteartiger Bodensatz, während die überstehende Flüssigkeit gewöhnlich klar bleibt. In einer Gelatine-Stichkultur treten gläserbürstenartige, vom Stichrand ausgehende Ausstrahlungen mit langsam fortschreitender Gelatineverflüssigung auf.

■ **Kultur-biochemische Eigenschaften** (Abb. 63)
Sie sind für die Bestimmung von *Bac. anthracis* von untergeordneter Bedeutung. Aus Glucose, Lävulose, Maltose, Saccharose, Trehalose und Dextrin wird Säure gebildet, die VPR ist positiv, Nitrate werden zu Nitriten reduziert.
▷ Eigelbreaktion: Es handelt sich um einen Lecithinasenachweis, der bei *Bac. anthracis* und *Bac. cereus* positiv, bei den anderen Bazillen negativ ausfällt.
▷ Perlschnurtest: Wenn *Bac. anthracis* auf einem festen Nährboden gezüchtet wird, der 0,5 IE Penicillin/ml enthält, nehmen die Bazillen nach einigen Stunden eine kugelige Gestalt an, so daß sie wie eine Perlschnur aussehen. Der Test kann zur schnellen Erkennung von Milzbrandbazillen beitragen.
Weitere Merkmale zur Differentialdiagnose der Bazillen siehe GIBSON & GORDON (5), SEIDEL (18), KRIEG (13).

■ **Serologischer Nachweis von Bac. anthracis-Antigenen**
Wenn Milzbrandbazillen in den Organen, z. B. aufgrund fortgeschrittener Fäulnis, mikroskopisch nicht mehr erfaßbar sind, kann die Thermopräzipitation nach ASCOLI (1) durchgeführt werden. Sie kann auch zur Bestimmung von Milzbrandstämmen benutzt werden. Die Methode beruht auf dem Nachweis gelöster spezifischer Milzbrandantigene durch die Präzipitation. Zur Durchführung der Reaktion werden 2 bis 3 g zerkleinertes Organmaterial kurz aufgekocht und durch Papierfilter klar filtriert. In kleinen Präzipitationsröhrchen wird zuerst das präzipitierende Milzbrandserum mit einer Kapillare auf den Röhrchenboden gebracht und dann der klare Extrakt auf das Serum geschichtet. Im positiven Falle bildet sich innerhalb weniger Minuten an der Berührungsfläche ein Präzipitationsring. Die Reaktion kann auch als Agargelpräzipitation nach OUCHTERLONY durchgeführt werden (16). Die Thermopräzipitation ist nicht zur Untersuchung

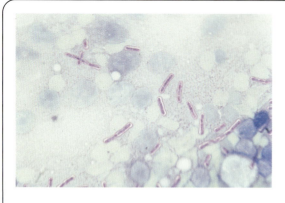
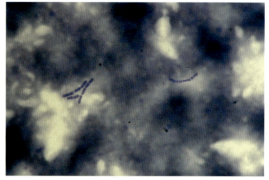
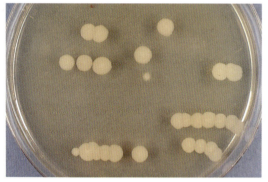
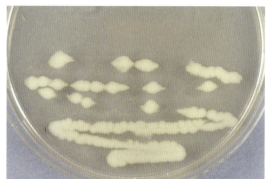

▲ Fig. 59: *Bacillus anthracis*, smear from the spleen of a mouse, capsule stain after Foth, reddish capsule and blue bacillus. Magnification x 1000
▼ Fig. 61: *Bacillus anthracis*, pure culture on nutrient agar, 24 h, 37 °C. Magnification x 0.4

▲ Fig. 60: *Bacillus cereus*, blood smear from a horse, capsule stain of Foth, blue bacilli without capsule. Magnification x 1000
▼ Fig. 62: *Bacillus cereus*, pure culture on nutrient agar, 24 h, 37 °C. Magnification x 0.4

▲ Abb. 59: *Bacillus anthracis*, Milzausstrich von einer Maus, Kapselfärbung nach Foth, rötlich gefärbte Kapsel und blauer Bazillenleib, Abb.-M. 1000 : 1
▼ Abb. 61: *Bacillus anthracis*, Reinkultur auf Nähragar, 24 h, 37 °C, Abb.-M. 1 : 2,5

▲ Abb. 60: *Bacillus cereus*, Blutausstrich vom Pferd, Kapselfärbung nach Foth, blaugefärbte Bazillen ohne Kapsel, Abb.-M. 1000 : 1
▼ Abb. 62: *Bacillus cereus*, Reinkultur auf Nähragar, 24 h, 37 °C, Abb.-M. 1 : 2,5

■ **Animal experiment**
White mice are the animals of choice, and they are infected subcutaneously. This induces a general infection which is fatal within 2 to 4 days. A gelatinous oedema develops at the injection site. Animal inoculation can also be used for the primary isolation of *Bac. anthracis*. If the bacilli and spores are numerous in the test material, then it should be

■ **Tierversuch**
Bevorzugt werden weiße Mäuse benutzt, die sbk. infiziert werden. Es entsteht eine Allgemeininfektion, die innerhalb von 2 bis 4 Tagen zum Tode führt. An der Injektionsstelle bildet sich ein sulziges Ödem. Der Tierversuch kann auch zur Erstisolierung von *Bac. anthracis* benutzt werden. Handelt es sich um ein keimreiches und sporenhaltiges Unter-

von Futtermitteln und Knochenmehl geeignet (10).

heated to 80 °C for 10 to 30 minutes. Guinea pigs may be used for the detection of anthrax bacilli in raw materials in which they are present.

■ Resistance and sensitivity to disinfectants

The vegetative forms have little resistance to chemical and physical agents. In culture the bacilli are killed within 10 to 15 minutes when heated to 55–58 °C. In a cadaver putrefying anaerobically, they will die in 2–3 days.

Unlike the vegetative forms, the spores of the anthrax bacillus are very resistant towards external influences, but not to the degree that one encounters in spores of some clostridia. They will survive in the open for several decades during which time they presumably turn occasionally into the vegetative form only to revert to spores again. It is therefore difficult to determine the maximum survival time. They are not killed by drying or by drying and salting skins or by pickling meat. The physical methods for killing anthrax spores include: boiling in water to which 0.5 % soda has been added, incineration, applying dry heat of between 120 and 140 °C for one to two hours.

Chemical disinfection is difficult. Exposure for 2

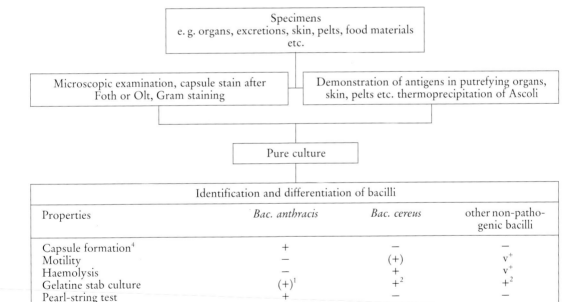

Properties	Bac. anthracis	Bac. cereus	other non-pathogenic bacilli
Capsule formation[4]	+	–	–
Motility	–	(+)	v[+]
Haemolysis	–	+	v[+]
Gelatine stab culture	(+)[1]	+[2]	+[2]
Pearl-string test	+	–	–
Yolk reaction	+	+	–
Animal inoculation	+	(+)[3]	–
Ascoli reaction	+	–	–

[1] Bottle-brush growth and gradual crater-like liquefaction;
[2] Rapid liquefaction;
[3] Septicaemia after large dose;
[4] Only present in organ smears

Fig. 63: Test procedure for the detection of Bac. anthracis and its differentiation from Bac. cereus and other bacilli

hours to a 5% solution of formaldehyde is not certain to effect disinfection. Glutaraldehyde (2% for 2 hours) and hydrogen peroxide (3% for 1 hour) are effective. Particularly efficient is peracetic acid, a 0.6% solution will kill the spores within 60 minutes (3, 7). LENSING & OEI (14) report the following substances as being effective: sodium dichlor-isocyanourate dehydrate (2400 ppm active chlorine per 30 minutes), glutaraldehyde (2% for 2 hours). The disparities in the literature reports are due to the differences in the test methods used.

1.2 Bacillus cereus
(Syn.: *Bac. pseudoanthracis*)

■ Incidence and veterinary significance
Bac. cereus is generally considered non-pathogenic, yet severe illnesses have been reported in man, with pulmonary oedema, haemorrhagic pleurisy, spleen and liver enlargement and meningitis. Similarly it can cause severe, even fatal general infections in animals.

Bac. cereus also causes food poisoning (9). A bacterial phospholipase (lecithinase) develops in the food materials which hydrolyses lecithin and this in turn gives rise to enteric phosphocholin causing the food poisoning. A similar form of food poisoning can occur in cats and dogs and can be induced experimentally in these animals (2, 17). *Bac. cereus* has also been identified as one cause of bovine mastitis, and the bacillus can spread from the udder to cause a severe generalized condition (4, 6, 8).

■ Morphology
This bacillus, measuring 3 to 5 μm is very similar to *Bac. anthracis* and it forms short and long chains, but the organism is non-motile and it does not have a capsule (fig. 60).

■ Culture
Bac. cereus grows on all the usual media. The appearance of the colonies varies considerably from strain to strain. They can either be large, flat and compact (fig. 62) or they may be rough with numerous outgrowth. Haemolysis develops on blood agar (fig. 65). A selective medium, such as that of MOSSEL; Merck, may be used to isolate *Bac. cereus* from food materials. These include polymyxin to suppress contaminants and egg yolk as an indicator of *Bac. cereus* because a white precipitate is formed

Verbrennen, trockene Hitze von 120 bis 140 °C/120 bis 60 min, gesättigter Wasserdampf von 100 °C/ 15 min, gespannter Wasserdampf/5 min.

Die chemische Desinfektion ist schwierig. Eine 5%ige Formaldehydlösung bewirkt innerhalb von 2 h keine sichere Desinfektion. Wirksam sind Glutaraldehyd (2%/2 h), Wasserstoffperoxid (3%/1 h). Besonders gut wirksam ist Peressigsäure, die als 0,6%ige Lösung Sporen innerhalb von 60 min abtötet (3, 7). LENSING & OEI (24) geben folgende Substanzen als wirksam an: Natriumdichlorisocyanurat-dihydrat (2400 ppm aktives Chlor/30 min), Peressigsäure (0,25%/30 min), Formaldehyd (4%/ 2 h), Glutaraldehyd (2%/2 h). Die unterschiedlichen Literaturangaben ergeben sich aus unterschiedlichen Prüfungsmethoden.

1.2 Bacillus cereus
(Syn.: *Bac. pseudoanthracis*)

■ Vorkommen und medizinische Bedeutung
Bac. cereus gilt vorwiegend als apathogen, es sind jedoch beim Menschen schwere Erkrankungen mit Lungenödem, hämorrhagischer Pleuritis, Milztumor, Leberschwellung und Meningitis beschrieben worden. In ähnlicher Weise kann es zu schweren, teilweise tödlich verlaufenden Allgemeininfektionen bei Tieren kommen.

Ferner verursacht *Bac. cereus* Lebensmittelvergiftungen (9). Dabei entsteht in den Lebensmitteln eine bakterielle Phospholipase C (Lecithinase), die Lecithin hydrolysiert, aus dem dann enteral Phosphocholin entsteht, das zu Lebensmittelvergiftungen führt. Eine ähnliche Futtermittelvergiftung kann bei Katzen und Hunden auftreten oder läßt sich bei diesen Tieren experimentell auslösen (2, 17). Außerdem wurde *Bac. cereus* als Mastitiserreger beim Rind festgestellt, dabei kann der Bazillus vom Euter ausgehend zu schwerer Allgemeinerkrankung führen (4, 6, 8).

■ Morphologie
Das etwa 3–5 μm große Stäbchen ähnelt sehr *Bac. anthracis* und bildet kurze oder längere Fäden, jedoch im Organismus keine Kapseln und ist beweglich (Abb. 60).

■ Kultur
Bac. cereus wächst auf allen üblichen Nährböden. Das Aussehen der Kolonien variiert bei den einzelnen Stämmen sehr. Es kann sich um große, flache, kompakte Kolonien (Abb. 62) oder um rauhe Kolonien mit zahlreichen Ausläufern handeln. Auf Blutagar tritt eine Hämolyse auf (Abb. 65). Für die Isolierung von *Bac. cereus* aus Lebensmitteln kann ein Selektivnährboden benutzt werden (z. B. nach MOSSEL; Merck), der zur Unterdrückung der Begleitflora Polymyxin enthält und zur Erkennung

around the colonies by the action of lecithinase. They also contain mannitol, because *Bac. cereus* is mannitol-negative and therefore the contaminant colonies are yellow (the colour indicator is phenol red).

■ **Biochemical properties**
See figure 63.

■ **Animal experiments**
This bacillus is usually non-pathogenic, but a fatal septicaemia can be induced in mice with large doses.

1.3 Bacillus larvae

■ **Incidence and veterinary significance**
Bac. larvae causes foul brood of bees. The infected bee larvae and pupae are transformed into a tangled mass in which the bacilli are present.

■ **Morphology**
It is a rod, measuring $0.5-0.6 \times 1.5-6\,\mu m$, which has peritrichous flagella. The coccoid spores are situated either centrally or terminally dilating the body of the cell.

■ **Culture**
Bac. larvae does not grow on the ordinary media, but requires thiamine and various amino acids. Blood agar (with or without the addition of glucose) or casein peptone-yeast extract glucose agar (19) have been found useful.

1.4 Bacillus alvei

Is responsible for the so-called European foul brood.

1.5 Group of Gram-positive, non-pathogenic, aerobic, spore-forming bacilli
(Mesentericus-subtilis group)

■ **Incidence and significance**
Besides the named types, the genus *Bacillus* contains more than 40 other species which are non-pathogenic, occur ubiquitously in the soil, in dust, the air and are found as contaminants during bacteriological examinations. It may be necessary to differentiate them from *Bac. anthracis* (fig. 63).
The most important species are:
▷ *Bac. subtilis* (*Bac. mesentericus*) see figures 66 and 67.
▷ *Bac. pumilus*

von *Bac. cereus* Eigelb (weißes Präzipitat um Kolonie durch Lecithinasewirkung) sowie Mannit. *Bac. cereus* ist mannitnegativ, somit färbt sich die mannitpositive Begleitflora gelb (Farbindikator Phenolrot).

■ **Kulturell-biochemische Eigenschaften**
Siehe Abb. 63.

■ **Tierversuch**
Meistens apathogen, mit hohen Infektionsdosen kann es bei Mäusen zu einer tödlichen Septikämie kommen.

1.3 Bacillus larvae

■ **Vorkommen und medizinische Bedeutung**
Bac. larvae ist Ursache der bösartigen Faulbrut der Bienen. Er kommt in der fadenziehenden Masse vor, in die Larven und Puppen der Bienen unter der Erregereinwirkung verwandelt werden.

■ **Morphologie**
Es handelt sich um $0{,}5-0{,}6 \times 1{,}5 \times 6\,\mu m$ große, peritrich begeißelte Stäbchen. Die ovoiden Sporen liegen zentral oder subterminal und treiben den Bazillenleib auf.

■ **Kultur**
Bac. larvae wächst nicht auf einfachen Nährböden, sondern verlangt Thiamin und verschiedene Aminosäuren. Bewährt hat sich Blutagar mit oder ohne Glucosezusatz oder Caseinpepton-Hefeextrakt-Glucose-Agar (18).

1.4 Bacillus alvei

Ursache der sog. europäischen Faulbrut, die die Larven vor und nach der Verdeckelung befällt und tötet.

1.5 Gruppe der grampositiven, apathogenen, aeroben Sporenbildner
(Mesentericus-Subtilis-Gruppe)

■ **Vorkommen und Bedeutung**
Neben den genannten Arten enthält die Gattung *Bacillus* noch über 40 andere Arten, die apathogen sind, ubiquitär im Erdboden, Staub und Luft vorkommen und oft als Kontaminanten bei bakteriologischen Untersuchungen auftreten. Ihre differential-diagnostische Abtrennung von *Bac. anthracis* kann erforderlich sein (Abb. 63).
Die wichtigsten Arten sind:
▷ *Bac. subtilis* (*Bac. mesentericus*) (Abb. 66 u. 67),
▷ *Bac. pumilus*,

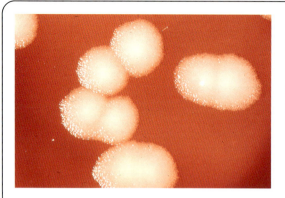
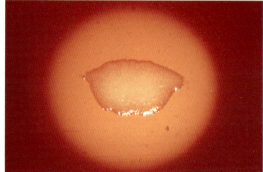
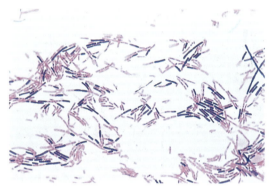
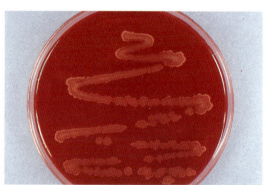

▲ Fig. 64: *Bacillus anthracis*, pure culture on blood agar, no haemolysis, 24 h, 37 °C. Magnification x 2
▼ Fig. 66: *Bacillus subtilis*, culture smear, Gram stain, Gram-variable reaction. Magnification x 1000

▲ Abb. 64: *Bacillus anthracis*, Reinkultur auf Blutagar, keine Hämolyse, 24 h, 37 °C, Abb.-M. 2 : 1
▼ Abb. 66: *Bacillus subtilis*, Kulturausstrich, Gram-Färbung, gramlabiles Verhalten, Abb.-M. 1000 : 1

▲ Fig. 65: *Bacillus cereus*, pure culture on blood agar, distinct, strong haemolysis, 24 h, 37 °C. Magnification x 2
▼ Fig. 67: *Bacillus subtilis*, pure culture on blood agar, 48 h, 37 °C. Magnification x 0.33

▲ Abb. 65: *Bacillus cereus*, Reinkultur auf Blutagar, deutliche und kräftige Hämolyse, 24 h, 37 °C, Abb.-M. 2 : 1
▼ Abb. 67: *Bacillus subtilis*, Reinkultur auf Blutagar, 48 h, 37 °C, Abb.-M. 1 : 3

▷ *Bac. megaterium*
▷ *Bac. stearothermophilus*.

▷ *Bac. megaterium,*
▷ *Bac. stearothermophilus*.

■ **Bacteriological properties**
These rods measure 0.2–2.2 × 1.2–7.0 µm, all of which form endospores. The spores are cylindrical, ellipsoidal or spherical and their position in the cell may be central, terminal or subterminal. In some species the cells swell up during spore formation. The bacilli are Gram-positive, Gram-variable or

■ **Bakteriologische Eigenschaften**
Es handelt sich um 0,2–2,2 × 1,2–7,0 µm große Stäbchen, die alle Endosporen bilden. Die Sporen sind zylindrisch, ellipsoid oder sphärisch und liegen in der Zelle zentral, subterminal oder terminal. Bei einigen Arten schwillt die Zelle durch die Sporenbildung an. Die Bazillen verhalten sich grampositiv,

even Gram-negative. Usually they are motile. The optimal temperature for growth varies not only from species to species but even from one strain to another. Usually it lies between 30 °C and 37 °C, in thermophilic species e. g. *Bac. stearothermophilus*, however, it is 55 °C.

gramlabil oder selten gramnegativ, sie sind meistens beweglich. Die optimale Vermehrungstemperatur schwankt von Art zu Art, aber auch innerhalb einer Art von Stamm zu Stamm, sie beträgt meistens 30–37 °C, bei den thermophilen (z. B. *Bac. stearothermophilus*) 55 °C.

Bibliography / Literatur

1. Ascoli, A. (1911): Die Präzipitation bei Milzbrand. Zbl. Bakt. I. Orig. **58**, 63–70.
2. Chastain, C. B., & D. L. Harris (1974): Association of Bacillus cereus with food poisoning in dogs. J. Am. Vet. Med. Ass. **164**, 489–490.
3. Dietz, P., & R. Böhm (1980): Ergebnisse der experimentellen Desinfektionsmittelprüfung an Milzbrandsporen. Hyg. u. Med. **5**, 103–107.
4. Gedek, W. (1986): Bacillus-cereus-Mastitiden beim Rind als Folge einer Arzneimittelkontamination. Tierärztl. Umschau **41**, 526–530.
5. Gibson, T., & R. E. Gordon (1974): Bacillus. In: Bergey's manual of determinative bacteriology, 8. Aufl., S. 529–550. Baltimore: Williams & Wilkins.
6. Gloos, H. (1968): Die Cereus-Mastitis des Rindes. Schweiz. Arch. Tierhk. **110**, 63–80.
7. Hussaini, S. N., & K. R. Ruby (1976): Sporicidal activity of peracetic acid against B. anthracis spores. Vet. Rec. **98**, 257–259.
8. Jones, T. D., & P. C. B. Turnbull (1981): Bovine mastitis caused by Bacillus cereus. Vet. Rec. **108**, 272–274.
9. Katsaras, K., & G. Hildebrandt (1979): Ursachen bakterieller Lebensmittelvergiftungen: Bacillus-cereus-Toxine. Fleischwirtsch. **59**, 668–676.
10. Illner, F. (1980): Milzbrand. In: J. Beer (Hrsg.): Infektionkrankheiten der Haustiere. 2. Aufl., S. 571–580. Jena: VEB Gustav Fischer.
11. Kauker, E. (1965): Globale Verbreitung des Milzbrandes um 1960. Sitzungsberichte der Heidelberger Akademie der Wissenschaften. Heidelberg: Springer.
12. Kauker, E., & K. Zettl (1963): Milzbrand in der Welt (1955–1961). Berliner Münchener tierärztl. Wschr. **76**, 172–174, 194–197.
13. Krieg, A. (1970): Über die Differenzierung aerober Sporenbildner unter besonderer Berücksichtigung von Bacillus anthracis und Bac. thuringiensis. Zbl. Bakt. I. Orig. **213**, 63–68.
14. Lensing, H. H., & H. L. Oei (1984): Untersuchungen über die Wirksamkeit von Desinfektionsmitteln gegen Milzbrandsporen. Tijdschr. Diergeneeskd. **109**, 557–563.
15. Mayer, H., K. Ehrhardt & D. Lorenz (1975): Über das Vorkommen sporadischer Milzbrandfälle bei Schweinen in Nordwürttemberg. Tierärztl. Umschau **30**, 543–549.
16. Mathois, H. (1962): Zur Anwendung der Agardoppeldiffusion in der Milzbranddiagnostik. Mh. Tierhk. **14**, 407–412.
17. Nikodemusz, I. (1967): Die enteropathogene Wirkung von Bacillus cereus bei Hunden. Zbl. Bakt. I. Orig. A, **202**, 533–538.
18. Seidel, G. (1965): Die aeroben Sporenbildner unter besonderer Berücksichtigung des Milzbrandbazillus. »Beiträge zur Hygiene und Epidemiologie«, Heft 17. Leipzig: Joh. Ambrosius Barth.
19. Stehle, G., & S. Braun (1981): Gesetzliche Bekämpfung der Bienenseuchen. Berlin, Hamburg: Paul Parey.
20. Wagener, K., & W. Bisping (1971): Milzbrand. In: Das öffentliche Gesundheitswesen. Bd. 2, Teil A, S. 478–488. Stuttgart: Georg Thieme.

2 Genus: Clostridium (Cl.)

This genus includes Gram-positive, and in older cultures also Gram-variable or Gram-negative rods which are motile by virtue of their peritrichous flagella. They form round to oval spores which distend the vegetative form in most species. Growth is strictly anaerobic.

Clostridia are found in the soil, in beds of rivers and other bodies of water and in the intestinal tract of man and animals. More than 300 species have been described, some of which have not been finally classified, however, and some are of no veterinary importance. The pathogens cause gas gangrene, enterotoxaemia or intoxications such as tetanus and botulism.

2 Gattung: Clostridium (Cl.)

Die Gattung umfaßt grampositive, in älteren Kulturen auch gramlabile bis -negative, meistens aufgrund einer peritrichen Begeißelung bewegliche Stäbchen. Sie bilden runde bis ovale Sporen, die die vegetative Form bei den meisten Arten auftreiben. Das Wachstum ist streng anaerob.

Clostridien kommen regelmäßig im Erdboden, in den Bodenschichten der Gewässer und im Darmkanal von Mensch und Tier vor. Es sind mehr als 300 Arten beschrieben worden, die aber teilweise nicht endgültig bestimmt sind oder für die Veterinärmedizin keine Bedeutung besitzen. Als Krankheitserreger verursachen sie entsprechend den im Vordergrund stehenden Symptomen in erster Linie Gasödeme, Enterotoxämien oder Intoxikationserkrankungen, wie z. B. Tetanus und Botulismus.

Specimens
Muscles, organs, wound swabs, soil, dust etc.

Microscopic examination: large, plump rods, spores not always present

Aerobic culture: for assessment of contaminants

Anaerobic culture
1. Preparation of the test sample, necessary in heavy contamination: heating to 80 °C for 15 to 30 mins. or placing into methylated spirits; within 24 hours, marked reduction in aerobic contaminants (28)
2. Nutrient media
   solid media: Zeissler agar, selective media,
   fluid media: liver broth, thioglycollate broth, with 5 % glucose, cooked meat broth
3. Anaerobic culture procedure
   fluid media: addition of subtances to lower redox potential (e. g. sodium thioglycollate, cystein HCl, organ parts like pieces of liver, pulped brain etc.)
   Addition of small amounts of agar (0.1 %), which retards the uptake of oxygen,
   boiling media for 15–20 min.
   before inoculation overlay tubes with liquid paraffin,
   solid media: deep agar
   Fortner method.
   Evacuate culture vessels, if necessary repeat after filling with inert gases,
   anaerobic method with catalytic oxidation of H_2 to H_2O (commercial anaerobic jars with gas generator, catalyst and anaerobic indicator see page 267)

Identification of clostridia in pure culture

1. Biochemical properties

	Haemolysis	Spore position[2]	Cell swelling[1]	Proteolysis	Gelatinolysis	Nitrate	Indole	Glucose	Lactose	Saccharose	Salicin	H_2S	Lecithinase
Cl. chauvoei	+	s	–	–	+	+	–	+	+	+	–	+	–
Cl. septicum	+	s	+	–	+	+	–	+	+	–	–	v	–
Cl. perfringens	+	cst	–	–	+	+	–	+	+	+	–	v	+
Cl. novyi (A, B)	+	cs	+	–	+	+	v	+	–	–	–	+	+
Cl. sordellii	+	cs	–	+	+	v	+	+	–	–	+	+	+
Cl. bifermentans	+	cst	+	+	+	–	+	+	–	–	v	+	+
Cl. sporogenes	+	s	+	+	+	+	–	+	–	–	–	+	–
Cl. histolyticum	+	st	–	+	+	+	–	–	–	–	–	+	–

[1] swelling caused by spore within cell body; [2] c = central, t = terminal, s = subterminal position of spore

2. Evaluation of colony form on Zeissler plate or other medium, result unreliable because atypical forms are common (Tab. 14)

3. Motility test, all clostridia except Cl. perfringens are motile, but on exposure to oxygen they can rapidly lose their motility

4. Toxin neutralization in laboratory animals. Detection of toxins for identification of Cl. perfringens types see figure 81

5. Pathogenicity test in laboratory animals, inject 1 ml liver broth under the skin of abdomen of guinea pig, induces gas oedema
   pathological assessment:
   Cl. chauvoei: haemorrhagic gas oedema,
   Cl. septicum: sero-haemorrhagic gas oedema,
   Cl. perfringens: large vesicle with gas and fluid,
   Cl. novyi: gelatinous gas oedema

6. Differentiation on the basis of fatty acid formation with the aid of gas chromatography see table 16

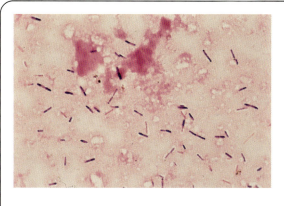 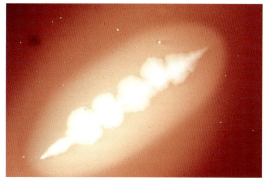

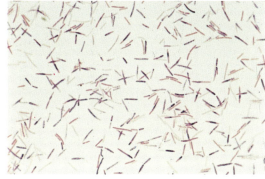 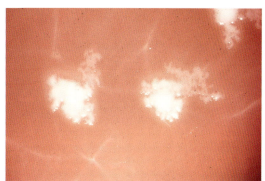

▲ Fig. 69: *Clostridium chauvoei*, impression smear from the liver of an experimentally infected guinea pig, rods lying singly, Gram stain. Magnification x 1000
▼ Fig. 71: *Clostridium novyi*, culture smear, Gram stain, Gram-positive to Gram-variable rods, 2–8 µm in length. Magnification x 1000

▲ Abb. 69: *Clostridium chauvoei*, Abklatschpräparat von der Leber eines experimentell infizierten Meerschweinchens, einzeln liegende Stäbchen, Gram-Färbung, Abb.-M. 1000 : 1
▼ Abb. 71: *Clostridium novyi*, Kulturausstrich, Gram-Färbung, grampositive bis gramlabile, lange (2–8 µm) Stäbchen, Abb.-M. 1000 : 1

▲ Fig. 70: *Clostridium chauvoei*, pure culture on Zeissler plate, incubated in the "Gaspak" system, the pearl-string or grey vine-leaf-like confluent colonies are surrounded by a zone of haemolysis, 48 h, 37 °C. Magnification x 2
▼ Fig. 72: *Clostridium novyi*, pure culture on Zeissler plate, greyish-white colonies with thick curl-like processes, 48 h, 37 °C. Magnification x 2

▲ Abb. 70: *Clostridium chauvoei*, Reinkultur auf Zeißler-Platte, gezüchtet im Gaspak-System, perlmutterartige bis graue, weinblattförmige, geschlossene Kolonien, die von einer Hämolysezone umgeben sind, 48 h, 37 °C, Abb.-M. 2 : 1
▼ Abb. 72: *Clostridium novyi*, Reinkultur auf einer Zeißler-Platte, grauweiße Kolonien mit dicken, lockenförmigen Ausläufern, 48 h, 37 °C, Abb.-M. 2 : 1

◀ Fig. 68: Detection and identification of clostridia as causes of malignant oedema

◀ Abb. 68: Nachweis und Bestimmung von Clostridien als Gasödemerreger

2.1 Clostridia as cause of blackleg and wound clostridiosis
(gas oedema, gas gangrene, malignant oedema)

2.1.1 Clostridium chauvoei
(Syn.: *Cl. feseri*, *Cl. sarcoemphysematos*)

The cause of blackleg of cattle and sheep. In Germany blackleg has a distinct geographical distribution. In cattle it occurs especially along the North Sea coast and in the south in the mountain regions (high and middle range). But central Germany is the main distribution area for blackleg of sheep. The bovine disease is due to oral infection (meadow, food materials etc.), while sheep contract blackleg mainly through wound infection.

2.1.2 Clostridia as causes of wound infections

Dirty wounds are often infected by a variety of bacteria. Beside an aerobic flora there are often several different species of clostridia. The clinical signs differentiate between severe and usually fatal generalized infections and localized wound infections. The following clostridia invariably cause wound infections; they are listed roughly in descending order of frequency and pathogenicity:
▷ *Cl. septicum*, the cause of false blackleg of man and animals including poultry (33).
▷ *Cl. novyi* Type A, cause of malignant oedema of man and animals.
▷ *Cl. histolyticum*, this organism occurs to a moderate extent in the soil and is thus relatively rare in malignant oedema of man and animals.
▷ *Cl. perfringens* is the most important cause of human gas gangrene, but such diseases are rare in animals. Its importance in enterotoxaemias is discussed on page 89.
▷ *Cl. sporogenes*, can be found in benign gas oedema infections, usually together with other clostridia and a flora of aerobes.
▷ *Cl. sordellii* can be of similar significance in wound infections as *Cl. sporogenes*. Both biochemically and in its cultural properties it closely resembles *Cl. bifermentatis* but, since the latter is non-pathogenic, it is important to differentiate between the two (17).

■ **Morphology** (figs. 69, 71, 73, 74 and 77)
These are large rods, about 3–8 μm in length, sometimes even larger. They are motile with the excep-

Table 14: The cultural behaviour of clostridia on the Zeissler plate and the clinical picture in experimentally infected guinea pigs

Tabelle 14: Das kulturelle Verhalten von Clostridien auf der Zeißler-Platte und das Krankheitsbild bei der experimentellen Infektion des Meerschweinchens

Clostridium	Growth form	Appearance of colony	Clinical signs in experimentally infected guinea pigs
chauvoei	IV	round to vine-leaf or pearl-string shaped colonies, slight haemolysis (fig. 20)	haemorrhagic oedema
septicum	III	veil-like diffuse growth, delicate simple projections (simple arabescs), slight haemolysis (figs. 75, 76)	sero-haemorrhagic oedema
novyi A, B	II	interwoven, curl-like coils, which weave in and out of the colony, parallel protrusions (double arabescs), weak haemolysis (fig. 72)	gelatinous oedema without gas formation
histolyticum	VIII	very small, round colonies, sunk into the medium, colourless to grey, slight haemolysis	tissue lysis
perfringens	I	round, raised, ochre-coloured, opaque colonies, greenish in oxygen, disc-shaped haemolysis	gas oedema, large bubbles, toxin detection (fig. 81)
sporogenes	VI	small, hard, wart-like colony with circular, intensive haemolysis	slight oedema
sordellii	II	round to irregular, grey colonies, 1–2 mm diameter	haemorrhagic oedema, proteolysis
bifermentans	II	discrete or diffuse colonies of variable haemolysis	non-pathogenic, large doses cause transient oedema
tetani	III/IV	diffuse growth with delicate proceses (form III) or round confluent colonies, slight haemolysis	tetanus
botulinum	II	flat, slightly arched, smooth or floccular, rough colonies, distinct haemolysis (fig. 80)	botulism

tion of *Cl. perfringens*, but in cultures this motility may be lost within 6–24 hours upon exposure to oxygen or if the flagella are lost (62).

■ **Spore formation**

The capacity for spore formation can vary from species to species, but also between strains. Spores are best demonstrated with special spore stains (e. g. Rackette, fig. 79); the spores are not stained by the ordinary methods used for bacteria. Sporulation media are discussed on page 93.

■ **Culture**

The test routine is given in figure 68. When the culture is to be made from material to which oxygen can easily gain access (such as a swab), one should invariably make use of a transport medium (e. g. Stuart's) to avoid damaging the clostridia in transit.
▷ Selective media: Clostridia may have to be isolated from heavily contaminated material and in such cases media can be used that incorporate selective agents such as neomycin, kanamycin, polymyxin, oleandomycin, sodium azide, crystal violet or sulphadiazine. Such media are commercially available in various formulation as ready-poured plates. However, since the resistance of the different clostridia to additives varies, the actual harvest of clostridia may be less on these than on media without inhibitors (16, 20, 40, 50, 59).

Cl. perfringens beweglich. Die Beweglichkeit kann jedoch in Kulturen nach Zutritt von Sauerstoff oder nach Geißelabstoßung innerhalb von 6–24 h (62) verlorengehen.

■ **Sporenbildung**

Das Ausmaß der Sporenbildung kann von Art zu Art, aber auch von Stamm zu Stamm sehr variieren. Ihr Nachweis geschieht am besten durch Sporenfärbungen (z. B. nach Rakette, s. Abb. 79), bei den üblichen Bakterienfärbungen bleibt die Spore ungefärbt. Sporulationsmedien s. S. 93.

■ **Kulturelle Isolierung**

Der Untersuchungsgang ist in der Abb. 68 dargestellt. Handelt es sich um Untersuchungsmaterialien, in die leicht Sauerstoff eintreten kann (z. B. Tupfer), sollte grundsätzlich ein Transportmedium (z. B. nach Stuart) benutzt werden, um eine Schädigung der Clostridien beim Transport zu vermeiden.
▷ Selektivmedien: Müssen die Clostridien aus einem stark kontaminierten Material angezüchtet werden, können Medien mit selektiven Zusätzen, wie z. B. Neomycin, Kanamycin, Polymyxin, Oleandomycin, Natriumacid, Kristallviolett, Sulfadiazin benutzt werden. Solche Nährmedien werden in unterschiedlicher Zusammensetzung als Fertignährböden im Handel angeboten. Da die einzelnen Clostridienarten aber eine unterschiedliche Resistenz gegenüber den Zusätzen aufweisen können, kann

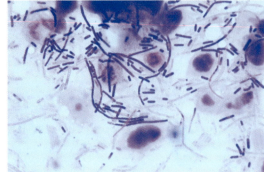
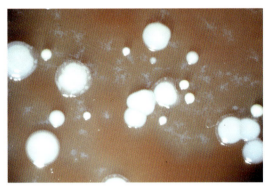
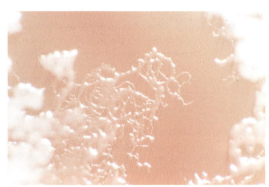

▲ Fig. 73: *Clostridium septicum*, smear from the muscle of an ox with false blackleg, Gram stain, Gram-positive rods beginning to form spores. Magnification y 1000
▼ Fig. 75: *Clostridium septicum*, direct culture from the muscle of an ox with false blackleg, mixed culture on a Zeissler plate, besides *E. coli* and other contaminants (large white colonies) the *Cl. septicum* is in the form of a delicate lawn-like colonies with weak haemolysis, 48 h, 37 °C. Magnification x 2

▲ Fig. 74: *Clostridium septicum*, impression smear from the liver of an experimentally infected guinea pig, Gram stain, Gram-positive and Gram-variable rods lying in long filaments. Magnification x 1000
▼ Fig. 76: *Clostridium septicum*, pure culture on a Zeissler plate, lawn-like growth with delicate processes, 48 h, 37 °C. Magnification x 7

▲ Abb. 73: *Clostridium septicum*, Ausstrich aus der Muskulatur eines Rindes mit Pararauschbrand, Gram-Färbung, grampositive Stäbchen mit beginnender Sporenbildung, Abb.-M. 1000 : 1
▼ Abb. 75: *Clostridium septicum*, Direktkultur aus der Muskulatur eines Rindes mit Pararauschbrand, Mischkultur auf Zeißler-Platte, neben *E. coli* und anderen Kontaminanten (große weiße Kolonien) *Cl. septicum* in Form eines zarten rasenförmigen Wachstums mit einer schwachen Hämolyse, 48 h, 37 °C, Abb.-M. 2 : 1

▲ Abb. 74: *Clostridium septicum*, Abklatschpräparat von der Leber eine experimentell infizierten Meerschweinchens, Gram-Färbung, grampositive und gramlabile, in Fäden liegende Stäbchen, Abb.-M. 1000 : 1
▼ Abb. 76: *Clostridium septicum*, Reinkultur auf Zeißler-Platte, rasenförmiges Wachstum mit zarten Ausläufern, 48 h, 37 °C, Abb.-M. 7 : 1

The migration of motile clostridia on solid media can be very undesirable and may be reduced by pre-drying the plates in the incubator.

■ **Identification on the basis of morphological and cultural properties**
If the clostridia are present in pure culture, then they can be identified by their characteristics as

die Ausbeute an Clostridien geringer als auf den hemmstofffreien Medien sein (16, 20, 40, 50, 59).
Das Ausschwärmen der beweglichen Clostridien aus festen Nährböden kann sehr störend sein, dies kann durch eine Vortrocknung der Platten im Wärmeschrank verringert werden.

■ **Identifizierung nach morphologischen und kulturellen Eigenschaften**
Liegen die isolierten Clostridien in Reinkultur vor, kann ihre Bestimmung nach den Eigenschaften er-

Table 15: Differentiation between *Cl. chauvoei* and *Cl. septicum* (44)

Property	Cl. chauvoei	Cl. septicum
Form of colony on Zeissler agar	confluent colonies (fig. 70)	diffuse growth (fig. 75 and 76)
Lethal toxins 1	+	+
2	−	+
Toxin neutralization with		
Cl. chauvoei antiserum	+	−
Cl. septicum antiserum	+	+
Immunofluorescence with		
Cl. chauvoei antiserum	+	−
Cl. septicum antiserum	−	+
Liver impression smear from experimentally infected guinea pigs	rods lying singly (fig. 69)	long filaments (fig. 74)
Saccharose fermentation	v^+	v^-
Salicin fermentation	v^-	v^+

shown in figure 68. The appearance of the colonies on the Zeissler plate can vary according to the medium, its moistness, the agar content, the type of blood and the strain of clostridium. The typical colony forms, as described by ZEISSLER et al. (74) are summarized in table 14. An indication as to the species can be obtained not only from the classical colony forms on the Zeissler plate but also from the appearance of colonies grown on the semi-solid glucose-cysteine agar (HEICKEN & BELLINGER, 31).

■ **Biochemical properties**

The biochemical properties of some clostridia are summarized in figure 68. A characteristic feature of clostridia is the strong tendency towards gas formation, which results from the fermentation of carbohydrates and proteolysis (in particular H_2S). A comprehensive review of the spectrum of activity can be found in SMITH & HOBBS (66). A further adjunct to the identification procedure is the analysis by gas chromatography of lower fatty acids (tab. 16), that are produced by some species (22, 72).

Certain methods have been described for a differentiation between *Cl. chauvoei* and *Cl. septicum*; some of these are listed in table 15, others are described below.

▷ Haemolysis test: 3 ml of a 2 % suspension of bovine or sheep blood are mixed with 0.15 ml of a 24 hour liver broth culture. This is either incubated or held at room temperature and with most strains of *Cl. chauvoei* haemolysis takes place in 10 to 30, at the most 60 minutes. Strains of *Cl. septicum* on the

Table 16: Differentiation of the medically important clostridia, on the basis of fatty acid production (71, 72)

A) Formation of acetic acid:
    Cl. histolyticum
B) Formation of acetic and butyric acid:
    Cl. septicum
    Cl. chauvoei
    Cl. botulinum
      (non-proteolytic strains of types B, E and F)
C) Formation of acetic, propionic and butyric acid:
    Cl. perfringens A–C)
    Cl. botulinum (C, D and E)
    Cl. novyi
    Cl. tetani
D) Formation of acetic, propionic, isobutyric, butyric, isovaleric and isocapronic acid:
    Cl. botulinum (proteolytic strains of types A, B and F)
    Cl. sporogenes

other hand, produce no haemolysis, even after 2 to 3 hours (28).

▷ Hydrolysis of aesculin (p. 31): This reaction is negative in *Cl. chauvoei* but positive in *Cl. septicum*.

■ Immunofluorescence

Cl. chauvoei and *Cl. septicum* can be readily differentiated with fluorescent antibodies, and cross reactions are said not to occur (49).

■ Antigenic structure

In clostridia we can identify both O- and H-antigens by means of agglutination, complement fixation and precipitation tests (62). However, they are of no practical consequence in the identification of the organism causing gas oedema.

■ Toxins

Toxins are produced by the various clostridia responsible for malignant oedema. Each species forms several toxins which may exert a lethal action in mice, a necrotizing effect in guinea pigs upon intradermal injection or cause haemolysis on blood agar. The demonstration of the lethal factors by means of the neutralization test in mice or guinea pigs can be employed as a means of distinguishing

Table 17: Neutralization of the toxins of the most important causal agents of gas oedema

			Antitoxic serum		
Toxins	*Cl. chauvoei*	*Cl. septicum*	*Cl. novyi* A	*Cl. novyi* B	*Cl. sordellii*
Cl. chauvoei	+	+	–	–	–
Cl. septicum	–	+	–	–	–
Cl. novyi A	–	–	+	+	–
Cl. novyi B	–	–	+	+	–
Cl. sordellii	–	–	–	–	+

+: neutralization; –: no neutralization

clostridial species (tab. 17). Types A and B of *Cl. novyi* produce cross reactions because both possess the lethal factor. According to BEER & AL-KHATIB (12), they can be differentiated with the lecitho-vitellin test, because they produce type-specific lecithinases (α and β). The neutralization of the lethal factors of *Cl. perfringens* is presented in figure 81.

These are exotoxins, which are formed in the cell and can either be secreted continuously, or be stored in the cell, so that larger amounts of toxin are liberated when the vegetative cell is lysed or destroyed.

■ Animal experiments

Guinea pigs are particularly susceptible to the organisms responsible for gas oedema. The subcutaneous injection of 1 ml of liver broth culture will usually kill within 24 to 48 hours. But the severity of the clinical gas oedema varies in the different clostridial types (tab. 14).

■ Resistance and sensitivity to disinfectants

There is a fundamental difference in the sensitivity between the spores and the vegetative forms, which are no less sensitive (apart from their susceptibility to oxygen) than other bacteria. The heat resistance of the spores to live steam can vary considerably between and within types and range from a few minutes to several hours. Usually, however, they are killed within 10 minutes (62). Consistent exceptions are the potent exotoxin producers such as *Cl. perfringens, Cl. tetani* and *Cl. botulinum*. But since the strain-linked heat resistance of the spores is generally unknown, one must subject them to saturated steam under pressure at 120 °C in order to be certain that the spores are dead. Higher temperature are thus required than are necessary for anthrax spores.

Chemical disinfection is very problematic. Most of the disinfectants either do not work at all, or they only prevent the spores from germinating. Chemical disinfectants, and this refers particularly to aldehyde based ones (48, 59, 64), would have to be used in such high concentrations that they are out of the question as practical disinfectants. For this reason one must use physical measures (see above) in order to be certain of killing clostridial spores.

Clostridien benutzt werden (Tab. 17). *Cl. novyi* Typ A und B zeigen Überkreuzreaktionen, weil beide den α-Letalfaktor enthalten. Sie können nach BEER & AL-KHATIB (12) durch den Lezithovitellintest unterschieden werden, weil sie typenspezifische Lezithinasen bilden (α u. β). Über die Neutralisation der Letalfaktoren bei *Cl. perfringens* siehe Abb. 81.

Es handelt sich um Ektotoxine, die in der Zelle gebildet werden. Sie werden entweder kontinuierlich nach außen abgegeben oder können auch in der Zelle gespeichert werden, dann werden mit der Auflösung oder Zerstörung der vegetativen Zellen größere Toxinmengen frei.

■ Tierversuch

Das Meerschweinchen ist gegenüber den Gasödemerregern besonders empfänglich. Die sbk. Infektion mit 1 ml Leberbouillonkultur führt meistens innerhalb von 24 bis 48 h zum Tode. Die Ausprägung des Gasödems weist bei den einzelnen Clostridienarten Unterschiede auf (Tab. 14).

■ Tenazität und Desinfektionsmittelempfindlichkeit

Es besteht ein grundsätzlicher Unterschied zwischen der Empfindlichkeit der vegetativen Formen, die sich (abgesehen von der Sauerstoffempfindlichkeit) von anderen Bakterien nicht unterscheidet, und der der Sporen. Die Hitzeresistenz der Sporen gegenüber strömendem Wasserdampf kann zwischen und innerhalb der Arten großen Schwankungen unterliegen und Minuten bis Stunden betragen. Meistens werden sie jedoch innerhalb von 10 min abgetötet (62). Regelmäßige Ausnahmen bilden starke Ektotoxinbildner wie *Cl. perfringens, Cl. tetani* und *Cl. botulinum*. Da jedoch meistens die stammgebundene Hitzeresistenz der Sporen nicht bekannt ist, muß zur sicheren Abtötung gespannter gesättigter Wasserdampf von 120 °C/20 min angewendet werden. Damit sind höhere Erhitzungstemperaturen erforderlich als bei den Milzbrandsporen.

Die chemische Desinfektion ist sehr problematisch, die meisten Desinfektionsmittel wirken nicht oder hemmen nur die Auskeimung der Sporen. Chemische Desinfektionsmittel, diskutiert werden insbesondere solche auf Aldehydbasis (48, 59, 64), müßten in so hohen Konzentrationen und über so lange Zeiten angewendet werden, daß sie für eine praktische Desinfektion nicht in Betracht kommen. Eine sichere Abtötung von Clostridiensporen ist deswegen nur durch physikalische Verfahren (s. o.) zu erreichen.

2.2 Clostridium septicum, cause of braxy
(Nordic Bradsot)

This is a peracute disease of lambs which is characterized by haemorrhagic inflammation and ulceration of the mucosa of the abomasum.

The diagnosis is based on the pathological lesions and the demonstration with the Gram stain of *Cl. septicum* filaments in the mucosa. Toxins are detected in the mouse lethal test and the toxin is specifically neutralized by *Cl. septicum* antiserum. The bacteriological properties of the organism are given on p. 85.

2.3 Clostridium novyi type B, cause of Infectious Necrotic hepatitis
(Black Disease, German Bradsot)

Necrotic hepatitis is a peracute, fatal intoxication of sheep. *Cl. novyi* type B is found in the liver necroses, in which it produces the toxin. This type is distinctly larger than types A, C and D *(Cl. gigas)*. A prerequisite for accurate typing is the identification of the toxins, which is difficult. At least 8 toxin fractions are known (OAKLEY & WARRACK, 54). In practice the diagnosis is based on the demonstration of the causal organism in the necrotic lesions of the liver, in which immunofluorescence can be useful, and in the detection of toxins in the liver lesions by means of the mouse lethal test.

2.4 Clostridium novyi type D (Cl. haemolyticum) cause of bacillary haemoglobinuria

An acute or subacute disease of cattle, less frequently sheep, which is common particularly in America and Australia. It is characterized by haemolysis, haemoglobinuria and jaundice. *Cl. novyi* type D, the causal organism, is typical because it produces large quantities of a haemolysin (β lecithinase).

2.5 Clostridium novyi type C, cause of an osteomyelitis

A disease that has been described mainly in buffalo in East Asia.

2.2 Clostridium septicum als Ursache des Labmagenpararauschbrandes
(Nordische Bradsot)

Es handelt sich um eine perakut verlaufende Erkrankung der Jungschafe, die durch eine hämorrhagische Entzündung der Schleimhaut des Labmagens mit Geschwürbildung gekennzeichnet ist.

Die Diagnose erfolgt unter Berücksichtigung der pathologisch-anatomischen Veränderungen durch den mikroskopischen Erregernachweis in der Schleimhaut in Form von *Cl. septicum*-Fäden (Gramfärbung). Ein Toxinnachweis kann im Mäuseletalitätstest erfolgen, das Toxin ist durch *Cl. septicum*-Antiserum spezifisch neutralisierbar. Bakteriologische Eigenschaften des Erregers s. S. 85.

2.3 Clostridium novyi Typ B als Ursache der nekrotischen Hepatitis
(Deutsche Bradsot)

Es handelt sich um eine perakut und tödlich verlaufende Intoxikation der Schafe. *Cl. novyi* Typ B findet sich in Lebernekroseherden, in denen es das Toxin produziert. Der Typ ist deutlich größer als die Typen A, C und D *(Cl. gigas)*. Die genaue Typbestimmung setzt die schwierige Toxinbestimmung voraus, insgesamt sind mindestens 8 Toxinfraktionen bekannt (OAKLEY & WARRACK, 54). Die praktische Diagnose stützt sich auf den Erregernachweis in den nekrotischen Leberherden, der auch durch die immunfluoreszenzmikroskopische Untersuchung geführt werden kann, sowie auf den Toxinnachweis aus den Leberherden im Mäuseletalitätstest.

2.4 Clostridium novyi Typ D (Cl. haemolyticum) als Erreger der »bazillären Hämoglobinurie«

Es handelt sich um eine akut bis subakut verlaufende Erkrankung des Rindes und seltener des Schafes, die besonders in Amerika und Australien vorkommt. Sie ist insbesondere durch Hämolyse, Hämoglobinurie und Ikterus gekennzeichnet. Der Erreger zeichnet sich durch die hochgradige Bildung eines Hämolysins aus (β-Lezithinase).

2.5 Clostridium novyi Typ C als Erreger einer Osteomyelitis

Die Erkrankung ist zur Hauptsache bei Büffeln in Ostasien beschrieben worden.

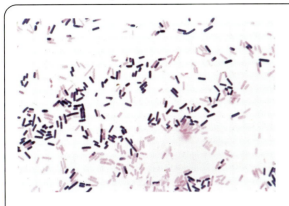
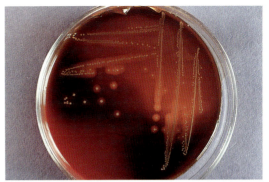
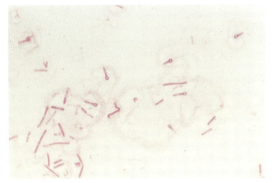
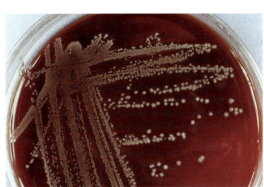

▲ Fig. 77: *Clostridium perfringens*, culture smear, Gram stain, Gram-positive to Gram-variable, plump, briquette-shaped rods. Magnification x 1000
▼ Fig. 79: *Clostridium tetani*, culture smear, spore stain after Rakette, terminal spore formation. Magnification x 1000

▲ Fig. 78: *Clostridium perfringens*, pure culture on a Zeissler plate, typical circular ("target-shaped)", haemolysis, 24 h, 37 °C. Magnification x 0.33
▼ Fig. 80: *Clostridium botulinum*, pure culture on a Zeissler plate, the bacterium has no special nutrient requirements and grows as relatively large, greyish-white floccular colonies, 48 h, 37 °C. Magnification x 0.4

▲ Abb. 77: *Clostridium perfringens*, Kulturausstrich, Gram-Färbung, grampositive bis gramlabile, plumpe, „brikettförmige" Stäbchen, Abb.-M. 1000 : 1
▼ Abb. 79: *Clostridium tetani*, Kulturausstrich, Sporenfärbung nach Rakette, terminale Sporenbildung, Abb.-M. 1000 : 1

▲ Abb. 78: *Clostridium perfringens*, Reinkultur auf Zeißler-Platte, typische kreisförmige („schießscheibenförmige") Hämolyse, 24 h, 37 °C, Abb.-M. 1 : 3
▼ Abb. 80: *Clostridium botulinum*, Reinkultur auf Zeißler-Platte, das Bakterium stellt keine besonderen Nährbodenansprüche und wächst in relativ großen, grauweißen, asbestflockenartigen Kolonien, 48 h, 37 °C, Abb.-M. 1 : 2,5

2.6 Clostridium perfringens cause of enterotoxaemias, food poisoning and some other diseases
(Syn.: *Bac. phlegmenes emphysematosae, Cl. welchii*)

■ Incidence and veterinary significance
On the basis of their toxin production types A to E have been identified within this species, and they

2.6 Clostridium perfringens als Ursache von Enterotoxämien, Lebensmittelvergiftungen und einigen anderen Erkrankungen
(Syn.: *Bac. phlegmones emphysematosae, Cl. welchii*)

■ Vorkommen und medizinische Bedeutung
Aufgrund der Bildung verschiedener Toxine werden innerhalb dieser Spezies die Typen A bis E

Table 18: Summary of the most important clinical conditions caused by Cl. perfringens

Tabelle 18: Übersicht zu den wichtigsten durch *Clostridium perfringens* verursachten Krankheitsbildern

Type	Clinical picture
A	Gas oedema in man and, rarely, in animals (mainly in dogs and horses) Food poisoning in man and animals Enterotoxaemia in animals (rare) Necrotizing mastitis in ewes and cows (46, 47, 57, 65) Enteritis in the dog (19) Necrotizing enteritis in fowls
B (*Bac. agni*)	Lamb dysentery (suckling lambs up to 2 weeks) (52) Enterotoxaemia of young animals (11) Dysentery of foals
C (*Bac. paludis*)	Struck in yearling sheep Haemorrhagic enterotoxaemia of suckling calves Necrotic enteritis of suckling pigs (34, 42, 46) Ulcerative enteritis of quail, quail disease (61)
D (*Bac. ovitoxicus*)	Pulpy kidney disease (enterotoxaemia) in lambs over 15 days old and sheep up to a year (13, 51) Enterotoxaemia of calves and piglets (43)
E	Enterotoxaemia in sheep and cattle

initiate different clinical manifestations (tab. 18). At the same time they occur in the intestine of healthy animals, type A being the most common (5, 24, 46). Sheep and goats are most vulnerable to the toxins of *Cl. perfringens*, followed in susceptibility by cattle and pigs (47).

■ **Morphology**
The various types are similar in appearance; they are short, squat, non-motile rods measuring 0.6–0.8 × 1.2–4 µm. Usually they are found lying singly and in the host's body they possess a capsule (fig. 77).

■ **Culture**
Cl. perfringens is an anaerobe which is not especially sensitive to atmospheric oxygen. On a Zeissler plate *Cl. perfringens* forms characteristic colonies (fig. 78).

■ **Biochemical properties**
For details on the fermentation of carbohydrates see figure 68. It is often difficult to differentiate between types B and C by means of the neutralization test but BEER & AL-KHATIB (12) claim that the demonstration of hyaluronidase has proved useful;

■ **Morphologie**
Mikroskopisch sehen die einzelnen Typen gleich aus. Es handelt sich um kurze, gedrungene, 0,6–0,8 × 1,2–4 µm große, unbewegliche Stäbchen, die in der Regel einzeln liegen und im Tierkörper eine Kapsel bilden (Abb. 77).

■ **Kultur**
Cl. perfringens ist ein Anaerobier, der jedoch nicht hochempfindlich gegenüber Luftsauerstoff ist. Auf der Zeißler-Platte bildet *Cl. perfringens* charakteristische Kolonien (Abb. 78).

■ **Kulturell-biochemische Eigenschaften**
Spaltung von Kohlenhydraten siehe Abb. 68. Für die Unterscheidung der Typen B und C, die im Neutralisationstest oft schwierig ist, hat sich nach BEER & AL-KHATIB (12) der Hyaluronidasenachweis bewährt, der beim Typ B positiv und beim

Table 19: The major toxins of *Cl. perfringens* types

Tabelle 19: Die Majortoxine der *Cl. perfringens*-Typen

Type:	A	B	C	D	E
Toxin:	α	α, β, ϵ	α, β	α, ϵ	α, ι

it is positive with type B and negative with type C (decapsulation test with *Sc. equi*, p. 20).

Typ C negativ ausfällt (Dekapsulationstest mit *Sc. equi*; s. S. 20).

■ Toxins

Cl. perfringens produces at least 20 different toxins and »aggressins«, which can be neutralized with antitoxins. For the differentiation between the various types A to E four major toxins are used, the remaining toxins are either lethal to experimental animals, or haemolytic or they are collagenases,

■ Toxine

Cl. perfringens bildet mindestens 20 Toxine und aggressive Fermente, die durch Antitoxine neutralisierbar sind. Für die Unterscheidung der Typen A bis E dienen 4 Majortoxine, die restlichen Toxine wirken im Tierversuch entweder letal, hämolysierend oder sind Kollagenasen, Proteinasen oder Des-

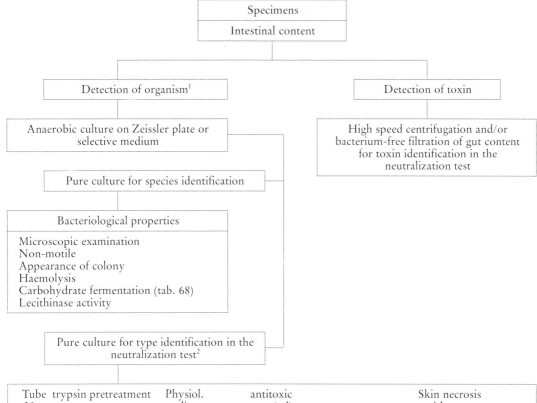

Tube No.	trypsin pretreatment		Physiol. saline (ml)	antitoxic sera (ml)				Skin necrosis with types				
				A	C	D	E	A	B	C	D	E
1	−	Control	0.3	−	−	−	−	+	+	+	v	+
2	−	A-serum	0.2	0.1	−	−	−	−	+	+	v	v
3	−	A-C-serum	0.1	0.1	0.1	−	−	−	v	−	v	v
4	−	A-C-D-serum	−	0.1	0.1	0.1	−	−	−	−	−	v
5	+	Control	0.3	−	−	−	−	v	+	v	+	+
6	+	A-serum	0.2	0.1	−	−	−	−	+	v	+	+
7	+	A-C-serum	0.1	0.1	0.1	−	−	−	v	v	−	+
8	+	A-C-D-serum	−	0.1	0.1	0.1	−	−	−	−	−	+
9	+	A-E-serum	0.1	0.1	−	−	0.1	−	+	v	+	−

[1] The general cultural demonstration of *Clostridium perfringens* is of little consequence, because all types, and especially type A, can occur in the gut of healthy animals;
[2] The neutralization test can be carried out as intradermal test in albino guinea pigs or as a mouse lethal test

[1] Der alleinige kulturelle Nachweis von *Clostridium perfringens* ist von geringer Aussagekraft, da alle Typen, insbesondere aber Typ A, im Darm gesunder Tiere vorkommen können;
[2] Der Neutralisationstest kann als Intrakutantest am Albinomeerschweinchen oder als Mäuseletalitätstest durchgeführt werden

Fig. 81: Test routine for diagnosis of *Cl. perfringens* enterotoxaemias

Abb. 81: Untersuchungsgang für die Diagnose von Enterotoxämien durch *Clostridium perfringens*

proteinases or desoxyribonucleases. Table 19 shows the distribution of the 4 major toxins in the 5 types of clostridia.

The α- and β-toxins are present in the culture fluid as complete toxins and by the addition of trypsin their effect can be reduced or abolished, while the ε- and ι-toxins are protoxins which are activated by trypsin.

Typing is performed either by the intracutaneous test in guinea pigs, using the dermonecrotic action of the toxin or in the mouse lethal test (12, 29, 35, 38, 54). The instructions of the manufacturer should be followed for the quantitative lay-out of the test. As example, the procedure of the guinea pig intracutaneous test is shown in figure 81. The following steps are necessary:
▷ Production of the toxin by incubation for 6 to 7 hours in the most suitable fluid medium (e. g. 0.5 % meat broth with glucose and minced horse meat, casein-hydrolysate-dextrose broth; cooked meat medium [Oxoid]; Katsaras and Hartwigk, 40). It might be of advantage if the strain that is to be tested is first activated by culture passage (liver broth) or animal passage (in guinea pigs or pigeons).
▷ High speed centrifugation and/or bacteria-free filtration of the fluid medium.
▷ Trypsin is added to one portion of the filtrate and allowed to interact for 1 hour at 37 °C.
▷ Except for the controls, the untreated and the trypsin-treated filtrates are mixed with antisera (fig. 81) and allowed to stand for 30 to 60 minutes at 20 °C.
▷ The intracutaneous injections are carried out on an albino guinea pig whose back and flanks have been previously depilated.
▷ The reaction is assessed after 24 and 48 hours as shown in figure 81.

The neutralization test does not always produce the expected results because toxin production is often uncertain (particularly in type A), the ε-toxin is not always present as the protoxin and may be active even without the trypsin treatment and the effects of the α- and β-toxins are not invariably completely countered by trypsin (29).

The mouse lethal test can be employed instead of the guinea pig intradermal test. In this case the culture filtrates and the culture filtrate-antiserum mixtures are injected intravenously in doses of 0.3 to 0.5 ml. Fink (25) is of the opinion that intraperitoneal injection is preferable, because it is technically simpler and less subject to biological variation than the intravenous method.
▷ Detection of toxin in the gut: A bacteria-free filtrate is prepared from the intestinal content, depending on its consistency. If necessary it can be treated several times with the high speed centrifuge. A considerable toxin loss can occur by the filtration. The presence of toxin is then demonstrated in the mouse lethal or the guinea pig intradermal test.

oxyribonukleasen. Die Verteilung der Majortoxine auf die 5 Typen zeigt die Tab. 19.

Das α- und β-Toxin liegen in fertiger Form in der Kulturflüssigkeit vor, ihre Wirkung kann durch Trypsin verringert oder aufgehoben werden. Dagegen liegen ε- und ι-Toxin als Protoxin vor und werden durch Trypsin aktiviert.

Die Typisierung erfolgt entweder im Intrakutantest am Meerschweinchen unter Ausnutzung der dermonekrotischen Wirkung der Toxine oder im Mäuseletalitätstest (12, 29, 35, 38, 54). Der quantitative Ansatz richtet sich zweckmäßigerweise nach den Angaben des Antitoxinherstellers. Als Beispiel ist in der Abb. 81 die Durchführung des Intrakutantestes am Meerschweinchen zusammengestellt. Folgende Arbeitsvorgänge sind erforderlich:
▷ Toxinproduktion in einem flüssigen, optimalen Nährboden (z. B.: Fleischbouillon mit 0,5 % Glucose und gehacktem Pferdefleisch, Casein-Hydrolysat-Dextrin-Bouillon; cooked-meat-medium [Oxoid]; Katsaras & Hartwigk, 40), evtl. nach Aktivierung des zu bestimmenden Stammes durch Kultur- (Leberbouillon) oder Tierpassagen (Meerschweinchen, Taube). Bebrütungsdauer 6 bis 7 h.
▷ Hochtourige Zentrifugation oder (und) keimfreie Filtration der Kulturflüssigkeit.
▷ Ein Teil des Filtrates mit Trypsin versetzen und 1 h bei 37 °C einwirken lassen.
▷ Unbehandeltes und trypsinbehandeltes Filtrat wird bis auf die Kontrollen mit antitoxischen Seren versetzt (Abb. 81) und 30 bis 60 min bei 20 °C gehalten.
▷ Intrakutane Injektion an einem Albinomeerschweinchen, dessen Rücken und Flanken vorher enthaart worden sind.
▷ Die Reaktion wird nach 24 und 48 h entsprechend Abb. 81 beurteilt.

Der Neutralisationstest führt nicht immer zu den zu erwartenden Ergebnissen, da die Toxinbildung oft unregelmäßig ist (besonders beim Typ A), das ε-Toxin nicht immer als Protoxin vorliegt, sondern auch ohne Trypsinbehandlung wirksam sein kann und die α- und β-Toxinwirkung nicht immer durch Trypsin vollständig aufgehoben wird (29).

An Stelle des Intrakutantestes am Meerschweinchen kann auch der Mäuseletalitätstest durchgeführt werden. Dabei werden die Kulturfiltrate und Kulturfiltrat-Antiserum-Gemische in einer Menge von 0,3 bis 0,5 ml iv. injiziert (38). Nach Fink (25) ist die ip. Injektion vorzuziehen, da sie technisch einfacher durchzuführen ist und eine geringere biologische Schwankungsbreite besitzt als die iv. Injektion.
▷ Toxinnachweis im Darm: Je nach Konsistenz wird der Darminhalt keimfrei filtriert oder, wenn erforderlich, mehrmals hochtourig zentrifugiert. Mit der Filtration kann ein erheblicher Toxinverlust auftreten. Der Toxinnachweis erfolgt dann im Mäuseletal- oder im Intrakutantest am Meerschweinchen.
▷ Enterotoxin: Neben den erwähnten Typtoxinen

▷ Enterotoxin: Apart from the above-mentioned type toxins, *Cl. perfringens* also produces an enterotoxin which is responsible for food poisoning in man (KATSARAS & HILDEBRANDT, 39; HAUSCHILD 30). It is formed most commonly by type A, rarely by type C. The enterotoxin is formed during sporulation and is liberated by lysis of the sporangia. More than 10^6 bacteria have to be taken up in order to elicit food poisoning. The clostridia multiply and sporulate in the gut, causing the enterotoxin to be liberated. A prerequisite for the *in vitro* detection of enterotoxin is a plentiful sporulation of the clostridia in special sporulation media (e. g. ELLNER's, 23, or the one of DUNCAN & STRONG, 21). The demonstration of enterotoxins can be performed biologically (mouse lethal test, guinea pig intradermal test, gut ligature test) or serologically (agar gel diffusion test, indirect passive haemagglutination test). Details of these methods can be found in KATSARAS (38), KATSARAS & HARTWIGK (40), KATSARAS & SIEMS (41) and HARTWIGK (29).

■ **Resistance of spores**
The resistance of spores and the effect of disinfectants on them has been discussed on p. 87. Enterotoxin-producing spores can be very resistant to heat and survive exposure to 120 °C for 2 hours (KATSARAS & SIEMS, 41).

2.7 Clostridium sordellii, cause of enteritis and toxaemia

Isolated instances have been reported where this clostridium was found to be responsible for haemorrhagic and necrotic enteritis and for enterotoxaemia of cattle (2, 12), sheep (4) and foals (32). Experimental oral administration of bacteria-free toxin filtrates has also led to the development of intestinal disorders (3). Finally a generalized toxaemia of sheep may occur on rare occasions (60).

2.8 Clostridium difficile, cause of intestinal disorders

The significance of *Cl. difficile* as a causal agent of intestinal infections in animals is still not completely understood. It was first described as the cause of human enterocolitis which had been initiated by antibiotics, and later it was also found in hamsters, rabbits and guinea pigs. In pigs it has been described in swine dysentery (45); and it has been associated with natural infections accompanied by diarrhoea in pigs (37) and dogs (15).

bildet *Cl. perfringens* ein Enterotoxin, das beim Menschen Lebensmittelvergiftungen verursacht (KATSARAS & HILDEBRANDT, 39; HAUSCHILD, 30). Es wird meistens vom Typ A, selten vom Typ C gebildet. Das Enterotoxin entsteht während der Sporulation und wird durch die Lysis der Sporangien freigesetzt. Für die Auslösung der Lebensmittelvergiftung müssen über 10^6 Clostridien/g Lebensmittel aufgenommen werden. Die Clostridien vermehren sich und versporen im Darm, anschließend wird das Enterotoxin frei. Der in-vitro-Nachweis des Enterotoxins setzt somit für die Toxinproduktion eine gute Versporung der Clostridien in speziellen Sporulationsmedien (z. B. nach ELLNER, 23, oder DUNCAN & STRONG, 21) voraus. Der Enterotoxinnachweis läßt sich biologisch (Mäuseletaltest, Intrakutantest beim Meerschweinchen, Darmligaturtest) oder serologisch (Agargeldiffusionstest, umgekehrte passive Hämagglutination) führen. Einzelheiten über die Methoden s. bei KATSARAS (38), KATSARAS & HARTWIGK (40), KATSARAS & SIEMS (41), HARTWIGK (29).

■ **Tenazität der Sporen**
Hinsichtlich der Tenazität und Desinfizierbarkeit, der Sporen s. S. 87. Die Hitzeresistenz der Sporen von enterotoxinbildenden Stämmen kann sehr hoch sein und bei 120 °C über 2 h betragen (KATSARAS & SIEMS, 41).

2.7 Clostridium sordellii als Ursache von Darmerkrankungen und Toxämien

Das Clostridium ist in Einzelfällen als Ursache von hämorrhagischen bis nekrotisierenden Enteritiden, von Enterotoxämien beim Rind (2, 12), beim Schaf (4) sowie beim Fohlen (32) nachgewiesen worden. Orale Infektionsversuche und die Verabreichung von bakterienfreien Toxinfiltraten führten ebenfalls zu Darmerscheinungen (3). Ferner wurden selten toxische Allgemeinerkrankungen beim Schaf beobachtet (60).

2.8 Clostridium difficile als Ursache von Darmerkrankungen

Die Bedeutung von *Cl. difficile* als Darminfektionserreger beim Tier ist noch unzureichend bekannt. Es wurde zunächst als Ursache einer durch Antibiotika induzierten Enterocolitis beim Menschen beschrieben, später auch bei Hamstern, Kaninchen und Meerschweinchen (58). Beim Schwein wurde es im Zusammenhang mit der Schweinedysenterie beschrieben (45). Natürliche Infektionen, die einen solchen Zusammenhang nicht aufwiesen, wurden im Zusammenhang mit Diarrhöen beim Schwein (37) und beim Hund (15) gefunden.

2.9 Clostridium spiroforme infections

In rabbits, guinea pigs and hamster *Clostridium spiroforme* has been described as the cause of a spontaneous colitis or one that had been induced by clindamycin. It was possible to demonstrate the presence of a toxin in the gut, which could be neutralized by *Cl. perfringens* type E (iota)-antitoxin (18, 55).

2.10 Clostridium tetani

■ **Incidence and veterinary significance**
Responsible for tetanus in man and animals.

■ **Morphology**
A slim rod, 0.5–1.1 × 2.5–5.0 µm in size, with terminal round spores and peritrichous flagella. *Cl. tetani* becomes Gram-variable to Gram-negative after 2 to 3 days in culture. When the spores are fully developed they are in diameter twice as large as the

I. Examination of wound specimens for *Clostridium tetani*		
Microscopic examination for Cl. with drumstick form with Gram stain is of little importance because the organism is not often found and other clostridia of similar form may occur (*Cl. tetanomorphum*, *Cl. tetanoides*)	Cultural examination perhaps after heating sample to 80 °C/ 20 min. Liver broth, cooked meat broth, thioglycollate broth, after 2–3 days subculture to solid media, after 4–6 days demonstration of toxin in animal test, microscopic check of broth, in young cultures *Cl. tetani* is Gram-positive, later -variable to -negative	Animal experiment, wound material is implanted into a skin pocket of mice near the root of the tail, or fluid material or suspension is injected subcutaneously. In positive tests symptoms of tetanus.

II. Demonstration of toxin from a) patient's serum b) culture filtrate	
Animal experiment	
Test procedure	Test results
1. Several mice (if possible) are injected subcutaneously with 0.5–1.0 ml of patient's serum or culture filtrate	Mice fall sick (»seal position«) within 1 to 3 days
2. Mice are injected subcutaneously with 1.0 ml patient's serum or 0.5 ml culture filtrate and 500 I. U. antitoxin	No illness
3. Mice are injected subcutaneously with patient's serum or culture filtrate that has been heated to 100 °C/30 min. Any toxin present was destroyed by the heating	No illness

Fig. 82: Test procedure for the detection of *Clostridium tetani* and tetanus toxin

vegetative forms; they are best demonstrated with a special spore stain such as that of Rakette (p. 336 and fig. 79).

■ **Culture**
On Zeissler plates they appear as round, colourless to grey colonies (growth type VIII of Zeissler) with irregular borders. The organisms have the tendency, especially on moist media, to spread diffusely. They are heamolytic. Because of their great oxygen sensitivity they can only be isolated on solid media under strict anaerobic conditions. Figure 82 provides information of culturing *Cl. tetani* from animal material.

■ **Biochemical properties**
The demonstration of the toxin is more important for the identification of this clostridium than the determination of its biochemical properties. *Cl. tetani* liquefies gelatine, turns brain pulp black, it does not ferment the usual carbohydrates, forms gas in liver broth and neither lipase nor lecithinase are produced.

■ **Toxin**
Tetanus toxin consists of several biologically distinct fractions. The clinical picture of »lockjaw« is due to tetanospasmin, while tetanolysin is an oxygen-sensitive haemolysin. The demonstration of the toxins plays an important role in diagnostic investigations and in the identification of *Cl. tetani* (fig. 82).

2.11 Clostridium botulinum

■ **Incidence and veterinary significance**
Responsible for botulism in man and animals. It produces several toxins and on the basis of these, types A to G have been identified (tab. 20). In Germany, animals most frequently succumb to type C while in man type B is the commonest cause of botulism, types E or A are less often involved. Type E has been isolated regularly from water, mud and soil and from the gut of both fresh- and salt-water fish (8, 9, 10).

■ **Morphology**
A straight rod measuring 0.9–1.2 × 4–6 µm with peritrichous flagella and less commonly terminal spores. Gram-variable forms appear on older cultures, particularly of types B, E and F.

■ **Culture**
Cl. botulinum is a strict anaerobe, even small traces of oxygen will inhibit growth. Temperatures between 18 °C and 38 °C are recommended for incuba-

doppelten Durchmesser der Stäbchen auf und lassen sich am besten mit einer Sporenfärbung nachweisen, z. B. nach Rakette (S. 336 und Abb. 79).

■ **Kultur**
Auf der Zeißler-Platte entstehen runde, farblose bis graue Kolonien (Wuchsform VIII nach Zeißler) mit unregelmäßigem Rand. Besonders auf feuchten Nährböden können die Clostridien rasenförmig ausschwärmen. Es tritt eine Hämolyse auf. Die Isolierung auf festen Nährböden gelingt aufgrund der hohen Sauerstoffempfindlichkeit nur bei strenger Anaerobiose. Den Einsatz der Kultur zur Isolierung von *Cl. tetani* aus Patientenmaterial zeigt Abb. 82.

■ **Kulturell-biochemische Eigenschaften**
Für die Identifizierung ist der Toxinnachweis wichtiger als die Feststellung des biochemischen Leistungsspektrums. *Cl. tetani* verflüssigt Gelatine, schwärzt Hirnbrei, greift die üblichen Kohlenhydrate nicht an. In Leberbouillon kommt es zu einer Gasbildung, Lipase und Lezithinase werden nicht gebildet.

■ **Toxin**
Das Tetanustoxin besteht aus mehreren biologisch unterschiedlich wirksamen Fraktionen. Das Bild des Starrkrampfes wird durch das Tetanospasmin bedingt, das Tetanolysin ist ein sauerstoffempfindliches Hämolysin. Bei den diagnostischen Untersuchungen und bei der Identifizierung von *Cl. tetani* spielt der Toxinnachweis eine wichtige Rolle (Abb. 82).

2.11 Clostridium botulinum

■ **Vorkommen und medizinische Bedeutung**
Erreger des Botulismus bei Mensch und Tier. Aufgrund der Bildung verschiedener Toxine werden die Typen A bis G unterschieden (Tab. 20). Erkrankungen von Tieren sind in Deutschland meistens durch den Typ C, von Menschen durch den Typ B und selten durch den Typ E oder A bedingt. Der Typ E ist besonders häufig aus Wasser-, Schlamm- und Erdproben sowie aus dem Darmkanal von Süß- und Seewasserfischen isoliert worden (8, 9, 10).

■ **Morphologie**
0,9–1,2 × 4–6 µm großes, gerades, peritrich begeißeltes Stäbchen mit subterminaler und seltener terminaler Sporenbildung. In älteren Kulturen treten insbesondere bei den Typen B, E und F gramlabile Formen auf.

■ **Kultur**
Cl. botulinum ist ein strenger Anaerobier, schon geringe Sauerstoffspuren hemmen das Wachstum. Zur Bebrütung wurden Temperaturen von 18 bis

tion, but the optimum lies between 30 °C and 37 °C. The optimum pH is in the neutral range or slightly above (7.0–7.6). *Cl. botulinum* will grow in the usual media recommended for clostridial multiplication such as liver broth, glucose broth, cooked meat medium, producing a uniform turbidity and occasionally a floccular deposit. Media of defined composition are preferred for the production of toxins, because the addition of animal tissues whose quality varies, results in insufficient and uneven toxin levels. Numerous media additives have been described (for summary see SONNENSCHEIN, 67), such as casein hydrolysate, corn steep liquor, glucose, yeast extract, trypticase, glycerol. The most favourable incubation time for toxin harvest lies, according to SONNENSCHEIN (67), between 4 (types A, E), 5 (types B, C) and 10 days (type D).

On solid media growths may vary in appearance. The colonies may be slightly domed with ragged edges, they may be flat and rough (fig. 80) or, in fact, the growth may resemble a veil-like film. With exception of the opaque core, the colonies are transparent with a greyish-white, dull or slightly shiny surface. Most strains are haemolytic. ZELLER (73) recommends liver blood agar for their culture, because glucose-containing media induce a rapid breakdown of clostridia. The diagnostic culture methods are summarized in figure 83.

38 °C angegeben, die optimale Temperatur liegt zwischen 30–37 °C. Der optimale pH-Wert liegt im neutralen Bereich oder leicht darüber (7,0–7,6). *Cl. botulinum* wächst in den üblichen für Clostridienvermehrung benutzten flüssigen Nährböden wie Leberbouillon, Glucosebouillon, cooked meat medium mit gleichmäßiger Trübung des Mediums und vereinzelter Flockenbildung. Für die Toxinproduktion werden Medien mit definierter Zusammensetzung bevorzugt, da der Zusatz von tierischen Gewebeteilen aufgrund deren unterschiedlicher Qualität zu einer unzureichenden und ungleichmäßigen Toxinbildung führen kann. Es sind eine Vielzahl von Nährbodenzusätzen beschrieben worden (Zusammenstellung s. SONNENSCHEIN, 67), z. B.: Caseinhydrolysat, corn steep liquor, Glucose, Hefeextrakt, Trypticase, Glycerin. Die optimale Bebrütungsdauer für die Toxinausbeute liegt nach SONNENSCHEIN (67) zwischen 4 (Typ A, E), 5 (Typ B, C) und 10 Tagen (Typ D).

Das Wachstum auf festen Nährböden kann unterschiedlich aussehen, es können flach gewölbte Kolonien mit gefranstem Rand, flache, rauhe Kolonien (Abb. 80) oder hauchartige Schleier auftreten. Die Kolonien sind mit Ausnahme des opaken Zentrums durchscheinend und besitzen eine grauweiße, matte oder leicht glänzende Oberfläche. Bei den meisten Stämmen tritt eine Hämolyse auf. ZELLER

Table 20: The toxins of *Clostridium botulinum* and their distribution (67)

Tabelle 20. Die Toxintypen von *Clostridium botulinum* und ihre Verbreitung (67)

Type	Toxin	Distribution	Intoxication source	Particularly susceptible
A	A	West USA, USSR (Ukraine)	Plant foods, meat, fish and wounds?	Man, fowl, mink
B	B	Central & East USA, North & Central Europe	Meat and meat products (usually from pigs), wounds	Man, cattle, horse, fowl
C	C_α C_1, C_2 D	North & South America, South Africa, Australia, Europe	Lucilia larvae, plants, putrefying mud	Aquatic birds
C	C_β C_2	Australia, South Africa, Europe	Spoiled food, carcasses	Cattle, horse, mink
D	D C_1, C_2	South Africa, USSR[2]	Carcasses	Cattle
E	E	North Europe, USSR, Canada, Alaska, Japan	Fish and fish products	Man
F	F	Scotland, USA, Denmark, USSR	Liver paste, fish	Man
G	G	Argentine	—	—[1]

[1] Natural intoxications are unknown in man and animals;
[2] A type D intoxication has been described by HAAGSMA and TER LAAK (27) in cattle in Netherlands

[1] natürliche Intoxikationen bei Mensch und Tier sind nicht bekannt;
[2] eine Typ D-Intoxikation bei Rindern ist von HAAGSMA & TER LAAK (27) in den Niederlanden beschrieben worden

Genus: Clostridium (Cl.)

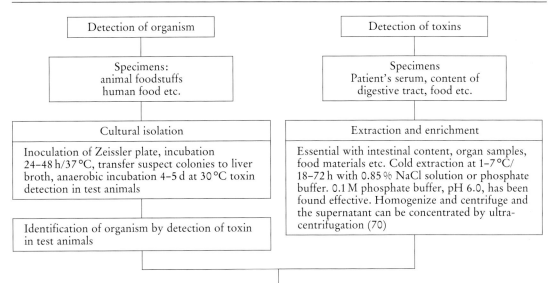

Fig. 83: Test procedure for the demonstration of *Cl. botulinum* and its toxin

Abb. 83: Untersuchungsgang zum Nachweis von *Clostridium botulinum* und Botulinustoxin

[1] The intravenous administration does not increase the reliability;
[2] Particularly Type E toxin is activated by trypsin, so that the injection material my have to be pretreated accordingly

[1] die Injektion erhöht die Nachweissicherheit nicht;
[2] insbesondere das Typ E-Toxin wird durch Trypsin aktiviert, so daß eine entsprechende Vorbehandlung des Injektionsmaterials notwendig sein kann.

(73) empfiehlt zur Züchtung Leberblutagar, da glucosehaltige Nährböden einen raschen Zerfall der Clostridien bewirken. Über die diagnostische Anwendung der Kulturmethoden siehe Abb. 83.

■ **Biochemical properties**

These can vary even within one type. They are of minor importance in diagnosis, because the detection of the toxins is of primary interest for identification of the types. Basically we differentiate between those strains that do and those that do not break down protein. All the strains of type A as well as some from types B, C, D and F are proteolytic. Fatty acids (acetic, butyric, and propionic)

■ **Kulturell-biochemische Eigenschaften**

Die biochemischen Eigenschaften können auch innerhalb eines Typs sehr variieren. Sie sind diagnostisch von untergeordneter Bedeutung, da für die Identifizierung der Toxinnachweis im Vordergrund steht. Grundsätzlich werden eiweißabbauende und eiweißnichtabbauende Stämme unterschieden. Zu den proteolytischen gehören alle Stämme vom Typ A sowie einzelne Stämme der Typen B, C, D und F.

Toxins

The various types of *Cl. botulinum* are characterized by their toxins. Type C comprises two subtypes, Cα and Cβ, (tab. 20). The identification of the toxins is of great diagnostic importance, not only for the identification of the clostridial type but also in the examination of patients' serum, food materials etc. The basis for this lies in the neutralization test, using small laboratory animals (mouse, guinea pigs); the test sequence is described in figure 83. Cross-neutralizations can occur between types C and D. Cα antitoxin will neutralize both Cα and Cβ toxins, while Cβ antitoxin neutralizes only Cβ toxin.

Besides the neutralization test one can also employ serological methods for the determination of the toxins. In this connection the precipitation test and passive haemagglutination test are of significance (68, 69).

Resistance of spores

The claims for the heat resistance of the spores vary a great deal. For dry heat the range lies between 120 °C for 120 minutes and 180 °C for 5–10 minutes, for moist heat it is between 105 °C for 120 minutes and 120 °C for 20 minutes. The spores of types A and F are particularly heat resistant and this decreases from types B to E. Thus, the following claims have been made for type E: 100 °C for 10 minutes, 77 °C for 2 minutes, 80 °C for 10 minutes (summary in SONNENSCHEIN, 67).

Chemical disinfection is very problematic (p. 87), because chemical substances are usually incapable of destroying the spores, but only prevent them from germinating (SONNENSCHEIN, 67).

Bibliography / Literatur

1. AL-KHATIB, G. (1968): Über den Nachweis und die Differenzierung von Clostridium perfringens und seiner Toxine im Darminhalt verendeter Haustiere. Mh. Vet. Med. 23, 593–597.
2. AL-MASHAT, R. R., & D. J. TAYLOR (1983): Bacteria in enteric lesions of cattle. Vet. Rec. 112, 5–10.
3. AL-MASHAT, R. R., & D. J. TAYLOR (1983): Production of diarrhoea and enteric lesions in calves by the oral inoculation of pure culture of Clostridium sordellii. Vet. Rec. 112, 141–146.
4. AL-MASHAT, R. R., & D. J. TAYLOR (1983): Clostridium sordellii in enteritis in an adult sheep. Vet. Rec. 112, 19.
5. AMTSBERG, G., W. BISPING, P. KRABISCH & I. MATTHIESEN (1977): Zum Vorkommen und zur pathogenen Bedeutung von Clostridium perfringens beim Kalb. 1. Mitt.: Quantitative bakteriologische Untersuchungen zum Cl.-perfringens-Keimgehalt in Kot und Darminhalt von gesunden und erkrankten Kälbern. Zbl. Vet. Med. B, 24, 104–113.
6. BACH, R., & G. MÜLLER-PRASUHN (1971): Teichforellen als Träger von Clostridium botulinum. Arch. Lebensmittelhyg. 22, 64–68, 91–95.
7. BALJER, G., S. CHORHERR, R. HOFFMANN, H. KNÖPPLER & H. WIEDEMANN (1974): Clostridium-botulinum-Toxin vom Typ C als Ursache eines Vogelsterbens in einem oberbayerischen See. Tierärztl. Prax. 2, 191–197.
8. BAUMGART, J. (1972): Vorkommen und Nachweis von Clostridium botulinum Typ E bei Seefischen. Arch. Lebensmittelhyg. 23, 34–39.
9. BAUMGART, J. (1970): Nachweis von Clostridium botulinum Typ E bei handelsfertigen Forellen. Fleischwirtschaft 50, 1545–1546.
10. BAUMGART, J. (1970): Nachweis von Clostridium botulinum Typ E. I. Mitt.: Toxinnachweis bei Plattfischen. Arch. Lebensmittelhyg. 21, 102–104.

11. Beer, J., G. Al-Khatib & H. Pilz (1968): Enterotoxämie der Kälber durch Clostridium perfringens Typ B. Mh. Vet. Med. 23, 18–24.
12. Beer, J., & G. Al-Khatib (1968): Zum Nachweis und zur Differenzierung pathogener Clostridien und ihrer Toxine. Mh. Vet. Med. 23, 709–714.
13. Behrens, H. (1954): Zur Enterotoxämie (Clostridium welchii Typus D-Intoxikation) der Schafe. Dtsch. tierärztl. Wschr. 61, 1–4.
14. Berg, J. N., W. H. Fales & C. M. Scanlan (1979): Occurrence of anaerobic bacteria in diseases of the dog and cat. Amer. J. Vet. Res. 40, 876–881.
15. Berry, A. P., & P. N. Levett (1986): Chronic diarrhoea in dogs associated with Clostridium difficile infection. Vet. Rec. 118, 102–103.
16. Blender, D. C., & C. P. Merilan (1961): Isolation of clostridia by crystal violet inhibition of aerobic spore-forming bacteria. Amer. J. Vet. Res. 22, 944–947.
17. Brooks, M. E., & M. Sterne (1956): Occurrence of Clostridium sordellii in Great Britain. Vet. Rec. 68, 121–122.
18. Carman, R. J., & S. P. Borriello (1983): Laboratory diagnosis of Clostridium spiroforme-mediated diarrhoea (Jota-enterotoxaemia) of rabbits. Vet. Rec. 113, 184–185.
19. Carman, R. J., & J. C. M. Lewis (1983): Recurrent diarrhoea in a dog associated with Clostridium perfringens type A. Vet. Rec. 113, 342–343.
20. Döll, W., & H. Schmidt (1969): Die Keimausbeute von Clostridien auf selektiven und nichtselektiven Anaerobier-Nährböden, dargestellt an Reinkulturen von verschiedenen Clostridien-Species. Zbl. Bakt. I. Orig. A 212, 109–114.
21. Duncan, C. L., & D. H. Strong (1968): Improved medium for sporulation of Clostridium perfringens. App. Microbiol. 16, 82–86.
22. Ellender, R. D., Jr. Hildalgo & L. C. Grunbles (1970): Characterization of five clostridial pathogens by gas liquid chromatography. Am. J. Vet. Res. 31, 1863–1866.
23. Ellner, P. D. (1956): A medium promoting quantitative sporulation in Clostridium perfringens. J. Bact. 71, 495–501.
24. Elter, B., & E. Scharner (1968): Zum Vorkommen von Clostridium perfringens bei gesunden Schlachtrindern. Z. ges. Hyg. 14, 766–768.
25. Fink, C. N. (1971): Vergleich des Intrakutantestes beim Meerschweinchen mit dem iv.- und dem ip.-Test (Letaltest) an der Maus bei Verwendung von alpha-toxinhaltigen Kulturfiltraten des Clostridium perfringens Typ A. Vet. Med. Diss. FU Berlin.
26. Haagsma, J., & E. A. ter Laak (1979): Eerste geval van botulismus typ D bij runderen in Nederland vastgesteld. Tijdsch. Diergeneesk. 104, 609–613.
27. Haagsma, J., & E. A. ter Laak (1978): Een geval van botulismus bij runderen, veroozaakt door de voedering van kuilgras. Tijdschr. Diergeneesk. 103, 910–912.
28. Harms, F. (1943): Die bakteriologische Unterscheidung von Rauschbrand und Pararauschbrand mit neueren Verfahren. Berl. Münch. tierärztl. Wschr., 198–200.
29. Hartwigk, H. (1970): Zur Technik der Isolierung und Differenzierung des Clostridium (Cl.) welchii (perfringens). Schlacht- u. Viehhof-Ztg., 70, 468–473.
30. Hauschild, A. H. W. (1972): Das Enterotoxin von Clostridium perfringens und seine Rolle bei Lebensmittelvergiftungen. Fleischwirtsch. 52, 873–875.
31. Heicken, K., & H. Bellinger (1962): Experimentelle Untersuchungen zum Catgutproblem. Zbl. Bakt. I. Orig. 184, 493–530.
32. Hibbs, C. M., D. R. Johnson, K. Reynolds & R. Harrington (1977): Clostridium sordellii isolated from foals. Vet. Med. Small Anim. Clin. 72, 256–258.
33. Hinz, K. H. (1975): Gasödemerkrankung bei Broilern. Dtsch. tierärztl. Wschr. 82, 307–310.
34. Hogh, P. (1969): Infektiöse nekrotisierende Enteritis bei Saugferkeln, verursacht von Clostridium Typ C. IV. Bakteriologische Diagnose. Acta vet. scand. 10, 57–83.
35. Hösli, J., Ph. Seifert, F. Ehrensberger & R. Weilenmann (1980): Zur Diagnostik der Clostridien-Enterotoxämie der Schafe. Schweiz. Arch. Tierhk. 122, 137–150.
36. Jansen, B. C., & P. C. Knoetze (1977): The taxonomic position of Clostridium botulinum type C. Onderstepoort J. Vet. Res. 44, 53–54.
37. Jones, M. A., & D. Hunter (1983): Isolation of Clostridium difficile from pigs. Vet. Rec. 112, 253.
38. Katsaras, K. (1980): Clostridium perfringens-Toxine. Arch. Lebensmittelhyg. 31, 121–125.
39. Katsaras, K., & G. Hildebrandt (1979): Ursachen bakterieller Lebensmittelvergiftungen: Enterotoxin von Clostridium perfringens Typ A. Fleischwirtschaft 59, 954–958.
40. Katsaras, K., & H. Hartwigk (1976): Nachweismethoden der Toxine des Clostridium perfringens unter besonderer Berücksichtigung der Enterotoxine. Zbl. Bakt. I. Ref. 249, 97–111.
41. Katsaras, K., & H. Siems (1974): Enterotoxin-Nachweis bei hitzeresistenten Clostridium perfringens-Typ A Stämmen aus einer Lebensmittelvergiftung. Zbl. Bakt. I. Orig. 229, 409–420.
42. Köhler, B., Z. Zabke, R. Sondermann, H. Pulst & H. J. Rummler (1979): Untersuchungen zur nekrotisierenden Enteritis der Saugferkel (Clostridium-perfringens-Typ-C-Enterotoxämie) in industriemäßig produzierenden Sauenzuchtanlagen. 4. Mitt.: Epizootiologie. Arch. exp. Vet. med. 33, 505–619.
43. Köhler, B., & R. Stander (1973): Untersuchungen zum Vorkommen von Clostridium perfringens und seiner Toxine und zur Clostridium-perfringens-Enterotoxämie beim Rind. Arch. exp. Vet. med. 27, 29–47.
44. Köhler, B. (1980): Klostridien-Infektionen und -Intoxikationen. In: J. Beer (Hrsg.): Infektionskrankheiten der Haustiere. 2. Aufl., S. 581–622. Jena: VEB Gustav Fischer.
45. Lyons, R. J., G. A. Hall, R. M. Lemcke, J. Bew & P. D. Luther (1980): Studies of organism possibly implicated in swine dysentery. Proceed. 6th Inter. Pig. Vet. Soc. Congr., Copenhagen, 231.
46. Köhler, B., J. Beer, B. Reschke, H. Gayer & M. Jonas (1970): Untersuchungen zum Vorkommen von Clostridium perfringens und seiner Toxine im Darmkanal und über seine Bedeutung als Krankheitserreger beim Schwein. Arch. exp. Vet. med. 24, 1325–1346.
47. Köhler, B. (1971): Klostridienintoxikationen beim Schwein. Mh. Vet. Med. 26, 69–74.
48. Koppsteiner, G., & H. Mrozek (1973): Die sporizide Wirkung chemischer Desinfektionsmittel. Arch. Lebensmittelhyg. 6, 125–131.
49. Martig, J. (1966): Zur Differentialdiagnose zwischen Rauschbrand und Pararauschbrand mit Hilfe der Immunofluoreszenz. Schweiz. Arch. Tierhkd. 108, 303–324.
50. Mette, H. (1980): Das Vorkommen von Clostridien in Produkten von Tierkörperbeseitigungsanstalten mit einem Beitrag zur Eignung von Selektivnährböden zum Clostridiennachweis. Vet. med. Diss. Hannover.
51. Mitscherlich, E., C. Sebetic & H. Behrens (1954): Die Enterotoxämie der Schafe (Clostridium welchii Typus D-Intoxikation) in Deutschland. Dtsch. tierärztl. Wschr. 61, 4–7.
52. Mitscherlich, E., S. Gürtück & H. Köhler (1953): Die Lämmerruhr (Cl. welchii-Intoxikation) in Deutschland. Berl. Münch. tierärztl. Wschr. 66, 1–3.
53. Oakley, C. L., & G. H. Warrack (1959): The soluble antigens of Clostridium oedematiens type D (Cl. haemolyticum). J. Path. Bact. 78, 543–551.
54. Oakley, C. L., & G. H. Warrack (1953): Routine typing of Clostridium welchii. J. Hyg. 51, 102–107.
55. Peeters, J. E., R. Geeroms, R. J. Carman & T. D. Wilkens (1986): Significance of Clostridium spiroforme in the enteritis-complex of commercial rabbits. Vet. Microbiol. 12, 25–31.

56. PRESCOTT, J. F., J. A. JOHNSON, J. M. PATTERSON & W. S. BULMER (1978): Haemorrhagic gastroenteritis in the dog associated with Clostridium welchii. Vet. Rec. 103, 116–117.
57. RENK, W. (1962): Mastitiden bei Infektionen mit Clostridium perfringens. Berl. Münch. tierärztl. Wschr. 75, 162–165.
58. REHG, J. E., & Y. S. LU (1982): Clostridium difficile typhlitis in hamsters not associated with antibiotic therapy. J. Am. Vet. Med. Ass. 181, 1422–1423.
59. REUTER, G. (1968): Erfahrungen mit Nährböden für die selektive mikrobiologische Analyse von Fleischerzeugnissen. Arch. Lebensmittelhyg. 19, 84–89.
60. RICHARDS, S. M., & B. W. HUNT (1982): Clostridium sordellii in lambs. Vet. Rec. 111, 22.
61. SCHNEIDER, J. (1971): Untersuchungen zur ulcerösen Enteritis bei Hühnerküken. Arch. Geflügelkd. 35, 10–13.
62. SCHOOP, G. (1980): Clostridien der Haustiere. In: H. BLOBEL & TH. SCHLIESSER: Handbuch der bakteriellen Infektionen der Tiere. Bd. 6, S. 555–666. Jena: VEB Gustav Fischer.
63. SCHOOP, G. (1961): Nachweis von Clostridium botulinum Typ C bei Rindern. Dtsch. tierärztl. Wschr. 68, 71–72.
64. SCHULZE TEMMING-HANHOFF, W. (1974): Experimentelle Untersuchungen zur Desinfektion von Clostridium perfringens- und Clostridium botulinum-Sporen mit Formaldehyd. Vet. Med. Diss. Hannover.
65. SENF, W. (1983): Zur Clostridium-perfringens-Enterotoxämie beim Rind. Mh. Vet. Med. 38, 528–534.
66. SMITH, L. D., & G. HOBBS (1974): Clostridium. In: Bergey's manual of determinative bacteriology, 8. Aufl., S. 551–572. Baltimore: Williams & Wilkins.
67. SONNENSCHEIN, B. (1980): Clostridium botulinum. In: H. BLOBEL & TH. SCHLIESSER: Handbuch der bakteriellen Infektionen bei Tieren. Bd. 2, S. 691–745. Jena: VEB Gustav Fischer.
68. SONNENSCHEIN, B. (1978): Der Nachweis der Botulinustoxine A, B und E mit Hilfe der passiven Hämagglutination. Zbl. Bakt. I. Orig. A 240, 221–234.
69. SONNENSCHEIN, B. (1974): Zum Nachweis und zur Typisierung von Clostridium-botulinum-Toxinen durch die Agargelpräzipitation. Arch. Lebensmittelhyg. 25, 53–58.
70. SONNENSCHEIN, B., & W. BISPING (1976): Extraktion und Anreicherung von Clostridium botulinum-Toxinen aus dem Untersuchungsmaterial. Zbl. Bakt. I. Orig. A 234, 247–259.
71. WERNER, H. (1972): Anaerobendifferenzierung durch gaschromatographische Stoffwechselanalysen. Zbl. Bakt. I. Orig. A 220, 446–451.
72. WERNER, H. (1985): Anaerobierinfektionen. 2. Aufl. Stuttgart: Georg Thieme.
73. ZELLER, M. (1959): Ein Beitrag zur Botulismusdiagnose. Arch. Lebensmittelhyg. 10, 265–268.
74. ZEISSLER, J., C. KRAUSPE & L. RASSFELD-STERNBERG (1958/60): Die Gasödeme des Menschen. Bd. 1–3. Darmstadt: Steinkopff.

Actinomyces, Dermatophilus, Nocardia

These micro-organisms are true Gram-positive, rod-shaped bacteria, that possess the ability of forming branching filaments. It is because of this property that they are close to fungi, although they show all the characteristics of prokaryotic cells.

1 Actinomyces (Ac.)

Five species are recognized within this genus:
▷ *Ac. bovis* (animals)
▷ *Ac. israelii* (man)
▷ *Ac. naeslundii* (man)
▷ *Ac. odontolyticus* (man)
▷ *Ac. viscosus* (dog)

Ac. bovis is the cause of actinomycosis of animals (tab. 21). Actinomycosis is usually diagnosed clinically, but this does not allow for the differential diagnosis against granulomata of other aetiology (e.g. nocardiae, staphylococci). A bacteriological diagnosis can be made by the microscopic and cultural identification of the organism (4, 5, 7, 14).

■ Microscopic examination
Tissue samples or abscess smears are examined for the presence of sulphur granules, measuring 1–2 mm which can either be soft, whitish and friable or hard and granular. Smears are prepared from these and stained by Gram. The actinomycetes are Gram-positive rods or branched filaments, which can show club-shaped thickened ends that stain Gram-negatively (fig. 88).

■ Culture
The biopsy material is spread onto brain heart infusion blood agar and incubated anaerobically

(5% CO_2, 95% N_2) at 37°C. These sulphur granules, washed in sterile saline, are particularly well suited for this. An aerobic culture should be set up simultaneously as control. Flat granular colonies develop after 2–5 days which appear white and soft after 7 days (fig. 88). In exceptional cases *Ac. bovis* can also occur in the R-form.

auf brain-heart-infusion-Blutagar ausgestrichen und anaerob (5% CO_2, 95% N_2) bei 37°C bebrütet. Zur Kontrolle können gleichzeitig aerobe Kulturen angelegt werden. Nach 2–4 d entstehen zunächst flache, granulierte und nach 7 d glatte, weiße, weiche Kolonien (Abb. 88). Ausnahmsweise können bei *Ac. bovis* auch R-Formen auftreten.

■ **Biochemical properties**
For details see PIER & FICHTNER (14).

■ **Kulturell-biochemische Eigenschaften**
Siehe PIER & FICHTNER (14).

Table 21: Differentiation between the genus *Actinomyces*, *Nocardia* and *Dermatophilus* as well as the *Actinomyces* spp.

Tabelle 21. Unterscheidungsmerkmale der Gattungen *Actinomyces*, *Nocardia* und *Dermatophilus* sowie der *Actinomyces*-Arten

I. Generic characters of Actinomyces, Nocardia and Dermatophilus

Genus	Veterinary importance	Pathogen reservoir	O_2 dependence	Acid fast	Aerial mycelium	Growth on fungal media
Actinomyces	cause of focal or systemic disease, with characteristic granulomas in skin, subcutis, organs and bones	upper digestive tract, endogenous infection	anaerobic to microaerophilic	−	−	−
Nocardia		soil	aerobic	partial[1]	+	+
Dermatophilus	Dermatophilosis, skin disease of animals and man	skin parasite	aerobic, better anaerobic to microaerophil.	−	−	−

II. Characters of Actinomyces spp.

	A. bovis	A. israelii	A. odontolyticus	A. naeslundii	A. viscosus
Catalase formation	−	−	−	−	+
Urease formation	−	−	−	+	+
Gelatinolysis	−	−	−	−	v
Nitrate reduction	−	v⁺	+	v⁺	v⁺
Mannitol fermentation	−	v⁺	−	−	−
Lactose fermentation	+	v⁺	v⁺	+	+
Saccharose fermentation	+	+	+	+	+
Salicin fermentation	−	v⁺	−	v	v⁺
Glycerol fermentation	−	−	−	−	v
Arabinose fermentation	−	v⁻	v⁻	−	−
Xylose fermentation	−	v⁺	v	−	−
Raffinose fermentation	−	v⁺	−	+	+

[1] Staining by Kinyon's method with Carbol fuchsin and decolourized with 1% H_2SO_4 without alcohol addition

[1] Färbung nach Kinyon mit Karbolfuchsin und Entfärbung mit 1%iger H_2SO_4 ohne Alkoholzusatz

2 Nocardia (N.)

Three pathogenic species are recognized in this genus:
▷ *N. asteroides*, world-wide distribution,
▷ *N. brasiliensis*, Central and South America,
▷ *N. caviae*, distribution still largely unknown.

The soil is the natural reservoir of all three species and they can cause disease in man and animals. Nocardiosis may be acute to chronic, leading to the formation of abscess-like lesions in the skin, the serous membranes and the internal organs. The organisms are facultative pathogens. *N. asteroides* is by far the most common type seen.

N. asteroides
The most important diseases caused in animals by this bacterium are:

Bovine mastitis, acute to chronic forms, which are not infrequently iatrogenic, following intramammary treatment (8, 12). Other organ systems are less commonly involved but abortion and generalized infections can occur (1, 2, 3, 9, 10, 16).

Systemic nocardiosis of dogs which usually originates from a pulmonary infection may progress to a sero-purulent pleurisy and spread further even to include the central nervous system (15).

Cutaneous nocardiosis of cattle
This is a granulomatous purulent inflammation of the subcutaneous tissue and its lymph vessels. The disease is seen mainly in tropical countries. Apart from cattle, it can also affect dogs and human beings. In the latter the disease is most frequently caused by *N. brasiliensis*.

The diagnosis is confirmed by demonstration of the causal organism.

The usual test materials are exudate, pus and samples of diseased tissues. As with actinomycosis, these can contain rice grain-sized, white microcolonies that may be soft or hard; they are especially suitable for the examination.

■ **Microscopic examination** (figs. 84 and 85)
In Gram stained smears one will find, side by side, Gram-positive filaments, rods and coccoid froms. They are partially acid-fast (staining by KINYON's method with carbol fuchsin, decolouration with 1% H_2SO_4).

2 Nocardia (N.)

Innerhalb der Gattung werden 3 pathogene Arten unterschieden:
▷ *N. asteroides*, weltweit verbreitet,
▷ *N. brasiliensis*, Mittel- und Südamerika,
▷ *N. caviae*, Verbreitung noch weitgehend unbekannt.

Alle 3 Arten haben ihr natürliches Reservoir im Erdboden und können bei Mensch und Tier zu Erkrankungen führen. Nocardiosen verlaufen akut bis chronisch und führen zur Ausbildung abszeßähnlicher Gebilde in der Haut, auf den serösen Häuten und in den inneren Organen. Die Erreger sind fakultativ pathogen. Weitaus am häufigsten wird *N. asteroides* festgestellt.

N. asteroides
Die wichtigsten beim Tier vorkommenden Erkrankungsformen sind:

Bovine Mastitis, akut bis chronisch verlaufende Form, die als iatrogene Infektion nach einer intramammären Behandlung beobachtet werden kann (8, 12, 13, 21). Seltener kann es auch zu anderen Organerkrankungen, zu Aborten und Generalisationen kommen (1, 2, 3, 9, 10, 16).

Systemische Nokardiose bei Hunden, die meistens ihren Ausgang von Lungeninfektionen nimmt und in deren Verlauf es zu einer seropurulenten Pleuritis kommen kann. Es kann zu einer weiteren Ausbreitung im Organismus mit Einschluß des ZNS kommen (15).

Hautnocardiose des Rindes
Es handelt sich um eine granulomatös-eitrige Entzündung der Unterhaut und ihrer Lymphgefäße. Die Krankheit tritt hauptsächlich in tropischen Ländern auf. Neben dem Rind können auch Hund und Mensch erkranken, beim Menschen sind die Erkrankungen in Mittel- und Südamerika hauptsächlich durch *N. brasiliensis* verursacht.

Eine sichere Diagnose einer Nocardiose setzt den Nachweis des Erregers voraus.

Als Untersuchungsmaterial kommen Exsudate, Eiter und Proben der erkrankten Gewebe in Frage. In diesen können, ähnlich wie bei der Aktinomykose, etwa reiskorngroße weiche Mikrokolonien oder feste Gewebsgranula vorhanden sein, die sich für die Untersuchung besonders eignen.

■ **Mikroskopische Untersuchung** (Abb. 84 u. 85)
Bei der Gram-Färbung treten nebeneinander grampositive Fäden, Stäbchen und kokkoide Formen auf. Es besteht eine partielle Säurefestigkeit (Färbung nach KINYON mit Karbolfuchsin, die Entfärbung erfolgt mit 1%iger H_2SO_4).

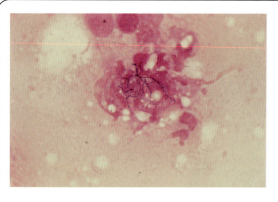
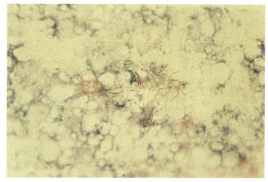
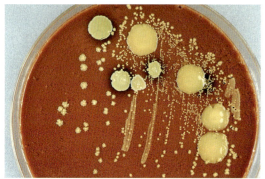
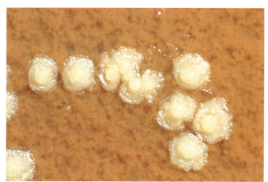

▲ Fig. 84: *Nocardia asteroides*, smear from milk of bovine mastitis, Gram stain, Gram-positive bacterial filaments. Magnification x 1000
▼ Fig. 86: *Nocardia asteroides*, mixed culture on chocolate agar, inoculated with milk from bovine mastitis, besides large colonies (contaminants) there are delicate greyish-white nocardia colonies, some have serrated edges, 48 h, 37 °C, aerobic incubation. Magnification x 0.4

▲ Fig. 85: *Nocardia asteroides*, smear from pus of a fistula in a dog, Kinyon stain, acid-fast bacteria. Magnification x 1000
▼ Fig. 87: *Nocardia asteroides*, pure culture on chocolate agar, greyish-white, irregular colonies, 48 h, 37 °C. Magnification x 5

▲ Abb. 84: *Nocardia asteroides*, Ausstrich von einer Mastitismilch eines Rindes, Gram-Färbung, grampositive Bakterienfäden, Abb.-M. 1000 : 1
▼ Abb. 86: *Nocardia asteroides*, Mischkultur auf einer Kochblutplatte, die mit Mastitismilch von einem Rind beimpft wurde, neben großen Kolonien (Kontaminanten) feine, grauweiße Nocardia-Kolonien, teilweise mit gezacktem Rand, 48 h, 37 °C, aerobe Bebrütung, Abb.-M. 1 : 2,5

▲ Abb. 85: *Nocardia asteroides*, Ausstrich von Fisteleiter eines Hundes, Färbung nach Kinyon, säurefeste Bakterien, Abb.-M. 1000 : 1
▼ Abb. 87: *Nocardia asteroides*, Reinkultur auf Kochblutagar, grauweiße, unregelmäßig geformte Kolonien, 48 h, 37 °C, Abb.-M. 5 : 1

■ **Culture** (figs. 86 and 87)
Many media are suitable for growing nocardiae, for instance: brain heart infusion blood agar or Sabouraud's dextrose agar. After 3–4 days aerobic incubation at 25–37 °C white to orange, wax-like colonies, 1–2 mm in size and firmly adherent to the medium. There is usually a small amount of aerial mycelium. After 2 to 7 days the filaments break down into coccoid or rod-like elements.

■ **Kulturelle Untersuchung** (Abb. 86 u. 87)
Es sind zahlreiche Medien verwendbar, wie z.B. brain-heart-infusion-Blutagar oder Dextroseagar nach Sabouraud. Nach aerober Bebrütung bei 25–37 °C bilden sich nach 3–4 d kleine, 1–2 mm große, dem Nährboden anhaftende, weiß bis orange gefärbte, wachsartige Kolonien, die meistens ein geringes Luftmyzel ausbilden. Die Fäden zerfallen nach 2–7 d in kokkoide und stäbchenförmige Elemente.

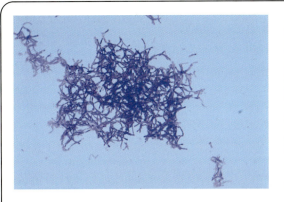
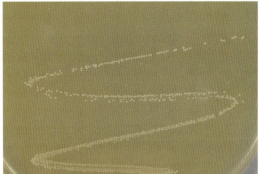
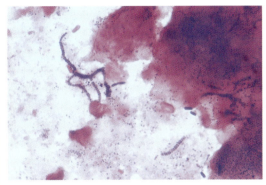
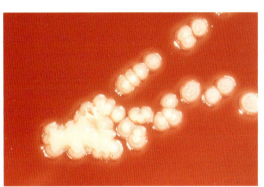

▲ Fig. 88: *Actinomyces bovis*, smear of brain-heart infusion broth, Gram stain, Gram-positive branching filaments. Magnification x 1000
▼ Fig. 90: *Dermatophilus congolensis*, smear from skin lesion of a horse, Gram stain, Gram-positive bacteria with micro-organisms arranged in rouleaux form. Magnification x 1000

▲ Fig. 89: *Actinomyces bovis*, pure culture on brain-heart infusion agar, smooth white colonies, anaerobic incubation, 6 d, 37 °C. Magnification x 0.5
▼ Fig. 91: *Dermatophilus congolensis*, pure culture on blood agar, firmly adherent, greyish-white to yellowish colonies with irregular surfaces and haemolysis, anaerobic incubation, 48 h, 37 °C. Magnification x 2

▲ Abb. 88: *Actinomyces bovis*, Ausstrich von einer Brain-Heart-Infusion-Bouillon, Gram-Färbung, grampositive Fäden mit Verzweigungen, Abb.-M. 1000 : 1
▼ Abb. 90: *Dermatophilus congolesis*, Ausstrich aus Hautveränderungen eines Pferdes, Gram-Färbung, grampositive Bakterien mit geldrollenförmig hintereinander gelagerten Mikroorganismen, Abb.-M. 1000 : 1

▲ Abb. 89: *Actinomyces bovis*, Reinkultur auf Brain-Heart-Infusion-Agar, glatte, weiße Kolonien, anaerob brütet, 6 d, 37 °C, Abb.-M. 1 : 2
▼ Abb. 91: *Dermatophilus congolensis*, Reinkultur auf Blutagar, fest anhaftende, grauweiße bis gelbliche Kolonien mit unregelmäßiger Oberfläche und Hämolyse, anaerob brütet, 48 h, 37 °C, Abb.-M. 1 : 2

3 Dermatophilus (D.)

Dermatophilus congolensis belongs to this genus.

D. congolensis is responsible for a dermatitis in man and many animals. The causal organism grows in the epidermis and develops mycelial filaments, causing massive exudation with stratified scabs in which it can survive for a long time. Certain predisposing factors must be present for the disease to

3 Dermatophilus (D.)

Die Gattung enthält als Spezies *Dermatophilus congolensis*.

D. congolensis verursacht bei vielen Tierarten und beim Menschen eine Dermatitis. Der Erreger wächst in der Epidermis zu myzelartigen Fäden aus und verursacht eine massive Exsudation mit Ausbildung lamellär geschichteter Borken, in denen er

Table 22: Biochemical behaviour of *Dermatophilus congolensis* (19)

Tabelle 22: Kulturell-biochemisches Verhalten von *Dermatophilus congolensis* (19)

Motility	+	Dul	−
Glu	+	Ind	−
Lac	−	MR	−
Sac	v	VPR	−
Gal	v	Ure	+
Sor	−	Gel	+
Fru	+	Nit	−
Man	−	Cat	+

develop, these include lowered resistance of the skin, injuries, other skin conditions, climatic influences.

In Germany the disease has been described, in horses, cattle, sheep and other animals (11, 17, 18, 19, 20). In sheep one differentiates between »lumpy wool disease« (encrustation and matting of the wool) and »strawberry foot rot« (scabs and erosions on the head and distal parts of the limbs, which bear no wool) (11).

The bacteriological diagnosis is based on the demonstration of the organism.

■ **Microscopical examination** (fig. 90)

Gram-positive coccoid bacteria are to be seen in the crushed scabs, some may be found lying one behind the other in the typical rouleaux form. Cell division in two planes results in groups of four.

■ **Culture** (fig. 91)

This organism grows best under microaerophilic (increased CO_2 content) to anaerobic conditions. A gas mixture consisting of 95 % N_2 and 5 % CO_2, has been found effective and an aerobic atmosphere can slow growth considerably.

Dry, greyish-yellow, distinctly haemolytic colonies, 1–2 mm in size and firmly adherent to the medium develop within 1–2 days. On further incubation these colonies turn yellowish-orange and mucoid, producing drawn out threads when touched (11, 19, 20). *Dermatophilus* will not grow on the usual fungal media (Sabouraud's, Kimmig etc.).

■ **Biochemical properties**

Are summarized in table 22.

■ **Mikroskopische Untersuchung** (Abb. 90)

In den zermörserten Sekretkrusten finden sich grampositive, kokkoide Bakterien, die teilweise in einer typischen Geldrollenform aneinandergereiht liegen. Durch Teilung in 2 Ebenen können Vierergruppen gebildet werden.

■ **Kulturelle Untersuchung** (Abb. 91)

Der Keim wächst am besten unter mikroaerophilen (Erhöhung der CO_2-Konzentration) bis anaeroben Bedingungen, bewährt hat sich ein Gasgemisch aus 95 % N_2 und 5 % CO_2. Unter aeroben Verhältnissen kann das Wachstum stark verzögert sein.

Innerhalb von 1–2 d bilden sich 1–2 mm große, dem Nährboden fest anhaftende, trockene, graugelbliche Kolonien mit einer deutlichen Hämolyse. Bei weiterer Bebrütung werden die Kolonien gelborange, schleimig und fadenziehend (11, 19, 20). Auf den üblichen Pilznährböden (Sabouraud, Kimmig u. a.) wächst Dermatophilus nicht.

■ **Kulturell-biochemische Eigenschaften**

Siehe Tabelle 22.

Bibliography / Literatur

1. BEERWERTH, W. (1960): Generalisierte Aktinomykose (Nocardiose) beim Rind. Mhefte Tierhk. **12**, Sonderteil Rindertuberkulose und Brucellose **9**, 1–9.
2. DOGUER, M. (1962): Ein pathogener Mikroorganismus (Nocardia) isoliert aus den Lungen eines Kalbes. Zbl. Bakt. I. Orig. **185**, 395–397.
3. FEY, H., P. HOLM & E. TEUSCHER (1954): Nocardiosen. Kasuistische Mitteilung über einen Fall von septischer Nocardiose beim Hund und zwei Fälle von Nocardia-Abortus beim Rind. Schweiz. Arch. Tierhk. **96**, 642–648.

4. Franke, F. (1973): Die mikrobiologische Diagnostik der Gesäugeaktinomykose der Schweine. Berl. Münch. tierärztl. Wschr. **86**, 428–432.
5. Franke, F. (1973): Untersuchungen zur Ätiologie der Gesäugeaktinomykose des Schweines. Zbl. Bakt. I. Orig. A **223**, 111–124.
6. Franke, F. (1971): Untersuchungen über die in vitro-Empfindlichkeit von aus aktinomykotischen Gesäugen von Sauen isolierten mikroaerophilen Aktinomyzeten gegen Antibiotika. Dtsch. tierärztl. Wschr. **78**, 574–576.
7. Grässer, R. (1962): Mikroaerophile Actinomyceten und Gesäugeaktinomykose des Schweines. Zbl. Bakt. I. Orig. **184**, 478–492.
8. Hillermark, K. (1960): Nocardia asteroides als Ursache boviner Mastitis. Acta vet. scand. **1**, 281–293.
9. Lindt, S., H. König & H. Fey (1961): Nocardiosen beim Rind. Schweiz. Arch. Tierhk. **103**, 468–478.
10. Monga, D. P., M. P. Kapur & S. N. Dixit (1978): Bovine abortion caused by Nocardia asteroides. Mykosen **21**, 152–153.
11. Mumme, J., & R. Supper (1982): Dermatophilose in einer Schafherde. Tierärztl. Praxis **10**, 153–161.
12. Nassal, J. (1967): Akute Nocardia-Mastitis beim Rind. Dtsch. tierärztl. Wschr. **74.**, 434–437.
13. Pier, A. C., M. J. Mejia & E. H. Willers (1961): Nocardia asteroides as a mammary pathogen of cattle. I. The disease in cattle and the comparative virulence of 5 isolates. Amer. J. Vet. Res. **22**, 502–517.
14. Pier, A. C., & R. E. Fichtner (1985): Actinomyces, Dermatophilus, Nocardia. In: H. Blobel & T. Schliesser (Hrsg.): Handbuch der bakteriellen Infektionen bei Tieren. Bd. V, S. 532–551. Jena: VEB Gustav Fischer.
15. Swerczek, T. W., B. Schiefer & S. W. Nielsen (1968): Canine actinomycosis. Zbl. Vet. med. B **15**, 955–970.
16. Wall, G. v. d. (1964): Lungen-Nocardiose beim Kalb. Dtsch. tierärztl. Wschr. **71**, 11–16.
17. Weber, A. (1978): Die Dermatophilose bei Mensch und Tier. Berl. Münch. tierärztl. Wschr. **91**, 341–345.
18. Weber, A., K. Frese & O. Reitz (1975): Eine Hauterkrankung beim Rind, hervorgerufen durch Dermatophilus congolensis. Tierärztl. Praxis **3**, 175–179.
19. Weber, A., & T. Schliesser (1971): Mikrobiologische Untersuchungen an zwei Stämmen von Dermatophilus congolensis van Saceghem 1915. Zbl. Vet. Med. B, **18**, 546–556.
20. Weiss, R., K. H. Böhm & P. Witzmann (1976): Dermatitis bei Pferden, hervorgerufen durch Dermatophilus congolensis Saceghem 1915. Berl. Münch. tierärztl. Wschr. **89**, 109–112.
21. Zureck, F. (1963): Nocardia asteroides als Ursache einer Euterentzündung beim Rind. Zbl. Bakt. I. Orig. **188**, 377–383.

Mycobacteria
Mykobakterien

Genus Mycobacterium (M.) of the family Mycobacteriaceae; acid-fast bacteria.

The genus contains a multitude of species of varying pathogenicity (tab. 23), all of which have the following properties in common: They are rods of various lengths, non-motile and non-sporulating. Because of their particular biochemical make-up they are difficult to stain, but once the stains are taken up they are difficult to remove, even with acid alcohol; they are acid-fast.

1 Tubercle bacilli and atypical mycobacteria

■ **Incidence and veterinary importance**
The susceptibility of animals to experimental subcutaneous injection is shown in table 24.

The natural aetiological conditions are produced in table 25. In veterinary medicine the typical tubercle bacilli are *M. bovis* and *M. avium* (despite their special taxonomic position) and for some animals *M. tuberculosis*. The other mycobacteria may induce disease in some instances, they are opportunists (atypical mycobacteria).

■ **Morphology and microscopic identification**
The typical tubercle bacilli are slender rods $0.2–0.5 \times 1–4$ μm.

In veterinary medicine a direct smear is usually prepared from the test material to demonstrate their presence. From some such materials it is difficult to prepare a smear, (e.g. caseous tissues, tenacious mucus from the lungs) and this can be pre-treated enzymically (pancreatin, trypsin, papain) or with alkaline solutions.

The staining methods make use of the property of acid-fastness.

Genus *Mycobacterium* (M.) der Familie *Mycobacteriaceae*; säurefeste Bakterien.

Die Gattung enthält eine Vielzahl von Arten unterschiedlicher Pathogenität (Tab. 23), die in folgenden Eigenschaften übereinstimmen: unterschiedlich lange Stäbchen, unbeweglich, keine Sporenbildung, wegen der besonderen biochemischen Struktur schwer anfärbbar, einmal aufgenommene Farbstoffe werden auch in salzsaurem Alkohol nur schwer abgegeben (säurefeste Bakterien).

1 Tuberkelbakterien und atypische Mykobakterien

■ **Vorkommen und medizinische Bedeutung**
Die experimentelle Empfindlichkeit von Tieren (nach sbk. Infektion) ist in der Tab. 24 zusammengestellt.

Unter natürlichen Verhältnissen bestehen die in Tab. 25 dargelegten ätiologischen Verhältnisse. Als typische Tuberkuloseerreger müssen in der Veterinärmedizin *M. bovis*, *M. avium* (trotz der besonderen taxonomischen Stellung) und für einige Tierarten *M. tuberculosis* gelten. Die übrigen Mykobakterien können in Einzelfällen zu Erkrankungen führen, sie verhalten sich opportunistisch (atypische Mykobakterien).

■ **Morphologie und mikroskopischer Nachweis**
Bei den typischen Tuberkelbakterien handelt es sich um schlanke, $0,2–0,5 \times 1–4$ μm lange Stäbchen.

Bei ihrem Nachweis werden in der Veterinärmedizin von dem Untersuchungsmaterial meistens Direktausstriche angefertigt. Schwer ausstreichbares Material (z. B. verkästes Gewebe, zäher Lungenschleim) kann enzymatisch (Pankreatin, Trypsin, Papain) oder mit alkalischen Lösungen vorbehandelt werden.

Die Färbeverfahren nutzen die Säure-Alkohol-Festigkeit aus.

Table 23: Summary of the recognized Mycobacteria spp. (after SCHLIESSER, 26)

Tabelle 23. Zusammenstellung anerkannter Mykobakterienarten (nach SCHLIESSER, 26)

Group	Mycobacterium species	
Tuberculosis complex, slow growing	tuberculosis (typ. humanus) bovis (typus bovis)	africanum[1] microti (muris, vole bacillus)[2]
I (after Runyon) slow growing photochromogenic	asiaticum kansasii (lucriflavum)	marinum (balnei, platypoecilus) simiae (habana)
II (after Runyon) slow growing scotochromogenic	flavescens (acapulcensis) gordonae (aquae)	scrofulaceum (marianum) szulgai
III (after Runyon) slow growing non-chromogenic	avium (typus gallinaceus) gastri haemophilum intracellulare (Battey bacillus, brunense) malmoense nonchromogenicum	terrae (Radish bacillus, novum) triviale ulcerans (buruli) xenopi (littorale)
IV (after Runyon) rapid growing	aurum chelonei, (abscessus, borstelense, friedmanii, runyonii) chitae duvalii farcinogenes (Nocardia farcinica?) fortuitum (giae, minetti, peregrinum, ranae, salmoniphilum)	gadium gilvum komossense neoaurum parafortuitum (diernhoferi?) phlei (grass bacillus, timothy bacillus, moelleri) senegalense (Nocardia farcinica?) smegmatis (aquae, butyricum, friburgensis, lacticola) thermoresistibile vaccae
Others	paratuberculosis leprae lepraemurium	

( ) older or synonymous names; [1] does not occur in animals; [2] natural host is the field mouse

( ) = ältere oder synonyme Bezeichnung; [1] kommt bei Tieren nicht vor; [2] natürlicher Wirt Feldmaus

▷ Bright-field microscopy: Ziehl-Neelsen stain (p. 337; fig. 93). The mycobacteria appear red on a blue background. Such a microscopic demonstration is possible if bacteria are present in the material at the rate of 5×10^4/ml. The mycobacteria often appear irregularly stained (beaded).
▷ Fluorescence microscopy: The preparation is stained with fluorescent dyes (fluorochrome). This method is used relatively rarely in veterinary work, but it has the advantage that, because of the greater resolution, objectives with a magnifying power of only 20–50 times, can be used. A larger field can thus be searched. Other dyes are auramine and acridine orange.

▷ Hellfeldmikroskopie: Ziehl-Neelsen-Färbung (s. S. 337; Abb. 93). Die Mykobakterien erscheinen rot auf blauem Untergrund. Ein mikroskopischer Nachweis wird möglich, wenn 5×10^4 Bakterien/ml im Material vorhanden sind. Die Mykobakterien erscheinen oft ungleichmäßig (granuliert) gefärbt.
▷ Fluoreszenzmikroskopie: Dabei werden die Präparate mit fluoreszierenden Farbstoffen (Fluorochrome) gefärbt. Die Färbemethode, die in der Veterinärmedizin relativ selten benutzt wird, hat den Vorteil, daß infolge des höheren Auflösungsvermögens eine Untersuchung mit 20- bis 50fach vergrößernden Objektiven erfolgen kann, so daß ein größeres Gesichtsfeld durchmustert werden kann. Als Farbstoffe kommen Auramin und Akridinorange in Frage.

Table 24: Susceptibility of animals to subcutaneously administered tubercle bacilli (26)

Species	M. bovis	M. tuberculosis	M. avium
Monkey (rhesus)	+++	+++	(+)
Ape (chimpanzee)	+++	+++	–
Ox	++	–	+
Sheep	++	–	+
Goat	++	–	+
Pig	++	++	(+)
Horse	(+)	–	(+)
Dog	(+)	(+)	–
Cat	+	(+)	(+)
Guinea pig	+++	+++	+
Rabbit	+++	–	++
Mouse	(+)	(+)	+
Rat	–	–	–
Poultry	–	–	+++

– not susceptible; (+) slightly susceptible; + local reaction; ++ susceptible; +++ highly susceptible

■ Demonstration of mycobacteria by culture

The following procedures are required for demonstrating the organism by means of culture:
▷ Preparation of the test material in particular the killing off of contaminants,
▷ inoculation and incubation of the media,
▷ evaluation of the cultures and identification of the mycobacteria.

The test routine is illustrated in figure 92. The elimination of contaminants is possible, because mycobacteria are more resistant to acid and alkaline solutions than other bacteria. The prescribed exposure times must be carefully adhered to in order to avoid damage of the mycobacteria.

For samples of animal origin, which are frequently contaminated, the pre-treatment with sulphuric acid has been found effective (fig. 92). Other decontamination agents are 3 % HCl, 4 % NaOH, 20–30 % papain solution (26). The choice of agent depends largely on the degree of contamination and the type of test material. BEERWERTH (1, 2) has recommended the successive treatment first with 4 % NaOH for 20 minutes, followed by 5 % oxalic acid for another 20 minutes.

Numerous media have been described for the isolation of mycobacteria, however, the most successful are the egg-based media, such as Petragnani's (also in Witte's modification) and Löwenstein-Jensen medium (composition in table 26). All these can be obtained ready made, and they contain malachite green for the suppression of contaminants.

The media are in the form of »slopes«, that is to say they are poured into test tubes and solidify in sloping position so as to present a larger area for inoculation. The stopper must allow the necessary

gaseous exchange and prevent desiccation. This can be achieved with rubber stoppers that have spiral shaped perforations, with screw caps etc.

For optimum results it is desirable to meet the varying requirements of different mycobacteria for glycerol and oxygen. Thus, the human, avian and most of the atypical mycobacteria have an absolute requirement for glycerol and the opportunity for gaseous exchange if optimum growth is to be obtained on primary culture. Bovine strains, on the other hand, grow best in air-tight containers on glycerol-free media.

Taking these requirements into consideration and making use of two selective media (pyromucin hydrazide 10 µg/ml, and toluidin blue 0.03 %), NASSAL (17, 18) developed a satisfactory system for

Die Nährmedien werden in Schrägform in Reagenzröhrchen abgefüllt. Der Verschluß muß den erforderlichen Gasaustausch gewährleisten und eine Austrocknung verhindern. Dies ist z. B. mit spiralförmig durchbohrten Gummistopfen, mit Schraubverschlüssen u. ä. erreichbar.

Für optimale Kulturergebnisse ist es erforderlich, dem unterschiedlichen Glycerin- und Sauerstoffbedürfnis der Mykobakterien zu entsprechen. So benötigen humane und aviäre Stämme sowie die meisten atypischen Mykobakterien für ein optimales Wachstum in der Erstkultur unbedingt Glycerin und die Möglichkeit eines Gasaustausches, während bovine Stämme am besten auf glycerinfreien und luftdicht abgeschlossenen Nährböden wachsen.

Nach NASSAL (17, 18) hat sich unter Berücksich-

Table 25: Incidence and significance of the most important mycobacteria in animals

Tabelle 25. Vorkommen und Bedeutung der wichtigsten Mykobakterien bei Tieren

Group of Runyon	Mycobacteria	Incidence and significance	Literature References
	M. tuberculosis- M. bovis complex	tuberculosis in mammals and man	27, 28
I photochromogenic	M. kansasii-group M. simiae	saprophyte, rarely mycobacteriosis in man, infections in animals very rare (ox, pig)	1, 2, 8, 9, 28
	M. marinum	tuberculosis of fish & amphibia (other mycobacteria, especially from group IV can be the cause)	28
II scotochromogenic	M. gordonae M. scrofulaceum	ubiquitous saprophyte, especially in meadow land, rarely cause of human mycobacteriosis, generally non-pathogenic in animals. It can occasionally induce lesions in intestinal lymph nodes (ox, pig), dermatitis nodosa (ox) or other changes	28, 29, 31
III non-chromogenic	M. avium serotypes 1–3	tuberculosis of poultry, isolated cases of intestinal tuberculosis in pigs and other mammals. Generalized form rare in mammals, e. g. bovine abortion. Serotype 2 is the most common in Germany. Rare cause of human mycobacteriosis	7, 21, 28, 30, 38
	M. intracellulare more than 20 serotypes (4–28)	saprophyte of soil and water, cause of avian tuberculosis and less commonly of mammalian infections. Especially in pigs cause of an intestinal lymph node tuberculosis, which is often due to contaminated sawdust used for bedding (especially serotype 8 [Davis])	3, 6, 12, 13, 28, 32, 33, 38
	M. terrae M. triviale	saprophyte in soil and water, mainly non-pathogenic to animals, occasionally lymph node infection and »skin lesions«	1, 2, 28
IV rapidly growing	M. fortuitum-group of: M. fortuitum M. chelonei M. phlei M. smegmatis M. vaccae	saprophyte living in soil, water and on plants, found regularly in the gut of ruminants, pigs and other animals, occasionally pathogenic, bovine mastitis and nodular thelitis, nodular dermatitis, lesions in the intestinal lymph nodes	1, 7, 16, 28, 29

Differentiation of mycobacteria grown in culture

Mycobacteria are identified largely by virtue of their biochemical properties. A multitude of characteristics have been described, but these could only be fully utilized in the course of very specialized investigation. Under diagnostic laboratory conditions the primary question to be answered is whether the isolated organism is a genuine cause of tuberculosis. The methods which can be used to answer this question are shown in figures 92 and 97 and in table 27 (17, 18, 20, 26).

Differenzierung der isolierten Mykobakterien

Die Bestimmung eines Mykobakterienisolates erfolgt wesentlich über kulturell-biochemische Eigenschaften. Es sind eine Vielzahl von Merkmalen beschrieben worden, deren erschöpfende Ausnutzung nur im Rahmen spezieller Fragestellungen erforderlich ist. Unter den Bedingungen eines diagnostischen Laboratoriums muß primär entschieden werden, ob es sich bei dem Isolat um einen echten Tuberkuloseerreger handelt. Die für die Beantwortung dieser Frage geeigneten Untersuchungsmethoden siehe Abb. 92, 97 und Tab. 27 (17, 18, 20, 26).

Specimens
Organs, pus, lymph nodes, punctates, milk etc.

Microscopic examination
Staining with Ziehl-Neelsen, red mycobacteria on blue background (fig. 93). Minimum search time: 5 to 10 minutes

Examination by culture
1. Preparation of the test material: about 25 g of the organ material is ground mechanically and homogenized after the addition of 50 ml physiological saline. Fluid material is centrifuged at 3000 RPM for 15–20 mins.
2. Decontamination: the homogenized material or the sediment is mixed with 4 to 6 times its volume of acid (e. g. 3–6 % H_2SO_4) and left to stand for 10 (–15) minutes and again centrifuged for 10 (–15) minutes.
3. Nutrient media: egg medium of Hohn, Petragnani or Löwenstein-Jensen (some obtainable commercially as ready tubes). Glycerol-containing media for the isolation of M. bovis.
4. Inoculation of media: vigorous strokes with the loop or Pasteur pipette, starting in the condensation fluid at the bottom of the tube and covering the whole of the surface of the slope. At lest 2-3 different media should be inoculated per test sample.
5. Incubation: aerobically at 37 °C for a maximum of 8–12 weeks.
6. Assessment of cultures: cultures should be read once a week and Ziehl-Neelsen stained smears should be prepared from suspicious colonies. The rapidity of growth provides the first indication as to the type of mycobacterium present. If visible colonies appear: in less than 5 days: rapidly growing mycobacteria (group IV Runyon) in more than 5 days: group of tubercle bacilli or groups I-III of Runyon (further differentiation is shown in figure 97 and table 27).

Demonstration of organism by animal inoculation
This would only be considered for the identification of M. tuberculosis or *M. bovis*. The sulphuric acid added previously is removed by twice washing with physiological saline and about 2 ml are injected subcutaneously into the knee fold of a guinea pig. Test period is 6–8 weeks. Any animals that die before or are killed at the end of this period are examined *post mortem* and the iliac and subiliac lymph nodes are cultured and examined microscopically for the presence of tubercle bacilli.

Fig. 92: Bacteriological demonstration of tubercle bacilli

Abb. 92: Bakteriologischer Nachweis von Tuberkelbakterien

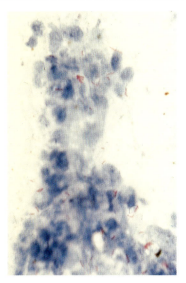
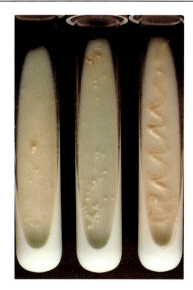
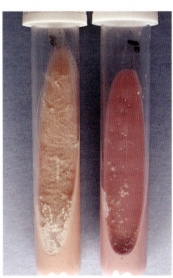
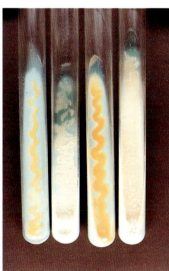

▲ Fig. 93: *Mycobacterium bovis*, smear from a bovine lymph node, Ziehl-Neelsen stain, red acid-fast rods. Magnification x 1000
▼ Fig. 95: Growth of *M. tuberculosis* and *M. bovis* on bromcresol purple medium, left tube: *M. tuberculosis*, eugonic growth with climbing phenomenon and discolouration of the medium, right tube: *M. bovis*, dysgonic growth without climbing phenomenon or discolouration of the medium. 8 weeks, 37°C. Magnification x 0.4

▲ Fig. 94: Mycobacteria, cultures on Hohn's medium, left tube eugonic growth of *M. tuberculosis* in dry firm colonies, middle tube dysgonic growth of *M. bovis*, right tube eugonic growth of *M. avium* in moist, waxy colonies. 8 weeks at 37°C. Magnification x 0.4
▼ Fig. 96: Atypical mycobacteria, from right to left: *M. vaccae, M. smegmatis, M. fortuitum* and *M. scrofulaceum*. Various incubation times. Magnification x 0.4

▲ Abb. 93: *Mycobacterium bovis*, Ausstrich aus einem Lymphknoten eines Rindes, Ziehl-Neelsen-Färbung, rote säurefeste Stäbchen, Abb.-M. 1000:1
▼ Abb. 95: Wachstum von *M. tuberculosis* und *M. bovis* auf Bromkresolpurpur-Nährboden, linkes Röhrchen: *M. tuberculosis*, eugones Wachstum mit Kletterphänomen und Verfärbung des Nährbodens, rechtes Röhrchen: *M. bovis*, dysgones Wachstum ohne Kletterphänomen und ohne Verfärbung des Nährbodens, 8 Wochen, 37°C, Abb.-M. 1:2,5

▲ Abb. 94: Mykobakterien, Kultur auf Nährboden nach Hohn, linkes Röhrchen eugones Wachstum von *M. tuberculosis* in trockenen, festen Kolonien, mittleres Röhrchen dysgones Wachstum von *M. bovis*, rechtes Röhrchen eugones Wachstum von *M. avium* in feuchten, schmierigen Kolonien, 8 Wochen, 37°C, Abb.-M. 1:2,5
▼ Abb. 96: Atypische Mykobakterien, von rechts nach links: *M. vaccae, M. smegmatis, M. fortuitum* und *M. scrofulaceum*, unterschiedliche Bebrütungszeiten, Abb.-M. 1:2,5

Table 26: Isolation and initial differentiation of mycobacteria (after NASSAL, 18; NEUSCHULZ, 20)

Petragani media				Mycobacterium, initial identification		
with glycerol		no glycerol		with glycerol and gas exchange		
with gas exchange	No gas exchange	with gas exchange	no gas exchange	with PMH	with toluidine blue	
++	+	(+)	−	+	−	M. tuberculosis
(+)	+	+	++	−	−	M. bovis
++	+	+	+	+	+	atypical Mycobacteria

− no growth; (+) to ++ degrees of growth; PMH = pyromucin hydrazide

Tabelle 26. Isolierung und vorläufige Unterscheidung von Mykobakterien (nach NASSAL, 18; NEUSCHULZ, 20)

− kein Wachstum; (+) bis ++ Grad des Wachstums; PMH = Brenzschleimsäurehydrazid

▷ Growth intensity: Eugonic growth: rapid, luxuriant colonies which are visible after 2 to 3 weeks, *M. tuberculosis*, *M. avium*;

dysgonic growth: slow, sparse colonies visible after 4 weeks, *M. bovis*.

▷ Colony form (fig. 94): *M. tuberculosis*: dry, cauliflower-like, yellowish colonies that are difficult to break up;

M. bovis: small, roundish, flat, whitish colonies with a moist sheen, that break up easily;

M. avium: whitish, sticky, honey-like film or crater-shaped colonies that break up readily.

▷ Pigment formation (fig. 96): This is tested on Löwenstein-Jensen medium and serves to characterize atypical mycobacteria: photochromogenic strains grow in the dark without pigment. To demonstrate photochromogenicity young, well developed colonies should be exposed in electric light (100 watt clear bulb) for at least 1 hour at a distance of 50 cm and then incubated again in darkness for a further 1–3 days (MEISSNER, 15).

Scotochromogenic strains develop yellowish-orange colonies in the dark.

The rapidly growing mycobacteria produce colourless or greyish-red colonies.

▷ Temperature requirements: This is also tested on Löwenstein-Jensen medium and a water bath should be used at temperatures above 37 °C.

▷ Acid production from glycerol (fig. 95): Either the bromcresol purple medium of WAGENER & MISCHERLICH (36) or the phenol red-malachite green medium of NASSAL (18) are used to test for acid production.

Bromcresol purple — uninoculated medium: purple

M. tuberculosis — colour change to yellow

M. bovis — no colour change

M. avium — purple becomes slightly lighter

Phenol red-malachite green — uninoculated medium: green

M. tuberculosis — colour change to light yellow

M. bovis — no colour change

▷ Wachstumsintensität: Eugonisches Wachstum: schnell, üppig, sichtbare Kolonien nach 2 bis 3 Wochen, *M. tuberculosis*, *M. avium*;

dysgonisches Wachstum: langsam, spärlich, sichtbare Kolonien nach 4 Wochen, *M. bovis*.

▷ Kolonieform (Abb. 94): *M. tuberculosis*: trocken, »blumenkohl- oder streuselkuchenförmig«, gelblich, schwer verreibbar;

M. bovis: klein, rundlich, flach, feucht-glänzend graugelb, leicht verreibbar;

M. avium: schmierig-honigartig, goldgelbe Beläge oder kraterförmige Kolonien, leicht verreibbar.

▷ Pigmentbildung (Abb. 96): Sie wird auf Löwenstein-Jensen-Medium geprüft und dient der Charakterisierung der atypischen Mykobakterien: Photochromogene Stämme wachsen im Dunkeln pigmentlos. Zum Nachweis der Photochromogenität sollen junge, gut gewachsene Kolonien mindestens 1 h von elektrischem Lampenlicht (100 Watt-Birne mit durchsichtigem Glas) in einer Entfernung von 50 cm angestrahlt und dann weiter im Dunkeln 1 (bis 3) d bebrütet werden (MEISSNER, 15).

Skotochromogene Stämme wachsen im Dunkeln gelb-orange.

Die schnellwachsenden Mykobakterien wachsen farblos oder grau rötlich bis orange.

▷ Temperaturverhalten: Prüfung auf Löwenstein-Jensen-Medium, bei Temperaturen über 37 °C soll ein Wasserbad benutzt werden.

▷ Säurebildung aus Glycerin (Abb. 95): Die Feststellung erfolgt entweder auf dem Bromkresolpurpurnährboden nach WAGENER & MITSCHERLICH (36):

Farbe des unbeimpften Nährbodens: violett,

M. tuberculosis: Farbumschlag nach gelb,

M. bovis: kein Farbumschlag,

M. avium: leichte Aufhellung der violetten Farbe, oder auf dem Phenolrot-Malachitgrün-Nährboden nach NASSAL (18):

Farbe des unbeimpften Nährbodens: rot,

M. tuberculosis: Farbumschlag nach hellgelb,

M. bovis: kein Farbumschlag,

M. avium — colour change to yellowish-brown or yellowish-orange

▷ Niacin test: Especially well suited for the recognition of *M. tuberculosis*

Test material — heavy growth of pure culture on Löwenstein-Jensen medium

Extraction of Niacin: The culture is flooded with 1–2 ml of distilled water; tubes are inclined and the extraction time is 20–30 minutes;

Reaction — to 1 ml of extraction fluid pipetted off, 1 ml of 10% BrCN solution and 1 ml of an alcoholic aniline solution are added. A positive result is shown by an intense yellow colour within 5 minutes. For reasons of safety the reaction should be carried out in a fume cupboard. After the test has

M. avium: Farbumschlag nach gelbbraun bis gelborange.

▷ Niazintest: Der Test ist zur Erkennung von *M. tuberculosis* besonders geeignet.

Ausgangsmaterial: gut bewachsende Reinkultur (Löwenstein-Jensen-Medium),

Extraktion von Niazin: Übergießen der Kultur mit 1–2 ml Aqua dest. Extraktionszeit in Schräglage 20–30 min;

Reaktion: Zu 1 ml der abpipettierten Extraktionsflüssigkeit werden 1 ml einer 10%igen BrCN-Lösung und 1 ml einer 4%igen alkoholischen Anilinlösung gegeben. Im positiven Fall tritt innerhalb von 5 min eine intensive Gelbfärbung auf. Die Aktion muß aus Sicherheitsgründen unter dem Abzug

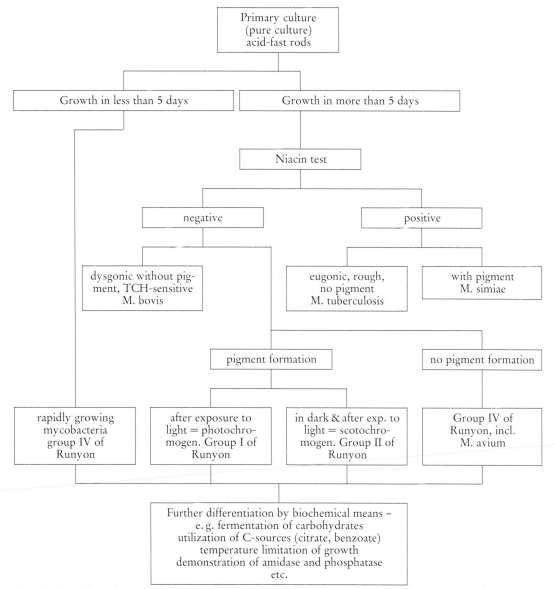

Fig. 97: Simplified schedule for identification of mycobacteria (after SCHLIESSER, 26)

Abb. 97: Vereinfachtes Schema zur Identifizierung von Mykobakterien (nach SCHLIESSER, 26)

been read the same quantity of NaOH is added in order to prevent the formation of dangerous HCN gas (5, 14, 18).

The Peknice test is safer and need not be carried out under fume extraction. To 1 ml of extract 1 ml of a 1 % solution of KCN or NaCN is added and 1 ml of a 5 % solution of chloramine-T. A few drops of 10 % NaOH are added before the test is discarded for autoclaving (5).

▷ Inhibitor tests: One can use either pyromucin hydrazide (PMH) or Thiophen-2-carbonic acid hydrazide (TCH) to differentiate between *M. bovis* and *M. tuberculosis*. As a rule these substances are added to the Löwenstein-Jensen medium before it sets; the final concentration is 10 µg/ml. The growth of *M. bovis* strains is inhibited (except the INAH-resistant strains). *M. avium* can be identified with the toluidine blue medium of NASSAL (17) (0.023 % in the Petragnani-Witte medium, table 26).

▷ Nitrate reduction: The $NaNO_3$ solution must be made up fresh before the test: 0.085 g $NaNO_3$ is dissolved in 100 ml M/45 phosphate buffer, pH 7.0 = 3.024 g KH_2PO_4 + 3.156 g Na_2HPO_4 each in 1 l of distilled water. 2 ml of the sterile $NaNO_3$ solution is inoculated with a loopful of mycobacteria and incubated at 37 °C for 4 hours. This is followed by the addition of 1 ml each of 50 % HCl solution, 0.2 % aqueous sulphonamide solution and

Table 27: Biochemical differentiation between the tubercle bacilli of animals (after SCHLIESSER, 26)

Characters	M. tuberculosis	M. bovis	M. avium
Growth rate	>5 d	>5 d	>5 d
Growth type and colony form on glycerol-containing media	eugonic cauliflower-like firmly adherent colonies from which no homogeneous suspension can be made	dysgonic small, flat, moist, glistening, round colonies, easily broken up	eugonic moist, whitish fairly profuse film, easily broken up crater formation
Pigment formation	–	–	–
Upper temp. limit	42 °C	42 °C	44 °C
Gylcerol requirement	+	–	+
Gylcerol acid formation	+	–	v
Niacin test	+	–	–
TCH-inhibited (10 µg/ml)	–	+	–
Toluidine blue inhibited	+	+	–
Nitrate reduction	+	–	–
Urease	+	+	–
Nicotinamidase	+	–	+
Pyrazineamidase	+	–	+

Table 28: Serotypes of *M. avium* and *M. intracellulare* (after SCHLIESSER, 26)

M. avium		*M. intracellulare*	
1 (I)	4 (IV)	13 (Chance)	21
2 (II)	5 (V)	14 (Boone)	22
3 (III)	6 (VI)	15 (Dent)	23 (Brockett)
	7 (VII)	16 (Yandle)	24
	8 (Davis)	17 (Wilson)	25
	9 (Watson)	18 (Altman)	26 (Cox)
	10 (III a)	19 (Darden)	27 (Harrison)
	11 (III b)	20 (Arnold)	28
	12 (Howell)		

( ) older designation

0.1% aqueous N-ethylene diamine dihydrochloride solution. A pink to red colour appears if the test is positive. A negative control test should be run alongside (34).

Other biochemical reactions are reviewed by SCHLIESSER (26), e.g. demonstration of amidase after Bönecke (4, 26), demonstration of phosphatase (11, 26), hydrolysis of Tween 80 (26, 37), demonstration of aryl sulphatase (26).

▷ Climbing phenomenon: Provided the moisture content of a solid sloped medium is maintained, a film of bacterial growth may rise up the glass tube from the condensation fluid at the bottom. This climbing phenomenon is a constant characteristic of *M. tuberculosis* and *M. avium* (WAGENER et al., 35).

■ **Antigenic structure and serological diagnosis**

In animals the demonstration of humoral antibodies has achieved no practical diagnostic significance, although many methods have been tested.

An exception to this is avian tuberculosis, where the rapid slide agglutination can be used in diagnosis usually with serotype 2 of *M. avium* as antigen.

Serotyping of mycobacterial strains, especially from group III of Runyon, (*M. avium*, *M. intracellulare*), has been carried out and can be used as an aid in the classification of isolates and may help to answer epidemiological questions. The method of choice is the agglutination test developed by SCHAEFER (24), which has since been employed by a number of investigators (3, 19, 21, 23, 32, 38). The serotypes we recognize today are listed in table 28. In Germany the majority of strains of *M. avium* isolated from poultry or cattle belong to serotype 2.

Table 29: Identification of tubercle bacilli by animal inoculation (18, 26)

Experimental animal[1]	M. tuberculosis	M. bovis	M. avium
Guinea pig (0.01 mg/subcutaneous)	++	++	+/−
Rabbit (0.01 mg/intravenous)	+[2]	++[3]	++[4]
Fowl (0.1 mg/intravenous)	−	−	++[4]

− no tuberculosis; ++ generalized tuberculosis; + focal tuberculosis

[1] in order to obtain comparable results, the bacterial dose has to be weighed out exactly;
[2] pulmonary tuberculosis with no lesions in other organs;
[3] usually tuberculosis of Villemin strain (miliary tubercles);
[4] usually tuberculosis of Yersin type (spread of the mycobacteria throughout the whole body, swelling of the parenchymatous organs without the formation of grossly discernible tubercles)

■ **Animal inoculation**

Diagnostic animal inoculations are performed on guinea pigs and this is considered to be the most reliable method of identifying *M. tuberculosis* and *M. bovis*. This should be restricted to laboratories that have optimum culture facilities. But for aesthetic and economic reasons, and because of the risk of infection to laboratory staff animal inoculation should not become routine but be reserved for special cases (22, 26). Today tubercle bacilli can be differentiated by means of numerous biochemical tests, so that animal inoculations are almost obsolete for this purpose. The basis of animal inoculation tests is the variation in the pathogenicity of tubercle bacilli for the different laboratory animals (table 29).

Bibliography / Literatur

1. BEERWERTH, W. (1967): Die Züchtung von Mykobakterien aus dem Kot der Haustiere und ihre Bedeutung für die Epidemiologie und Bekämpfung der Tuberkulose. Praxis der Pneumologie 21, 189–202.
2. BEERWERTH, W., & U. KESSEL (1976): Mykobakterien in der Umwelt von Mensch und Tier. Zbl. Bakt. I. Orig. A 235, 177–183.
3. BEERWERTH, W., & K. POPP (1971): Zur epizootiologischen Bedeutung der Sägemehleinstreu für das Auftreten der Schweinetuberkulose. Zbl. Vet. med. B, 18, 634–645.
4. BÖNICKE, R. (1961): Die Bedeutung der Acylamidasen für die Identifizierung und Differenzierung der verschiedenen Arten der Gattung Mycobacterium. Jb. Tbk.-Forsch. Inst. Borstel 5, 7–87.
5. BÖNICKE, R., & B. P. LISBOA (1959): Neuere chemische Verfahren zum Nachweis der Niazinbildung der Tuberkelbakterien und ihre Bedeutung für die Typendifferenzierung. Tuberk.-Arzt 12, 380.
6. DALCHOW, W., & J. NASSAL (1979): Mykobakteriose beim Schwein durch Sägemehleinstreu. Tierärztl. Umschau 34, 253–261.
7. GRIEGER, K., K. WENDT, H. W. FUCHS & J. BORETIUS (1984): Atypische Mykobakterien als Erreger enzootisch verlaufender Mastitiden. Mh. Vet. Med. 39, 727–730.
8. HUMMEL, P. (1966): Über das Vorkommen von atypischen Mykobakterien bei Hund und Katze. Zbl. Vet. med. B., 13, 51–61.
9. JARNAGIN, J. H., E. M. HIMES & W. RICHARDS (1983): Mycobacterium kansasii from lymph nodes of cattle in the United States. Am. J. Vet. Res. 44, 1853–1855.
10. KÄPPLER, W. (1965): Zur Differenzierung von Mykobakterien mit dem Phosphatase-Test. Beitr. Klin. Tuberk. 130, 223–226.
11. KÄPPLER, W. (1964): Über die Differenzierung von Mycobacterium tuberculosis und Mycobacterium bovis mit in-vitro-Methoden. Prax. Pneumol. 18, 671–680.
12. KAUKER, E., & W. RHEINWALD (1972): Untersuchungen über das Vorkommen atypischer Mykobakterien der Gruppe 3 nach Runyon in Einstreu (Sägemehl) und Futter von Schweinen in Nordhessen. Berl. Münch. tierärztl. Wschr. 85, 384–387.
13. KAZDA, J. (1969): Die Bedeutung der atypischen Mykobakterien in der Veterinärmedizin. Wiener tierärztl. Mschr. 56, 424–428.

14. Konno, K. (1956): New chemical method of differentiate human type tubercel bacillus from other mycobacteria. Science **124**, 985.
15. Meissner, G. (1961): Vorkommen und Eigenschaften (bakteriologisch und tierexperimentell) von atypischen Mycobakterien. Jahresberichte Borstel **5**, 408–480.
16. Ménard, L., C. Vanasse, C. Diaz & G. Rivard (1983): Mycobacterium cheloni mastitis in a Quebec dairy herd. Can. Vet. J. **24**, 305–307.
17. Nassal, J. (1970): Isolierung und Differenzierung von Mykobakterien. 2. Sympos. Lebensmittelmikrobiol. der Dtsch. Vet. Ges., Berlin, S. 110–115.
18. Nassal, J. (1961): Experimentelle Untersuchungen über die Isolierung, Differenzierung und Variabilität der Tuberkulosenbakterien. Beiheft 2 zum Zbl. Vet. Med.
19. Neumeier, U. (1974): Serologische Typendifferenzierungen aviärer Mykobakterienstämme isoliert von Tieren. Vet. Med. Diss. Gießen.
20. Neuschulz, J. (1970): Möglichkeiten der bakteriologischen und biochemischen Differenzierung von Mykobakterien im Routinebetrieb. 2. Sympos. Lebensmittelmikrobiol. der Dtsch. Vet. Ges., Berlin, S. 116–117.
21. Piening, C., A. Anz & G. Meissner (1972): Serotyp-Bestimmungen und ihre Bedeutung für epidemiologische Untersuchungen bei der Schweinetuberkulose in Schleswig-Holstein. Dtsch. tierärztl. Wschr. **79**, 316–321.
22. Rotter, M., E. Olbrich & W. Kovac (1984): Zum Stellenwert des Tierversuches im Rahmen der Tuberkulose-Diagnostik. Hyg. u. Med. **9**, 65–67.
23. Saxegaard, F. (1981): Serological investigations of Mycobacterium avium and Mycobacterium avium-like bacteria isolated from domestic and wild animals. Acta vet. scand. **22**, 153–161.
24. Schaefer, W. B. (1965): Serologic identification and classification of the atypical mycobacteria by their agglutination. Am. Rev. Resp. Dis. **92**, 85–83.
25. Schaefer, W. B., & Z. Reggiardo (1963): Serologic identification and classification of the mycobacteria other than M. tuberculosis encountered in human disease. Am. Rev. Resp. Dis. **88**, 111.
26. Schliesser, T. (1985): Mycobacterium. In: H. Blobel & T. Schliesser (Hrsg.): Handbuch der bakteriellen Infektionen bei Tieren. Bd. V, S. 155–280. Jena: VEB Gustav Fischer.
27. Schliesser, T. (1978): Aktuelle Probleme der Mykobakterien (einschließlich Tuberkulose) bei Tieren. Wiener tierärztl. Wschr. **65**, 77–83.
28. Schliesser, T. (1976): Vorkommen und Bedeutung von Mykobakterien bei Tieren. Zbl. Bakt. I. Orig. A, **235**, 184–194.
29. Schliesser, T. (1967): Atypische Mykobakterien bei Tieren. Ztschr. Tuberkulose, **127**, 101–108.
30. Schmittdiel, E. (1964): Zum Vorkommen aviärer Mykobakterien in den Plazenten von abortierenden Rindern. Tierärztl. Umschau **19**, 395–397.
31. Seeger, J. (1969): Vorkommen und Bedeutung atypischer Mykobakterien der Gruppe II nach Runyon bei Schweinen, Hühnern und Hunden. Zbl. Bakt. I. Orig. **210**, 517–524.
32. Stoll, L. (1973): Vorkommen von aviären Mykobakterien vom Serotyp Davis bei der Lymphknotentuberkulose des Schweines in Südhessen. Dtsch. tierärztl. Wschr. **80**, 548–550.
33. Uhlemann, J., R. Held, K. Müller, H. Jahn & H. Dürrling (1975): Schweinetuberkulose in einem Mastkombinat nach Einstreu von Hobel- und Sägespänen. Mh. Vet. Med. **30**, 175–180.
34. Virtanen, S. (1960): A study of nitrate reduction by mycobacteria. Acta tuberc. scand. Suppl. **48**, 32.
35. Wagener, K., W. Thiel & L. Hensel (1956): Das Kletter-Phänomen, ein kulturelles Art- und Typenmerkmal der Tuberkelbakterien. Zbl. Bakt. I. Orig. **167**, 291–297.
36. Wagener, K., & E. Mitscherlich (1951): Fortschritte in der kulturellen Differenzierung der Tuberkelbakterientypen. Zbl. Bakt. I. Orig. **157**, 87–96.
37. Wayne, L. G., J. R. Doubek & R. L. Russel (1964): Classification and identification of mycobacteria. Tests employing Tween 80 as substrate. Am. Rev. Resp. Dis. **90**, 588–597.
38. Weber, A., T. Schliesser, I. M. Schultze & U. Bertelsmann (1976): Serologische Typendifferenzierung aviärer Mykobakterienstämme isoliert von Schlachtrindern. Zbl. Bakt. I. Orig. **235**, 202–206.
39. Whitheas, J. E. M., P. Wildy & H. C. Engbaek (1953): Arylsulphatase activity of mycobacteria. J. Path. Bact. **65**, 451–460.

2 Mycobacterium paratuberculosis

■ **Incidence and veterinary significance**

Paratuberculosis is a chronic enteritis of cattle, sheep, goats and other ruminants. Non-ruminants (horses, donkeys, pigs and dogs) are very rarely affected. Cattle between 2 and 6 years show the disease most commonly, but the incubation period may extend to several years. The animals are infected as calves from contact with infected faeces, through the milk or even in the uterus. The pathological changes occur mostly in the ileum and caecum and they consist of severe thickening of the mucosa, leading to the formation of longitudinal and transverse folds, somewhat reminiscent of the gyri of the brain. This is accompanied by swelling of the mediastinal lymph nodes. Other organs such as the liver, hepatic lymph nodes and the udder, may also become involved. Not infrequently, this is a clinically latent disease. The organism can be

2 Mycobacterium paratuberculosis

■ **Vorkommen und medizinische Bedeutung**

Die Paratuberkulose ist eine chronische Enteritis, die bei Rind, Schaf, Ziege und anderen Wiederkäuern auftritt, sehr selten können Spontanerkrankungen auch bei Nichtwiederkäuern (z. B. Pferd, Esel, Schwein, Hund) auftreten. Rinder erkranken am häufigsten im Alter von 2–6 Jahren, die Inkubationszeit kann mehrere Jahre betragen. Die pathologisch-anatomischen Veränderungen betreffen zur Hauptsache Ileum und Caecum und bestehen in einer starken Schwellung der Schleimhaut, die gehirnwindungsähnliche Längs- und Querfalten bei gleichzeitiger Schwellung der Darmlymphknoten aufweist. Auch andere Organe können infiziert sein (Leber, Leberlymphknoten, Euter). Nicht selten verläuft eine Infektion klinisch latent. Der Erreger wird überwiegend bereits im Kälberalter durch Kontakt mit infiziertem Kot, durch Milch oder

Table 30: The diagnosis of paratuberculosis Tabelle 30. Diagnose der Paratuberkulose

I. Isolation of organism

Test material: faeces, smears from intestinal mucosa, mesenteric lymph nodes or other organs.

Microscopic examination: Ziehl-Neelsen stain: bacteria red in nests or compact clusters (fig. 99). Only about 30 % of affected animals are recognized by means of microscopic examination. The success rate can be improved by pre-treating the faecal samples with sodium hypochlorite (Desmecht, 3). Nevertheless, in view of the difficulty of growing these bacteria, the microscopic method remains the easiest and most reliable (2).

Culture methods: The procedure is costly and is therefore not always used for diagnosis. However, with the best medium, it provides reliable results. Mesenteric lymph nodes and the jejunum are most suitable for the isolation of bacteria. Pre-treatment: The addition of 5 % oxalic acid (if necessary in combination with a solution of caustic soda) will reduce the contaminants — allow this to act for 30 minutes at 37 °C. Nutrient media: Several media have been described for primary isolation, these are summarized on p. ■. Extracts of mycobacteria are added to the media, most commonly *M. phlei*. Smith's medium has been found to be successful, because it is transparent and allows the early recognition of colonies. Incubation time is 4–8 weeks.

Animal inoculation: The injection of guinea pigs or other small laboratory animals is usually negative, apart from the development of not very obvious granulomata at the injection site and occasional enlargement of the iliac and subiliac lymph nodes (5).

II. Serological/allergic diagnosis

Complement fixation test (CFT): the complement fixation test can confirm a tentative diagnosis of clinical disease in 90 % of cases. But a latent infection in only 30 % (4, 5, 7, 9).

Allergic intradermal test: Either paratuberculin (johnin) or avian tuberculin can be used. The disease can be confirmed in 70 % of clinically suspect cattle and in about 34 % of latent cases. When combined with the CFT the intradermal test will identify about 80 % of latent infections (9).

ELISA: By current experience the ELISA test is more sensitive than the CFT and is probably the method of choice.

The specificity of the serological methods and the intradermal test is limited, because infections with tubercle or other mycobacteria can lead to non-specific reactions.

---

excreted both by diseased animals and those that carry a latent infection.

■ Morphology

M. paratuberculosis is a Gram-positive, non-motile, strictly aerobic rod of $0.3–2 \times 0.3–0.5\,\mu m$ in size. The best stain is Ziehl-Neelsen. See table 30 for the demonstration of paratuberculosis bacteria and the serological/allergic diagnosis.

bereits intrauterin übertragen. Sowohl klinisch kranke als auch latent infizierte Tiere können den Erreger ausscheiden.

■ Morphologie

M. paratuberculosis ist ein $0.3–2 \times 0.3–0.5\,\mu m$ großes, gram-positives, unbewegliches, strikt aerobes Stäbchen. Die Färbung geschieht am besten nach Ziehl-Neelsen. Diagnostischer Nachweis der Paratuberkulosebakterien sowie serologisch/allergische Diagnose siehe Tab. 30.

Bibliography / Literatur

1. BEERWERTH, W. (1961): Die Paratuberkulose des Rindes. Die Blauen Hefte für den Tierarzt, 519–527.
2. BERGMANN, A., I. S. CAMARA & A. VOIGT (1981): Neuere Erkenntnisse zur Paratuberkulose. Mh. Vet. Med. 36, 471–477.
3. DESMECHT, M. (1977): Rendement comparé de diverses methodes de diagnostic de la paratuberculose. Ann. Med. Vet. 121, 421–426.
4. HOLE, N. H. (1953): The diagnosis of Johne's disease. Proc. XV Inter. Vet. Congr. 1, 272.
5. RANKIN, J. D. (1970): Die Paratuberkulose. In: Mykobakterien und mykobakterielle Krankheiten. Teil VII, S. 323–354. Jena: VEB Gustav Fischer.
6. RANKIN, J. (1958): The complement-fixation test in the diagnosis of Johne's disease in cattle. Vet. Rec. 70, 383–385.
7. ROSENBERGER, G., & D. KRAUSE (1955): Die Diagnose der Paratuberkulose des Rindes mittels der Komplementbindungsreaktion nach Hole. Dtsch. tierärztl. Wschr. 62, 161–164.
8. SCHAAF, E. E. (1957): Zur Züchtung und Identifizierung des M. paratuberculosis. Vet. Diss. Gießen.
9. SCHAAF, J., & W. BEERWERTH (1960): Die allergische und serologische Diagnose der Paratuberkulose. Mhefte Tierhk. 12, Sonderteil: »Rindertuberkulose und Brucellose« 9, 103–114.
10. SMITH, H. W. (1953): Modification of Dubos' media for the cultivation of Mycobacterium johnei. J. Path. Bact. 66, 375–381.

Gram-negative, aerobic or micro-aerophilic or facultatively anaerobic rods, with simple cultural requirements

Gramnegative, aerob oder mikroaerophil oder fakultativ anaerob wachsende, in der Kultur anspruchslose Stäbchen

This group includes a large number of bacteria which are often encountered in samples of animal origin either as pathogens or as part of the normal flora. Their identification still presents the bacteriologist with difficulty and the results of the identification tests are often unsatisfactory.

Many of the bacteria are of veterinary interest; they have the following properties:

Gram-negative, non-sporulating rods;

moderate in their cultural requirements, that is to say, the bacteria grow on simple media, on blood agar and on culture media designed for intestinal bacteria;

aerobic, rarely micro-aerophilic or facultatively anaerobic. Members of this group are listed in table 31.

These bacteria can be subdivided into two reaction groups, depending on whether they possess the respiratory enzyme oxidase (tab. 31) and each of these is subdivided into three further reaction types on the basis of their glucose metabolism by means of the oxidation-fermentation test:
▷ Reaction group I: oxidase-positive
reaction type I a: fermentation of glucose in the absence of oxygen
reaction type I b: oxidative glucose breakdown
reaction type I c: inactive type (glucose is not broken down)

Die Gruppe umfaßt eine sehr große Anzahl von Bakterien, die entweder als Krankheitserreger oder als Angehörige der normalen Körperflora oft in tierischen Untersuchungsstoffen nachgewiesen werden. Ihre Unterscheidung stellt den Bakteriologen immer noch vor schwierige Aufgaben, das Ergebnis der Identifizierungsbemühungen ist oft unbefriedigend.

In dieser Gruppe sollen veterinärmedizinisch interessante Bakterien mit folgenden Eigenschaften zusammengefaßt werden:

gramnegative, sporenlose Stäbchen;

in der Kultur anspruchslos, d.h. die Bakterien wachsen auf Nährböden einfacher Zusammensetzung, auf Blutagar und oft auf Nährböden für Darmbakterien;

aerobes, selten mikroaerophiles oder fakultativ anaerobes Wachstum. Die hierzu gehörenden Bakterien sind aus den Tab. 31 und 32 ersichtlich.

Diese Bakterien lassen sich durch An- oder Abwesenheit des respiratorischen Enzyms Oxidase in 2 Reaktionsgruppen (Tab. 31) und aufgrund des Glucosestoffwechsels innerhalb jeder Reaktionsgruppe mit dem Oxidations-Fermentations-Test (OF-Test) in je drei Reaktionstypen einteilen, nämlich:
▷ Reaktionsgruppe I: oxidasepositiv
Reaktionstyp I a: fermentativer Abbau von Glucose in Abwesenheit von Sauerstoff
Reaktionstyp I b: oxidativer Glucoseabbau
Reaktionstyp I c: Glucose wird nicht abgebaut (inaktiver Typ)

Table 31: Classification by means of the oxidase and OF test of Gram-negative, nonfastidious, aerobic or microaerophilic rods of veterinary interest

Tabelle 31: Einteilung gramnegativer, anspruchsloser, aerober oder mikroaerophiler Stäbchen von veterinärmedizinischem Interesse mittels des Oxydase- und OF-Testes

Reaction group I: oxidase-positive		
Reaction type I a glucose breakdown by fermentation	**Reaction type I b** glucose breakdown by oxidation	**Reaction type I c** no glucose breakdown
Pasteurella Actinobacillus Vibrio Aeromonas	Pseudomonas Flavobacterium	Alcaligenes faecalis Bordetella bronchiseptica Moraxella Campylobacter
Reaction group II: oxidase-negative		
Reaction type II a glucose breakdown by fermentation	**Reaction type II b** glucose breakdown by oxidation	**Reaction type II c** no glucose breakdown
Enterobacteriaceae	Acinetobacter calcoaceticus var. glucidolyticus (syn. A. anitratum, Herellea)	Acinetobacter calcoaceticus var. aglucidolyticus (syn. A. lwoffii, Mima)

Table 32: Biochemical differentiation between Gram-negative, culturally aerobic or micro-aerophilic bacteria with simple cultural requirements

Tabelle 32: Kulturell-biochemische Unterscheidung gramnegativer, kulturell anspruchsloser, aerober oder mikroaerophiler Bakterien

Reaction group	O/F test	Bacterium genus species	Growth on selective plate[1]	Bipolar staining	Motility
I	F	Pasteurella	−	+	−
		Actinobacillus	+	−	−
		Aeromonas	+	−	+
oxidase-positive	O	Pseudomonas	+	−	+
		Flavobacterium	v$^+$	−	+
	./.	Bordetella bronchiseptica	+	−	+
		Moraxella bovis	−	−	−
		Alcaligenes faecalis	+	−	+
		Campylobacter	−	−	+
II	F	Enterobacteriaceae	+	−	v
		Yersinia	+	v	+
		Chromobacterium	−	−	+
oxidase-negative	O	Actinobacter calcoaceticus var. glucocidolyticus	+	−	−
		Pseudomonas maltophilia	+	−	+
	./.	Acinetobacter calcoaceticus var. aglucidolyticus	+	−	−

▷ Reaction group II: oxidase-negative
  reaction type II a: fermentation of glucose
  reaction type II b: oxidative breakdown of glucose
  reaction type II c: glucose is not broken down

The classification of the different species of bacteria into these reaction forms is given in table 32.

1 Oxidase-positive and fermentative bacteria

(reaction type I a, table 32)

1.1 Genus: Pasteurella (P.)

■ Taxonomic position:
Family: *Pasteurellaceae*
Genera: *Pasteurella*
          Haemophilus (p. 232)
          Actinobacillus (p. 135)

There is a close relationship between bacteria belonging to these three genera so that they were classed together in the Haemophilus-Pasteurella-

---

Table 32: Continued

Gluc S	G	Lac	Sac	Ind	H$_2$S	LDC	ODC	Ure	Cit	Nit	Gel	Cat	Pigment	Hae
+	−	−	+	v	−	−	v	−	−	+	−		−	v
+	−	+	+	−	+	−	−	+	−	+			−	v
+	v$^+$	v	v	v	−	−	−	−	v	+	+		−	v
+	−	−	v	−	v			v	+	+	v$^+$		v$^+$	v
v$^+$	−	−	−	+	−			−	−	−	+		+	
−	−	−	−	−	−			+	+	+	−	+	−	−
−	−	−	−	−	−			−	v	−	+	v	−	
−	−	−	−	−	−			v$^+$	v	+	−		−	−
−	−	−	−	−	v			−	−	−	−	+	−	−
+	v	v	v	v	v	v	v	v	v	+	v		−	v
−	−	−	−	−	−		−	+	−	+	−		−	−
−	−	−	−	−	−			−	+	+	(+)		+	
+	−	−	−	−	−			v	+	−	v	+	−	v
−	−	−	−	−	+		−	−	+	v	+	+	+	
−	−	−	−	−	−			−	v	−	−	+	−	v

[1] e.g.: MacConkey agar, Gassner plate
F: glucose breakdown by fermentation; O: glucose breakdown by oxidation; ./.: no glucose breakdown

Table 33: Properties of the genera *Pasteurella*, *Actinobacillus*, *Aeromonas* and *Vibrio*

Tabelle 33: Eigenschaften der Gattungen *Pasteurella*, *Actinobacillus*, *Aeromonas* und *Vibrio*

Properties	Pasteurella	Actinobacillus	Aeromonas	Vibrio
Morphology	ovoid, short rods, 0.4 × 1.0–1.4 µm long, bipolar staining, especially in smears from organs	ovoid or rod-shaped, 0.4 × 1.0 µm long, though longer forms possible, coccoid inclusions, often at the ends of the bacteria	Rods with rounded ends, to coccoid, 1.0 × 4.4 µm singly, in pairs or in short threads	comma-shaped to straight rods, 0.5 × 2.4 µm sometimes »S« or spiral in shape
Oxidase	+	+	+	+
Motility	–	–	+[1]	+
Colony form	S: smooth, translucent, flat. M: moist, opaque, drawing threads when colony is touched. R: rough	sticky, adherent to the surface of the medium	grey to colourless, medium size, like enterobacteria, some β-haemolysis	colourless to slightly yellowish colonies or growth in a film
Temperature optimum	37 °C	37 °C	20–28 °C	25 °C[3]
Glucose	fermentative, no gas formed	fermentative, no gas formed	fermentative, often gas formation[2]	fermentative, no gas formation
Nitrate	+	+	+	+
Urease	v	+	–	–
Catalase	+	v[+]	+	+
Gelatinase	–	v	+	+
Sensitive to O/129[4]			–	+

[1] non-motile: *A. salmonicida*;
[2] no gas formation: *A. hydrophila* spp. *anaerogenes*;
[3] Exceptions: *V. metschnikovi*, *V. parahaemolyticus*;
[4] Vibriostatic agent O/129, Schubert, see table 41

[1] unbeweglich: *A. salmonicida*;
[2] keine Gasbildung: *A. hydrophila* ssp. *anaerogenes*;
[3] Ausnahmen: *V. metschnikovi*, *V. parahaemolyticus*;
[4] Vibriostaticum O/129, Schubert, s. Tab. 41

Actinobacillus group by KILIAN & FREDERIKSEN (35) and by MANNHEIM (40).

The genus includes Gram-negative, non-motile, facultatively anaerobic, short coccobacilli, which are catalase- and oxidase-positive and which produce acid but no gas during the fermentation of various carbohydrates. An exception is *P. aerogenes*. These bacteria demonstrate a distinct tendency towards bipolar staining, especially in organ smears (fig. 100), but this is no specific characteristic. The pasteurellae are frequently pleomorphic, and form long chains chiefly in passage cultures.

The taxonomic classification of the genus is not yet absolute and liable to changes. The following are listed in Bergey's manual:
P. multocida
P. haemolytica
P. pneumotropica
P. ureae

unter der Bezeichnung Haemophilus-Pasteurella-Actinobacillus-Gruppe zusammengefaßt wurden.

Die Gattung umfaßt gramnegative, unbewegliche, fakultativ anaerobe, katalase- und oxidasepositive, kokkoide Kurzstäbchen, die bei der Fermentation verschiedener Kohlenhydrate Säure, aber kein Gas (Ausnahme *P. aerogenes*) bilden. Insbesondere bei Organausstrichen zeigen die Bakterien eine deutliche Neigung zu bipolarer Färbung (Abb. 100), die aber kein spezifisches Merkmal ist. Die Pasteurellen sind oft pleomorph und bilden besonders nach Kulturpassagen lange Formen aus.

Die taxonomische Gliederung der Gattung ist nicht endgültig, sondern unterliegt Wandlungen. Nach Bergey's manual werden unterschieden:
P. multocida
P. haemolytica
P. pneumotropica
P. ureae

P. aerogenes
P. gallinarum

A different system has been proposed for the genus *Pasteurella* (48, 49). This is based primarily on the basis of the genetical relationship and involves 11 different species, some of which are listed together with their phenotypical properties in table 34.

The pasteurellae, especially those of avian origin, vary greatly in their phenotypic properties. As a result they are often difficult to identify as members of the above species (3).

According to this re-classification suggested by MUTTERS et al. (49), *P. haemolytica* and *P. pneumotropica* (biotypes Jawetz and Heyl) and *P. ureae* do not belong to the genus *Pasteurella*, but are apparently more closely related to the actinobacilli. The taxonomic position of *P. aerogenes* and *P. piscida* are unknown, but they are not pasteurellae.

P. aerogenes
P. gallinarum

Insbesondere auf der Grundlage des genetischen Verwandtschaftsgrades ist eine neue Gliederung des Genus *Pasteurella* vorgeschlagen worden, die 11 verschiedene Arten berücksichtigt, von denen einige mit ihren phänotypischen Eigenschaften in der Tab. 34 zusammengestellt sind (48, 49).

Insgesamt zeigen die Pasteurellenstämme, besonders solche, die von Vögeln stammen, eine große Variabilität in ihren phänotypischen Eigenschaften, so daß eine Bestimmung und Zuordnung zu den genannten Arten oft schwierig ist (3).

Nach dem in der Tab. 34 zusammengestellten Reklassifizierungsvorschlag von MUTTERS et al. (49) gehören u. a. *P. haemolytica* und *P. pneumotropica* (Biotypen Jawetz und Heyl) und *P. ureae* nicht zum Genus *Pasteurella*, sondern sind offenbar mit den Actinobazillen enger verwandt. Die taxonomische Stellung von *P. aerogenes* und *P. piscida* ist unbekannt, es handelt sich aber um keine Pasteurellen.

Table 34: Differentiation between species of *Pasteurella* (after MUTTERS et al., 49)

Tabelle 34: Differenzierung von Arten der Gattung *Pasteurella* (nach MUTTERS et al., 49)

Species	NAD requirement	ODC	Ind	Ure	Tre	Mal	D-Xyl	L-Ara	Man	Sor	Dul	Species affected
P. multocida												
ssp. multocida	−	+	+	−	v	−	v	−	+	+	−	mammals, birds and man
ssp. septica	−	+	+	−	+	−	+	−	+	−	−	
ssp. gallicida	−	+	+	−	−	−	+	v	+	+	+	
P. dagmatis	−	−	+	+	+	+	−	−	−	−	−	dog, cat, transmitted through bites to man
P. gallinarum	−	−	−	−	+	+	−	−	−	−	−	poultry
P. canis	−	+	v	−	v	−	v	−	−	−	−	biotype 1 (Indole +): dog, cat and man biotype 2 (Indole −): calf
P. stomatis	−	−	+	−	+	−	−	−	−	−	−	respiratory tract of dog and cat
P. anatis	−	−	−	−	+	−	+	−	+	−	−	duck
P. langaa	−	−	−	−	−	−	−	−	+	−	−	fowl
P. avium	v	−	−	−	+	−	v	−	−	−	−	poultry, previous name Haemophilus avium
P. volantium	+	v	−	−	+	+	v	−	+	v	−	poultry, previous name Haemophilus avium

1.1.1 Pasteurella multocida
(Syn.: *Bact. bipolare multocidum, Pasteurella septica*)

■ Incidence and veterinary significance

P. multocida occurs in practically all warm-blooded animals. The most important clinical manifestations are summarized in table 35. Latent infections are widely distributed, especially on the mucosa of the respiratory tract. Occasional infections of man can result from animal bites (dogs and cats) (46, 65).

■ Culture (figs. 101 and 102)

P. multocida grows aerobically on blood agar and other media which contain protein, such as tryptose agar, and less intensely also on nutrient agar. There is no growth on Gassner or MacConkey media.

KNIGHT et al. (36) have described a selective medium, containing clindamycin, gentamicin, potassium tellurite and amphotericin B. DE JONG & BORST (31) describe another medium which permits the simultaneous selective primary culture of *P. multocida* and *Bordetella bronchiseptica* in atrophic rhinitis of the pig.

Table 35: Pathogenic significance of *Pasteurella multocida*

Antigen type	Animal species	Clinical picture and incidence
B E (Africa)	Cattle buffalo	haemorrhagic septicaemia, especially South-east Asia, Central and East Africa, Southern and Eastern Europe, Near and Middle East (2, 10, 50)
B	Pig	haemorrhagic septicaemia, Asia, rare, does not occur in Central Europe (13, 47)
B	Cattle	acute pasteurellosis, apparently differentiated from haemorrhagic septicaemia on epidemiological grounds and because of its low tendency to spread (34, 58)
5: A 8 a: A	Poultry, especially fowl & turkey	fowl cholera, world-wide distribution
A A, D	Calf, Pig	pulmonary pasteurellosis of the »enzootic pneumonia« complex, world-wide (6, 10, 30, 50, 56), atrophic rhinitis of pigs (43)
A	Sheep	acute to chronic pleuro-pneumonia, world-wide
A, D	Rabbit	acute to chronic respiratory disease, including rhinitis (26, 27, 28, 29, 64), world-wide
D	Poultry	chronic pasteurellosis, fowl cholera, pneumonia, rhinitis, sinusitis, world-wide distribution
A	Dog	clinically latent infection of the mucous membranes of the pharynx and tonsils, world-wide

```
                           ┌─────────────┐
                           │  Specimens  │
                           └─────────────┘
         ┌──────────────────────┼──────────────────────┐
```

Microscopic examination	Culture methods	Animal inoculation
Smear preparation, monochromatic staining with methylene blue, bipolar staining	Blood agar, aerobic incubation 37 °C, 24–48 h, colony forms: S-form: small, smooth, round colonies. M-form: large mucoid colonies. R-form: rough form, rare	Mice injected intraperitoneally with 0.5 ml of supernatant of organ suspension. After death recover pasteurella from the organs

Character	P. multocida	P. haemolytica	P. pneumotropica	P. ureae	P. aerogenes	P. gallinarum
Oxidase	+	+	+	+	+	+
Catalase	+	+	+	+	+	+
Glucose	+	+	+	+	+[1]	+
Nitrate	+	+	+	+	+	+
Methyl red	−	−	−	−	−	−
Voges-Proskauer	−	−	−	−	−	−
Lysine decarboxylase	−	−	−	−	−	−
Arginine dehydrogenase	−	−	−	−	−	−
Haemolysis	−	+(β)	−	−	−	−
Indole	+	−	+	−	−	−
Urease	−	−	+	+	+	−
H_2S	+	v	v⁺	−	+	v⁺
Mannitol	+[2]	+	−	+	−	−
Lactose	−	v	v	−	−	−
Growth on MacConkey	−	+	+	−	+	−

Results on pasteurella strains isolated from cattle suffering pulmonary disease (6):
157 P. multocida strains: Indole: + (100 %), Haemolysis: − (100 %), Maltose: − (100 %), Saccharose: + (98.7 %), Mannitol: + (96.8 %), Urease: − (100 %), Growth on MacConkey agar: − (100 %).
35 P. haemolytica strains: Indole: − (100 %), Haemolysis: + (100 %), Maltose: + (89.2 %), Saccharose: + (89.2 %), Mannitol: − (81.1 %), Urease: − (100 %), Growth on MacConkey agar: + (54.1 %).

[1] with gas formation;
[2] canine and feline strains may be negative

[1] Mit Gasbildung;
[2] Stämme von Hund und Katze können negativ sein

Fig. 98: Demonstration and identification of *Pasteurella multocida* and its differentiation from other pasteurella species

Abb. 98: Nachweis und Differenzierung von *Pasteurella multocida* und ihre kulturell-biochemische Unterscheidung von anderen Pasteurella-Arten

There is considerable variation in the appearance of the colonies, which has led to the differentiation of M-, S- and R-forms (tab. 36). It has been suspected that there may be a relationship between the colony form and the virulence of the organism, and the S-form is reputed to be particularly virulent. Mucoid forms are apparently more common in the upper respiratory tract of calves than in calf pneumonia (56); they are often found in rabbits (26, 29).

The capsule, which is particularly well developed in type A strains, can be demonstrated in the hyaluronidase test (p. 20 and tab. 36).

■ **Biochemical properties**
See figure 98.

Die Kolonien zeigen in ihrer Gestalt eine große Vielgestaltigkeit, die zur Unterscheidung von M-, S- und R-Formen geführt hat (Tab. 36). Zwischen der Kolonieform und der Virulenz sind Zusammenhänge vermutet worden, dabei gilt die S-Form als besonders virulent. Mukoid wachsende Formen finden sich beim Kalb offenbar häufiger als Besiedler des oberen Respirationstraktes und seltener bei Pneumonien (56), sie kommen ferner häufig beim Kaninchen vor (26, 29).

Die Kapsel (Tab. 36), die besonders deutlich bei den Typ A-Stämmen ausgebildet ist, läßt sich im Hyaluronidasetest nachweisen (S. 20 und Tab. 36).

■ **Kulturell-biochemische Eigenschaften**
Siehe Abb. 98.

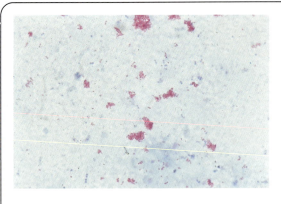
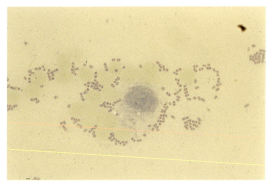
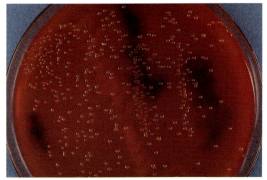
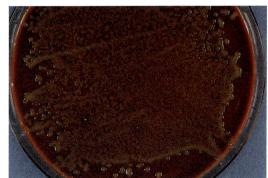

▲ Fig. 99: *Mycobacterium paratuberculosis*, smear from mesenteric lymph node of the ox, Ziehl-Neelsen stain, acid-fast bacteria in groups. Magnification x 1000
▼ Fig. 101: *Pasteurella multocida*, isolated from the lung of a pig. Pure culture on blood agar, 24 h, 37 °C. Magnification x 0.4

▲ Abb. 99: *Mycobacterium paratuberculosis*, Ausstrich vom Darmlymphknoten eines Rindes, Ziehl-Neelsen-Färbung, säurefeste Bakterien in Haufen gelagert, Abb.-M. 1000:1
▼ Abb. 101: *Pasteurella multocida*, isoliert aus der Lunge eines Schweines, Reinkultur auf Blutagar, 24 h, 37 °C, Abb.-M. 1:2,5

▲ Fig. 100: *Pasteurella multocida*, rabbit blood smear, methylene blue stain, bipolar staining of the pasteurella organisms. Magnification x 1000
▼ Fig. 102: *Pasteurella multocida*, isolated from a pig's lymph node, mucoid growth on chocolate agar, 24 h, 37 °C. Magnification x 0.4

▲ Abb. 100: *Pasteurella multocida*, Ausstrich von Kaninchenblut. Methylenblaufärbung, bipolare Färbung der Pasteurellen, Abb.-M. 1000:1
▼ Abb. 102: *Pasteurella multocida*, isoliert aus dem Lymphknoten eines Schweines, schleimiges Wachstum auf Kochblutagar, 24 h, 37 °C, Abb.-M. 1:2,5

■ **Toxins**

Toxic substances have been demonstrated in strains of *P. multocida* derived from cases of atrophic rhinitis. Such toxins are especially potent in culture filtrates and produce inflammation after intradermal injections in guinea pigs (31, 59, 69). In tissue culture they cause cell damage (55). BHI broth is a suitable medium for toxin production.

■ **Toxine**

Im Zusammenhang mit der *Rhinitis atrophicans* sind insbesondere im Kulturfiltrat von aus diesem Krankheitsbild stammenden *P. multocida*-Stämmen toxische Stoffe nachgewiesen worden, die bei der intrakutanen Injektion in die Meerschweinchenhaut zu Entzündungen führen (31, 59, 68). In der Zellkultur führen diese Toxine zu Zellschädigungen (55). Als flüssiges Medium für die Toxinproduktion ist die BHI-Bouillon geeignet.

Table 36: Colony forms of *Pasteurella multocida* (9, 16, 26, 30)

Colony type	Appearance of colony	Broth culture	Capsule[1]	Typing by haem-agglut.	Acriflavin test[2]	Direction of dissociation
M mucoid	moist, mucoid, pulls threads diameter 2–5 mm	slight turbidity with thread-pulling sediment	+	–	mucoid precipitate	
S smooth	smooth, fluorescent or iridescent, diam. 1–3 mm	uniform turbidity	+	+	cells remain in suspension	
	smooth little fluorescence	uniform turbidity	+	+	some delicate flocculation	
	smooth, non-fluorescent	sediment	+	–	flocculation	
R rough	rough (rare)	sediment	–	–	flocculation	↓

[1] demonstrable in the hyaluronidase test (p. 20);
[2] 0.5 ml acriflavin solution (1 : 1000) is added to the sediment from 2 ml broth, and shaken up. Flocculation occurs within 5 minutes

Antigenic structure

The antigenic structure of *P. multocida* is not uniform, and various serotypes have been identified. Initially, ROBERTS (54) found four immunological variants (I–IV) in mice. This was followed by CARTER (8, 9) who used the indirect haemagglutination test to demonstrate the capsular antigens A, B, D and E. The method has been described in detail by MEYERINGH (43). NAMIOKA & MURATA (51) were able to detect the same capsular antigens with the slide agglutination method. The same authors succeeded in demonstrating O-antigens by means of agglutination. The relationships between K- and O-antigens are listed in table 37. The O-antigens 1, 2, 6, and 8 are particularly common in strains originating from pigs (57). Further experiments with serological typing were performed by LITTLE & LYON (39) using slide agglutination and HEDDLESTON et al. (25), with the gelprecipitation test. The contradictory results obtained are discussed by BROGDEN & PACKER (7).

The identified serotypes can be linked to certain forms of clinical disease (tab. 35). For instance, of the pasteurella strains which originate from bovine respiratory diseases, 70.1 % have capsule antigen A, 10.8 % capsule antigen D and 1.3 % capsule antigen B (6). Rhinitis atrophicans strains from the pig have been found to be mostly type D, less frequently type A and rarely type B (43).

In some strains only O-antigens can be demon-

Table 37: O-antigens and their relationship to K-antigen types, after CARTER (8)

K-antigen types	O-antigens	Serotypes
A[1]	1	1 : A
	3	3 : A
	5	5 : A
	7	7 : A
	8	8 : A
	9	9 : A
B	6	6 : B
	11	11 : B
D[2]	1	1 : D
	2	2 : D
	3	3 : D
	4	4 : D
	10	10 : D
E	6	6 : E

[1] Hyaluronidase is generally produced by strains of type A;
[2] Strains of type D are usually positive in the acriflavin test

strated and not K-antigens (50). The success rate of typing pasteurellae by their K-antigens is increased by treatment with hyaluronidase (33).

■ **Animal inoculation**

The small laboratory animals, particularly pigeons, rabbits and mice and to a lesser extent guinea pigs, are susceptible to *P. multocida*. Parenteral injection usually leads to a fatal generalized infection, yet virulence varies in the different species and it depends on the antigen type, the number of subcultures etc. According to the investigations of SCHIMMEL et al. (56), the fatal dose for the mouse was 10^1 to 10^8 bacteria. Strains B originating from cattle are apparently particularly virulent for mice (34).

1.1.2 Pasteurella haemolytica

■ **Incidence and veterinary importance**

This bacterium was first described in connection with mastitis of ewes (»Dammann-Freese bacterium«, 1907). According to MRÁZ (45), it is identical with *P. haemolytica*. Subsequently *P. haemolytica* has been reported in other species, mainly in pneumonia and other organ diseases of calves and young cattle (23, 58), horses, pigs, sheep (19, 61)

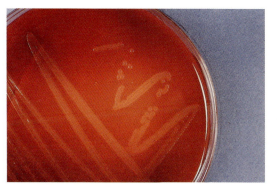
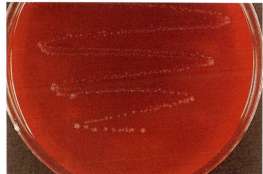
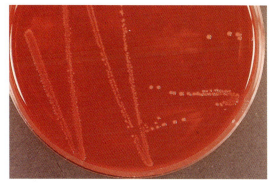
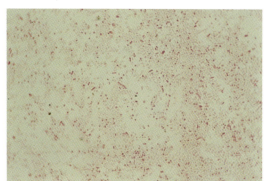

▲ Fig. 104: *Pasteurella haemolytica*, pure culture on Columbia blood agar, distinct haemolysis, 24 h, 37 °C, Magnification x 0.4
▼ Fig. 106: *Actinobacillus equuli*, pure culture on blood agar, 24 h, 37 °C. Magnification x 0.4

▲ Abb. 104: *Pasteurella haemolytica*, Reinkultur auf Columbia-Blutagar, deutliche Hämolyse, 24 h, 37 °C, Abb.-M. 1 : 2,5
▼ Abb. 106: *Actinobacillus equuli*, Reinkultur auf Blutagar, 24 h, 37 °C, Abb.-M. 1 : 2,5

▲ Fig. 105: *Actinobacillus lignieresii*, pure culture on blood agar, 24 h, 37 °C. Magnification x 0.4
▼ Fig. 107: *Actinobacillus suis*, culture smear, Gram stain, Gram-negative, pleomorphic rods. Magnification x 1000

▲ Abb. 105: *Actinobacillus lignieresii*, Reinkultur auf Blutagar, 24 h, 37 °C, Abb.-M. 1 : 2,5
▼ Abb. 107: *Actinobacillus suis*, Kulturausstrich, Gram-Färbung, gramnegative, pleomorphe Stäbchen, Abb.-M. 1000 : 1

and poultry (21, 41). Septicaemic conditions also occur, in lambs and poultry for instance. Usually, the animals must have a lowered resistance before the infection can become established, but latent infections of the mucous membranes do occur.

The uncertainty of the taxonomic position of these bacteria is discussed on page 125.

61), Geflügel (21, 41) und bei anderen Tierarten beschrieben worden. Auch septikämische Erkrankungen (z. B. Schaflämmer, Geflügel) sind möglich. In der Regel setzt die Erkrankung eine Resistenzminderung des Organismus voraus. Latente Schleimhautinfektionen kommen verbreitet vor.

Über die unsichere taxonomische Stellung des Bakteriums s. S. 125.

Table 38: Differentiation between biotypes A and T of *P. haemolytica*

Tabelle 38: Unterscheidung der Biotypen A und T von *P. haemolytica*

Character	Biotype A	Biotype T
Arabinose fermentation	+	−
Xylose fermentation	+	−
Trehalose fermentation	−	+
Penicillin	sensitive	resistant
Capsule antigens	1, 2, 5, 6, 7, 8, 9, 11, 12, 13, 14	3, 4, 10, 15
Somatic antigens	A, B	C, D
Cultures die off	rapidly	slowly
Pathogenicity	pneumonia in cattle and sheep, septicaemia in newborn lambs	septicaemia in older lambs, more than 3 months
Latent infection	nasopharynx of ox & sheep	

■ Morphology
The microscopic appearance corresponds to that of *P. multocida*.

■ Culture
Growth is poor on plain nutrient agar, but on blood agar, round, moist greyish colonies develop in 24 hours, with a diameter of 1 to 3 mm. A distinct haemolysis is shown on blood agar and bovine blood is particularly suitable (fig. 104).

■ Biochemical properties (cf. fig. 98)
Two biotypes A and T can be differentiated, their various properties are shown in table 38. More than 90 % of strains fall into biotype A (4, 17, 63).

■ Antigenic structure
A classification on the basis of antigenic structure can be carried out as in *P. multocida*. CARTER (11) first demonstrated surface antigens by means of the indirect haemagglutination test and BIBERSTEIN et al. (5), using the agglutination test, showed that somatic antigens were also present. The distribution of the antigens is shown in table 38. Sheep very frequently harbour the type A 1 (17, 19).

■ Animal inoculation
P. haemolytica is decidedly less pathogenic to laboratory animals than *P. multocida*. Nevertheless, a varying percentage of mice die following the intravenous or intraperitoneal injection. Rabbits, on the other hand, withstand cultures administered intravenously without harm, but not intraperitoneally (45). More than 10^8 bacteria are required for a fatal infection of mice, whereas 10^1 to 10^8 were needed to kill a mouse with *P. multocida* (56).

■ Morphologie
Das mikroskopische Aussehen entspricht *P. multocida*.

■ Kultur
Auf einfachem Nähragar tritt nur ein schwaches Wachstum auf. Auf Blutagar bilden sich nach 24 h runde, feuchte, graue Kolonien mit einem Durchmesser von 1 bis 3 mm. Auf Blutagar, besonders geeignet ist Rinderblut, wird eine deutliche Hämolyse gebildet (Abb. 104).

■ Kulturell-biochemische Eigenschaften
Siehe Abb. 48. Es lassen sich die zwei Biotypen A und T unterscheiden, deren verschiedene Eigenschaften zeigt Tab. 38. Über 90 % der Stämme gehören dem Biotyp A an (4, 17, 63).

■ Antigenstruktur
Eine Antigendifferenzierung läßt sich in ähnlicher Weise wie bei *P. multocida* durchführen. CARTER (11) wies erstmalig mittels der indirekten Hämagglutination Oberflächenantigene nach, BIBERSTEIN et al. (5) konnten zusätzlich mit der Agglutination somatische Antigene nachweisen. Die Verteilung der Antigene zeigt Tab. 38. Bei Schafen wurden die Typen A 1 und A 2 besonders oft gefunden (17, 19).

■ Tierversuch
Im Vergleich zu *P. multocida* ist *P. haemolytica* deutlich geringer versuchstierpathogen, jedoch sterben Mäuse in unterschiedlichen Prozentsätzen nach iv. oder ip. Infektion, Kaninchen vertragen iv. Kulturinjektionen ohne Schaden, nicht jedoch die ip. Infektion (45). Für die tödliche Infektion der Maus sind über 10^8 Keime (*P. multocida* 10^1–10^8 Keime/Maus) erforderlich (56).

1.1.3 Pasteurella pneumotropica

P. pneumotropica is found mainly as a commensal on the mucous membranes of rodents and, as a facultative pathogen it can participate in diseases, particularly of the respiratory organs. In this respect it is of significance when keeping laboratory animals (1, 37, 38, 62). It has also been isolated from the nasopharynx of dogs and can be transmitted to man through bites.

Its growth in culture corresponds to the nonmucoid forms of *P. multocida*. The biochemical properties are listed in figure 98 and the uncertainty of its taxonomic position is discussed on page 125.

1.1.4 Pasteurella ureae

This organism has been described as a cause of abortion and foetal deaths in pigs and other species (1, 15, 66). Only occasionally do the pleomorphic rods give the bipolar staining reaction. It grows well on blood agar, producing a viridans haemolysis. The biochemical properties are shown in figure 98.

1.1.5 Pasteurella gallinarum

P. gallinarum is a commensal of the respiratory mucosa of poultry and possesses little pathogenicity. It can, however, participate as the cause of respiratory diseases and it has been found in fowl cholera and keratoconjunctivitis (24). The biochemical properties are summarized in figure 98.

1.1.6 Pasteurella aerogenes

This is found mainly in the pig as a normal inhabitant of the gut; it is rarely seen in other animals. The biochemical properties are listed in figure 98 (14, 42, 67).

1.1.7 Pasteurella anatipestifer
(Syn.: *Pfeifferella anatipestifer*, *Moraxella anatipestifer*)

P. anatipestifer causes serositis of ducks (»new duck disease«), a septicaemic disease of ducklings up to 2 weeks of age (29). The bacterium produces grey, mucoid, non-haemolytic colonies. Carbohydrates are not fermented, but gelatine is liquefied; it is indole and urease negative and catalase positive. The taxonomic position of the bacterium is uncertain.

1.1.3 Pasteurella pneumotropica

P. pneumotropica kommt hauptsächlich als Kommensale auf den Schleimhäuten von Nagetieren vor, kann sich als fakultativ pathogenes Bakterium an Erkrankungen besonders der Atmungsorgane beteiligen und besitzt insofern eine Bedeutung für die Versuchstierhaltung (1, 37, 38, 62). Es ist ferner vom Nasopharynx von Hunden isoliert worden und kann durch Bisse auf den Menschen übertragen werden.

Das kulturelle Wachstum entspricht den nichtmukoiden Kolonien von *P. multocida*. Kulturellbiochemische Eigenschaften zeigt Abb. 98. Über die taxonomisch unsichere Stellung siehe S. 125.

1.1.4 Pasteurella ureae

Das Bakterium ist als Ursache von Aborten und Totgeburten beim Schwein und bei anderen Tierarten beschrieben worden (1, 15, 66). Die pleomorphen Stäbchen färben sich nur gelegentlich bipolar. Das Bakterium wächst gut auf Blutagar, dabei bildet sich eine vergrünende Hämolyse aus. Kulturellbiochemische Eigenschaften vergleiche Abb. 98.

1.1.5 Pasteurella gallinarum

P. gallinarum ist ein Kommensale auf den Schleimhäuten des Respirationstraktes beim Geflügel und von geringer Pathogenität. Sie kann sich ursächlich an Erkrankungen des Respirationstraktes beteiligen und bei der Läppchenkrankheit und bei Keratokonjunktivitis nachgewiesen werden (24). Kulturellbiochemische Eigenschaften siehe Abb. 98.

1.1.6 Pasteurella aerogenes

Das Bakterium wird hauptsächlich beim Schwein als normaler Darmbewohner und selten bei anderen Tierarten gefunden. Kulturell-biochemische Eigenschaften siehe Abb. 98 (14, 42, 67).

1.1.7 Pasteurella anatipestifer
(Syn.: *Pfeifferella anatipestifer*, *Moraxella anatipestifer*)

Ursache der infektiösen Serositis der Enten (»new duck disease«), eine septikämische Erkrankung der Jungenten bis zu 2 Wochen (20). Das Bakterium wächst in schleimigen, grauen Kolonien ohne Hämolyse. Kohlenhydrate werden nicht fermentiert, Gelatine wird verflüssigt, indol- und ureasenegativ, katalasepositiv. Die taxonomische Stellung des Bakteriums ist unsicher.

Bibliography / Literatur

1. ACKERMAN, J. I., & J. G. FOX (1981): Isolation of Pasteurella ureae from reproductive tracts of congenic mice. J. clin. Microbiol. 13, 1049–1053.
2. BAIN, R. V. S. (1963): Hemorrhagic septicaemia. FAO Agricultural Studies. Rome, No. 62.
3. BEICHEL, E. (1986): Differenzierung von 130 X- und V-Faktor-unabhängigen aviären Bakterienstämmen der Familie Pasteurellaceae Pohl 1981 unter besonderer Berücksichtigung neuer taxonomischer Erkenntnisse. Vet. Med. Diss. Hannover.
4. BIBERSTEIN, E. L., & C. K. FRANCIS (1968): Nucleic acid and homologies between the A and T Types of Pasteurella haemolytica. J. Med. Microbiol. 1, 105–108.
5. BIBERSTEIN, E. L., M. GILL & H. KNIGHT (1960): Serological types of Pasteurella haemolytica. Cornell Vet. 50, 283–300.
6. BLOBEL, H., J. BRÜCKLER, K. K. BAXI & A. AMEND (1985): Eigenschaften von Pasteurellen aus Atemwegserkrankungen vom Rind. Tierärztl. Umschau 40, 860–864.
7. BROGDEN, K. A., & R. A. PACKER (1979): Comparison of Pasteurella multocida serotyping systems. Am. J. Vet. Res. 40, 1332–1335.
8. CARTER, G. R. (1963): Proposed modification of the serological classification of Pasteurella multocida. Vet. Rec. 75, 1264–1265.
9. CARTER, G. R. (1957): Studies on Pasteurella multocida. II. Identification of antigenic characteristics and colonial variants. Am. J. Vet. Res. 18, 210–213.
10. CARTER, G. R. (1957): Studies on Pasteurella multocida. III. A serological survey of bovine and porcine strains from various parts of the world. Am. J. Vet. Res. 18, 437–440.
11. CARTER, G. R. (1956): A serological study of Pasteurella haemolytica. Canad. J. Microbiol. 2, 483–488.
12. CARTER, G. R. (1955): Studies on Pasteurella multocida. I. A haemagglutination test for the identification of serological types. Am. J. Vet. Res. 16, 481–484.
13. CHANDRASEKARAN, S., & P. C. YEAP (1982): Pasteurella multocida in pigs: the serotypes and the assessment of their virulence in mice. Brit. Vet. J. 138, 332–336.
14. CHLADEK, D. W., & R. P. ELLIS (1979): Serologic study of Pasteurella aerogenes sp. n. Am. J. Vet. Res. 40, 446–448.
15. CORKISH, J. D., & R. D. NAYLOR (1982): Abortion in sows and the isolation of Pasteurella ureae. Vet. Rec. 110, 582.
16. DAO TRONG DAT, W. BATHKE & D. SCHIMMEL (1973): Die Bedeutung der Pasteurelleninfektion bei Erkrankungen des Respirationstraktes der Kälber. I. Mitt. Isolierung und Charakterisierung der Pasteurellen. Arch. exp. Vet. Med. 27, 909–924.
17. FODOR, L., J. VARGA, I. HAJTOS & G. SZEMEREDI (1984): Serotypes of Pasteurella haemolytica isolated from sheep, goats and calves. Zbl. Vet. Med. B 31, 466–469.
18. FOX, M. L., R. G. THOMSON & S. E. MAGWOOD (1971): Pasteurella haemolytica of cattle: Serotype, production of beta-galactosidase and antibacterial sensitivity. Can. J. Comp. Med. 35, 313–317.
19. FRASER, J., N. J. GILMOUR, S. LAIRD & W. DONACHIE (1982): Prevalence of Pasteurella haemolytica serotypes from ovine pasteurellosis in Britain. Vet. Rec. 110, 560–561.
20. GERLACH, H. (1970): Pasteurella anatipestifer-Infektion bei Entenküken. Dtsch. tierärztl. Wschr. 77, 541–542.
21. GERLACH, A. (1977): Die Bedeutung von Pasteurella haemolytica in Hühnerbeständen. Prakt. Tierarzt 58, 324–328.
22. GHONIEM, N., G. AMTSBERG & W. BISPING (1973): Vergleichende Darstellung des biochemischen Reaktionsspektrums von Pasteurella multocida-Stämmen von Hund und Schwein. Zbl. Vet. Med. B 20, 310–317.
23. GIBBS, H. A., M. H. ALLAN, A. WISEMAN & I. E. SELMAN (1983): Pneumonic pasteurellosis in housed, weaned, single suckled calves. Vet. Rec. 112, 87.
24. HALL, W. J., K. L. HEDDLESTON, D. H. LENGENHAUSEN & R. W. HUGHES (1955): Studies on pasteurellosis. I. A new species of Pasteurella encountered in chronic fowl cholera. Am. J. Vet. Res. 16, 598–603.
25. HEDDLESTON, K. L., J. E. GALLAGHER & P. A. REBERS (1972): Fowl cholera: gel diffusion precipitin test for serotyping Pasteurella multocida from avian species. Avian Dis. 16, 925–936.
26. HELLMANN, E. (1959): Zur kulturellen und morphologischen Differenzierung der Pasteurella multocida. Zbl. Vet. med. B 6, 781–795.
27. HENNING, J. (1971): Typisierung von Pasteurella multocida mit Hilfe des indirekten Hämagglutinationstestes. Zbl. Bakt. I. Orig. A 216, 414–417.
28. HIPPE, W. (1982): Zur ätiologischen Bedeutung von Pasteurellen und Bordetellen für den Ansteckenden Schnupfen des Kaninchen. Tierärztl. Umschau 37, 284–290.
29. HIPPE, W., & T. SCHLIESSER (1981): Kulturelle und serologische Untersuchungen an Pasteurella-multocida-Stämmen von Kaninchen mit Erkrankungen der oberen Atemwege. Zbl. Vet. Med. B 28, 645–653.
30. JENTSCH, K. D. (1961): Vergleichende kulturelle, biochemische und serologische Untersuchungen an Pasteurella multocida-Stämmen aus gesunden und entzündeten Schweinelungen. Zbl. Vet. med. B 8, 1158–1169.
31. JONG, M. F. DE, H. L. OEI & G. J. TETENBURG (1980): AR-pathogenicity tests for Pasteurella multocida isolates. Int. Pig Vet. Soc. Congr. Copenhagen. S. 211.
32. JONG, M. F. DE, & G. H. A. BORST (1985): Selective medium for the isolation of P. multocida and B. bronchiseptica. Vet. Rec. 116, 167.
33. JORDACHE, A., C. UNGUREANU, U. FIERLINGER, F. CARASU, V. PADURARU, D. SCHIMMEL & P. KIELSTEIN (1981): Identifizierung der Pasteurella-Serotypen durch indirekte Hämagglutination. Archiv. Vet. (Bukarest) 15, 57–64.
34. KIELSTEIN, P., & D. SCHIMMEL (1983): Durch Pasteurellen bedingte Pneumonien des Kalbes und Möglichkeiten ihrer experimentellen Übertragung. Mh. Vet. Med. 38, 83–87.
35. KILIAN, M., W. FREDERIKSEN & E. L. BIBERSTEIN (1981): Haemophilus, Pasteurella and Actinobacillus. London: Academic Press.
36. KNIGHT, D. P., J. E. PAINE & D. C. E. SPELLER (1983): A selective medium for Pasteurella multocida and its use with animal and human specimens. J. clin. Path. 36, 591–594.
37. KRÜGER, M., F. HORSCH & E. SCHUBERT (1980): Pasteurella-pneumotropica-Infektion bei Albinoratten. Mh. Vet. Med. 35, 193–195.
38. KUNSTÝR, I., H. HACKBARTH, H. NEUMANN, S. RODE & H. MÜLLER (1980): Pasteurella-pneumotropica-Infektion in einer Barrieren-Ratten-Zuchteinheit. Zschr. Versuchstierkd. 22, 303–308.
39. LITTLE, P. A., & B. M. LYON (1943): Demonstration of serological types within the nonhemolytic Pasteurella. Am. J. Vet. Res. 4, 110–112.
40. MANNHEIM, W. (1981): Taxonomic implications of DNA relatedness and quinone patterns. In: KILIAN, M., W. FREDERIKSEN & E. L. BIBERSTEIN (eds.): Haemophilus, Pasteurella, and Actinobacillus. London: Academic Press.
41. MATTHES, S., H. CH. LÖLIGER & H. J. SCHUBERT (1969): Enzootisches Auftreten der Pasteurella haemolytica beim Huhn. Dtsch. tierärztl. Wschr. 76, 94–95.
42. McALLISTER, H. A., & G. R. CARTER (1974): An aerogenic Pasteurella-like organism recovered from swine. Am. J. Vet. Res. 35, 917–922.
43. MEYERINGH, H., C. DIRKS, P. SCHÖSS & H. SCHIMMELPFENNIG (1977): Untersuchungen zur Ätiologie der

Rhinitis atrophicans des Schweines. Dtsch. tierärztl. Wschr. **84**, 266–268.
44. MEYERINGH, H. (1975): Untersuchungen zur Ätiologie der Rhinitis atrophicans des Schweines, serologische Bestimmung der Kapselantigene von Pasteurella multocida-Kulturen und Untersuchungen zur Kontagiosität experimentell erzeugter Pasteurella multocida-Rhinitiden. Vet. Med. Diss. Hannover.
45. MRÁZ, O. (1969): Pasteurella haemolytica Newsom and Cross, 1932. Zbl. Bakt. I. Ref. **215**, 267–280.
46. MÜLLER, H. E., & E. RASCHKE (1969): Zur Pasteurella multocida-Infektion beim Menschen. Münch. med. Wschr. **111**, 19–23.
47. MURTY, D., & R. K. KAUSCHIK (1965): Studies on an outbreak of acute swine pasteurellosis due to Pasteurella multocida type B. Vet. Rec. **77**, 411.
48. MUTTERS, R., K. PIECHULLA, K. H. HINZ & W. MANNHEIM (1985): Pasteurella avium (Hinz and Kunjara 1977) comb. nov. and Pasteurella volantium sp. nov. Int. J. System. Bact. **35**, 5–9.
49. MUTTERS, R., P. IHM, S. POHL, W. FREDERIKSEN & W. MANNHEIM (1985): Reclassification of the genus Pasteurella Trevisan 1887 on the basis of deoxyribonucleic acid homology, with proposals for the new species Pasteurella dagmatis, Pasteurella canis, Pasteurella stomatis, Pasteurella anatis, and Pasteurella langaa. Int. J. System. Bact. **35**, 309–322.
50. NAMIOKA, S., & D. W. BRUNER (1963): Serological studies on Pasteurella multocida. IV. Type distribution of the organisms on the basis of their capsule and O-groups. Cornell Vet. **53**, 41–53.
51. NAMIOKA, S., & M. MURATA (1961): Serological studies on Pasteurella multocida. I. A simplified method for capsule typing of the organism. Cornell Vet. **51**, 498–507.
52. NAMIOKA, S., & M. MURATA (1961): Serological studies on Pasteurella multocida. II. Characteristics of somatic (O) antigen of the organism. Cornell Vet. **51**, 507–521.
53. NAMIOKA, S., & M. MURATA (1961): Serological studies on Pasteurella multocida. III. O antigenic analysis of cultures isolated from various animals. Cornell Vet. **51**, 522–528.
54. ROBERTS, R. S. (1947): An immunological study of Pasteurella septica. J. comp. Path. **57**, 261–278.
55. RUTTER, J. M., & P. D. LUTHER (1984): Cell culture assay for toxigenic Pasteurella multocida from atrophic rhinitis of pigs. Vet. Rec. **114**, 393–396.
56. SCHIMMEL, D., P. KIELSTEIN, W. BRUER, R. PUTSCHE & R. SLUCKA (1983): Isolierung und Differenzierung von Pasteurellen aus dem Respirationstrakt des Kalbes. Mh. Vet. Med. **38**, 81–83.
57. SCHIMMEL, D., U. FIERLINGER, A. JORDACHE, R. PUTSCHE & C. UNGUREANU (1981): Zur serologischen Typisierung von P. multocida. Archiv. Vet. (Bukarest) **15**, 65–68.
58. SCHIMMEL, D., & P. KIELSTEIN (1980): Bedeutung bakterieller Infektionen im enzootischen Pneumonie-Komplex der Kälber und Maßnahmen zu ihrer Bekämpfung. Mh. Vet. Med. **35**, 30–31.
59. SCHÖSS, P., C. P. THIEL & H. SCHIMMELPFENNIG (1985): Rhinitis atrophicans des Schweines: Untersuchungen über das Vorkommen toxinbildender Stämme von Pasteurella multocida und Bordetella bronchiseptica. Dtsch. tierärztl. Wschr. **92**, 316–319.
60. SMITH, G. R. (1960): Virulence and toxicity of Pasteurella haemolytica in the experimental production of ovine septicemia. J. comp. Path. **70**, 429–436.
61. SMITH, G. R. (1960): The pathogenicity of Pasteurella haemolytica for young lambs. J. comp. Path. **70**, 326–328.
62. SHEPHERD, A. J., A. P. LEMAN & R. J. BARNETT (1982): Isolation of Pasteurella pneumotropica from rodents in South Africa. J. Hyg. **89**, 79–87.
63. SMITH, G. R. (1959): Isolation of two types of Pasteurella haemolytica from sheep. Nature **183**, 1123–1133.
64. SPANOGHE, L., & G. OKERMANN (1978): Die infektiösen und nichtinfektiösen Ursachen des enzootischen Schnupfens bei Schlachtkaninchen. Prakt. Tierarzt **59**, 20–24.
65. STILLE, W., L. STOLL & E. HELM (1969): Infektionen mit Pasteurella multocida nach Tierbissen. Dtsch. med. Wschr. **94**, 1816–1820.
66. SUZUKI, T. (1980): Die Isolierung von Pasteurella ureae im Zusammenhang mit Totgeburten bei Schweinen. J. Jap. Vet. Med. Ass. **33**, 219–222.
67. THIGPEN, J. E., M. E. CLEMENTS & B. N. GUPTA (1978): Isolation of Pasteurella aerogenes from the uterus of a rabbit following abortion. Lab. Anim. Sci. **28**, 444–447.
68. THIEL, C. P. (1983): Untersuchungen über das Vorkommen toxinbildender Pasteurella multocida- und Bordetella bronchiseptica-Stämme bei der Rhinitis atrophicans des Schweines. Vet. Med. Diss. Hannover.
69. WARD, G. E., R. MOFFAT & E. OLFERT (1978): Abortion in mice associated with Pasteurella pneumotropica. J. clin. Microbiol. **8**, 177–180.
70. WRAY, C., & J. R. A. MORRISON (1983): Antibiotic resistant Pasteurella haemolytica. Vet. Rec. **113**, 143.

1.2 Genus: Actinobacillus (Act.)

This genus includes Gram-negative, non-motile, ovoid to rod-shaped bacteria, that measure $0.4 \times 1.0 \mu m$. They can be pervaded by coccoid elements, which often accumulate at the ends, giving the rods a characteristic »morse-code« form. Occasionally filaments are produced.

Actinobacilli are aerobic or facultatively anaerobic.

The colonies tend to be of a tacky to mucoid consistency, especially on primary culture, and they are difficult to lift off the medium.

The biochemical properties used in the determination of genus and species are presented in table 33 and figure 103.

1.2 Gattung: Actinobacillus (Act.)

Die Gattung umfaßt gramnegative, unbewegliche, $0,4 \times 1,0 \mu m$ große, ovale bis stäbchenförmige Bakterien, die mit kokkoiden Elementen durchsetzt sein können, die oft an den Enden liegen und den Stäbchen eine charakteristische »Morsecode-Form« geben können. Gelegentlich werden Fäden gebildet.

Aktinobazillen sind aerob und fakultativ anaerob.

Besonders bei Erstisolierungen neigen die Kolonien zu zähklebrigem bis schleimigem Wachstum, so daß sie von der Nährbodenoberfläche schwer abzuheben sind.

Die kulturell-biochemischen Eigenschaften zur Gattungs- und Artbestimmung sind in der Tab. 33

Specimens

Microscopic demonstration of the granules (drusen) in suspected infection with Act. lignieresii

The colonies (0.3–0.4 mm in size) can be demonstrated in the pus either after pre-treatment with 15–20% KOH or staining with an iodine-potassium iodine solution with glycerol-picro carmine or Ziehl-Neelsen and careful decolourization in 1% H_2SO_4 (colonies lightly acid-fast)

Culture

Blood agar: after 24–48 h, greyish-white, tenacious colonies, adherent to the surface of the medium. This characteristic is dependent on the composition of the medium and may be lost in subcultures

Biochemical differentiation

1. Generic properties

Oxidase	+	Oxidation/fermentation	F
Glucose	+	Dulcitol	−
Lactose	+	Laevulose	+
Maltose	+	Nitrate	+
Xylose	+	Indole	−
Urease	+	Methyl red	−
Motility	−	Voges-Proskauer	−

2. Species characters

Character	Actinobacillus lignieresii	equuli	suis
Haemolysis	v⁻	v⁻	v⁺
Arabinose	−	−	+
Cellobiose	−	−	+
Mannitol	+	+	−
Melibiose	−	+	+
Raffinose	−	+	+
Salicin	−	−	+
Trehalose	−	−	+
Aesculin	−	−	+

Fig. 103: Demonstration and differentiation of actinobacilli

Abb. 103: Nachweis und Differenzierung von Aktinobazillen

According to Bergey's manual the genus contains the following species of veterinary interest:
▷ *Act. lignieresii*,
▷ *Act. equuli*,
▷ *Act. suis*,
▷ *Act. capsulatus* (cause of arthritis in rabbits).

Species of uncertain classification:
▷ *Act. seminis* which is described, particularly in Australia and South Africa as the cause of ovine, more rarely bovine, epididymitis (5, 14, 20, 21).
▷ *Act. salpingitidis*, isolated from hens affected with salpingitis (12), but hybridization experiments would indicate that it does not belong to the genus *Actinobacillus*.

und der Abb. 103 zusammengestellt.

Nach Bergey's manual werden innerhalb der Gattung folgende veterinärmedizinisch interessierende Arten unterschieden:
▷ *Act. lignieresii*,
▷ *Act. equuli*,
▷ *Act. suis*,
▷ *Act. capsulatus* (Arthritiserreger beim Kaninchen).

Arten mit unsicherer Zuordnung:
▷ *Act. seminis*, der insbesondere in Australien und Südafrika als Ursache oviner und seltener boviner Epididymitiden beschrieben wurde (5, 14, 20, 21).
▷ *Act. salpingitidis*, aus Hennen mit Salpingitis isoliert (12), scheint aufgrund von Hybridisierungsversuchen nicht zu dieser Gattung zu gehören.

1.2.1 Actinobacillus lignieresii

■ **Incidence and veterinary significance**
In cattle and sheep, and very rarely in horses, dogs and cats. *Act. lignieresii* causes actinomycosis-like changes in soft tissues, (such as the tongue, lymph nodes) and also in internal organs like the lungs, stomach and liver (18). Man is very rarely affected and the disease presents as a generalized or local infection. Purulent lesions develop with Gram-negative microcolonies (actinobacillosis). The organisms are commensals in the rumen and oral mucosa (14, 15).

■ **Culture**
See figure 105.

■ **Biochemical properties** (10, 11)
See table 33 and figure 103.

■ **Antigenic structure**
By means of agglutination and other reactions, it is possible to differentiate a number of types (14). There is an antigenic relationship between *Act. lignieresii*, *Ps. mallei* and the pasteurellae.

■ **Animal inoculation**
Contradictory reports have been published, some stating that *Ac. lignieresii* is non-pathogenic to guinea pigs and others claiming that massive intraperitoneal injections cause the Strauss phenomenon and produce orchitis.

1.2.2 Actinobacillus equuli
(Syn.: *Bact. nephritidis equi*, *Bact. viscosum equi*, *Shigella equirulis* etc.)

■ **Incidence and veterinary significance**
»Early paresis« of foals (paresis of foals, pyosepticaemia). A disease of the first few days of life, occurring as a rule between the 2nd and 5th days. It is rare in older foals. Characteristic features are polyarthritis and glomerulonephritis. Older horses can develop nephritis. *Act. equuli* is a commensal of the gut of healthy horses. Infections of pigs and dogs are less common.

■ **Culture**
See figure 106.

■ **Biochemical properties**
See table 33 and figure 103.

■ **Animal inoculation**
Act. equuli is non-pathogenic for small laboratory animals.

1.2.1 Actinobacillus lignieresii

■ **Vorkommen und medizinische Bedeutung**
Ursache aktinomykoseähnlicher Veränderungen der weichen Gewebe (z. B. Zunge, Lymphknoten), aber auch von inneren Organen wie Lunge, Magen, Leber (18) bei Rind und Schaf (2) sowie sehr selten bei Pferden, Hunden und Katzen (9). Sehr selten sind auch Infektionen beim Menschen in Form von Allgemein- oder Lokalinfektionen möglich (6), die vom Tier ausgehen können. Es entstehen eitrige Affektionen mit gramnegativen Drusen (Aktinobazillose). Kommensale im Pansen und auf der Mundschleimhaut (14, 15).

■ **Kultur**
Siehe Abb. 105.

■ **Kulturell-biochemische Eigenschaften**
Siehe Tab. 33 und Abb. 103 (10, 11).

■ **Antigenstruktur**
Es lassen sich mittels der Agglutination und anderer Reaktionen verschiedene Typen unterscheiden (14). Es bestehen Antigenverwandtschaften mit *Ps. mallei* und Pasteurellen.

■ **Tierversuch**
Es liegen widersprüchliche Mitteilungen vor, nach denen *Act. lignieresii* entweder für Meerschweinchen apathogen ist oder indem es nach massiver ip. Infektion zu Hodenentzündungen in Form des Strausschen Phänomens kommt.

1.2.2 Actinobacillus equuli
(Syn.: *Bac. nephritidis equi*, *Bact. viscosum equi*, *Shigella equirulis* u. a.)

■ **Vorkommen und medizinische Bedeutung**
»Frühlähme« der Fohlen (Fohlenlähme, Pyoseptikämie). Erkrankung in den ersten Lebenstagen (in der Regel 2.–5. d), selten bei älteren Fohlen. Charakteristisch sind Polyarthritis und Glomerulonephritis. Bei älteren Pferden kann eine Nephritis auftreten. Kommensale im Verdauungskanal gesunder Pferde. Seltener sind Infektionen beim Schwein und Hund.

■ **Kultur**
Siehe Abb. 106.

■ **Kulturell-biochemische Eigenschaften**
Siehe Tab. 33 und Abb. 103.

■ **Tierversuch**
Act. equuli ist für kleine Versuchstiere apathogen.

1.2.3 Actinobacillus suis

■ Incidence and veterinary significance
Act. suis causes diseases in pigs. In sucking piglets they are usually of septic character but in older piglets and weaners they mostly take a subacute to chronic course (arthritis, periarthritis, endocarditis, formation of multiple abscesses). In adult pigs the lesions tend to be more localized (e. g. kidneys) (3, 8, 13, 22, 23). Infections can also occur in other domestic animals (e. g. horse), but they are very rare.

■ Culture
A distinct haemolysis develops on blood agar within 24 hours, but the viability of the cultures is limited (22, 23).

■ Biochemical properties
See table 33 and figure 103. It is debatable whether *Act. suis* should be considered a different species from *Act. equuli* (because it is haemolytic, pathogenic to mice and mannitol is not fermented). MRÁZ (11) considers it to be merely a haemolytic variant of *Act. equuli*.

■ Animal inoculation
It is fatal to mice when injected intraperitoneally.

1.2.3 Actinobacillus suis

■ Vorkommen und medizinische Bedeutung
Ursache von Erkrankungen bei Schweinen, die bei Saugferkeln meistens septischen Charakter besitzen, bei älteren Ferkeln und Läufern überwiegend subakut bis chronisch verlaufen (Arthritis, Periarthritis, Endokarditis, multiple Abszeßbildung) und bei erwachsenen Schweinen Herdinfektionen (z. B. in der Niere) bilden können (3, 8, 13, 22, 23). Sehr selten können Infektionen auch bei anderen Haustieren vorkommen, z. B. beim Pferd (4).

■ Kultur
Auf der Blutplatte bildet sich nach 24 h eine deutliche Hämolyse. Die Lebensfähigkeit der Kulturen ist begrenzt (22, 23).

■ Kulturell-biochemische Eigenschaften
Siehe Tab. 33 und Abb. 103. Ob *Act. suis* im Vergleich zu *Act. equuli* als eigene Art (fehlender Mannitabbau, Hämolyse, Mäusepathogenität) gerechtfertigt ist, wird bestritten, nach MRÁZ (11) stellt er nur eine hämolytische Variante zu *Act. equuli* dar.

■ Tierversuch
Die ip. Infektion von Mäusen führt zum Tode.

Bibliography / Literatur

1. BAILIE, W. E., H. D. ANTHONY & K. D. WEIDE (1966): Infectious thromboembolic meningoencephalomyelitis in feedlot cattle. J. Am. Vet. Med. Ass. **148**, 162–166.
2. BEHRENS, H. (1983): Aktinobazillose des Schafes. Tierärztl. Umschau **38**, 633.
3. BOULEY, G. (1966): Étude d'une souche d'actinobacillus suis isolée en Normandie. Rec. Méd. Vét. **142**, 25–29.
4. CARMAN, M. G., & R. T. HODGES (1982): Actinobacillus suis infection of horses. New Zeal. Vet. J. **30**, 82–84.
5. ERASMUS, J. A., J. A. L. DE WET & L. PRZOZESKY (1982): Actinobacillus seminis infection in a Walrich ram. J. S. Afr. Vet. Med. Ass. **53**, 129.
6. FLAMM, H., & G. WIEDERMANN (1962): Infektionen durch den Actinobacillus lignieresii beim Menschen. Zsch. Hyg. **148**, 368–374.
7. JONES, T. H., K. J. BARRETT, L. W. GREENHAM, A. D. OSBORNE & R. R. ASHDOWN (1964): Seminal vesiculitis in bulls associated with infection by Actinobacillus actinoides. Vet. Rec. **76**, 24–28.
8. MAIR, N. S., C. J. RANDALL, G. W. THOMAS, J. F. HARBOURNE, C. T. MCCREA & K. P. COWL (1974): Actinobacillus suis infection in pigs: a report of four outbreaks and two sporadic cases. J. comp. Path. **84**, 113–119.
9. MAYER, H. (1981): Actinobacillus. In: H. BLOBEL & T. SCHLIESSER (Hrsg.): Handbuch der bakteriellen Infektionen bei Tieren. Bd. 3., S. 594–626. Jena: VEB Gustav Fischer.
10. MRÁZ, O. (1969): Vergleichende Studie der Arten Actinobacillus lignieresii und Pasteurella haemolytica. I. Mitt.: Actinobacillus lignieresii. Zbl. Bakt. I. Orig. **209**, 212–232.
11. MRÁZ, O. (1968): Actinobacillus lignieresii Brumpt 1910. Übersichtsreferat. Zbl. Bakt. I. Ref. **214**, 149–160.
12. MRÁZ, O., P. VLADÍK & J. BOHÁČEK (1976): Actinobacilli in domestic fowl. Zbl. Bakt. I. Orig. A **236**, 294–307.
13. PEDERSEN, K. B. (1977): Actinobacillus infections in swine. Nord. Vet. Med. **29**, 137–140.
14. PHILLIPS, J. E. (1967): Antigenic structure and serological typing of Actinobacillus lignieresii. J. Path. Bact. **93**, 463–475.
15. PHILLIPS, J. E. (1964): Commensal actinobacilli from the bovine tongue. J. Path. Bact. **87**, 442–444.
16. PHILLIPS, J. E. (1961): The commensal role of Actinobacillus lignieresii. J. Path. Bact. **82**, 205–208.
17. SMITH, T. (1918): A pleomorphic bacillus from pneumonic lungs of calves simulating Actinomyces. J. Exp. Med. **28**, 333–343.
18. TILL, D. H., & F. P. PALMER (1960): A review of actinobacillosis with a study of the causal organism. Vet. Rec. **72**, 527–534.
19. TONDER, E. M. VAN (1979): Actinobacillus seminis infection in sheep in the Republic of South Africa. Onderstepoort J. Vet. Res. **46**, 129–133, 141–148.
20. TONDER, E. M. VAN, & T. F. W. BOLTON (1970): The isolation of Actinobacillus seminis from bovine semen, a preliminary report. J. S. Afr. Vet. Med. Ass. **41**, 287–288.
21. WORTHINGTON, R. W., & P. P. BOSMAN (1968): Isolation of Actinobacillus seminis in South Africa. J. S. Afr. Vet. Med. Ass. **39**, 81–85.
22. ZIMMERMANN, T. (1965): Die Actinobazillose des Schweines. Tierärztl. Umschau **20**, 565–568.
23. ZIMMERMANN, T. (1969): Untersuchungen über die Actinobacillose des Schweines. 1. Mitt. Isolierung u. Charakterisierung der Erreger. Dtsch. tierärztl. Wschr. **71**, 457–461.

1.3 Family Vibrionaceae
1.3.1 Genus: Vibrio (V.)

The Campylobacter species were at one time classed under this genus. However, because of certain bacteriological properties, such as micro-aerophilic growth, considerable inactivity towards carbohydrates and a different cytosine/guanine content of the DNA, they have now been classified separately. The genus *Vibrio* has thus lost much of its erstwhile importance to mammals and it practically includes only species which are pathogenic to birds and fish.

1.3.1.1 Vibrio metschnikovi

This bacterium has been described in rare cases as the cause of a cholera-like gastro-enteritis of birds (KUJUMGIEV, 19; KRAUSE & WINDRATH, 18; GAMELÉIA, 8). Many of the isolations of *V. metschnikovi* reported in recent years were probably due to *Campylobacter* (page 224).

V. metschnikovi is a comma-shaped bacterium which cannot be differentiated under the microscope from *V. cholerae*. It will grow aerobically on the simplest media and forms smooth edged or rough, transparent colonies 2–4 mm in diameter.

■ **Biochemical properties**
See tables 33 and 39.

1.3.1.2 Vibrio anguillarum

This is the cause of infection in many species of fish (20), especially those which inhabit salt or brackish water. *V. anguillarum* requires high salt concentrations, the optimum concentration being between 1.5 and 3.5 %.

Table 39: Biochemical properties of *V. metschnikovi* (20)

Broth containing					
3.5 % salt	+	Gal	+	Sac	+
Ind	+	Lev	+	Sor	−
Ara	−	Mal	+	Xyl	−
Glu	+	Man	+		

Table 40: Biochemical properties of *V. anguillarum* (20, 28)

Feature	V. anguillarum		
	Type A	Type B	Type C
Ind	+	−	−
H₂S	−	−	−
Ara	+	+	−
Cel	+	+	−
Glu	+	+	+
Gly	+	+	−
Man	+	−	+
Sac	+	−	+
Tre	+	+	+
Amy	−	−	+
Lit	R	R	R

The most important infectious disease caused by *V. anguillarum* affects salt water eels. The clinical signs are patches of skin necrosis, primarily in the head region and the development of red areas on the skin. The infection becomes generalized and mortality is high (27). The disease was first described in eels, but has since been seen in a number of bony fishes.

V. anguillarum is a Gram-negative, curved bacterium with monotrichous flagellation. Simple media with the salt content increased to 1–1.5 % will grow visible colonies within 2 days at 20 °C. The biochemical properties are listed in table 40. *V. anguillarum* is very sensitive to the vibriostatic agent O/129. With this test it is possible to differentiate vibrios from other Gram-negative rods, especially aeromonads, which are resistant to O/129 (34). Blood agar can be used for this in the form of a disc test (Oxoid discs with 10 or 150 µg). Incubation 24 h at 37 °C.

Several biotypes and serotypes can be differentiated in this species (tab. 40).

V. piscium is identical with *V. anguillarum*, according to Bergey's manual (SHEWAN & VÉRON, 34), and it has been observed in infections of pike and carp (5). It is probable that *V. piscium var. japonicum* is a fresh water variant that is responsible for a furunculosis-like disease of rainbow trout (14, 15).

Unter den Infektionskrankheiten steht die Salzwasseraalseuche (Rotseuche) im Vordergrund. Die Krankheitssymptome bestehen in flächigen Hautnekrosen, besonders in der Kopfregion, und fleckenartiger Rotfärbung der Haut, gleichzeitig besteht eine Allgemeininfektion mit teilweise hoher Sterblichkeit (27). Die Krankheit wurde zuerst bei Aalen beobachtet, inzwischen aber auch bei einer Vielzahl von Knochenfischen festgestellt.

V. anguillarum ist ein gramnegatives, monotrich begeißeltes, gebogenes Bakterium. Auf einfachen Nährböden mit einem erhöhten Kochsalzgehalt von 1 bis 1,5 % tritt bei 20 °C innerhalb von 2 d sichtbares Koloniewachstum auf. Kulturell-biochemische Eigenschaften zeigt Tab. 40. *V. anguillarum* ist gegenüber dem Vibriostatikum O/129 empfindlich. Dadurch lassen sich diese Vibrionen von anderen gramnegativen Stäbchen, insbesondere Aeromonaden, die resistent sind, abgrenzen (34). Die Untersuchung kann auf Blutagar mit dem Blättchentest (Oxoid-Blättchen mit 150 bzw. 10 µg) geführt werden. Bebrütung 24 h/37 °C.

Innerhalb der Art lassen sich verschiedene Bio- und Serotypen unterscheiden (Tab. 40).

Identisch mit *V. anguillarum* ist nach Bergey's manual (SHEWAN & VÉRON, 34) *V. piscium*, der bei Infektionen von Hechten und Karpfen gefunden wurde (5). Bei *V. piscium var. japonicum* handelt es sich vermutlich um eine Süßwasservariante, die eine furunkuloseähnliche Erkrankung bei Regenbogenforellen verursacht (14, 15).

1.3.1.3 Vibrio parahaemolyticus

It was first described in Japan in 1961, as the cause of food poisoning following the consumption of raw sea fish and mussels. The bacterium occurs normally in sea water and can be found on salt water fish and their products. Two biotypes have been differentiated, only one haemolyzes human blood, but not the other (alginolyticus). Both have been found in Germany in the Baltic region (21, 22) and in other European countries (11), but their pathogenicity to man has not been proved.

1.3.1.3 Vibrio parahaemolyticus

Erstmals in Japan (1961) als Ursache einer Nahrungsmittelvergiftung nach Aufnahme von rohen Meeresfischen und Muscheln beschrieben. Das Bakterium kommt normalerweise im Seewasser, auf Seefischen und Seefischprodukten vor. Es lassen sich 2 Biotypen unterscheiden, von denen der eine Menschenblut hämolysiert, der andere nicht (alginolyticus). Beide Typen wurden in Deutschland im Ostseeraum (21, 22) und anderen europäischen Ländern (11) nachgewiesen, ihre Pathogenität für den Menschen ist jedoch noch ungeklärt.

1.3.2 Genus: Aeromonas (A.)

This genus, together with the genus *Vibrio* belongs to the family *Vibrionaceae*. The habitat of the aeromonads is primarily water, and they play a special role as fish pathogens. They are psychrophilic bacteria, but members of the »hydrophila« group will also grow at 37 °C and can therefore adapt to man and the warm-blooded domestic animals, where they may occasionally cause disease or a latent infection of the organs.

1.3.2 Gattung: Aeromonas

Die Gattung gehört zusammen mit der Gattung *Vibrio* zu der Familie der *Vibrionaceae*. Es handelt sich bei den Aeromonaden in erster Linie um Wasserbewohner, so daß sie als Erreger von Fischkrankheiten eine besondere Rolle spielen und psychrophile Bakterien sind. Die Vertreter der »hydrophila«-Gruppe wachsen jedoch auch bei 37 °C und können sich daher dem Menschen und den warmblütigen Haustieren anpassen und bei diesen gele-

Table 41: Classification and differentiation of Aeromonads (25) (cf. table 33)

Tabelle 41: Einteilung und Differenzierung der Aeromonaden (25), siehe auch Tab. 33

Generic characters			
Oxi	+		optimum temperature 22–28 °C
OF	+/+		Resistant to vibriostatic
Cat	+		agent O/129[1]
Nit	+		

Species characters						
Biochemical features	A. hydrophila	A. caviae	A. sobria	A. salmonicida subsp.		
				salmonicida	achromogenes	masoucida
Motility	+	+	+	−	−	−
Coccoid, pairs chains, clusters	−	−	−	+	+	+
Rods, single or pairs	+	+	+	−	−	−
Brown pigment formation	−	−	−	+	−	−
Growth in broth at 37 °C	+	+	+	−	−	−
Ind (1 % peptone water)	+	+	+	−	+	+
Amino acids as sole source of carbon						
L-arginine	+	+	+	−	−	−
L-histidine	+	+	+	−	−	+
Gas from Glu	+	−	+	+	−	+
VPR	+	−	v	−	−	+
H$_2$S (2.5 % peptone water)	+	−	+	−	−	+

[1] 2,4-diamino-6,7-diisopropylpteridine, disc test with 10 µg dissolved in dioxan (33)

[1] 2,4-Diamino-6,7-Diisopropylpteridin, Blättchentest, mit 10 µg gelöst in Dioxan (33)

The classification of the genus *Aeromonas* into species and subspecies has gone through numerous changes in recent years. The following system appears in Bergey's manual (25):
▷ Motile aeromonads
   A. hydrophila
   A. caviae
   A. sobria
▷ Non-motile aeromonads
   A. salmonicida with the subspecies
      salmonicida
      achromogenes
      masoucida

The most important differentiating features are listed in table 41.

1.3.2.1 Aeromonas hydrophila, A. caviae and A. sobria (motile aeromonads)

According to Bergey's manual, the motile aeromonads are classified into three species (tabs. 41 and 42).

■ **Incidence and veterinary significance**

The motile aeromonads are ubiquitous in water,

gentlich Erkrankungen auslösen oder zu einer latenten Besiedlung der Organe führen.

Die Einteilung der Gattung *Aeromonas* in Arten und Unterarten hat in den letzten Jahren vielfache Wandlungen erfahren. In Bergey's manual (25) ist folgende Einteilung vorgenommen worden:
▷ bewegliche Aeromonaden
   A. hydrophila
   A. caviae
   A. sobria
▷ unbewegliche Aeromonaden
   A. salmonicida, mit den Subspecies *salmonicida, achromogenes, masoucida*.

Die wichtigsten Unterscheidungsmerkmale sind in der Tab. 41 zusammengestellt.

1.3.2.1 Aeromonas hydrophila, A. caviae und A. sobria (bewegliche Aeromonaden)

Nach Bergey's manual (25) werden bei den beweglichen Aeromonaden drei Arten unterschieden (Tab. 41 u. 42).

■ **Vorkommen und medizinische Bedeutung**

Die beweglichen Aeromonaden sind ubiquitäre

142 Gram-negative, aerobic or microaerophilic or facultatively anaerobic rods, with simple cultural requirements

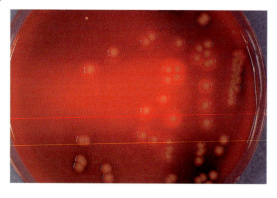
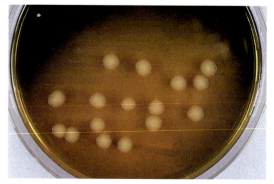
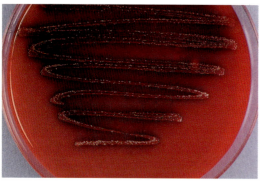
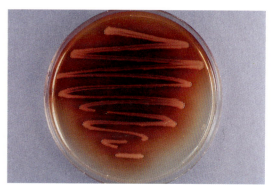

▲ Fig. 108: *Aeromonas sp.* isolated from the organs of a snake. Pure culture on blood agar. 48 h, 37 °C. Magnification x 0.4
▼ Fig. 110: *Aeromonas salmonicida, subsp. salmonicida,* pure culture on blood agar, weak haemolysis, 48 h, 37 °C. Magnification x 0.4

▲ Abb. 108: *Aeromonas sp.,* isoliert aus den Organen einer Schlange. Reinkultur auf Blutagar, 48 h, 37 °C, Abb.-M. 1 : 2,5
▼ Abb. 110: *Aeromonas salmonicida subsp. salmonicida,* Reinkultur auf Blutagar, schwache Hämolyse, 48 h, 25 °C, Abb.-M. 1 : 2,5

▲ Fig. 109: *Aeromonas sp.* isolated from the organs of a snake. Pure culture on Gassner plate, 48 h, 37 °C. Magnification x 0.4
▼ Fig. 111: *Aeromonas salmonicida, subsp. salmonicida,* pure culture on furunculosis agar. Formation of brown pigment, 48 h, 37 °C. Magnification x 0.25

▲ Abb. 109: *Aeromonas sp.,* isoliert aus den Organen einer Schlange. Reinkultur auf Gaßner-Platte, 48 h, 37 °C, Abb.-M. 1 : 2,5
▼ Abb. 111: *Aeromonas salmonicida subsp. salmonicida,* Reinkultur auf Furunculosis-Agar, Bildung von braunem Pigment, 48 h, 25 °C, Abb.-M. 1 : 4

their occurrence correlates with the content of organic substances in the water and thus they are part of the normal bacterial flora of fresh water fish. *A. caviae* and *A. sobria* are generally considered to be non-pathogenic. But strains that are pathogenic to fish do occur in the *A. hydrophila* group, although they cannot be related to any specific disease. They are probably more important in secondary infections (27). As such they are encountered as

Wasserbakterien, ihr Vorkommen korreliert mit dem Gehalt des Wassers an organischer Substanz. Sie gehören deswegen zur natürlichen Bakterienflora der Süßwasserfische. *A. caviae* und *A. sobria* gelten allgemein als apathogen. Innerhalb der *A. hydrophila*-Gruppe kommen fischpathogene Stämme vor, doch können sie keiner bestimmten Fischkrankheit zugeordnet werden. Sie spielen deswegen eher die Rolle von Sekundärerregern (27). In diesem

Table 42: Biochemical properties of motile Aeromonads (35)

Tabelle 42: Biochemisches Verhalten der beweglichen Aeromonaden (35)

Aeromonas sp.	Gas from Glu	H$_2$S	VPR	Aes	Sal
A. hydrophila	+	+	+	+	+
A. caviae	−	−	−	+	+
A. sobria	+	+	v	−	−

causes of disease in poikilothermic animals:
▷ infectious ascites of cyprinids, following a primary virus infection;
▷ »fresh water eel disease«;
▷ skin lesions in pike, Coregonus sp., cyprinids etc.;
▷ swim bladder inflammation in pike and grass carp;
▷ »red leg disease« of frogs.

A. hydrophila is a particular species that can grow in temperatures above 30 °C, and therefore it also occurs in diseases of warm-blooded animals (31). Injections of *A. hydrophila* can kill mice (4), but spontaneous diseases appear to be very rare. It has been reported in a septicaemia of the dog (24) and turkey (10), in bovine abortion (38) and mastitis (1), as well as in diarrhoea of pigs (6). Coincidental latent infections by these aeromonads can occur in the gut and they are also encountered as food contaminants (17). For a report on human infections see CASELITZ (3). Enteric conditions in man (food poisoning) may be due to the production of enterotoxins (39).

Zusammenhang werden sie bei folgenden Erkrankungen wechselwarmer Tiere gefunden:
▷ Infektiöse Bauchwassersucht der Cypriniden nach primärer Virusschädigung;
▷ Süßwasseraalseuche;
▷ Fleckenseuche des Hechtes, der Maräne, der Cypriniden u. a.;
▷ Rotseuche der Aale;
▷ Schwimmblasenentzündung bei Hechten, Zander, Graskarpfen; red leg disease bei Fröschen.

Da insbesondere *A. hydrophila* sich auch bei Temperaturen über 30 °C vermehren kann, kommen auch Infektionen bei warmblütigen Tieren vor (31). In Infektionsversuchen an Mäusen kann *A. hydrophila* zu Todesfällen führen (4). Spontane Erkrankungen scheinen sehr selten zu sein, es wird u. a. über septikämische Erkrankungen beim Hund (24) und bei Putcn (10), über einen Abort beim Rind (38) und Mastitis (1) sowie über Diarrhoe beim Schwein (6) berichtet. Gleichzeitig kommen diese Aeromonaden in Form von latenten Infektionen im Darm oder als Kontaminanten von Lebensmitteln vor (17). Über Infektionen des Menschen berichtete CASELITZ (3). Darmerkrankungen des Menschen (Lebensmittelvergiftungen) können durch Enterotoxine bedingt sein (39).

■ Culture

It will grow in nutrient and blood agar (fig. 108) and on selective media for *Enterobacteriaceae* as relatively large, grey to colourless colonies. Some strains are haemolytic.

Biochemical differentiation of aeromonads see table 42.

■ Kultur

Wachstum auf Nähr- und Blutagar (Abb. 108) sowie auf Selektivplatten für *Enterobacteriacae* (Abb. 109) in relativ großen, grauen bis farblosen Kolonien. Ein Teil der Stämme wächst hämolytisch.

Biochemische Unterscheidung der beweglichen Aeromonaden vergleiche Tab. 42.

1.3.2.2 Aeromonas salmonicida (non-motile aeromonads)

The following subspecies have been identified:
Subsp. salmonicida, which includes strains that originate from salmonid fishes and are biochemically characteristic,
subsp. achromogenes and *subsp. masoucida* which encompass two biochemically atypical strains isolated from salmonids.

1.3.2.2 Aeromonas salmonicida (unbewegliche Aeromonaden)

Innerhalb dieser Art werden unterschieden:
subsp. salmonicida, die biochemisch typische, von Salmoniden stammende Stämme umfaßt,
subsp. achromogenes und *subsp. masoucida,* die beide biochemisch untypische, von Salmoniden stammende Stämme umfassen.

Bei der Erythrodermatitis (chronische oder Ge-

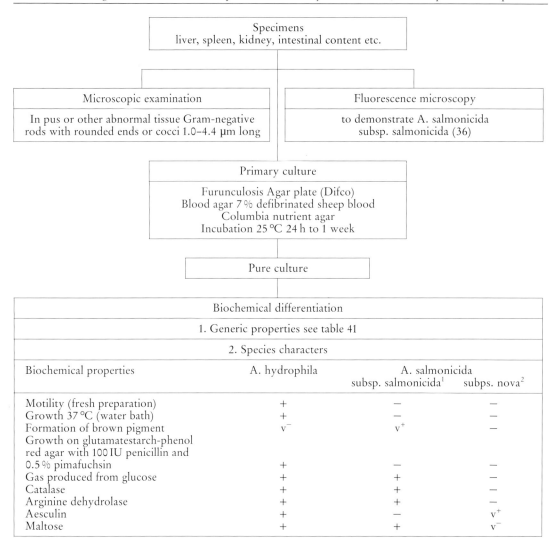

Fig. 112: Isolation and differentiation of aeromonads pathogenic to fish.

Abb. 112: Isolierung und Differenzierung fischpathogener Aeromonaden

Another related bacterium *A. salmonicida subsp. nova* has been isolated from erythrodermatitis of carp (chronic or ulcerative form of infectious ascites) (7, 37).

■ Incidence and veterinary significance
A. salmonicida subsp. salmonicida causes furunculosis of salmonids, especially in trout, which is characterized by dermatitis, particularly at the base of the fins and tail. Scales are lost and the gills are inflamed and haemorrhagic. Ulceration of the skin and catarrhal, even haemorrhagic enteritis develops affecting mainly the end gut (16).

■ Culture (figs. 110 and 111)
The optimum incubation temperature is around

schwürsform der Infektiösen Bauchwassersucht) der Karpfen ist ein weiteres verwandtes Bakterium *(A. salmonicida subsp. nova)* isoliert worden (2, 37).

■ Vorkommen und medizinische Bedeutung
A. salmonicida subsp. salmonicida ist der Erreger der Furunkulose der Salmoniden, insbesondere der Forellen, die gekennzeichnet ist durch Hautentzündungen im Bereich der Flossenansätze und an der Schwanzbasis, Schuppenverluste, Entzündungen und Blutungen im Kiemenbereich, Hautulcera und katarrhalische, teils hämorrhagische Enteritis, bevorzugt im Enddarm (16).

■ Kultur (Abb. 110 u. 111)
Die optimale Bebrütungstemperatur liegt um 25 °C.

25 °C. The *subspecies salmonicida* form small colonies on blood agar and produce haemolysis after 2 days. Brown pigments develop on Furunculosis Agar (Difco) and usually also on nutrient agar. The subspecies *nova* grows more slowly than the other aeromonads. After 48 hours delicate colonies develop which are initially colourless and then turn greyish-white and crumbly after 2 days.

Auf Blutagar bildet die Subspecies *salmonicida* kleine Kolonien und nach 2 d eine Hämolyse aus. Auf Furunculosis-Agar (Difco) und meistens auch auf Nähragar entsteht ein braunes Pigment. Die Subspecies *nova* zeigt im Vergleich zu den anderen Aeromonaden verzögertes Wachstum. Es bilden sich nach 48 h zarte, zunächst farblose, nach weiteren 2 d grauweiße Kolonien von krümeliger Konsistenz.

■ **Biochemical properties**
See figure 112; the results of numerous other reactions are reported by FUHRMANN (7), WIEDEMANN (37), KRABISCH & WIEDEMANN (16) and other. Hottinger broth with 1 % sugar is suitable for demonstrating the fermentation of glucose.

■ **Kulturell-biochemische Eigenschaften**
Siehe Abb. 112; über den Ausfahll zahlreicher weiterer Reaktionen haben FUHRMANN (7), WIEDEMANN (37), KRABISCH & WIEDEMANN (16) sowie andere berichtet. Für den Nachweis des Glucoseabbaus eignet sich Hottinger-Bouillon mit 1 % Zucker.

Bibliography / Literatur

1. BERMANN, A., W. SEFFNER & S. BUSCH (1981): Zur Beteiligung von Aeromonas hydrophila an einem Mastitisgeschehen. Mh. Vet. Med. **36**, 548–553.
2. BOOTSMA, R., & J. BLOMMAERT (1977): Zur Ätiologie der Erythrodermatitis beim Karpfen Cyprinus carpio. Fisch u. Umwelt, Heft 5, S. 20–27. Stuttgart: Gustav Fischer.
3. CASELITZ, F. H. (1966): Pseudomonas — Aeromonas und ihre humanmedizinische Bedeutung. Jena: VEB Gustav Fischer.
4. CASELITZ, F. H., & D. KREBS (1962): Über die Tierpathogenität von Aeromonasstämmen. Zbl. Bakt. I. Orig. **187**, 56–64.
5. DAVID, H. (1927): Über eine durch choleraähnliche Vibrionen hervorgerufene Fischseuche. Zbl. Bakt. I. Orig. **102**, 46–60.
6. DOBRESCU, L. (1978): Enterotoxigenic Aeromonas hydrophila from a case of piglet diarrhoea. Zbl. Vet. Med. B **25**, 713–718.
7. FUHRMANN, H. (1983): Vorkommen und Bedeutung fischpathogener Erreger in Fischhaltungen Nordwestdeutschlands. Vet. Med. Diss. Hannover.
8. GAMELÉIA, M. N. (1888): Vibrio metschnikovi son mode naturel d'infection. Ann. Inst. Pasteur **2**, 552–557.
9. GAMALÉIA, M. N. (1888): Vibrio metschnikovi (n. sp.) et ses raports avec le microbe du choléra asiatique. Ann. Inst. Pasteur **2**, 482–488.
10. GERLACH, H., & K. BITZER (1971): Infektion mit Aeromonas hydrophila bei Jungputen. Dtsch. tierärztl. Wschr. **78**, 606–608.
11. GJERDE, J., & B. BOE (1981): Isolation and characterization of Vibrio alginolyticus and Vibrio parahaemolyticus from the Norwegen coastal environment. Acta vet. scand. **22**, 331–343.
12. HAASTEIN, T., & G. HOLT (1972): The occurrence of vibrio disease in wild Norwegian fish. J. Fisch. Biol. **4**, 33–37.
13. HODGKISS, W., & J. M. SHEWAN (1950): Pseudomonas infection in a plaice. J. Path. Bact. **62**, 655–657.
14. HOSHINA, T. (1957): Further observations on the causative bacteria of the epidemic disease like furunculosis of rainbow-trout. J. Tokyo Univ. Fish, **43**, 59–66.
15. HOSHINA, T. (1956): An epidemic disease affecting rainbow-trout in Japan. J. Tokyo. Univ. Fich. **42**, 15–16.
16. KRABISCH, P., & H. WIEDEMANN (1979): Diagnose und Vorkommen von Aeromonas salmonicida bei Salmoniden aus bayerischen Gewässern. Tierärztl. Prax., **77**, 81–90.
17. KIELWEIN, G., R. GERLACH & H. JOHNE (1969): Untersuchungen über das Vorkommen von Aeromonas hydrophila in Rohmilch. Arch. Lebensmittelhyg. **20**, 34–38.
18. KRAUSE, W., & H. WINDRATH (1919): Über eine durch einen Vibrio veranlaßte Seuche der Sonnenvögel (Leithrix luteus L., chinesische Nachtigall). Berl. Münch. tierärztl. Wschr. **35**, 468–469.
19. KUJUMGIEV, I. (1957): Prima segnalazione delle infezione da Vibrio metschnikovi (Paracolera aviario) nei tacchini e fagiani. Vet. ital. **8**, 1094–1102.
20. MITSCHERLICH, E. (1981): Campylobacter und Vibrio. In: H. BLOBEL & T. SCHLIESSER (Hrsg.): Handbuch der bakteriellen Infektionen bei Tieren. Bd. III, S. 1–74. Jena: VEB Gustav Fischer.
21. NAKANISHI, H., L. LEISTNER, H. HECHELMANN & J. BAUMGART (1968): Weitere Untersuchungen über das Vorkommen von Vibrio parahaemolyticus und Vibrio alginolyticus bei Seefischen in Deutschland. Arch. Lebensmittelhyg. **19**, 40–53.
22. NAKANISHI, H., L. LEISTNER & J. BAUMGART (1967): Nachweis von Vibrio parahaemolyticus und Vibrio alginolyticus bei Seefischen in Deutschland. Arch. Lebensmittelhyg. **18**, 201–203.
23. NEUMANN, W., & W. PLÖGER (1980): Prüfung einiger aus Karpfen isolierter Aeromonas-Stämme der Hydrophila-Punctata-Gruppe im Resistenztest. Dtsch. tierärztl. Wschr. **87**, 24–26.
24. PIERCE, R. L., C. A. DALEY, C. E. GATES & K. WOHLGEMUTH (1973): Aeromonas hydrophila septicemia in a dog. J. Am. Vet. Med. Ass. **162**, 469.
25. POPOFF, M. (1984): Genus III Aeromonas. In: Bergey's Manual of systematic bacteriology. Vol. 1, S. 545–548. Baltimore, London: Williams & Wilkins.
26. POPOFF, M., & M. VÉRON (1976): A taxonomic study of the Aeromonas hydrophila-Aeromonas punctata group. J. gen. Microbiol. **94**, 11–22.
27. REICHENBACH-KLINKE, H. H. (1980): Krankheiten und Schädigungen der Fische. S. 111–115. Stuttgart: Gustav Fischer.
28. SCHÄPERCLAUS, W. (1934): Untersuchungen über die Aalseuchen in deutschen Binnen- und Küstengewässern. 7. Fischerei **32**, 191–217.
29. SCHUBERT, R. H. W. (1974): Genus Aeromonas. In: R. E. BUCHANAN & N. E. GIBBONS (Hrsg.): Bergey's Manual of Determinative Bacteriology, 8. Aufl., S. 345–348. Baltimore: Williams & Wilkins.
30. SCHUBERT, R. H. W. (1969): Zur Taxonomie von Aeromonas salmonicida subsp. achromogenes (Smith 1963) Schubert 1967 and Aeromonas salmonicida subsp. masoucida Kimura 1969. Zbl. Bakt. I. Orig. **211**, 413–417.

31. Schubert, R. H. W. (1967): Die Pathogenität der Aeromonaden für Mensch und Tier. Arch. Hyg. Bakt. 150, 709–716.
32. Schubert, R. H. W. (1964): Zur Taxonomie der anaerogenen Aeromonaden. Zbl. Bakt. I. Orig. 193, 343–352.
33. Schubert, R. H. W. (1962): Zur Technik der Differenzierung von Vibrionen und Pseudomonaden mit dem Vibriostaticum O/129. Zbl. Bakt. I. Orig. 184, 560–561.
34. Shewan, S. M., & M. Véron (1974): Genus Vibrio. In: Bergey's manual of determinative bacteriology, 8. Aufl., S. 340–345. Baltimore: Williams & Wilkins.
35. Shewan, S. M., & W. Hodgkiss (1954): A method for the rapid differentiation of certain non-pathogenic asporogenous bacilli. Nature 63, 208–209.
36. Wiedemann, H. (1981): Direkte Immunfluoreszenz zum Nachweis der Aeromonas-salmonicida-Infektionen bei Süßwasserfischen. Berl. Münch. tierärztl. Wschr. 94, 153–155.
37. Wiedemann, H. (1979): Erythrodermatitis der Karpfen, zur Isolierung und Klassifizierung des Erregers. Dtsch. tierärztl. Wschr. 86, 176–181.
38. Wohlgemuth, K., M. S. Pierce & C. A. Kirkbride (1972): Bovine abortion associated with Aeromonas hydrophila. J. Am. Vet. Med. Ass. 160, 1001–1002.
39. Fehlhaber, K., G. Scheibner, V. Bergmann, L. F. Litzke & E. Nietiedt (1985): Virulenzuntersuchungen an Aeromonas-hydrophila-Stämmen. Mh. Vet. Med. 40, 829–832.

2 Oxidase-positive and oxidative bacteria

(reaction type I b)

2.1 Genus: Pseudomonas (Ps.)

To this genus belong Gram-negative, motile, obligate aerobic rods, which are oxidase-positive (except *Ps. maltophilia*), and catalase-positive. Carbohydrate breakdown is oxidative without formation of gas. The numerous species are almost exclusively saprophytic, and only a few have additional importance as pathogens.

2.1.1 Pseudomonas aeruginosa

(Syn.: *Bacterium pyocyaneum*)

■ **Incidence and veterinary significance** (tab. 43)
Ps. aeruginosa is a facultative pathogen, causing in-

2 Oxidasepositive und oxidative Bakterien

(Reaktionstyp I b)

2.1 Gattung: Pseudomonas (Ps.)

In die Gattung gehören gramnegative, bewegliche, obligat aerobe, oxydasepositive (Ausnahme *Ps. maltophilia*), katalasepositive Stäbchen. Der Kohlenhydratabbau ist oxydativ und ohne Gasbildung. Die sehr zahlreichen Arten leben meistens ausschließlich saprophytär, nur wenige besitzen zusätzlich eine Bedeutung als Krankheitserreger.

2.1.1 Pseudomonas aeruginosa

(Syn.: *Bacterium pyocyaneum*)

■ **Vorkommen und medizinische Bedeutung**
(Tab. 43)

Table 43: Veterinary importance of *Pseudomonas aeruginosa* (4, 21)

Tabelle 43: Veterinärmedizinische Bedeutung von *Pseudomonas aeruginosa* (4, 21)

Animal species	Disease
Ox	Generalized disease, mastitis, infection of the reproductive organs, respiratory diseases, enteritis, synovitis, lymphangitis, arthritis, lung and liver abscesses
Sheep, goat	Mastitis, pneumonia, lung abscesses
Horse	Infections of reproductive organs, associated with sterility, abortion and foal mortality; lung abscesses (12)
Pig	Enteritis[1], respiratory infections, otitis
Dog, cat	Generalized diseases, infections of the reproductive organs, pneumonia, otitis externa, endocarditis, conjunctivitis, urethroadenocystitis
Mink	Pneumonia, septicaemia (20, 32)
Chinchilla	Generalized infection with conjunctivitis, otitis, pneumonia, enteritis, infections of the reproductive organs
Laboratory animals	Generalized infections, pneumonia, enteritis (3)

[1] Enterotoxins can be involved in causation of the enteritis

[1] an der Entstehung können Enterotoxine beteiligt sein (3)

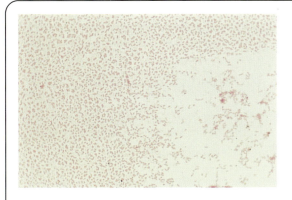
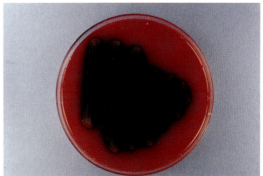
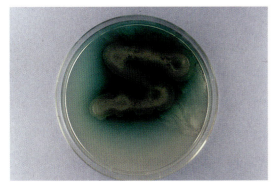
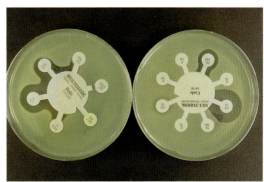

▲ Fig. 113: *Pseudomonas aeruginosa*, smear of a pure culture, Gram stain. Magnification x 1000
▼ Fig. 115: *Pseudomonas aeruginosa*, pure culture on nutrient agar, formation of the blue-green pigment pyocyanin, 48 h, 37 °C. Magnification x 0.25

▲ Abb. 113: *Pseudomonas aeruginosa*, Ausstrich von einer Reinkultur, Gram-Färbung, Abb.-M. 1000 : 1
▼ Abb. 115: *Pseudomonas aeruginosa*, Reinkultur auf Nähragar, Bildung des blau-grünen Pigmentes Pyocyanin, 48 h, 37 °C, Abb.-M. 1 : 4

▲ Fig. 114: *Pseudomonas aeruginosa*, pure culture on blood agar, haemolysis and formation of the blue-green pigment pyocyanin, 48 h, 37 °C. Magnification x 0.25
▼ Fig. 116: *Pseudomonas aeruginosa*, resistance test, total susceptibility (E) to gentamicin (CN) and neomycin (N), slight susceptibility (e) to Kanamycin (K) and polymyxin B (PB)

▲ Abb. 114: *Pseudomonas aeruginosa*, Reinkultur auf Blutagar, Bildung einer Hämolyse und des blaugrünen Pigmentes Pyocyanin, 48 h, 37 °C, Abb.-M. 1 : 4
▼ Abb. 116: *Pseudomonas aeruginosa*, Resistenztest, volle Empfindlichkeit (E) gegenüber Gentamicin (CN) und Neomycin (N), geringe Empfindlichkeit (e) gegenüber Kanamycin (K) und Polymyxin B (PB)

flammation and blue-green pus. Its presence in the animal body is mostly a flare-up of a latent infection, such as an invasion of the intestinal mucosa or the prepuce (2, 13, 28). Outside the body *Ps. aeruginosa* is encountered in water, soil and effluent. When involved in mastitis, it can become important in food hygiene with respect to untreated raw milk (19, 24, 25, 26).

Ps. aeruginosa ist ein fakultativ pathogener Entzündungserreger und Ursache des blaugrünen Eiters. Sein Vorkommen im tierischen Organismus ist meist Ausdruck einer latenten Infektion, so z. B. die Besiedlung der Schleimhäute des Darmkanals oder des Präputiums (2, 13, 28). Außerhalb des Organismus kommt *Ps. aeruginosa* im Wasser, Abwasser und im Erdboden vor. Mit der Mastitis kann ein lebensmittelhygienisch bedeutsames Vorkommen in der Rohmilch verbunden sein (19, 24, 25, 26).

Table 44: Differentiation of various pseudomonas species — Tabelle 44: Differenzierung verschiedener Pseudomonasarten

Pseudomonas	Fluorescence in UV light	Oxi	Mot	5°C	42°C	Gel	Ure	Glu	Lac	Mal	ADH	LDC	ODC
aeruginosa	+	+	+	−	+	+	+	v^+	−	−	+	−	−
fluorescens	+	+	+	+	−	+	v^+	+	−	−	+	−	−
putida	+	+	+	v^+	−	−	v^+	+	−	v^+	+	−	−
stutzeri	−	+	+	v^+	v^+	−	(+)	+	−	v^+	−	−	−
alcaligenes	−	+	+	−	+	−	−	−	−	−	−	−	−
cepacia	−	+	+	−	v^+	+	+	+	+	+	−	v^+	v
diminuta	−	+	+	−	−	+	−	−	−	−	−	−	−
maltophilia	−	−	+	−	−	+	−	v	−	+	−	+	−
pseudomallei	−	+	+	−	+	+	v^+	+	+	+	+	−	−
mallei	−	v^+	−	−	−	v^+	v^+	+	−	v^+	v^+	−	−

■ **Morphology** (fig. 113)
Slender rods, 0.5–0.8 × 1.5–3.0 µm, with 1–3 terminal flagella.

■ **Culture** (figs. 114 and 115)
This undemanding bacterium will grow on simple media as relatively large, usually greenish colonies. The various pigments diffuse into the surrounding medium. A characteristic odour appears and blood agar is haemolyzed. Besides the smooth, soft and shiny S-form, dry granular R-, and mucoid confluent, M-forms can occur.

■ **Biochemical properties**
(tab. 44)
▷ Pigment formation: Pyocyanin is a bluish-green pigment, characteristic of *Ps. aeruginosa*.
The pigments can be demonstrated with special media (e.g. Pseudomonas Agar, Merck) and they can be extracted from broth cultures with chloroform.
Fluorescin (pyoverdin), is a yellowish-green pigment which fluoresces under ultra-violet light. It is not specific for *Ps. aeruginosa* and is insoluble in chloroform and slightly soluble in water.
Pyorubin is a red pigment, which is rarely encountered in routine diagnosis. Other pigments are discussed by CASELITZ (7).
▷ Fermentation of carbohydrates: Carbohydrates breakdown is oxidative without gas formation. Acid production is weak and when using a medium with a relatively high peptone content, a result may be produced which appears negative, because the breakdown of peptone renders the medium alkaline (7).
Litmus milk is clotted, made alkaline and peptonized (18). Other properties will be found in table 44 and CASELITZ (7).

■ **Morphologie** (Abb. 113)
Schlanke, 0,5–0,8 × 1,5–3,0 µm große Stäbchen mit 1–3 polaren Geißeln.

■ **Kultur** (Abb. 114 u. 115)
Das anspruchslose Bakterium wächst auf einfachen Nährböden in relativ großen, meist grünlichen Kolonien. Die verschiedenen Farbstoffe diffundieren in das umgebende Medium. Es tritt ein charakteristischer Geruch auf. Auf Blutagar kommt es zu einer Hämolyse. Neben der glatten, glänzenden, weichen S-Form können die trockene, granulierte R- und die schleimige, konfluierende M-Form auftreten.

■ **Kulturell-biochemische Eigenschaften**
(Tab. 44)
▷ Farbstoffbildung: Pyocyanin, blau-grüner Farbstoff, für *Ps. aeruginosa* charakteristisch.
Der Farbstoff kann auf Spezialnährböden (z. B. Pseudomonas-Agar, Merck) nachgewiesen und aus Bouillonkulturen mit Chloroform ausgeschüttelt werden. Er wird nicht von allen Stämmen gebildet.
Fluorescein (Pyoverdin), gelbgrüner, im UV-Licht fluoreszierender Farbstoff, der nicht für *Ps. aeruginosa* spezifisch ist. Unlöslich in Chloroform, leicht löslich in Wasser.
Pyorubin, roter Farbstoff, der in der Routinediagnostik selten beobachtet wird. Weitere Farbstoffe s. CASELITZ (7).
▷ Spaltung von Kohlenhydraten: Der Kohlenhydratabbau erfolgt oxydativ und ohne Gasbildung. Die Säurebildung ist schwach, und bei Verwendung von Nährböden mit einem relativ hohen Peptongehalt kann ein negatives Ergebnis dadurch vorgetäuscht werden, daß infolge des Peptonabbaus eine Alkalisierung des Nährbodens eintritt (7).
Lackmusmilch wird zur Gerinnung, Alkalisierung und Peptonisation gebracht (18). Weitere Eigenschaften siehe Tab. 44 und CASELITZ (7).

■ **Antigenic structure**

By virtue of the presence of various O- and H-antigens, a number of serotypes can be differentiated (14). The investigations were carried out mainly on strains of human origin, but the same and other types can be found in animals (1, 16, 34).

2.1.2 Other pseudomonas species

Other pseudomonas are isolated from animal material with varying frequency, e.g.
▷ *Ps. fluorescens,*
▷ *Ps. cepacia,*
▷ *Ps. maltophilia,*
▷ *Ps. putida,*
▷ *Ps. stutzeri.*

They are similar in distribution to *Ps. aeruginosa,* but little is known to date about their pathogenic significance to animals. Their identification, which is usually disregarded in routine veterinary diagnosis, is costly and requires special procedures (see table 44 and 45). Various miniature identification systems are offered commercially. It is of veterinary interest, however, when these organisms occur in food materials of animal origin.

2.1.3 Pseudomonas mallei

The taxonomic position of this bacterium had been uncertain for a long time and therefore it had been assigned at various times to very different genera: *Pfeifferella, Loefflerella, Malleomyces, Actinobacillus.* It is classified as a pseudomonad because its bacteriological properties correspond most closely to those of that genus and there are close links with *Ps. pseudomallei* (antigenic relationship, phage sensitivity, nucleic acid composition). However, *Ps. mallei* deviates from the typical pseudomonads by its lack of motility, obligate parasitism and slow growth in culture.

Table 45: Differentiating characteristics of *Pseudomonas aeruginosa, fluorescens* and *putida*

Property	Behaviour and test result		
	Ps. aeruginosa	*Ps. fluorescens*	*Ps. putida*
Flagellation	polar monotrich	polar lophotrich	polar lophotrich
Growth at 22 °C	+	+	+
Growth at 37 °C	+	–	–
Growth at 42 °C	+	–	–
Pyocyanin	+	–	–
Fluorescin	+	+	+
Gelatinolysis	+	+	–

■ Incidence and veterinary significance

Ps. mallei is the cause of glanders, an infectious disease of soliped animals, which generally takes a chronic course and is characterized by the appearance of nodules and ulcers on the skin, mucous membranes and internal organs. Under natural conditions predatory cats and man can also succumb to this disease. Germany was free of glanders for the first time in 1914.

■ Morphology and microscopic examination

It is a Gram-negative, non-motile, pleomorphic rod, measuring $0.5 \times 1.5-4\,\mu$. It is easy to stain with carbol fuchsin (½ minute), often exhibiting a granular appearance due to the storage of poly-β-hydroxybutyrate. In contaminated material it is frequently impossible to differentiate the glanders bacilli from others.

■ Culture

Ps. mallei will grow aerobically but slowly on simple media so that small colonies can only be recognized after 48 hours. However, multiplication can be intensified by the use of richer media (heart infusion broth, trypticase-soya agar etc.) or by the addition of 1% glycerol (10, 27, 29). XIE et al. (35) have described a selective medium: 1000 units polymyxin E, 1250 units Bacitracin, 0.25 mg actidione added to 100 ml basic medium.

On this medium *Ps. mallei* will form round, convex, grey translucent colonies after 24–48 hours, 1–2 mm in size. They turn opaque with age, take on a granular surface and become yellowish or brownish. The colonies have a tendency towards mucoid confluence. On potato slopes they produce a typical growth (KITT, 1885) in the form of a honey-yellow layer (»honey dew« colonies), which later assume a brownish tinge.

■ Animal inoculation

It is possible to demonstrate *Ps. mallei* and obtain it in pure culture by means of animal inoculation, after STRAUSS. Guinea pigs are injected subcutaneously in the abdominal region with 0.5–1.0 ml of infected material. After 2–3 days a purulent inflammation of the testicular tunica vaginalis develops. The scrotum becomes red and swollen, pus, containing the bacteria, breaks through the skin and the animal dies in 1 to 5 weeks. Glanders nodules develop in the lung, liver and spleen. Bacteria can be cultured from the pus in the testes.

■ Indirect diagnosis of glanders

There are serological and allergic methods for the diagnosis in the living animal:

The serum agglutination test is usually positive

■ Vorkommen und medizinische Bedeutung

Ps. mallei ist der Erreger des Rotzes (Malleus), einer gewöhnlich chronisch verlaufenden Infektionskrankheit der Einhufer mit Knötchen- und Geschwürbildung in den Schleimhäuten, der Haut und den inneren Organen. Unter natürlichen Verhältnissen erkranken ferner Raubkatzen und der Mensch. Deutschland ist 1914 zum ersten Male frei von Rotz gewesen.

■ Morphologie und mikroskopische Untersuchung

Gramnegatives, unbewegliches, pleomorphes, $0.5 \times 1.5-4\,\mu m$ großes Stäbchen, das sich gut mit Karbolfuchsin (½ min) färbt und dabei häufig eine granulierte Beschaffenheit (Speicherung von Poly-β-hydrobutyrat) zeigt. In kontaminiertem Material können die Rotzbakterien oft nicht von anderen Bakterien unterschieden werden.

■ Kultur

Ps. mallei wächst aerob auf einfachen Nährböden langsam, so daß kleine Kolonien erst nach 48 h zu erkennen sind. Das Wachstum kann durch die Benutzung reichhaltiger zusammengesetzter Nährböden (heart-infusion-agar, trypticase-soy-agar u. ä.) sowie durch den Zusatz von 1% Glycerin intensiviert werden (10, 27, 29). XIE et al. (35) haben ein Selektivmedium beschrieben: 1000 E Polymyxin E, 1250 E Bacitracin, 0,25 mg Aktidion/100 ml Basismedium.

Auf diesen Nährböden bildet *Ps. mallei* nach 24–48 h 1–2 mm große, runde, konvexe, durchscheinend graue Kolonien, die mit zunehmendem Alter opak werden, eine fein granulierte Oberfläche erhalten und sich zentral gelblich oder bräunlich färben. Die Kolonien neigen zum schleimigen Zusammenfließen. Auf Kartoffelscheiben zeigt *Ps. mallei* ein typisches Wachstum (KITT, 1885) in Form eines honiggelben Belages (»honigtropfenartige« Kolonien), die später einen bräunlichen Farbton annehmen.

■ Tierversuch

Der Nachweis von *Ps. mallei* und seine Reinzüchtung kann im Tierversuch nach STRAUSS erfolgen. Dabei erhalten Meerschweinchen 0,5–1,0 ml Rotzmaterial sbk. unter die Bauchhaut injiziert. Nach 2–3 d entwickelt sich eine eitrige Entzündung der Tunica vaginalis der Testis. Das Skrotum ist gerötet und geschwollen, der bakterienhaltige Eiter bricht nach außen durch, der Tod der Tiere tritt nach 1–5 Wochen ein. In Lunge, Leber und Milz entwickeln sich Rotzknötchen. Aus dem Eiter des Hoden können die Bakterien kulturell isoliert werden.

■ Indirekte Malleusdiagnose

Der Diagnose am lebenden Tier dienen serologische und allergische Methoden:

Serumlangsamagglutination, wird meistens in der

during the first week after the infection, reaching its height on the 10th to 11th day. It then falls, to become negative after 6–9 weeks. The complement fixation test remains positive in horses even in the chronic stage.

In positive cases the mallein eye test produces reddening, swelling, conjunctivitis and sticking together of the eye lids.

For details of the performance of these tests see appropriate Government publication.

2.1.4 Pseudomonas pseudomallei

■ **Incidence and medical significance**

Ps. pseudomallei is the cause of melioidosis, which can affect mammals, especially soliped ungulates, birds and man. In the horse the clinical picture is very like that of glanders and it may appear in different forms: a peracute septicaemic form that rapidly leads to death; an acute form which is the most common and presents, among other signs, oedema of the limbs, and mild attacks of colic; the subacute to chronic form is characterized by emaciation, locomotor disturbances, oedema of the limbs, pulmonary symptoms and skin lesions.

Infection is by the oral route through bedding, food etc. Since the organism can survive for long periods in the soil (30), this is a sapronosis or geonosis.

The disease occurs mainly in the Far East, but it was first recorded in France in 1976 (6, 9, 11, 23). The causal agent is probably more widely distributed than is recognized at present.

■ **Morphology**
Gram-negative rod, 1.5 µm long, with lophotrichous flagella and bipolar staining.

■ **Culture**
Within 24 hours this organism will develop into relatively large (5–10 mm diameter), moist colonies which in 2–5 days appear to have radial folds and reddish or brown colour. Smooth or mucoid forms are occasionally encountered. Initially they smell putrid, then earthy (5, 27).

■ **Biochemical properties**
See table 44.

ersten Woche nach der Infektion positiv und erreicht ihren Höhepunkt am 10.–11. d. Sie sinkt anschließend wieder ab und wird nach 6–9 Wochen negativ; Komplementbindungsreaktion, bleibt auch bei chronisch erkrankten Pferden positiv;

Mallein-Augenprobe, im positiven Fall Rötung, Schwellung, Verklebung der Augenlider, eitrige Konjunktivitis.

Einzelheiten der Durchführung und Bewertung der Untersuchungsmethoden in den Richtlinien des Bundesministers für Ernährung, Landwirtschaft und Forsten zur Feststellung von Rotz (Malleus) bei Einhufern vom 7.5.1974.

2.1.4 Pseudomonas pseudomallei

■ **Vorkommen und medizinische Bedeutung**
Das Bakterium ist Ursache der Melioidose, die bei Säugetieren, insbesondere Einhufern, Vögeln und beim Menschen auftreten kann. Die Krankheitserscheinungen beim Pferd sind rotzähnlich. Nach dem Krankheitsverlauf kann man unterscheiden: perakute, septikämische Form, die in kurzer Zeit zum Tode führt; akute Form, die am häufigsten ist und bei der sich u. a. Ödeme an den Gliedmaßen und leichte Koliken entwickeln können; subakute bis chronische Form mit Abmagerung, Bewegungsstörungen, Ödemen an den Gliedmaßen, Lungenerscheinungen, Hautveränderungen.

Die Infektion erfolgt oral mit Einstreu, Futter usw. Es handelt sich um eine Sapronose bzw. Geonose, denn der Erreger kann sich im Boden lebensfähig halten (30).

Die Krankheit kommt hauptsächlich im Fernen Osten vor, sie ist aber erstmalig 1976 auch in Frankreich festgestellt worden (6, 9, 11, 23). Der Erreger kommt möglicherweise weiter verbreitet vor als z. Zt. bekannt ist.

■ **Morphologie**
Gramnegatives, 1,5 µm langes, lophotrich begeißeltes, bipolar anfärbbares Stäbchen.

■ **Kultur**
Das Bakterium bildet nach 24 h relativ große (Durchmesser 5–10 mm), feuchte Kolonien, die nach 2 bis 5 d mit einer radiären Struktur gefaltet erscheinen und sich rötlich bis braun verfärben. Gelegentlich können auch glatte oder mukoide Kolonien auftreten. Der Geruch der Kulturen ist zunächst faulig, später erdig (5, 27).

■ **Kulturell-biochemische Eigenschaften**
Siehe Tab. 44.

Bibliography / Literatur

1. ATHERTON, J. G., & T. L. PITT (1982): Types of Pseudomonas aeruginosa isolated from horses. Eq. Vet. J. **14**, 329–332.
2. BAIER, W., W. LEIDL, A. MAHRLA & M. SCHRÖDL

(1955): Über das Pyocyaneum-Problem in der künstlichen Besamung. Berl. Münch. tierärztl. Wschr. **68**, 141–143, 156–159.
3. Baljer, G., & J. T. Barret (1979): Nachweis von enterotoxinbildenden Pseudomonas aeruginosa-Stämmen im Darmligaturtest beim Ferkel. Zbl. Vet. Med. B **26**, 740–747.
4. Becker, K. H. (1981): Untersuchungen zur Abgrenzung von Pseudomonas mallei gegen andere mesophile Pseudomonaden mit neuzeitlichen diagnostischen Methoden. Vet. Med. Diss. Gießen.
5. Bergan, T. (1981): Human- and animal-pathogenic members of the genus Pseudomonas. In: M. P. Starr, H. Stolp, H. G. Trüper, A. Balows & H. G. Schlegel (Eds.): The Prokaryotes, Vol. I, S. 687. Berlin, Heidelberg, New York: Springer.
6. Bourrier, M. (1978): Melioidose équine en Mayenne dans une écurie de chevaux de selle. Bull. Mens. Soc. Vét. Pratiq. France **62**, 673–676, 678–679.
7. Caselitz, F. H. (1966): Pseudomonas/Aeromonas und ihre humanmedizinische Bedeutung. Jena: VEB Gustav Fischer.
8. Cox, H. U., & D. G. Luther (1980): Determination of antimicrobial susceptibility of Pseudomonas aeruginosa by disk diffusion and microdilution methods. Am. J. Vet. Res. **41**, 906–909.
9. Desbrosse, F., A. Dodin & M. Galimand (1978): La pseudomorve ou melioidose: maladie due au bacille de Whitmore, mise en évidence dans la région ouest-Parisienne. Bull. Mens. Soc. Vét. Pratiq. France **62**, 957–972.
10. Evans, D. H. (1966): Growth of Actinobacillus mallei in chemically defined media. Can. J. Microbiol. **12**, 617–623.
11. Galimand, M., & A. Dodin (1982): Repartition de Pseudomonas pseudomallei en France et dans le monde. La melioidose. Bull. Mens. Soc. Vét. Pratiq. France **66**, 651–667.
12. Garg, D., V. P. Manchanda & N. K. Chandiramani (1983): Pseudomonas aeruginosa-associated equine abortion, mare infertility and foal mortality. Ind. J. An. Sci. **53**, 36–40.
13. Getty, S. M., & D. J. Ellis (1967): The experimental use of bull semen contaminated with Pseudomonas aeruginosa. J. Am. vet. med. Ass. **151**, 1688–1691.
14. Habs, I. (1957): Untersuchungen über die O-Antigene von Pseudomonas aeruginosa. Zschr. Hyg. **144**, 218–228.
15. Hirsh, D. C., N. Wiger & S. J. Knox (1979): Susceptibility of clinical isolates of Pseudomonas aeruginosa to antimicrobial agents. J. Vet. Pharm. Therap. **2**, 275–278.
16. Hubrig, Th., & W. Köhler (1961): Über eine neue, im Genitaltrakt von Bullen vorkommende serologische Gruppe h bei Pseudomonas aeruginosa. Zuchthygiene **5**, 123–130.
17. Köhler, W. (1957): Zur Serologie der Pseudomonas aeruginosa. Zschr. Immun. Forsch. **114**, 282.
18. Kielwein, G. (1972): Klassifizierung der Gattungen Pseudomonas u. Aeromonas. Arch. Lebensmittelhyg. **23**, 281–284.
19. Kielwein, G. (1970): Untersuchungen über die milchhygienische Bedeutung von Pseudomonaden und Aeromonaden. Vet. Med. Habilitationsschrift, Gießen.
20. Long, G. G., & J. R. Gorham (1981): Field studies: Pseudomonas pneumonia in mink. Am. J. Vet. Res. **42**, 2129–2133.
21. Lusis, P. I., & M. A. Soltys (1971): Pseudomonas aeruginosa. Vet. Bull. **41**, 169–177.
22. Mannheim, W., & H. Bürger (1966): Über physiologische Merkmale und die Frage der systematischen Stellung des Rotz-Erregers. Zschr. Med. Mikrobiol. Immunol. **152**, 249–261.
23. Mayer, H. (1982): Zum Vorkommen von Pseudorotz (Melioidose) in Westeuropa. Tierärztl. Umschau **37**, 126–131.
24. Nicholls, T. J., M. G. Barton & B. P. Anderson (1981): An outbreak of mastitis in a dairy herd due to Pseudomonas aeruginosa contamination of dry-cow therapy at manufacture. Vet. Rec. **108**, 93–96.
25. Osborne, A. D., K. Armstrong, N. H. Catrysse, G. Butler & L. Versavel (1981): An outbreak of Pseudomonas mastitis in dairy cows. Can. Vet. J. **22**, 215–217.
26. Otte, I., G. Hahn & A. Tolle (1978): Vorkommen, Nachweis und Bedeutung von Ps. aeruginosa in Rohmilch und in der Umgebung von Milchtieren. Milchwissenschaft **33**, 737–739.
27. Redfearn, M. S., N. J. Palleronii & R. Y. Stanier (1966): A comparative study of Pseudomonas pseudomallei and Bacillus mallei. J. gen. Microbiol. **43**, 293–313.
28. Schwerdtner, H. (1971): Über das Vorkommen und die Bedeutung von Pseudomonas aeruginosa bei Besamungsbullen. Zuchthygiene **5**, 260–267.
29. Smith, P. B., & W. B. Cherry (1957): Identification of Malleomyces by specific bacteriophages. J. Bact. **74**, 668–672.
30. Thomas, A. D., & J. C. Forbes-Faulkner (1981): Persistence of Pseudomonas pseudomallei in soil. Austr. Vet. J. **57**, 535–536.
31. Thomas, A. D., J. C. Forbes-Faulkner & B. J. Duffield (1981): Susceptibility of Pseudomonas pseudomallei isolates of non-human origin to chemotherapeutic agents by the single disc sensitivity method. Vet. Microbiol. **6**, 367–374.
32. Trautwein, G., C. F. Helmboldt & S. W. Nielsen (1962): Pathology of Pseudomonas pneumonia in mink. J. Amer. Vet. Med. Ass. **140**, 701–704.
33. Weis, J., & J. Grosser (1981): Ein Beitrag zum Vorkommen von antibiotikaresistenten Staphylococcus aureus- und Pseudomonas aeruginosa-Stämmen. Tierärztl. Umschau **36**, 106, 108–109.
34. Wokatsch, M. G. (1964): Serologische Untersuchungen an Pseudomonas aeruginosa (Bact. pyocyaneus) aus verschiedenen Tierarten. Zbl. Bakt. I. Orig. **192**, 468–476.
35. Xie, X., H. F. Xu, R. X. Gong & X. W. Duan (1980): A new selective medium for isolation of glanders bacilli. Coll. Pap. Vet. Res. **6**, 83–90.

2.2 Flavobacterium

Members of this genus occur as saprophytes in soil and water and they are sometimes isolated as contaminants from samples of animals origin; they are non-pathogenic.

Flavobacteria are identified by the following characteristics: Gram-negative rods, 0.5 × 1.0–3.0 µm in size, non-motile, with aerobic growth on ordinary media, they produce pigments with varying intensity, are catalase-, oxidase- and

2.2 Flavobacterium

Angehörige dieser Gattung kommen saprophytär im Erdboden und Wasser vor und können deswegen gelegentlich als Kontaminanten eines tierischen Untersuchungsstoffes isoliert werden, ohne daß eine Pathogenität besteht.

Flavobakterien sind durch folgende Eigenschaften gekennzeichnet: gramnegativ, 0,5 × 1,0–3,0 µm große Stäbchen, unbeweglich, aerobes Wachstum auch auf einfachen Nährböden, Bildung eines gel-

phosphatase-positive and form acid from carbohydrates under aerobic conditions. Other properties are listed in table 32.

3 Oxidase-positive glucose-inactive bacteria
(Reaction type I c)

3.1 Genus: Alcaligenes (A.)

The taxonomic position of this species is not yet settled. The most important species is *A. faecalis*, but other types, such as *A. denitrificans* and various others of uncertain classification, are recognized. *A. faecalis* is found in soil, water, faeces, urine etc. and because of its ubiquity, it can occasionally be isolated from animal specimens, without it being associated with any disease. It has been claimed (1–5), that bacteria related to *A. faecalis* are responsible for respiratory diseases of poultry, particularly of turkeys (coryza). But the organism isolated from turkeys is probably identical with *B. avium* (p. 156).

The identification of *A. faecalis* requires a series of careful biochemical tests, because it is all too easy to confuse it with *Achromobacter* and *Pseudomonas*.

A. faecalis has the following properties:
Gram-negative, rod- to coccus-shaped, motile 0.5–2.0 × 0.5–2.6 µm in size. It grows aerobically and without pigment on simple media, is oxidase-, catalase- and indole-negative and carbohydrates are not fermented (tab. 32).

Bibliography / Literatur
1. BARNES, H. J., & S. M. HOFSTADT (1983): Susceptibility of turkey poults from vaccinated and unvaccinated hens to Alcaligenes rhinothracheitis. Av. Dis. **27**, 378–392.
2. GRAY, J. G., J. F. ROBERTS, R. C. DILLMAN & D. G. SIMMONS (1983): Pathogenesis of change in the upper respiratory tract of turkeys experimentally infected with an Alcaligenes faecalis isolate. Infect. Imm. **42**, 350–355.
3. HELLER, E. D., Y. WEISMAN & A. AHARONOVOVITCH (1984): Experimental studies on turkey coryza. Av. Path. **13**, 137–143.
4. MONTGOMERY, R. D., S. H. KLEVEN & P. VILLEGAS (1983): Observations on the pathogenicity of Alcaligenes faecalis in chickens. Av. Dis. **27**, 751–761.
5. RIMLER, R. B., & D. G. SIMMONS (1983): Differentiation among bacteria isolated from turkeys with coryza (rhinotracheitis). Av. Dis. **27**, 491–500.

3.2 Genus: Bordetella (B.)
3.2.1 Bordetella bronchiseptica

■ **Incidence and veterinary significance**

B. bronchiseptica is widely distributed among domestic and wild animals (17) and has a special affinity for the organs of respiration becoming attached to the ciliated epithelium of the airways.

Latent infections predominate, and especially in pigs the number of carriers is high. Conditions

which can be produced either by *B. bronchiseptica* alone or in association with other micro-organisms (bacteria, viruses, mycoplasmas) are:
▷ Atrophic rhinitis of pigs in which *Pasteurella multocida* participates as cause, in bronchopneumonias, principally of sucking piglets (7, 9, 14, 16);
▷ rhinitis and pneumonia in rabbits and other small rodents (1, 12, 13);
▷ bronchopneumonia (kennel cough) in dogs, less frequently in cats;
▷ respiratory diseases of turkeys and other types of poultry (4, 5).

■ **Morphology**

B. bronchiseptica is a Gram-negative, motile, coccoid to ovoid rod, 0.3–0.5 × 0.5–1.0 μm in size, lying singly, in pairs or small groups.

■ **Culture and biochemical characteristics**

See figures 117, 118 and 119.

B. bronchiseptica possesses capsule-like structures (outer membrane proteins) which are lost by passage (phase modulation). Thus one can differentiate between the virulent encapsulated phase I, from the

Specimens
Swabs from respiratory tract, lung tissue etc.

Isolation by culture
1. Nutrient media: will grow on the usual diagnostic culture media, especially on blood agar, but also on nutrient agar, Gassner agar, Endo agar, MacConkey agar etc.
2. Incubation: aerobic 37 °C, 24–72 hours
3. Culture morphology: after 24 h on blood agar colonies are just visible, after 48 h they are 1.5 mm, smooth, round and shiny (fig. 118). Haemolysis can occur with horse blood and acid pH.
4. Dissociation develops readily if incubation is continued, especially in subcultures. Phase modulation see p. 155.

Biochemical differentiation					
Oxidase	+	Citrate	+	Nitrate	+
Oxidation/fermentation	$-^1$	Urease	$+^2$	Gelatinase	−
Catalase	+	H$_2$S	−	Motility	+
Indole	−				

Serological identification
Slide agglutination test using specific serum pertussis serum can also be used

[1] with glucose and other carbohydrates;
[2] Strains isolated from turkeys and other types of poultry have no urease activity and do not reduce nitrate (*Bordetella avium* p. 156; 5, 6)

Fig. 117: Demonstration and identification of *Bordetella bronchiseptica*

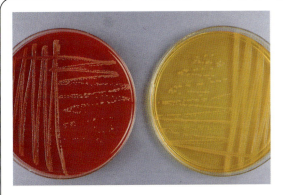
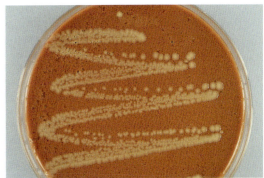
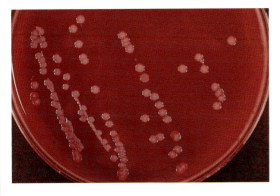
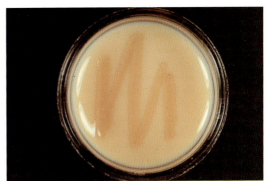

▲ Fig. 118: *Bordetella bronchiseptica*, pure culture on blood and Gassner agar, 48 h, 37 °C. Magnification x 0.17
▼ Fig. 120: *Moraxella bovis*, pure culture on blood agar, 48 h, 37 °C. Magnification x 0.4

▲ Fig. 119: *Bordetella bronchiseptica*, isolated from the nasal mucosa of a pig on chocolate agar, 48 h, 37 °C. Magnification x 0.4
▼ Fig. 121: *Moraxella bovis*, pure culture on Loeffler serum plate, serum liquefaction 48 h, 37 °C. Magnification x 0.4

▲ Abb. 118: *Bordetella bronchiseptica*, Reinkultur auf Blut- und Gaßner-Agar, 48 h, 37 °C, Abb.-M. 1 : 6
▼ Abb. 120: *Moraxella bovis*, Reinkultur auf Blutagar, 48 h, 37 °C, Abb.-M. 1 : 2,5

▲ Abb. 119: *Bordetella bronchiseptica*, Isolierung von der Nasenschleimhaut eines Schweines auf Kochblutagar, 48 h, 37 °C, Abb.-M. 1 : 2,5
▼ Abb. 121: *Moraxella bovis*, Reinkultur auf der Serumplatte nach Loeffler, Serolyse, 48 h, 37 °C, Abb.-M. 1 : 4

transition form phase II and the avirulent, non-capsulated form phase III. It is through phase modulation that the raised, shiny, white to greyish-white colonies of phase I change into the flat, irregularly outlined colonies of phase II. A selective medium has been described by HOMMEZ et al. (8).

■ Toxins
The heat-labile dermonecrotoxin (thioprotein, de-

Phase II (Übergangsform) und die avirulente, kapsellose Phase III unterscheiden. Mit der Phasenmodulation wandeln sich die erhabenen, glänzenden, weißen bis grauweißen Kolonie der Phase I zu flachen, unregelmäßig begrenzten Kolonien der Phase II. Ein Selektivmedium ist von HOMMEZ et al. (8) beschrieben worden.

■ Toxine
Pathogenetisch und immunbiologisch sind ein hit-

monstrable in the guinea pig skin and mouse lethal tests) and the haemagglutinin (localized in the fimbriae) are of significance from both the pathogenetic and the immunobiological points of view (2, 9).

■ **Antigenic structure**

Various serotypes can be differentiated on the basis of their K- and H-antigens as well as the thermostable O-antigens. 14 capsule antigens have been identified. All strains have the antigen O 1 and K 1. There is an antigenic relationship with *B. pertussis* and *B. parapertussis*. The strains isolated from pigs are largely serologically uniform, according to PEDERSEN (14), and they have antigens O: 1, 2 and K: 1, 2 ÉLIÁS et al. (2) are of the opinion that there are different combinations among the K-antigens.

■ **Animal inoculation**

B. bronchiseptica is pathogenic to mice. Intraperitoneal, intracerebral and intratracheal injection routes have been used to test virulence. With highly virulent strains, injected intracerebrally, the LD_{50} is 300, but 1000 organisms are required with the intratracheal route (2).

3.2.2 Bordetella avium

Bordetella avium is found mainly in turkeys, rarely in fowls, ducks and other birds. In turkeys it is a primary pathogenic agent, causing a highly contagious disease of the respiratory tract. The investigations of HINZ & GLÜNDER (6) indicate that *B. avium* can clearly be differentiated by biochemical means from *B. bronchiseptica*, since the former produces no urease, does not reduce nitrate and alkalizes media containing salts of various acids and amides (acetamide, formamide).

Bibliography / Literatur

1. ÉLIÁS, B., M. KRÜGER & M. GEHRT (1983): Untersuchungen zur Verbreitung und Diagnostik von Bordetella bronchiseptica in Meerschweinchenbeständen. Mh. Vet. Med. **38**, 385–387.
2. ÉLIÁS, B., M. KRÜGER & F. RÁTZ (1982): Epizootiologische Untersuchungen der Rhinitis atrophicans des Schweines. II. Biologische Eigenschaften der von Schweinen isolierten Bordetella bronchiseptica-Stämme. Zbl. Vet. Med. B, **29**, 619–635.
3. GENEGER, J. (1979): Untersuchungen zur Ätiologie der Rhinitis atrophicans des Schweines. Bakteriologische Untersuchungen an Bordetella-bronchiseptica-Stämmen verschiedener Tierarten. Vet. Med. Diss. Hannover.
4. GLÜNDER, G., K. H. HINZ & B. STIBUREK (1979): Zur therapeutischen Wirksamkeit von Tetracyclin-HCl und Sulfaquinoxalin/Trimethoprim bei der Puten-Bordetellose. Zbl. Vet. Med. B **26**, 591–602.
5. HINZ, K. H., G. GLÜNDER, B. STIBUREK & H. LÜDERS (1979): Experimentelle Untersuchungen zur Bordetellose der Pute. Zbl. Vet. Med. B **26**, 202–213.
6. HINZ, K. H., & G. GLÜNDER (1985): Zum Vorkommen von Bordetella avium sp. nov. und Bordetella bronchiseptica bei Vögeln. Berl. Münch. tierärztl. Wschr. **98**, 369–373.
7. HODGES, R. T., & G. W. YOUNG (1984): Prevalence and in-vitro antimicrobial sensitivity of Bordetella bronchiseptica in the nasal cavity of pigs. N. Z. Vet. J. **32**, 111–114.
8. HOMMEZ, J., L. A. DEVRIESE & F. CASTRYCK (1983): An improved selective medium for the isolation of Bordetella bronchiseptica. Vlaams Diergeneesk. Tijdschr. **52**, 199–201.
9. KRÜGER, M., & F. HORSCH (1983): Die Pathogenese und Immunprophylaxe der Bordetella-bronchiseptica-Infektion des Schweines (Übersichtsreferat). Mh. Vet. Med. **38**, 287–291.
10. KRÜGER, M., & F. HORSCH (1982): Untersuchungen zur Differenzierung von Bordetella-bronchiseptica-Stämmen. 1. Mitt.: Nachweis des hitzelabilen Exotoxins und des Hämagglutinins. Arch. exp. Vet. Med. **36**, 691–698.

11. MARTINEAU, G., & A. DEWAELE (1978): Sensibilité de Bordetella bronchiseptica à différents antibiotics et sulfamidés. Ann. Méd. Vét. **122**, 607–612, 687–691.
12. MEYER, H. (1971): Bordetellainfektionen, ein Problem der Massentierhaltung bei Kaninchen. Berl. Münch. tierärztl. Wschr. **84**, 273–274.
13. OLDENBURG, J., B. KÖHLER, H. W. FUCHS & F. HORSCH (1972): Vorkommen und Bedeutung von Bordetella bronchiseptica beim Kaninchen. Mh. Vet. Med. **27**, 738–743.
14. PEDERSEN, K. B., & K. BERFORD (1981): The aetiological significance of Bordetella bronchiseptica and Pasteurella multocida in atrophic rhinitis in swine. Nord. Vet. Med. **33**, 513–522.
15. PEDERSEN, K. B. (1975): The serology of Bordetella bronchiseptica isolated from pigs compared with strains from other animal species. Acta path. microbiol. scand. **83 B**, 590–594.
16. SCHÖSS, P. (1982): Bordetella-bronchiseptica-Infektion in einem SPF-Schweinebestand. Ein Beitrag zur Ätiologie der Rhinitis atrophicans. Dtsch. tierärztl. Wschr. **89**, 177–181.
17. SWITZER, W. P., C. J. MARÉ & E. D. HUBBARD (1966): Incidence of Bordetella bronchiseptica in wildlife and man in Iowa. Am. J. Vet. Res. **27**, 1134–1136.

3.3 Genus: Neisseria (N.)

The family *Neisseriaceae* includes the genus *Neisseria*, the genera *Moraxella* (p. 158) and *Acinetobacter* (p. 209), and ovoid, rod-shaped bacteria.

The cocci of the genus *Neisseria* are Gram-negative, non-motile, non-sporulating, and they are arranged in pairs (diplococci). Most of them are somewhat kidney-shaped. The features which differentiate them from the other genera of the family are presented in table 46.

Their medical significance affects man in the first instance (*N. gonorrhoeae*: gonorrhoea; *N. meningitidis*: transmissible cerebrospinal meningitis). There are other species which occur in man on mucous membranes particularly in the respiratory tract and these are of differential diagnostic importance.

It is difficult at present to assess the extent to which neisseria occur in animals, because the identification of this genus or the genus *Moraxella (Branhamella)* is uncertain (3). The neisseria which do occur in animals appear primarily to be non-pathogenic inhabitants of mucous membranes (1,

3.3 Gattung: Neisseria (N.)

Die Gattung *Neisseria* gehört zur Familie der *Neisseriaceae* (Tab. 46), die mit den Gattungen *Moraxella* (S. 158) und *Acinetobacter* (S. 209) auch ovoide stäbchenförmige Bakterien enthält.

Die Kokken der Gattung *Neisseria* sind gramnegativ, unbeweglich, sporenlos, sie liegen zu Paaren zusammen (Diplokokken) und haben meist eine nieren- oder semmelförmige Gestalt. Ihre Unterscheidungsmerkmale zu den anderen Gattungen der Familie zeigt Tab. 46.

Ihre medizinische Bedeutung betrifft hauptsächlich den Menschen (*N. gonorrhoeae*: Gonorrhoe; *N. meningitidis*: übertragbare Genickstarre). Weitere Arten kommen beim Menschen auf den Schleimhäuten insbesondere des oberern Respirationstraktes vor und haben differentialdiagnostische Bedeutung.

In welchem Umfang Neisserien beim Tier vorkommen, ist zur Zeit schwer zu beurteilen, da die Zuordnung zu dieser Gattung oder zur Gattung *Moraxella (Branhamella)* vielfach unsicher ist (3). Soweit Neisserien beim Tier vorkommen, dürfte es

Table 46: Members of the family *Neisseriaceae* occurring in animals

Tabelle 46: Übersicht zu den bei Tieren vorkommenden Bakterien aus der Familie der *Neisseriaceae*

Genus	Species	Morphology	Oxi	Glu	Cat	Hae	Nit	serum liquefaction	occurrence
Neisseria	N. canis	co[2]	+	−	+	−	+	−	dog
Moraxella subgenera:									
Moraxella	M. bovis	rod	+	−	v	v[+]	−	+	ox, horse
Branhamella	M. (B.) ovis	co	+	−	+	v[+]	v[+]	−	ox, sheep
	M. (B.) cuniculi	co	+	−	+	−	−	−	horse
	M. (B.) caviae	co	+	−	+	(+)	+	−	rabbit guinea pig
Acinetobacter	A. calcoaceticus	rod[2]	−	v[1]	+	v	−	−	soil, water, man, animals

co: cocci
[1] only acid formation; [2] often arranged in pairs

[1] nur Säurebildung; [2] oft paarweise gelagert

2). VEDROS (6) attributes *N. canis* to this genus; it is present in the pharyngeal region of cats and has been transmitted to man through bites.

A disease has been described in the reproductive organs of geese which was presumed to be due to neisseria, and had antigenic similarity with *N. gonorrhoeae* (4, 5).

Bibliography / Literatur

1. BERGER, U. (1962): Über das Vorkommen von Neisserien bei einigen Tieren. Z. Hyg. Infektionskr. **148**, 445–457.
2. BERGER, U. (1960): Neisseria animalis nov. spec. Z. Hyg. Infektionskr. **147**, 158–161.
3. DENT, V. E. (1982): Identification of oral Neisseria species of animals. J. appl. Bact. **52**, 21–30.
4. NALIVAIKO, L. I. (1983): A disease of the genital organs of geese caused by species of Neisseria. Veterinariya (Moskau) 60–61.
5. SZEP, J., M. PATAKY & J. BÖGRE (1979): Recent practical and experimental observations on the infectious inflammatory disease of cloaca and penis in geese. Acta vet. acad. hung. **27**, 195–202.
6. VEDROS, N. A. (1984): Genus Neisseria Trevisan 1885. In: Bergey's manual of systematic bacteriology. Vol. 1, S. 290–296. Baltimore, London: Williams & Wilkins.

3.4 Genus: Moraxella (M.)

Members of this genus are either rods *(subgenus Moraxella)*, or cocci *(subgenus Branhamella)*. The rods are usually very small (1.0–1.5 × 1.5–2.5 μm) and, in fact, similar to cocci, plump and arranged in pairs, rarely in short chains. The cocci are smaller (0.6–1.0 μm), and they occur either singly, in pairs with opposing sides flattened, or in tetrads. Other common features are: Gram-negative, aerobic growth as non-pigmented colonies, oxidase positive, no fermentation of carbohydrates and usually sensitive to penicillin.

There are 6 types of the *subgenus Moraxella* (BØVRE, 2) and most of these occur only in man. From the veterinary standpoint the most important are *M. bovis*, although *M. phenylpyruvica* has been isolated from animals in rare instances.

3.4.1 Subgenus: Moraxella
3.4.1.1 Moraxella bovis

■ **Incidence and veterinary significance**

M. bovis occurs mainly in cattle not only as a commensal in the mucosa of the upper respiratory tract and the conjunctiva of healthy animals, but also in infectious keratoconjunctivitis. As causal agent of this condition they are supported by other microorganisms, such as mycoplasms, chlamydiae, rickettsiae and viruses as well as by secondary environmental factors (UV-rays and mechanical irritation of the eyes). Thus the aetiological role of *M. bovis* fluctuates (1, 6). Chlamydiae appear to play an important part in this condition, so that *M. bovis* is

only of secondary importance (6). In rare instances *M. bovis* occurs in the horse *(M. equi)*.

■ **Morphology**
This is a Gram-negative, non-motile, small, plump rod, which is generally arranged in pairs or short chains.

■ **Culture** (figs. 120 and 121)
M. bovis will grow aerobically on the common media. Within 24–48 hours incubation at 37 °C it will develop shiny, greyish-white, 1–2 mm long colonies that sink slightly into the medium (S-form). There is distinct haemolysis on blood agar (apart from the strains originating from the horse, *M. equi*). R-forms can develop spontaneously in cultures and in this case the colonies are larger and not sunk into the medium. Most of the strains exhibit liquefaction on Loeffler's serum. Other properties are listed in table 46.

■ **Animal inoculation**
The intraperitoneal injection of haemolytic strains of *M. bovis* into mice and guinea pigs leads to a fatal disease. Abortion may also occur in experimental animals (3, 4, 5).

3.4.2 Subgenus Branhamella
3.4.2.1 Moraxella (Branhamella) ovis

Occurs on the respiratory mucosa of healthy sheep and, less frequently, cattle; it is also encountered in keratoconjunctivitis. *M. (Branhamella) ovis* are cocci which will grow on the usual media as greyish-white colonies of about 2.5 mm in diameter in 48 hours incubation. As a rule they haemolyze blood agar. For other properties see table 46.

3.4.2.2 Moraxella (Branhamella) cuniculi

It has been isolated from the oral cavity of healthy rabbits. Its bacteriological properties are listed in table 46.

3.4.2.3 Moraxella (Branhamella) caviae

It has been cultured from the upper digestive and respiratory tracts of healthy guinea pigs. Its properties are presented in table 46.

Rolle scheinen bei diesem Krankheitsbild Chlamydien zu spielen, so daß *M. bovis* dann nur die Bedeutung eines Sekundärerregers zukommt (6). Selten kommt *M. bovis* auch beim Pferd vor *(M. equi)*.

■ **Morphologie**
Es handelt sich um ein gramnegatives, unbewegliches, kleines, plumpes Stäbchen, das meistens als Diplobakterium oder in kurzen Ketten erscheint.

■ **Kultur** (Abb. 120 u. 121)
M. bovis wächst aerob auf den üblichen Nährböden. Es bilden sich innerhalb 24–48 h bei Bebrütung bei 37 °C 1–2 mm große, grauweiße, glatte Kolonien, die leicht in den Nährboden einsinken (S-Form). Auf Blutagar kommt es zu einer deutlichen Hämolyse (ausgenommen vom Pferd stammende Stämme, *M. equi*). In den Kulturen können spontan R-Formen mit größeren und nicht einsinkenden Kolonien entstehen. Auf der Serumplatte nach Loeffler führen die meisten Stämme zu einer Serolyse. Weitere Eigenschaften siehe Tab. 46.

■ **Tierversuch**
Hämolytische Stämme von *M. bovis* verursachen bei Mäusen und Meerschweinchen nach ip. Infektion eine tödliche Erkrankung. Ferner können bei Versuchstieren Aborte auftreten (3, 4, 5).

3.4.2 Subgenus: Branhamella
3.4.2.1 Moraxella (Branhamella) ovis

Kommt einerseits bei gesunden Schafen, seltener Rindern auf der Respirationsschleimhaut vor und andererseits bei der Keratokonjunktivitis. Mikroskopisch handelt es sich um Kokken, die auf den üblichen Nährböden in grauweißen, nach 48 h Bebrütung etwa 2,5 mm großen Kolonien wachsen, auf Blutagar entsteht meistens eine Hämolyse. Weitere Eigenschaften s. Tab. 46.

3.4.2.2 Moraxella (Branhamella) cuniculi

Wurde aus der Mundhöhle gesunder Kaninchen isoliert. Eigenschaften siehe Tab. 46.

3.4.2.3 Moraxella (Branhamella) caviae

Wurde aus den oberen Verdauungs- und Atmungswegen von gesunden Meerschweinchen isoliert. Eigenschaften zeigt Tab. 46.

3.4.2.4 Moraxella (Branhamella) catarrhalis

So far, this has only been found in guinea pigs.

Bibliography / Literatur

1. BAPTISTA, P. (1979): Infectious bovine keratoconjunctivitis. A review. Brit. Vet. J. **135**, 225–242.
2. BØVRE, K. (1984): Genus Moraxella Lwoff 1939. In: Bergey's manual of systematic bacteriology, Vol. 1, S. 296–303. Baltimore: Williams & Wilkins.
3. BUCZEK, J., J. KRZYZANOWSKI & H. MOUALLEM (1979): Isolation of Neisseria ovis from sheep with infectious keratoconjunctivitis. Med. Weteryn. **35**, 136–138.
4. FRASER, J., & N. J. L. GILMOUR (1979): The identification of Moraxella bovis and Neisseria ovis from the eyes of cattle and sheep. Res. Vet. Sci. **27**, 127–128.
5. NORMAN, J. O., & M. H. ELISSALDE (1979): Abortion in laboratory animals induced by Moraxella bovis. Infect. Imm. **24**, 427–433.
6. DIETZ, O., J. WEHR, R. THALMANN, A. POPP & W. BUSCHMANN (1983): Neue Untersuchungen zur Ätiologie und Therapie der infektiösen Keratokonjunktivitis des Rindes. Mh. Vet. Med. **38**, 843–847.

4 Oxidase-negative and fermentative bacteria

(reaction type II a)

4.1 Enterobacteriaceae

Members of this family are distributed world-wide, in the environment, as saprophytes and pathogens of man and animals.

For a biochemical definition of the family see table 47.

■ Biochemical differentiation of the species

The classification of the family *Enterobacteriaceae* into genera and species is based on biochemical characters (tab. 48). The majority of strains can be assigned to their respective genera without difficulty, but there are some with divergent features, whose classification is more problematic.

4.1.1 Genus: Escherichia (E.)
4.1.1.1 Escherichia coli

■ Incidence and veterinary significance

In warm-blooded animals *E. coli* is a commensal on the one hand and on the other the cause of the most

Table 47: Properties common to the bacteria of the family *Enterobacteriaceae*

Gram-negative rods
Motile (peritrichous flagella) or non-motile
No spore formation
Aerobic or facultative anaerobic growth
Growth on simple media, including selective media such as Gassner's agar
Metabolism respiratory and fermentative
Fermentation of glucose, acid with or without gas formation
No production of oxidase
Nitrates are reduced to nitrites

diverse diseases which are of considerable economic importance. The most important of these are: septicaemia and diarrhoea of calves; diarrhoea of sucking and weaning piglets; enterotoxaemia of weaners (oedema disease); mastitis in cows and other species, MMA-complex of sows; infections of lambs; colisepticaemia due to invasive strains of E. coli and coli diarrhoea; dysentery of rabbits; diarrhoea of dogs; infections in poultry (septicaemia, coli granulomatosis); infection of the mucosa of the urogenital and respiratory tracts etc.; wound infections, retarded healing.

A summary of the various clinical pictures is available in WILLINGER (55).

■ **Morphology** (fig. 122)
E. coli is a plump to coccoid, Gram-negative rod, measuring 1.1–1.5 × 2–6 µm. It can be either motile or non-motile and usually appears singly or in pairs and generally possesses a capsule.

■ **Culture** (figs. 123, 124, 125)
E. coli makes no special nutritional demands, growing at 37 °C on nutrient agar, blood agar and the selective media usually employed for the detection of Enterobacteriaceae (tab. 52). In the S-form the colonies are round, with smooth outline, greyish-white and shiny. Besides these, there are decidedly mucoid colonies and the R-forms grow as smaller, dry colonies with irregular outline. A proportion of strains, especially the pathogenic ones, are haemolytic.

■ **Biochemical properties**
The biochemical features on which the identification of E. coli is based are listed in table 48 and the quantitative results of the most important reactions are summarized in figure 126 (12, 22, 34).

■ **Antigenic structure**
E. coli has the following antigens:
O-antigens: This is a heat-stable surface antigen, a lipo-polysaccharide, and it forms the basis of the classification of E. coli into groups (more than 160). The identification is carried out with the tube agglutination or micro-titre plates, using rabbit sera. A slide agglutination may be used for the initial test. For the determination of the O-antigens a bacterial suspension is employed which is either heated for 1 hour to 100 °C to destroy the K-antigens or, if they possess any K (A)-antigens, it is heated for 2 hours to 120 °C. In order to conserve materials the agglutination can first be performed with mixed sera and then with the individual group sera. Cross reactions can occur between the individual O-groups.
K-antigens: Capsule or envelope antigens. These

verschiedenartiger Erkrankungen, die von erheblicher wirtschaftlicher Bedeutung sind. Die wichtigsten Krankheitsbilder sind: Septikämie und Diarrhoe (Coliruhr) des Kalbes; Diarrhoe der Saug- u. Absatzferkel; Enterotoxämie der Absatzferkel (Ödemkrankheit); Mastitis bei Kühen und anderen Tieren, MMA-Komplex bei Sauen; Infektionen bei Schaflämmern (Coliseptikämie durch invasive Colistämme und Colidiarrhoe); Dysenterie der Kaninchen; Diarrhoe bei Hunden; Infektionen des Geflügels (Septikämie, Coligranulomatose); Schleimhautentzündung im Urogenitaltrakt, Respirationstrakt u. ä.; Wundinfektionen, Wundheilungsstörungen.

(Zusammenfassung der verschiedenen Krankheitsbilder bei WILLINGER, 55.)

■ **Morphologie** (Abb. 122)
E. coli ist ein gramnegatives, plumpes bis kokkoides, 1,1–1,5 × 2–6 µm großes, bewegliches oder unbewegliches, einzeln oder paarweise gelegenes, meistens bekapseltes Stäbchen.

■ **Kultur** (Abb. 123, 124 u. 125)
E. coli stellt keine besonderen Nährbodenansprüche und wächst bei 37 °C auf Nähragar, Blutagar und den zum Nachweis von Enterobacteriaceae üblichen Selektivplatten (Tab. 52).

In der S-Form sind die Kolonien rund, grauweiß, glattrandig und glänzend. Daneben kommen Stämme mit einem deutlichen schleimigen Wachstum vor. R-Formen wachsen in kleineren, trockenen Kolonien mit unregelmäßigem Rand. Ein Teil der Stämme, insbesondere pathogene, bilden eine Hämolyse aus.

■ **Kulturell-biochemische Eigenschaften**
Die kulturell-biochemischen Eigenschaften als Grundlage der Bestimmungen von E. coli sind aus der Tab. 48 und zusammen mit dem quantitativen Ausfall der wichtigsten Reaktionen aus der Abb. 126 ersichtlich (12, 22, 34).

■ **Antigenstruktur**
E. coli besitzt folgende Antigene:
O-Antigen: Oberflächenantigen, Lipopolysaccharid, hitzestabil. Grundlage für die Einteilung von E. coli in Gruppen (über 160). Der serologische Nachweis wird mit der Langsamagglutination in Röhrchen oder Mikrotiterplatten mit Kaninchenseren geführt. Für orientierende Untersuchungen kann auch die Objektträgeragglutination benutzt werden. Für die O-Antigenbestimmung verwendet man Keimsuspensionen, die zur Zerstörung des K-Antigens entweder 1 h bei 100 °C oder, wenn sie K (A)-Antigen besitzen, 2 h bei 120 °C erhitzt worden sind. Zur Materialersparnis kann die Agglutination zuerst mit Mischseren und dann mit einzelnen Gruppenseren durchgeführt werden. Zwischen den einzelnen O-Gruppen können Kreuzreaktionen auftreten.

Table 48: Biochemical differentiation of the species of *Enterobacteriaceae* of veterinary importance (for common family characters see Tab. 47)

Tabelle 48: Biochemische Differenzierung der veterinärmedizinisch wichtigen Gattungen der *Enterobacteriaceae* (Gemeinsame Familieneigenschaften Tab. 47)

Tribe	Genus	Lac	Ure	Ind	LDC	VPR	H_2S	ODC	Mot	Dul	Mlo	Cit	Man	PAD	MR	Sac	Sal	Ado
Escherichieae	Salmonella	$-^1$	−	v^-	+	−	v^+	+	+	v^+	$-^1$	v	+	−	+	−	v^-	−
	Citrobacter	+/(+)	v	v^-	−	−	v^+	+	+	v	−	+	+	−	+	v	v^+	v
	Escherichia	$+^2$	−	+	+	−	−	+	v^+	v	−	−	+	−	+	v	v^+	v
	Shigella	−/(+)	−	v	−	−	−	−	−	v	−	−	v	−	+	v	−	−
Edwardsiellae	Edwardsiella tarda	−	−	+	+	−	+	+	+	−	−	−	−	−	+	−	−	−
Klebsielleae	Klebsiella	v^+	v^+	−	v^+	+	−	−	−	v	v	v^+	+	−	−	+	+	+
	Enterobacter	+	v	−	v	+	−	+	+	v	v	+	+	−	−	+	+	v
	Hafnia	−/(+)	−	−	+	37°C v 22°C +	−	+	37°C − 22°C +	−	v	37°C v 22°C +	+	−	+	−/(+)	−	−
	Serratia	−/(+)	−	−	v^+	+	−	v^+	+	−	v	v^+	+	v^-	−	+	v^+	v
Proteeae	P. vulgaris	−	+	+	−	−	+	−	+	−	−	v	−	+	+	+	+	−
	P. mirabilis	−	+	−	−	v	+	+	+	−	−	v	−	+	+	(+)	v	−
	Morganella	−	+	+	−	−	−	+	+	−	−	−	−	+	+	−	v	−
	Providencia	−	v	+	−	−	−	−	+	−	−	+	v	+	+	v	v	v
Yersinieae	Yersinia enterocolitica	−	+/(+)	−	−	37°C − 22°C +	−	+	+	−	−	−	+	−	37°C + 22°C −	+	v	−
Erwinieae	Erwinia³	v	−	−	−	v	−	−	+	−	v	+	+	v	v	+	v	−

[1] Arizona: + or (+) or −; [2] Alcalescens-dispar group: Lac (+) or −, Glu + without gas formation; [3] Yellow pigment

[1] Arizona: + oder (+) oder −; [2] Alcalescens-Dispar-Gruppe: Lact (+) oder −, Glu + ohne Gasbildung; [3] gelbes Pigment

lie on top of the O-antigens and prevent them linking with the O-antibodies, so that strains carrying K-antigens cannot be agglutinated with O-antisera. The following K-antigens have been identified:

▷ K (A)-antigens: are particularly heat resistant; they are destroyed after 2 hours at 120 °C and occur mainly in the O-groups 08, 09, 020, 0101. Chemically they are polysaccharides.

▷ K (B)-antigens: are destroyed by heating to 100 °C and they are chemically acid polysaccharides.

K-antigens are determined by means of agglutination with OK-sera, which are produced by immunizing rabbits with living bacteria. The determination is usually performed with the slide agglutination test, using live culture material direct from the culture plate, or with the tube agglutination test. Electrophoresis is used for particularly exact antigen analyses. This technique has led to the discovery of partial antigens in some of the K-antigens (e.g. ab, ac, ad).

▷ Fimbrial antigens (previously termed L-antigens): they are situated in the fimbriae (pili), which are filamentous protrusions of the cell wall and consist of protein. Like the K-antigens, they can prevent a strain from being identified by its O-antigenic structure. Among other characteristics they have adhesive properties, through which the bacteria attach themselves to the brush border of epithelial cell of the small intestine. (This is a pathogenicity factor in coli diarrhoea.)

The adhesion antigens are very important for the identification of the enteropathogenic strains of E. coli. They are demonstrated in a slide agglutination test or the ELISA test, using appropriate antisera. Its has not yet been completely established how many adhesion antigens there are, but examples are presented in table 49. The demonstration of the K99-antigen must follow the primary isolation of the bacteria on Minca medium.

H-antigens: These are flagellar antigens, protein and heat-labile. They are demonstrated with the tube agglutination test and they are of subordinate importance in diagnosis.

Individual serotypes are found more frequently in certain species and in certain disease conditions and these strains are then credited with a greater pathogenicity for that particular disease. Some important serotypes are listed in table 49.

Methodological details about the agglutination test for the identification of the various antigens are provided by the commercial firms who produce the antisera and by the following authors: 35, 45, 51, 52, 53, 56, 58, 60.

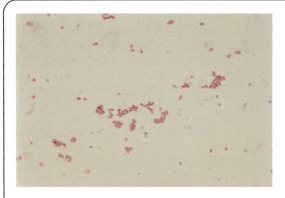
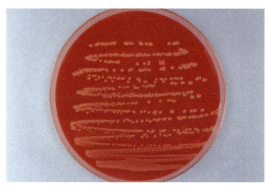
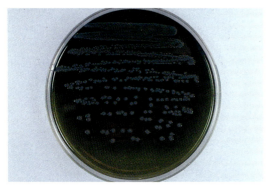
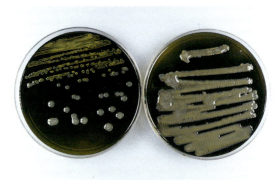

▲ Fig. 122: *Escherichia coli*, smear from urine sediment of a dog, about 10^6 organisms/ml, Gram stain. Magnification x 1000

▽ Fig. 124: *Escherichia coli*, pure culture on Gassner agar, colonies blue, medium without colonies is green, 24 h, 37 °C. Magnification x 0.25

▲ Fig. 123: *Escherichia coli*, pure culture on blood agar, 24 h, 37 °C. Magnification x 0.25

▽ Fig. 125: *Escherichia coli*, very mucoid form (left Petri dish) and *Klebsiella pneumoniae* (right Petri dish), pure culture on Gassner plates, the appearance of the colonies of mucoid *E. coli* cannot be differentiated from the klebsiella, 48 h, 37 °C. Magnification x 0.17

▲ Abb. 122: *Escherichia coli*, Ausstrich eines Harnsedimentes vom Hund, etwa 10^6 Keime/ml, Gram-Färbung, Abb.-M. 1000 : 1

▽ Abb. 124: *Escherichia coli*, Reinkultur auf Gaßner-Agar, Blauverfärbung der Kolonien und des unbewachsenen grünen Nährbodens, 24 h, 37 °C, Abb.-M. 1 : 4

▲ Abb. 123: *Escherichia coli*, Reinkultur auf Blutagar, 24 h, 37 °C, Abb.-M. 1 : 4

▽ Abb. 125: *Escherichia coli*, stark schleimig wachsende Form, (linke Petrischale) und *Klebsiella pneumoniae* (rechte Petrischale), Reinkulturen auf Gaßner-Platten, schleimig wachsende Colibakterien sind im Koloniebild von Klebsiellen nicht zu unterscheiden, 48 h, 37 °C, Abb.-M. 1 : 6

■ **Toxins**

The presence of enterotoxins, other than the adhesion antigens, has been described in *E. coli*.

▷ Enterotoxins: These are responsible for enterotoxic enteropathies of young animals (calves, piglets, lambs etc.) and they occur in the form of heat labile (LT) and heat stable (ST) enterotoxins. Two variants have been differentiated in ST, namely STa and STb. They are exotoxins. Strains which produce enterotoxin are termed »enterotoxic E. coli«

■ **Toxine**

Als Pathogenitätsfaktoren für die enteropathogenen *E. coli*-Stämme sind neben den adhäsiven Antigenen Enterotoxine beschrieben worden.

▷ Enterotoxine: Sie sind verantwortlich für enterotoxische Enteropathien der Jungtiere (Kalb, Ferkel, Lamm u. a.) und kommen als hitzelabiles (LT) und hitzestabiles (ST) Enterotoxin vor. Beim ST können 2 Varianten unterschieden werden (STa, STb). Ihrer Entstehungsweise nach handelt es sich um Exotoxi-

(ETEC). The majority of ETEC strains pathogenic to piglets produce both ST and LT, a small proportion only ST, and LT is never produced by itself. Strains pathogenic to calves and lambs usually form only ST.

Enterotoxin-forming strains of *E. coli* are rare in dogs, even in puppies suffering from enteritic conditions. None of the adhesion antigens known so far have yet been identified in dogs (38).

LT has similarities with cholera toxin, in respect of its mode of action and antigenic structure. By activation of the adenylate cyclase, which acts as catalyst raising the intracellular cAMP (cyclic adenosine-3′, 5′-monophosphate), and leads to an increase in the secretion of electrolytes, particularly

ne. Stämme, die Enterotoxin produzieren, werden als enterotoxische *E. coli* (ETEC) bezeichnet. Die Mehrzahl der ferkelpathogenen ETEC-Stämme produziert gleichzeitig ST und LT, ein geringerer Teil nur ST, LT wird nie alleine produziert. Die kälber- und lämmerpathogenen Stämme bilden meistens nur ST.

Bei Hunden, auch bei enteritiskranken Junghunden, sind enterotoxinbildende *E. coli*-Stämme selten. Die bisher bekannten Adhäsisonsantigene konnten noch nicht nachgewiesen werden (38).

Das LT besitzt hinsichtlich der Wirkungsweise und Antigenstruktur Beziehungen zum Choleratoxin. Es führt über die Aktivierung der Adenylatcy-

Table 49: The occurrence of O- and fimbrial-antigens in *Escherichia coli*

Tabelle 49: Das Vorkommen von O- und Fimbrien-Antigenen bei *Escherichia coli*

	I. O-antigens and their existence in animals		
Cattle	Sepsis of calves 078 K80 (B) 086 08 0115 09 0117 015 etc. 055	Calf diarrhoea 08 0101 09 etc. 020 these possess the K99-antigens, adhesion mechanism	Mastitis great heterogeneity in the O-groups, e.g.: 09 021 08 081 06 086 02
Pig	Coli dysentery of piglets 08 : K87 : K88 : H19 09 : K35 : K99 : H- 09 : K103 : K987P : H- 020 : K101 : K987P : H- 045 : K88 : H- 0101 : K30 : K99 : H-	0138 : K88 : (H14) 0139 : K82 : K88 : H1 0141 : K88 : (H4) 0147 : K88 : H19 0149 : K88 : H10 0157 : K88 : H19	Oedema disease 0138 : K81 (B) : H- 0139 : K82 : H1 0141 : K85 : (H4) & other less common types
Sheep	Sepsis of lambs 078 : K80 (B) 015, 020, 035 075, 0114, 0115 0125, 0137	Diarrhoea of lambs 09, 0101, 08 with the K99 antigen	
Dog	Enteritis: 04, 025, 042 & others		
Rabbit	Dysentery: 085, 02, 0101, 06, 018, 0128, 055, 044		
Horse	From the reproductive organs: 018, 02, 06, 0147, 0141		

	II. Fimbrial antigens and their haemagglutination	
Pig	K88 (ab, ac, ad) P987 K99 F41	No haemagglutination: P987 Mannose-resistant haemagglutination Antigens: Erythrocytes from species:
Ox	K99 F41	K88 guinea pigs, chicks K99 horse, sheep F41 man, sheep, horse, guinea pig CFA I man, ox, chick CFA II ox, chick
Sheep	K99	
Man	CFA I CFA II	

Na⁺ and Cl⁻, and water into the lumen of the small intestine.

The heat stability of ST has been variously stated (100 °C for 30 minutes, 80 °C for 30 minutes and 65 °C for 15 minutes). It is neither immunogenic nor acid stable, and it is sensitive to the activity of proteinases. The biological action sets in rapidly and is of short duration. The action mechanism differs from that of LT, as it activates guanyl cyclase in the intestinal epithelium (19, 23, 45, 57, 59).

The best known method for demonstrating enterotoxins (fig. 126) is the gut ligature test. During laparotomy, a 5–10 cm section of duodenum or jejunum is tied off, forming a sort of ampulla. Broth

clase, die den Anstieg von intrazellulärem cAMP (cyclischem Adenosin-3′, 5′-Monophosphat) katalysiert, zu einer Sekretionssteigerung von Elektrolyten, vor allem Na⁺ und Cl⁻, und Wasser in das Dünndarmlumen.

Die Hitzestabilität von ST wird unterschiedlich angegeben (100 °C/30 min, 80 °C/30 min, 65 °C/15 min). Es ist nicht immunogen, säurestabil und unempfindlich gegen Proteinasen. Die biologische Wirkung beginnt schnell und ist von kurzer Dauer. Der Wirkungsmechanismus ist von dem des LT verschieden und verläuft über eine Aktivierung der Guanylcyclase in den Darmepithelien (19, 23, 45, 57, 59).

Das bekannteste Verfahren zum Nachweis der Enterotoxine (Abb. 126) ist der Darmligaturtest.

Specimens
Intestinal content, faecal samples, organs, milk samples, etc.

Isolation by culture
a) Enrichment in broth. After 24 h incubation at 37 °C subculture onto lactose-containing selective media (tab. 52). the enrichment is often unnecessary. b) Direct culture on to lactose-containing selective media, incubation 24 h, 37 °C. *E. coli* produces lactose-positive colonies

Biochemical identification			
Motility	v	69.1 %[1]	Indole	+	98.6 %
Methyl red	+	99.9 %	Voges-Proskauer	−	0 %
Urease	−	0 %	Citrate	−	0.2 %
Lysine decarboxylase	v	88.7 %	Ornithine decarboxylase	v	64.2 %
Phenylalanine deaminase	−	0 %	H_2S	−	0 %
Gelatinase	−	0 %	Glucose	+	100.0 %
Gas produced from			
Glucose	+	91.9 %	Lactose	+	90.8 %
Saccharose	v	48.9 %	Mannitol	+	96.8 %
Dulcitol	v	49.5 %	Adonitol	−	5.6 %

Demonstration of enterotoxicity in strains isolated from faecal samples

a) Enteropathogenic strains are often haemolytic
b) Certain O-groups predominate among the enteropathogenic strains (tab. 49), in the pig, for instance, O 149, O 138, O 147, O 45, O 141, O 8, O 139. Slide agglutination test for a preliminary classification.
c) Demonstration of adhesion antigens: K 88, K 987P in pigs, K 99 in calves, by means of slide agglutination. This method is in very close agreement with the test for enterotoxins (24, 43).
d) Demonstration of enterotoxins
   LT and ST detection: gut ligature test is best performed on the same species from which the strain originated; most reliable but costly method, only possible, therefore, in isolated cases. Serious doubts on animal welfare grounds.
   LT test: Cell culture with good correlation to gut ligature test;
   ST test: suckling mice test, limited susceptibility because not all strains positive in the gut ligature test are recognized.

[1] Percentage of positive reactions

[1] Prozentsatz positiver Reaktionen

Fig. 126: Identification and differentiation of *Escherichia coli*

Abb. 126: Nachweis und Differenzierung von *Escherichia coli*

cultures or sterile filtrates of the strains to be tested are injected into this isolated segment. With enterotoxin-producing strains there is an increased fluid secretion, resulting in the distension of the ampulla in 8 hours (evidence of LT) up to 18 hours (indicative of ST) (4, 30, 31, 32, 44).

ST can also be demonstrated in a mouse test (suckling mouse assay). In the original method 4 day-old mice were injected through the skin into the stomach with the bacteria-free supernatant of broth cultures. According to AWAD-MASALMEH (4) the sterile filtrate is heated to 65 °C for 30 minutes and a 1 % solution of Evans blue is added. This can then be administered to the mice with a thin stomach tube. After 4 hours at 28 °C the animals are killed and the proportion of gut weight to the remaining body weight is determined. The quotient varies as the quantity of fluid in the gut is increased through the action of ST.

A simplified method was described by MOON et al. (29). The culture fluid is given orally to older mice and diarrhoea develops if ST is present (10).

Besides the gut ligature test, tissue culture methods have been developed for the demonstration of LT (Y1 adrenal cell test). It is based on the principle that the supernatant culture fluid containing LT will lead to a rounding of the originally spindle-shaped cells (incubation 18 h at 37 °C). The test is performed on micro titre plates (4, 11, 33, 45, 49).

The demonstration of enteropathogenicity, in as much as it is due to the action of enterotoxins, cannot be entirely justified as a routine procedure, in view of the cost and complexity of the method. A probable diagnosis may be arrived at by using other criteria of the isolated strain, such as haemolysis, demonstration of the O-group and/or the fimbrial antigen.

Apart from their toxic action, enteropathogenic strains may also cause inflammatory changes in the calf intestine, which extend into the propria and can be identified histologically (EIEC = entero-invasive *E. coli*; 18).

▷ Neurotoxins as cause of enterotoxaemia of pigs (Oedema disease): A neurotoxin (lipoprotein) is believed to be the cause of enterotoxaemia of pigs. It is formed by certain haemolytic strains of *E. coli* of the serogroups O139 : K82 (B), O141 : K85 (B), O138 : K81 (B) and others (table 49). This neurotoxin is thermolabile, insoluble at pH 4.0 and it can be neutralized with antitoxic sera. In mice it induces central nervous disturbances. These properties distinguish it fundamentally from endotoxin (39, 40).

▷ Endotoxins: Occur in all strains of coli. They are integral parts of the cell wall and form the O-antigen. Chemically they are protein-phospholipid-polysaccharide complexes, in which the polysaccharide determines the serological specificity and the lipoprotein component the toxicity. In septic conditions it is responsible for the intensely febrile

Dabei werden nach Laparotomie 5–10 cm lange Abschnitte des Duodenums und Jejunums ampullenförmig abgebunden. In diese Segmente werden Bouillonkulturen oder Sterilfiltrate der zu prüfenden Stämme eingespritzt. Bei enterotoxinbildenden Stämmen kommt es nach 8 (LT-Nachweis) bis 18 h (ST-Nachweis) zu einer starken Flüssigkeitssekretion und Auftreibung der Ampullen (4, 30, 31, 32, 44).

Der Nachweis von ST ist auch im Mäuseversuch (suckling mouse assay) möglich. Im Originalverfahren werden 4 d alten Mäusen bakterienfreie Kulturüberstände durch die Haut in den Magen injiziert. Nach AWAD-MASALMEH (4) kann das Sterilfiltrat nach Hitzeinaktivierung (65 °C/30 min) und Zugabe von Evans-Blue-Lösung (1 %ig) den Mäusen mit einer dünnen Magensonde verabreicht werden. Nach 4 h bei 28 °C werden die Tiere getötet und der Quotient aus Darm- und restlichem Körpergewicht bestimmt. Der Wert wird durch die Menge der durch ST in Darm abgegebenen Flüssigkeit bestimmt.

Ein vereinfachtes Verfahren wurde von MOON et al. (29) beschrieben, dabei wird älteren Mäusen die Kulturflüssigkeit oral verabreicht, bei vorhandenem ST tritt eine Diarrhoe ein (10).

Beim LT-Nachweis sind zusätzlich zum Darmligaturtest Nachweisverfahren mit der Zellkultur entwickelt worden (Y 1 adrenal cell test), die im Prinzip darin bestehen, daß LT enthaltende Überstände zu einer Abrundung der ursprünglich spindelförmigen Zellen führen (Bebrütung 18 h/37 °C). Der Test wird in Mikrotiterplatten durchgeführt (4, 11, 33, 45, 49).

Der Nachweis der Enteropathogenität, soweit diese durch die Enterotoxine bedingt ist, ist in der Routineuntersuchung aufgrund des methodischen Aufwandes nur teilweise arbeitstechnisch vertretbar. Unter Hinzuziehung weiterer Eigenschaften des isolierten Stammes (Hämolyse, Nachweis der O-Gruppe und [oder] des Fimbrienantigens) wird meistens nur eine Wahrscheinlichkeitsdiagnose zu stellen sein.

Neben der toxischen Wirkung können enteropathogene Colistämme teilweise auch histologisch erfaßbare Entzündungserscheinungen im Kälberdarm hervorrufen und in die Propia eindringen (EIEC = enteroinvasive *E. coli*; 18).

▷ Neurotoxine als Ursache der Enterotoxämie (Ödemkrankheit) des Schweines: Als Ursache der Enterotoxämie der Schweine wird ein Neurotoxin (Lipoproteid) angesehen, das von bestimmten hämolysierenden Colistämmen der Serogruppen O 139 : K82 (B), O 141 : K85 (B), O 138 : K81 (B) oder anderen (Tab. 49) gebildet wird. Es ist thermolabil, unlösbar bei pH 4,0, neutralisierbar mit antineurotoxischen Seren, verursacht bei Mäusen zentralnervöse Störungen. Durch diese Eigenschaften unterscheidet es sich grundsätzlich vom Endotoxin (39, 40).

clinical picture with more or less well developed signs of shock.

▷ Endotoxine: Kommen bei allen Colistämmen vor. Sie sind Bestandteil der Zellwand und bilden das O-Antigen. Chemisch handelt es sich um einen Protein-Phospholipid-Polysaccharid-Komplex, in dem das Polysaccharid die serologische Spezifität, der Lipidanteil die Toxizität bestimmt. Es verursacht bei septischen Infektionen ein hochfieberhaftes Krankheitsbild mit mehr oder weniger ausgeprägter Schocksymptomatik.

Bibliography / Literatur

1. AL-DABBAS, A. H. M., & H. WILLINGER (1986): Eigenschaften von aus diarrhöischen Saugkälbern isolierten E. coli-Stämmen. Wien. tierärztl. Wschr. 73, 217–222.
2. ASKAA, J., J. K. BONRUP & M. SØRENSEN (1978): Neonatal infections in puppies caused by Escherichia coli serogroups 04 and 025. Nord. Vet. Med. 30, 486–488.
3. AWAD-MASALMEH, M., H. WILLINGER, H. SAGMEISTER & F. KRISPEL (1985): Zur Immunprophylaxe der durch enteropathogene E. coli bedingten Krankheiten der Absatzferkel. Wien. tierärztl. Wschr. 72, 290–296.
4. AWAD-MASALMEH, M. (1983): Nachweis von Enterotoxinen bei pathogenen E. coli des Ferkels. Wien. tierärztl. Wschr. 70, 151–157.
5. AWAD-MASALMEH, M. (1982): Untersuchungen an enteropathogenen E. coli des Ferkels — Serologie und Chemoresistenz. Wien. tierärztl. Wschr. 69, 358–364.
6. BERTSCHINGER, H. U. (1970): Coli-Enterotoxämie beim Absatzferkel. Abhängigkeit der pathologisch-anatomischen Veränderungen vom Coli-Serotyp. Schweiz. Arch. Tierhk. 112, 374–384.
7. BOKHARI, S. M. H., & F. ØRSKOV (1952): O-grouping of E. coli strains isolated from cases of white scours. Acta path. microbiol. scand. 30, 87–89.
8. CHAREOSIRISUTHIGUL, T. (1978): Untersuchungen zur Biochemie, Serologie, Pathogenität und Antibiotikaresistenz an Escherichia-coli-Stämmen von gesunden und kranken Sauen (MMA-Komplex). Vet. Med. Diss. Hannover.
9. CIOSEK, D., & M. TRUSZCZYNSKI (1979): The evaluation of the O- and K-antigens as indicators of pathogenicity of E. coli strains isolated from swine coli-bacteriosis. Zbl. Vet. Med. B 26, 39–48.
10. DEAN, A. G., Y. C. CHING, R. W. WILLIAMS & L. B. HARDAN (1972): Test for Escherichia coli enterotoxin using infant mice. J. Infect. Dis. 125, 407–411.
11. DONTA, S. T., H. W. MOON & S. C. WHIPP (1974): Detection of heat-labile Escherichia coli enterotoxin with the use of adrenal cells in tissue culture. Science 183, 334–336.
12. EDWARDS, P. R., & W. H. EWING (1972): Identification of enterobacteriaceae. Minneapolis (Minnesota): Burgess.
13. FEY, H. (1972): Colibacillosis in calves. Stuttgart, Wien: Hans Huber.
14. FEY, H. (1957): Bakteriologie und Serologie der Colisepsis des Kalbes. 1. Mitt. Serologische und biochemische Untersuchungen. 2. Mitt. Die Bedeutung des Colityps 78 : 80 für die Kälberruhr. Zbl. Vet. med. 4, 309–318, 447–458.
15. FEY, H. (1955): Serologische, biochemische und biologische Untersuchungen an Stämmen aus boviner Colimastitis. Ergeb. Hyg. Bakt. 29, 394–474.
16. FOX, I. W., W. G. HOAG & J. STROUT (1965): Breed susceptibility, pathogenicity and epidemiology of endemic coliform enteritis in the dog. Lab. Anim. Care 15, 194–200.
17. GHONIEM, N., G. HANSCHKE, G. AMTSBERG & W. BISPING (1982): Vergleichende bakteriologische Untersuchungen und Antibiotikaresistenzbestimmung an Escherichia-coli-Stämmen von Kälbern aus Marokko und Nordwestdeutschland. Berl. Münch. tierärztl. Wschr. 95, 141–143.
18. GÜNTHER, H., F. SCHULZE & P. HEILMANN (1983): Zum pathogenetischen Verhalten verschiedener enterotoxinbildender Escherichia coli-Stämme im Darmkanal neugeborener Kälber. Mh. Vet. Med. 38, 96–103.
19. GYLES, C. L., & D. A. BARNUM (1969): A heat-labile enterotoxin from strains of Escherichia coli enteropathogenic for pigs. J. Infect. Dis. 120, 419–426.
20. HOFMANN, W., & A. WEBER (1979): Zur Behandlung der Enteritis neugeborener Kälber mit stallspezifischen E. coli-Vakzinen. Dtsch. Tierärztl. Wschr. 86, 47–50.
21. KAUFFMANN, F. (1972): Zur Klassifikation der Escherichia-K-Antigene. Zbl. Bakt. I. Orig. A 219, 66–68.
22. KAUFFMANN, F. (1966): The bacteriology of enterobacteriaceae. Copenhagen: Munksgaard.
23. KIRCHNER, A. (1981): Enteropathogene Escherichia coli, ihre Pathogenitätsfaktoren und deren Nachweisverfahren. Tierärztl. Umschau 36, 747–758.
24. LARIVIÈRE, S., R. LALLIER & M. MORIN (1979): Evaluation of various methods for the detection of enteropathogenic Escherichia coli in diarrheic calves. Am. J. Vet. Res. 40, 130–133.
25. MANSSON, I. (1962): Haemolytic Escherichia coli serotypes isolated from pigs, cattle, dogs, and cats. Acta vet. scand. 3, 65–78.
26. MANSSON, I. (1962): Isolations of haemolytic Escherichia coli from diseased and healthy animals on a particular premises. Acta vet. scand. 3, 163–173.
27. MATTHES, S. (1969): Die Darmflora gesunder und dysenteriekranker Jungkaninchen. Zbl. Vet. Med. B 16, 563–570.
28. MCDONALD, T. J., J. S. MCDONALD & D. L. ROSE (1970): Aerobic gram-negative rods isolated from bovine udder infections. Am. J. Vet. Res. 31, 1937–1941.
29. MOON, H. W., P. Y. FUNG, S. C. WHIPP & R. E. ISAACSON (1978): Effects of age and ambient temperature on the response of infant mice to heat-stable enterotoxin of Escherichia coli. Infect. Immun. 20, 36–39.
30. MOON, H. W., S. C. WHIPP, G. W. ENGSTROM & A. L. BAETZ (1970): Response of the rabbit ileal loop to cell-free products from Escherichia coli enteropathogenic for swine. J. Infect. Dis. 121, 182–187.
31. MOON, H. W., D. K. SORENSEN & J. H. SAUTTER (1966): Escherichia coli infection of the ligated intestinal loop of the newborn pig. Am. J. Vet. Res. 27, 1317–1325.
32. NIELSEN, N. O., & J. H. SAUTTER (1968): Infection of ligated intestinal loops with hemolytic Escherichia coli in the pig. Cand. Vet. J. 9, 90–97.
33. NIEMIALTOWSKI, M., Z. SZYNKIEWICZ, M. BINEK, B. KLIMUSZKO & L. KRZYZANOWSKA (1983): Evaluation of different cell cultures for the detection of heat-labile enterotoxins of Escherichia coli strains isolated from pigs. Vet. Quart. 5, 49–96.
34. ØRSKOV, F. (1974): Genus Escherichia. In: Bergey's manual of determinative bacteriology. 8th ed. Baltimore (USA): Williams & Wilkins.

35. ØRSKOV, F., & I. ØRSKOV (1979): Special Escherichia coli serotypes from enteropathies in domestic animals and man. Fortsch. Vet. Med. (Beiheft Zbl. Vet. Med.) 29, 7–14.
36. ØRSKOV, I., F. ØRSKOV, B. JAHN & K. JAHN (1977): Serology, chemistry, and genetics of O and K antigens of Escherichia coli. Bact. Reviews 41, 667–710.
37. RHOADES, H. E., S. P. SAXENA & R. C. MEYER (1971): Serological identification of Escherichia coli isolated from cats and dogs. Can. J. Comp. Med. 35, 218–223.
38. RICHTER, T., & E. HELLMANN (1985): Vorkommen und Eigenschaften enterotoxinbildender Escherichia coli-Stämme beim enteritiskranken Junghund. Zbl. Vet. Med. B 32, 446–453.
39. SCHIMMELPFENNIG, H., & R. WEBER (1979): Studies on the oedema disease producing toxin of Escherichia coli (E.-coli-Neurotoxin). Fortsch. Vet. Med. (Beihefte Zbl. Vet. Med.) 29, 25–32.
40. SCHIMMELPFENNIG, H. (1971): Zur Neutralisation des Neurotoxins von E. coli. 1. Mitt. Die Neutralisation des Toxins in vitro. Zbl. Vet. Med. B 18, 622–633.
41. SCHIMMELPFENNIG, H. (1970): Untersuchungen zur Ätiologie und Pathogenese der Ödemkrankheit des Schweines. Dtsch. tierärztl. Wschr. 27, 263–264.
42. SCHMITTDIEL, E., & R. STRITZINGER (1972): Vergleichende Untersuchungen über die Antibiotikaresistenz von E. coli-Stämmen, die in den Jahren 1965 und 1971 aus Organen von verendeten Kälbern isoliert wurden. Tierärztl. Umschau 27, 277–280.
43. SHERWOOD, D., D. R. SNODGRASS & G. H. K. LAWSON (1983): Prevalence of enterotoxigenic Escherichia coli in calves in Scotland and northern England. Vet. Rec. 113, 208–212.
44. SMITH, H. W., & S. HALLS (1967): Studies on Escherichia coli enterotoxins. J. Path. Bact. 93, 531–534.
45. SÖDERLIND, O., & R. MÖLLBY (1979): Enterotoxin, O-groups and K88 antigen in Escherichia coli from neonatal piglets with and without diarrhoea. Infect. Immun. 24, 611–616.
46. SÖDERLIND, O., & R. MÖLLBY (1978): Studies on Escherichia coli in pigs. V. Determination of enterotoxicity and frequency of O groups and K88 antigen in strains from 200 piglets with neonatal diarrhoea. Zbl. Vet. Med. B 25, 719–728.
47. SØGAARD, H. (1982): In vitro antibiotic susceptibility of E. coli isolated from acute and chronic bovine mastitis with reference to clinical efficacy. Nord. Vet. Med. 34, 248–254.
48. SOJKA, W. J., J. A. MORRIS & C. WRAY (1979): Enteric colibacillosis in lambs with special reference to passive protection of lambs against experimental infection by colostral transfer of antibodies from ewes vaccinated with K99. Fortsch. Vet. Med. (Beiheft Zbl. Vet. Med.) 29, 52–63.
49. TENNEY, J. H., T. F. SMITH & J. A. WASHINGTON (1979): Sensitivity, precision and accuracy of the Y1 adrenal cell enterotoxin assay. J. clin. Microbiol. 9, 197–199.
50. TRUSZCYNSKI, M. (1984): Escherichia coli-Infektionen beim Schaf. Mh. Vet. Med. 39, 813–816.
51. WEBER, A., & U. BERTELSMANN (1977): Serologische Untersuchungen der O-Antigene von E.-coli-Stämmen bei Pferden im Rahmen der deckhygienischen Überwachung. Berl. Münch. tierärztl. Wschr. 90, 52–55.
52. WEBER, A., & J. MANZ (1971): Serologische Untersuchungen der O-Antigene von E.-coli-Stämmen isoliert von Kaninchen. Berl. Münch. tierärztl. Wschr. 84, 441–443.
53. WILKS, S., G. AMTSBERG & C. MEIER (1982): Serotypisierung und Resistenzprüfung von Escherichia-coli-Stämmen aus gesunden und enteritiskranken Hunden. Berl. Münch. tierärztl. Wschr. 95, 271–275.
54. WILKENSON, G. T. (1974): O-groups of E. coli in the vagina and alimentary tract of the dog. Vet. Rec. 94, 105.
55. WILLINGER, H. (1981): Escherichia coli. In: H. BLOBEL & TH. SCHLIESSER (Hrsg.): Handbuch der bakteriellen Infektionen bei Tieren. Bd. 3, S. 257–343. Jena: VEB Gustav Fischer.
56. WILLINGER, H., & N. ILIADIS (1970): Serotypisierung hämolysierender aus Ferkeln isolierter Colibakterien. Wien. tierärztl. Mschr. 57, 340–342.
57. WILLINGER, H., J. TRĆKA & N. ILIADIS (1970): Die bakterielle Genese von Ferkeldurchfällen. Wien. tierärztl. Mschr. 57, 415–417.
58. WILLINGER, H., & H. MATHOIS (1965): Serologische Typisierung von Colisepsisstämmen beim Kalb. Wien. tierärztl. Mschr. 52, 155–159.
59. WITTIG, W. (1971): Neuere Erkenntnisse zur Pathogenese und Prophylaxe der Escherichia-coli-Infektion der Schweine. Mh. Vet. Med. 26, 75–78.
60. WITTIG, W. (1963): Untersuchungen über das Vorkommen verschiedener Escherichia-coli-Serogruppen bei der Coli-Enterotoxämie des Schweines. Arch. exp. Vet. med. 16, 461–482.

4.1.2 Genus: Citrobacter (C.)

Little is known about the pathogenic significance of *Citrobacter* in animals. Bacteria of this genus are found principally as part of the physiological microflora of the gut and consequently they can on occasion be isolated from animal specimens. An aetiological association has been reported in the literature between *C. freundii* and inflammation and hyperplasia of the colon and prolapse of the rectum in mice (2, 3, 4, 11).

Diseases attributed to *Citrobacter* have been described in the literature. In cattle (mastitis, 5, 8; abortion, 9; diarrhoea, 7), in pigs (MMA-complex, 1; diarrhoea, 6) and in sheep and goats (diarrhoea, 7). Other isolated reports claim the identification of *Citrobacter* in frogs, snakes and fishes (9).

4.1.2 Gattung: Citrobacter (C.)

Über die pathogene Bedeutung von *Citrobacter* für Tiere ist bisher wenig bekannt. Überwiegend kommen Bakterien dieser Gattung als Bestandteil der physiologischen Keimflora insbesondere des Darmes vor und können dann gelegentlich aus tierischen Untersuchungsstoffen isoliert werden. In der Literatur ist *C. freundii* mit Hyperplasie und Entzündung des Colons und *Prolapsus recti* bei Mäusen in ätiologischen Zusammenhang gebracht worden (2, 3, 4, 11).

Bei Haussäugetieren sind Erkrankungen beim Rind (Mastitis, 5, 8; Abort, 9; Diarrhoe, 7), beim Schwein (MMA-Komplex, 1; Diarrhoe, 6) und bei Schaf und Ziege (Diarrhoe, 7) beschrieben worden. Weitere vereinzelte Berichte betreffen das Vorkom-

Species	Lac	Ind	H_2S	ODC	Dul	Mlo	Ado
C. freundii[1]	v^-	−	+	v^-	v^+	−	−
C. amalonaticus[2]	v^+	+	−	+	v^-	−	−
C. diversus[3]	v^-	+	−	+	v	+	+

Table 50: Biochemical differentiation of *Citrobacter*

Tabelle 50: Biochemische Differenzierung von *Citrobacter*

[1] syn.: Bethesda-Ballerup group; [2] syn.: *Levinea amalonatica*; [3] syn.: *Citrobacter koseri*

The nomenclature of the genus *Citrobacter* is not uniform. Besides *C. freundii* (H_2S +, Ind −) and *C. intermedius* (H_2S −, Ind +), a third type is differentiated in the literature (tab. 50). *C. freundii* is the most important of these.

Innerhalb der Gattung *Citrobacter* ist die Nomenklatur nicht einheitlich. Neben der Unterscheidung von *C. freundii* (H_2S +, Ind −) und *C. intermedius* (H_2S −, Ind +) werden in der neueren Literatur drei Arten unterschieden (Tab. 50), von diesen ist *C. freundii* am wichtigsten.

■ **Culture** (figs. 129 and 130)
Citrobacter will grow on the usual media suitable for the detection of *Enterobacteriaceae* (tab. 52).

■ **Kultur** (Abb. 129 u. 130)
Citrobacter wächst auf den üblichen zum Nachweis von *Enterobacteriaceae* geeigneten Nährböden (Tab. 52).

■ **Biochemical properties**
The important characteristic is the utilization of citrate. Fermentation of lactose is positive, late positive or negative. The identification and differentiation is carried out according to the method given in table 50.

■ **Kulturell-biochemische Eigenschaften**
Charakteristisch ist, daß Citrate verwertet werden. Die Lactosespaltung ist positiv, verzögert positiv oder negativ. Die Identifizierung und Unterscheidung erfolgt nach den in Tab. 50 zusammengestellten Merkmalen.

■ **Antigenic structure**
More than 40 O-antigens and 90 H-antigens occur in *Citrobacter*. Cross-reactions can occur not only with salmonellae but also with *Escherichia*.

■ **Antigenstruktur**
Bei *Citrobacter* kommen mehr als 40 O- und 90 H-Antigene vor. Kreuzreaktionen sind sowohl mit Salmonellen als auch mit *Escherichia* möglich.

Fig. 127–130 see page 172.

Abb. 127–130 siehe Seite 172.

Bibliography / Literatur

1. Armstrong, C. H., B. E. Hooper & C. E. Martin (1968): Microflora associated with agalactia syndrome of sows. Am. J. Vet. Res. **29**, 1401–1407.
2. Barthold, S. W. (1980): The microbiology of transmissible murine colonic hyperplasia. Lab. Anim. Sci. **30**, 167–173.
3. Bennan, P. C., T. E. Fritz, R. J. Flynn & C. M. Poole (1965): Citrobacter freundii associated with diarrhea in laboratory mice. Lab. Anim. Care **15**, 266–275.
4. Bienik, H., & B. Tober-Meyer (1976): Zur Ätiologie der Colitis und des Prolapsus recti bei der Maus. Zschr. Versuchstierk. **18**, 337–348.
5. Jasper, D. E., J. D. Dellinger & R. B. Bushnell (1975): Herd studies on coliform mastitis. J. Am. Vet. Med. Assoc. **166**, 778–780.
6. Kabankov, J. S., & E. D. Kvasnikova (1980): (Bakteriologische Untersuchungen beim Ferkeldurchfall.) (russ.) Veterinarija, Moskva **7**, 32–34.
7. Kumar, A., & V. K. Sharma (1978): Enterobacteria of emerging pathogenic significance from clinical cases in man and animals, and detection of toads and wall lizards as their reservoirs. Antonie Leeuwenhoek J. Microbiol. Serol. **44**, 219–228.
8. McDonald, T. J., J. S. McDonald & D. L. Rose (1970): Aerobic gram-negative rods isolated from bovine udder infections. Am. J. Vet. Res. **31**, 1937—1941.
9. Renken-Zürner, A. (1985): Vorkommen und veterinärmedizinische Bedeutung von Bakterien aus der Familie der Enterobacteriaceae mit Ausnahme der Gattungen Escherichia und Salmonella sowie der Spezies Yersinia pestis. Vet. Med. Diss. Hannover.
10. Sharma, V. K. (1979): Enterobacteriaceae-Infektionen bei Mensch und Tier und deren natürliche Reservoire in Indien. Zbl. Bakt. I. Orig. A, **243**, 381–391.
11. Silverman, J., J. M. Chavannes, J. Rigotty & M. Ornaf (1979): A natural outbreak of transmissible murine colonic hyperplasia in A/J mice. Lab. Anim. Sci. **29**, 209–213.
12. Swiderski, M., & A. Jedrzejowski (1976): Infektiöse Antibiotikaresistenz und Virulenz eines Citrobacterstammes, der aus Erkrankungen von Schweinen isoliert wurde. Med. Veteryn. **32**, 665–668.

4.1.3 Genus: Salmonella (S.)

The biochemical definition of the genus *Salmonella* and its most important generic characters are shown in table 53.

The classification of the salmonella within this genus has undergone considerable changes in recent decades. Since there is a close relationship between the different salmonellae, the view of KAUFFMANN (15), that the serologically defined strains listed in the Kauffmann-White system are equivalent to species, can no longer be sustained. The classification suggested by LeMinor et al. (18) is more suitable for illustrating this relationship. This scheme recognizes only one species within the genus *Salmonella* and that is *S. choleraesuis*. However, within this species six subspecies are differentiated by genetical, biochemical and, in part, serological methods (tab. 51). These include, as serovars, all identifiable *Salmonella* and *Arizona* strains. Therefore, the correct designation for serovar *typhimurium* is: *S. choleraesuis subsp. choleraesuis serovar typhimurium*.

Since such a name is not practical, the following compromise is suggested (4):

Strains of the *subspecies choleraesuis* will be

4.1.3 Gattung: Salmonella (S.)

Die Gattung *Salmonella* ist biochemisch definiert, die wichtigsten Gattungsmerkmale sind in der Tab. 53 zusammengestellt.

Die Klassifikation der Salmonellen innerhalb der Gattung ist in den letzten Jahrzehnten sehr unterschiedlich gewesen. Da zwischen den einzelnen Salmonellen ein sehr enger Verwandtschaftsgrad besteht, kann die von KAUFFMANN (15) vertretene Ansicht, daß die im Kauffmann-White-Schema aufgeführten und serologisch definierten Stämme Arten darstellen, nicht aufrechterhalten werden. Für die Darstellung der verwandtschaftlichen Beziehungen ist die von LE MINOR et al. (18) vorgeschlagene Klassifikation geeigneter, die innerhalb der Gattung *Salmonella* nur eine Art unterscheidet, nämlich *S. choleraesuis*. Innerhalb dieser Spezies werden mit genetischen, biochemischen und z. T. serologischen Methoden sechs Subspezies unterschieden (Tab. 51). Diesen werden alle serologisch unterscheidbaren *Salmonella*- und *Arizona*-Stämme als Serovare zugeordnet. Die korrekte Bezeichnung für Serovar *typhimurium* lautet somit: *S. choleraesuis subsp. choleraesuis* Serovar *typhimurium*.

Da diese Bezeichnungen nicht praxisgerecht sind,

Table 51: Terminology and differentiation of the subspecies (subgenera) of the genus *Salmonella* (18)

Tabelle 51: Bezeichnung und Unterscheidung der Subspezies (Subgenera) der Gattung *Salmonella* (18)

Proposed designation	subsp. choleraesuis short name: I	subsp. salamae short name II	subsp. arizonae short identity: III a subsp. diarizonae short identity: III b	subsp. houtenae short identity: IV	subsp. bongori short identity: V
Previous designation	subgenus I	subgenus II	subgenus III a monophasic subgenus III b diphasic	subgenus IV	subgenus V
Primary occurrence					
warm-blooded animals	+	–	–	–	–
cold-blooded animals and environment	–	+	+	+	+
β-galactosidase					
(ONPG test)	–	–/(+)	+	–	+
Acid from Lac	–	–	+/(+)	–	–
Dul	+	+	–	–	–
Mucate	+	+	v	–	+
Galactouronate	–	+	v[1]	+	+
Utilization of					
Mal	–	+	+	–	–
d-tartrate	+	–(+)	–(+)	–/(+)	–
Gel	–	+	+	+	–

[1] Monophasic strains: negative, diphasic strains: positive

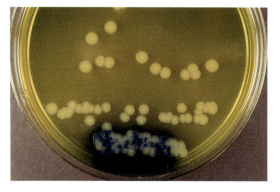
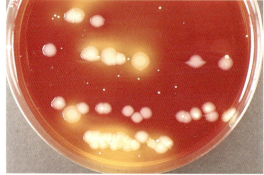
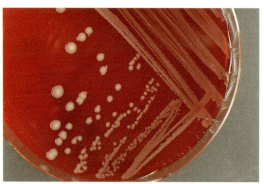
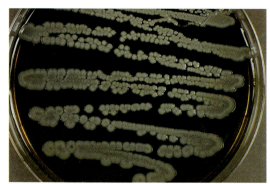

▲ Fig. 127: Salmonellae and *Escherichia coli*, mixed culture on Gassner agar, the colonies of coli bacteria and the area around them are coloured blue and salmonella colonies are yellow, 24 h, 37 °C. Magnification x 0.4
▼ Fig. 129: *Citrobacter diversus*, pure culture on blood agar, 24 h, 37 °C. Magnification x 0.4

▲ Fig. 128: Salmonellae and *Escherichia coli*, mixed culture on brilliant green-phenol red agar, colonies of coli bacteria and the area surrounding them are coloured yellow and salmonella colonies are red, 24 h, 37 °C. Magnification x 0.4
▼ Fig. 130: *Citrobacter diversus*, pure culture on Gassner agar, the weakly lactose-positive colonies are moist and mucoid, 24 h, 37 °C. Magnification x 0.4

▲ Abb. 127: Salmonellen und *Escherichia coli*, Mischkultur auf Gaßner-Agar, die Kolonien und ihre Umgebung verfärben sich bei den Colibakterien blau und bei den Salmonellen gelb, 24 h, 37 °C, Abb.-M. 1:2,5
▼ Abb. 129: *Citrobacter diversus*, Reinkultur auf Blutagar 24 h, 37 °C, Abb.-M. 1:2,5

▲ Abb. 128: Salmonellen und *Escherichia coli*, Mischkultur auf Brillantgrün-Phenolrot-Agar, die Kolonien und ihre Umgebung verfärben sich bei den Colibakterien gelb und bei den Salmonellen rot, 24 h, 37 °C, Abb.-M. 1:2,5
▼ Abb. 130: *Citrobacter diversus*, Reinkultur auf Gaßner-Platte, die schwach lactosepositiven Kolonien zeigen ein feuchtes bis schleimiges Wachstum, 24 h, 37 °C, Abb.-M. 1:2,5

named as before, e. g. *S. typhimurium*. Strains of the remaining subspecies will be identified by the short form listed in table 51, followed by the antigenic formula. For example: *Salmonella* III b 53 : r : Z 53. Serovars of this subspecies, which were isolated before 1963, and had therefore been given a name, can, for the sake of clarity, retain this name in square brackets, e. g. Salmonella IV [houten] 43 : Z 4 Z 23. Strains of the subspecies *arizona* (III a)

empfiehlt sich folgender Kompromiß (4):
Stämme der *Subspezies cholerae suis* werden wie bisher gekennzeichnet, z. B. *S. typhimurium;* Stämme der übrigen Subspezies werden mit der in der Tab. 51 angegebenen Kurzbezeichnung, gefolgt von der Antigenformel, bezeichnet, z. B.: *Salmonella* III b 53 : Z 53. Bei Serovaren dieser Unterarten, die vor 1963 isoliert wurden und deshalb noch einen Namen erhalten haben, kann zum besseren Ver-

and *diarizonae* (III b) are characterized purely by their antigenic formulae.

■ **Incidence and veterinary significance**
The following groups of salmonellae can be differentiated on the basis of their epidemiology and clinical significance to both man and animals.

a) Typhus-paratyphus group *(S. typhi, S. paratyphi)* as the cause of specific »typhoid« diseases of man. In animals *S. typhi* occurs as a result of environmental contamination mainly in birds, mussels, flies and very rarely in the domestic mammals.

S. paratyphi (generally B) is rare, but does occur in many domestic animals, where occasionally it may cause disease. Free-living birds, fishes, mussels, crabs, snails etc. can also be infected (10).

b) Salmonellae which occur in all useful animals and are transmissible to man. This includes the majority of salmonellae, the prototype being *S. typhimurium*. In all animals the infection is either latent (more usually) or it becomes clinically manifest. Young animals, especially calves, are very severely affected. These salmonellae cause food poisoning in man (»enteric salmonellae«). A survey of the possible condition in animals may be found in PIETZSCH (26).

c) Salmonellae which occur chiefly in animals and only rarely lead to human disease. These organisms have often become adapted to one particular animal species. The following are all part of this group, e. g.:

S. dublin, cause of salmonellosis of cattle, although it usually occurs in the form of latent infections. It is also encountered in many other species of animal.

S. gallinarum-pullorum, the agent of BWD (bacillary white diarrhoea) of chicks and fowl typhoid.

S. abortusovis, S. abortusequi, S. abortusbovis inducing abortion in the appropriate species.

S. choleraesuis, cause of enteritis in pigs and clinically latent invasion of the intestine. This is of no significance in the Federal Republic of Germany.

S. typhisuis causes a chronic enteritis of piglets and it is also of no importance in Germany.

S. typhimurium var. copenhagen is the cause of salmonellosis of pigeons. It is a serological minus variant of *S. typhimurium*, which is lacking the O-antigen 5. It is also found in many other species of animal.

The salmonellae most frequently identified in specimens of animal origin, including food material are:

S. typhimurium including *var. copenhagen*
S. dublin
S. gallinarum-pullorum
S. derby
S. infantis

ständnis dieser Name in eckiger Klammer angegeben werden, z. B. Samonella IV [houten] 43 : Z 4 Z 23. Stämme der Subspezies *arizonae* (III a) und *diarizonae* (III b) werden ausschließlich mit der Antigenformel charakterisiert.

■ **Vorkommen und medizinische Bedeutung**
Nach der Epidemiologie und klinischen Bedeutung bei Mensch und Tier lassen sich folgende Salmonellengruppen unterscheiden:

a) Typhus-Paratyphus-Gruppe *(S. typhi, S. paratyphi)* als Erreger spezifischer »typhöser« Erkrankungen des Menschen. Beim Tier kommt *S. typhi* als Folge der Umweltkontamination hauptsächlich bei Vögeln, insbesondere Möwen und anderen wassergebundenen Vögeln, bei Muscheln, Fliegen und sehr selten bei Haussäugetieren vor.

S. paratyphi (meistens B) kommt, wenn auch selten, bei vielen Haustieren vor und kann gelegentlich zu Erkrankungen führen. Ferner können freilebende Vogelarten, Fische, Muscheln, Krabben, Schnecken u. a. infiziert sein (10).

b) Salmonellen, die bei allen Nutztieren vorkommen und auf den Menschen übertragbar sind. Hierzu gehört die Mehrzahl der Salmonellen, Prototyp ist *S. typhimurium*. Bei Tieren verläuft die Infektion entweder klinisch latent (häufiger) oder manifest. Besonders häufig und schwer erkranken Jungtiere, insbesondere die Kälber. Beim Menschen führen diese Salmonellen zu Lebensmittelinfektionen (»enteritische« Salmonellen). Zusammenstellung der möglichen tierischen Erkrankungen bei PIETZSCH, 26).

c) Salmonellen, die hauptsächlich beim Tier vorkommen und nur selten zu Erkrankungen des Menschen führen. Diese Salmonellen haben sich oft einer Tierart besonders angepaßt. Zu dieser Gruppe gehören z. B.:

S. dublin, Erreger der Salmonellose des Rindes, das Bakterium kommt aber, meistens in Form von latenten Infektionen, auch bei vielen anderen Tierarten vor;

S. gallinarum-pullorum, Erreger von Kükenruhr/Hühnertyphus;

S. abortusovis, S. abortusequi, S. abortusbovis, Aborterreger bei den entsprechenden Tierarten;

S. choleraesuis, Enteritiserreger und klinische latente Darmbesiedlung beim Schwein, in der BR Deutschland ohne Bedeutung;

S. typhisuis, Erreger einer chronischen Enteritis beim Ferkel, in der BR Deutschland ohne Bedeutung;

S. typhimurium var. copenhagen, Ursache der Salmonellose der Tauben, es handelt sich um eine serologische Minusvariante von *S. typhimurium*, der das O-Antigen 5 fehlt, kommt auch bei vielen anderen Tierarten vor.

Die aus tierischen Untersuchungsstoffen einschließlich Lebens- und Futtermitteln am häufigsten nachgewiesenen Salmonellen sind:

S. agona
S. panama
S. enteritidis
S. heidelberg and others.

The incidence frequency of all these salmonellae may fluctuate from year to year, new types may be added, while some of the ones listed become less common.

It is of considerable epidemiological significance that many salmonellae can remain viable and retain their reproductive potential outside the living ani-

Preliminary enrichment
Necessary when the presence of small numbers of damaged salmonella anticipated. 0.1 % buffered peptone solution. Inoculation at the ratio of 1:10. Incubation ca 18 h at 37 °C, then mix with 10 ml peptone water and inoculate 100 ml selective broth

Specimens
Faecal or organ samples food materials etc.

Selective enrichment

Numerous, and frequently modified media have been developed for this. The following are proven:
 a) Tetrathionate enrichment
     e. g. sodium tetrathionate-brilliant green broth of Muller; potassium tetrathionate-crystal violet broth
 b) Enrichment with Rappaport-Vassiliadis medium,
 c) Selective enrichment
     e. g. Sodium selenite-lactose broth of Leifson,
         Sodium selenite-cystine broth
         Sodium selenite-brilliant green-mannitol broth,
 Inoculation usually at a ratio 1:10, with food materials about 25 g of sample. Incubation at 37 °C or with heavy contamination at 43 °C for 48 h. Subculture to selective solid medium after about 18–24 h and 42–48 h.

Isolation of salmonella on selective solid media
Two media are usually employed in parallel, namely: a) Brilliant green-phenol red-lactose (saccharose) agar,   b) Another medium of own choice (tab. 52).   Incubation 18 h at 37 °C, possibly extended to 42–48 h.   For procedure and assessment of cultures see table 52.

Differentiation of salmonella-suspect colonies

a) Preparation of pure culture,
 b) Identification of genus,
     serological: slide agglutination test with omnivalent or polyvalent salmonella sera (I, II, III),
     biochemical: test various metabolic properties,
 c) Determination of the serotype,
     serological: detection of O- and H-antigens by means of slide agglutination test,
     if necessary additional biochemical: test various metabolic properties.

Fig. 131: Demonstration and identification of salmonellae

mal in food materials, surface water, effluent, sewage sludge and numerous other substances.

Very many publications have appeared on the incidence and importance of salmonellae in animals, animal products and in the environment. Some of these are: 1, 2, 3, 5, 6, 7, 8, 10, 11, 12, 13, 16, 17, 21, 22, 23, 24, 25, 26.

■ Morphology

These are short, ovoid, Gram-negative rods 0.5–0.8 × 1–3.5 µm. Most of them are arranged singly. Their motility is due to peritrichous flagella. *S. pullorum-gallinarum* is normally non-motile.

■ Cultural demonstration

The diagnostic identification of salmonellae depends, in principle, on culture. There are three basic methods (fig. 131).

▷ Initial enrichment: This is necessary when it may be assumed that salmonellae are present in small numbers or damaged (e.g. through drying, heat, radiation or in medicated substrates).

▷ Fluid selective media: These can contain inhibitory substances which suppress the growth of contaminants, and at the same they should ensure suitable conditions for the salmonellae to multiply.

Numerous media have been devised and frequently modified for selective enrichment. It is recommended that tetrathionate and selenite enrichment media are used in parallel, because this greatly increases the yield.

Table 52: Selective plates for demonstrating *Enterobacteriaceae*

Selective plate	Inhibitor	Indicator	Colour of medium and colonies		
			uninoculated	lactose-negative bacteria	lactose-positive bacteria
Brilliant green phenol red lactose (saccharose) agar (fig. 128)	brilliant green	phenol red	yellowish-brown	red	yellowish-green
Gassner agar (fig. 127)	metachrome yellow	soluble blue	green	yellow	blue
Salmonella-shigella agar (SS agar)	brilliant green bile salts	neutral red	light brown	colourless, transparent, possibly black centres	pink to red
Desoxycholate citrate lactose agar (DCLS agar)	desoxycholate citrate	neutral red	weak reddish	colourless with transparent rim proteus: red	pink to red
Drigalski-Conradi plate	crystal violet	litmus	violet	blue	red
MacConkey agar	Bile salts crystal violet	neutral red	violet	colourless	red-violet

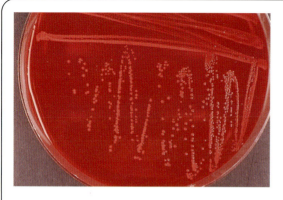
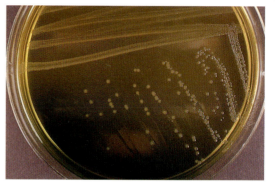
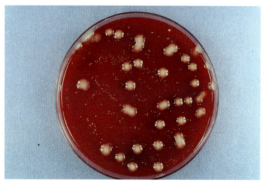
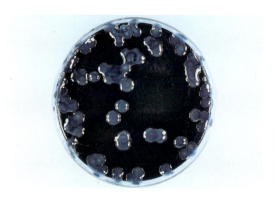

▲ Fig. 132: *Shigella spp.*, pure culture on blood agar, 24 h, 37 °C. Magnification x 0.4
▼ Fig. 134: *Klebsiella pneumoniae subsp. pneumoniae*, large mucoid colonies on blood agar, mixed culture with non-haemolytic streptococci, isolated from a cervix smear of a mare, 48 h, 37 °C. Magnification x 0.25

▲ Fig. 133: *Shigella spp.*, pure culture on a Gassner plate, 24 h, 37 °C. Magnification x 0.4
▼ Fig. 135: *Klebsiella pneumoniae subsp. pneumoniae*, pure culture on Gassner agar, mucoid, lactose-positive colonies, 48 h, 37 °C. Magnification x 0.25

▲ Abb. 132: *Shigella sp.*, Reinkultur auf Blutagar, 24 h, 37 °C, Abb.-M. 1 : 2,5
▼ Abb. 134: *Klebsiella pneumoniae subsp. pneumoniae*, Wachstum in großen, schleimigen Kolonien auf Blutagar, Mischkultur mit nichthämolysierenden Streptokokken, isoliert aus dem Cervixtupfer einer Stute, 48 h, 37 °C, Abb.-M. 1 : 4

▲ Abb. 133: *Shigella sp.*, Reinkultur auf einer Gaßner-Platte, 24 h, 37 °C, Abb.-M. 1 : 2,5
▼ Abb. 135: *Klebsiella pneumoniae subsp. pneumoniae*, Reinkultur auf einer Gaßner-Platte, schleimige, lactosepositive Kolonien, 48 h, 37 °C, Abb.-M. 1 : 4

The medium of RAPPAPORT/VASSILIADIS (28) has proved useful especially because of its effective inhibition of proteus. WEISS et al. (29) claims that a modified Rappaport medium, which in comparison with the tetrathionate broth had only a slight effect on the salmonella yield, showed distinct advantages in respect of the inhibition of lactose-negative bacteria. JONAS et al. (14) report on the use of this medium in the examination of food materials.

böden, da dadurch die Salmonellenausbeute gesteigert wird.

Bewährt hat sich das Medium nach RAPPAPORT-VASSILIADIS (28), vor allem wegen der guten Hemmung von Proteus. Ein modifiziertes Rappaport-Medium zeigte nach WEISS et al. (29) im Vergleich zur Tetrathionat-Bouillon in bezug auf die Salmonellenausbeute nur geringe, bezüglich der Hemmung lactosenegativer Bakterien deutliche Vorteile.

▷ Solid selective media: These normally depend on lactose as reagent (tab. 52) or on the precipitation of black sulphide compounds. The Wilson-Blair bismuth sulphite agar is one of the latter. Salmonella colonies, with the exception of those of S. paratyphi A and S. gallinarum-pullorum, have black centres. Another is the xylose lysine desoxycholate agar (XLD agar). The Gassner medium and the brilliant green-phenol red-lactose-saccharose plate have proved themselves in veterinary bacteriology. It is a fundamental principle that two different selective media should always be used.

Since about 70 % of the salmonellae of the Arizona group are lactose-positive, selective media containing sulphite as indicator are more suitable for their detection.

Some salmonellae which are specially adapted to certain animals (e. g. S. gallinarum-pullorum, S. abortusequi, S. abortusovis) grow very slowly on the selective plates, so that their incubation time should be extended to 48 hours. Even then, the colonies tend to be rather small.

The plates are incubated at 37 °C and/or 43 °C. The higher temperature is recommended when a heavy growth of contaminants is expected (e. g. effluent, sewage sludge etc.) where swarming proteus bacteria are present.

■ **Determination of the genus Salmonella**

Colonies which react on selective media as lactose-negative bacteria (tab. 52), or grow as black colonies due to the production of H_2S (e. g. bismuth sulphite agar), are suspect of being salmonella. Their subsequent differentiation relies on:
▷ the biochemical properties: the most important generic features are listed in table 48, particularly characteristic reactions will be found in table 53, together with their quantitative results;
▷ agglutination using omnivalent or polyvalent O-sera, the basis of this method is the O-antigen structure of the salmonellae.

The O-antigens (factors) are identified with arabic figures. Strains which have the same O-antigens are grouped together (A–Z, 51–67 no O-group 64, which is grouped with the O-group Y [= 048]). Thus, there are at present 51 serogroups (with their subgroups) (Kauffmann-White system, table 55).

If, besides the identifying O-antigen, a strain has other O-antigens, then subgroups are formed (e. g. C_1 to C_4; D_1 to D_3; E_1 to E_4; G_1 and G_2). The O-antigens and the classification into groups and subgroups resulting from it are the basis of the Kauffmann-White system (tab. 55).

Colonies that are grown on selective media and which are suspect of being salmonella are examined

Über die Anwendung des Mediums bei Lebensmitteluntersuchungen haben JONAS et al. (14) berichtet.
▷ Feste Selektivmedien: Diese arbeiten im wesentlichen mit Lactose als Reaktionskörper (Tab. 52) oder beruhen auf der Ausfällung von schwarzen Sulfidverbindungen. Zu den letzteren gehört der Wismut-Sulfit-Agar nach Wilson-Blair, auf dem die Salmonellen (mit Ausnahme von S. paratyphi A und S. gallinarum-pullorum) mit einem schwarzen Zentrum in der Kolonie wachsen sowie der Xylose-Lysin-Desoxycholat-Agar (XLD-Agar). In der Veterinärmedizin haben sich für den Nachweis anspruchsloser Salmonellen die Gaßner-Platte sowie die Brillantgrün-Phenolrot-Lactose-Saccharose-Platte bewährt. Grundsätzlich sollten stets zwei verschiedene Selektivplatten eingesetzt werden.

Da die Salmonellen der Arizona-Gruppe zu etwa 70 % lactosepositiv sind, eignen sich zu ihrem gezielten Nachweis Selektivplatten mit Sulfit als Indikator besser.

Einige der tierartlich besonders angepaßten Salmonellen (z. B. S. gallinarum-pullorum, S. abortusequi, S. abortusovis) wachsen auf den Selektivplatten sehr langsam, so daß ihre Bebrütungszeiten auf 48 h verlängert werden müssen, es ist auch dann mit dem Auftreten kleiner Kolonien zu rechnen.

Die Bebrütung erfolgt bei 37 °C und (oder) bei 43 °C. Die höhere Temperatur empfiehlt sich, wenn mit dem Vorkommen einer starken Begleitflora zu rechnen ist (z. B. Abwasser, Klärschlamm) und schwärmende Proteus-Bakterien vorhanden sind.

■ **Bestimmung der Gattung Salmonella**

Als salmonellenverdächtig werden Kolonien angesehen, die sich auf den lactosehaltigen Selektivplatten lactosenegativ verhalten (Tab. 52) oder infolge H_2S-Bildung in schwarzen Kolonien wachsen (z. B. Wismutsulfitagar). Ihre weitere Differenzierung erfolgt
▷ durch kulturell-biochemische Eigenschaften, die wichtigsten Gattungsmerkmale sind in der Tab. 48 zusammengestellt, besonders kennzeichnende Reaktionen mit ihrem quantitativen Ausfall in Tab. 53;
▷ durch Agglutination mit omni- oder polyvalenten O-Seren, Grundlage dieser Methode ist die O-Antigenstruktur der Salmonellen.

Die O-Antigene (Faktoren) werden mit arabischen Ziffern bezeichnet. Stämme mit gleichem O-Antigen werden in Gruppen zusammengefaßt (A–Z, 51–67 ohne O-Gruppe 64, die mit O-Gruppe Y [= 048] vereinigt wurde). Somit bestehen zur Zeit mit den Untergruppen 51 Serogruppen (Kauffmann-White-Schema, s. Tab. 55).

Haben Stämme neben dem bestimmenden O-Antigen noch andere O-Antigene, können Untergruppen gebildet werden (z. B. C_1 bis C_4; D_1 bis D_3; E_1 bis E_4; G_1 und G_2). Die O-Antigene und die aus ihnen resultierende Einteilung in Gruppen und Un-

Table 53: Biochemical properties of the genus *Salmonella* (percentage of positive reactions)

Tabelle 53: Biochemische Eigenschaften der Gattung *Salmonella* (Prozentsatz positiver Reaktionen)

Glu	+	100 %	Ind	−	1.1 %	Ado	−	0 %
gas from								
Glu	+	91.9 %[1]	Ara	v⁺	89.2 %	Ure	−	0 %
H$_2$S	+	91.6 %[4]	Sor	+	94.1 %	Cit	v⁺	80.1 %[6]
LDC	+	94.6 %[2]	Dul	v⁺	86.5 %[5]	MR	+	100 %
ODC	+	92.7 %[3]	Man	+	99.7 %	VPR	−	0 %

[1] *S. typhi* and *S. gallinarum* produce no gas; [2] *S. typhi* A; LDC negative; [3] *S. typhi* and *S. gallinarum*: ODC negative; [4] *S. paratyphi* A: H$_2$S negative; [5] *S. typhi, S. cholerae-suis, S. paratyphi* A, *S. gallinarum* Dul (+); [6] *S. typhi, S. paratyphi* A Cit negative, *S. cholerae-suis* Cit (+)

in slide tests with omnivalent or polyvalent sera to confirm that they belong to the genus *Salmonella* (tab. 54).

The positive agglutination test and the biochemical properties indicate the genus salmonella with sufficient accuracy.

However, one can support the genus identification by phage typing. Phage type 0–1 lyses about

tergruppen sind die Grundlage für die Aufstellung des Kauffmann-White-Schema (Tab. 55).

Die auf den Selektivplatten als salmonellenverdächtig beurteilten Kolonien werden mit omni- oder polyvalenten Seren mit der Objektträgeragglutination auf ihre Zugehörigkeit zur Gattung *Salmonella* untersucht (Tab. 54).

Die positive Agglutination und das biochemische

Table 54: Serological identification of salmonellae

Tabelle 54: Serologische Bestimmung von Salmonellen

Differentiation of salmonella-suspect (lactose-negative) bacteria
I. Agglutination with omni- or polyvalent O-sera

a) Omnivalent serum: selects group A–60
b) Polyvalent serum I   Polyvalent serum II   Polyvalent serum III
    Groups A–E$_4$ groups F–60   groups 61–65

The polyvalent sera give relatively strong cross-reactions between them and they also select some groups which do not fall within their selectivity range. Furthermore, since they partly share some antigens, they can react with members of other groups, such as Escherichia, Shigella, Citrobacter, Proteus.

II. Determination of the O-group

1. Group B   2. group D   3. group C   4. group E
    anti-O-serum 4, 5   anti-O-serum 9   anti-O-serum 6, 7, 8   anti-O-serum 3, 10, 15
if necessary test with other group-specific sera

III. Determination of subgroups

e.g. in group C: subgroup C$_1$ subgroup C$_2$
                    anti-O-serum 7   anti-O-serum 8
e.g. in group E: subgroup E$_1$ subgroup E$_2$
                    anti-O-serum 10   anti-O-serum 15

IV. Determination of H-antigens

1. e.g. within group D
    when suspecting *S. dublin*: anti-H-serum g, p
    when suspecting *S. enteritidis*: anti-H-serum g, m
    further differentiation within the enteritidis group using monovalent anti-H-sera p-q-t-s
2. e.g. within group B
    when suspecting *S. typhimurium*: anti-H-serum i and 1, 2

If the agglutination is negative one must try the identification by judiciously selecting anti-H-sera according to the Kauffmann-White system.

97% of salmonella strains (and some strains of coli). This test is particularly well suited for mass examinations; it is precise, economic and can be carried out quickly (FEY et al., 9).

■ **Identification of the serovar**

The primary method for further discrimination is serology, which may then be followed by biochemical examination and possibly phage typing.

a) Finding the O-group and the O-antigen structure: When the agglutination test with one of the polyvalent sera is positive the next step is to establish the group with single-factor O-sera. Since the salmonellae of veterinary importance occur mainly in groups B and D and in C and E, it is advisable to adopt the routine suggested in table 54.

If the agglutination with combined factor sera 6, 7, 8 (group C) or 3, 10, 15 (group E) is positive, the further break down of the groups must be carried out with single-factor O-sera (tab. 54).

b) Determination of H-antigens: The final identification of the serovar depends on the establishment of the H-antigens. The H-antigens (phases) are heat-, acid- and alcohol-labile proteins, which are localized in the flagella. A characteristic feature is the presence of two serologically distinguishable phases, namely (specific) phases 1 and (nonspecific) phase 2.

The H-antigens of phase 1 were initially identified with roman letters (a–z), but when the letters ran out, this was augmented with z_1, z_2 up to z_{57}. The H-antigens of phase 2 are identified with the numbers 1–7, which are distinct from those of the O-antigens. In part they bear small letters, that is to say that certain H-antigens, occurring in phase 1 are also found in phase 2.

Under natural conditions a strain of salmonella can be present in phase 1, i. e. flagella with the antigenic structure of phase 1 are in the majority. On the other hand, phase 2 can predominate or alternatively both phases may be equally represented in one strain. For phase variation see page 180.

When carrying out an H-antigen analysis time and expense can be saved, if the test sera are carefully selected from the antigen tables, so that the H-sera which indicate the most commonly occurring salmonellae are tried first. An example of such a test routine is presented in table 54.

Verhalten zeigen mit ausreichender Sicherheit die Zugehörigkeit zur Gattung *Salmonella* an.

Für die Gattungsdiagnose kann ferner die Lysotypie eingesetzt werden. Der Phage 0–1 löst etwa 97% der Salmonellenstämme (und einige Coli-Stämme). Der Test ist für Massenuntersuchungen besonders geeignet, präzis, wirtschaftlich und schnell durchführbar (FEY et al., 9).

■ **Bestimmung des Serovars**

Im Vordergrund für die weitere Bestimmung des Salmonellenstammes steht die serologische Untersuchung, danach kann auch die biochemische Untersuchung und eventuell die Lysotypie benutzt werden.

a) Ermittlung der O-Gruppe und der O-Antigenstruktur: Bei positivem Ausfall der Agglutination mit einem der polyvalenten Seren erfolgt als erstes die Gruppenbestimmung mit O-Seren. Da die veterinärmedizinisch wichtigen Salmonellen besonders in den Gruppen B und D und danach C und E vorkommen, empfiehlt sich zur Arbeitsersparnis die in Tab. 54 angegebene Reihenfolge.

Bei positiver Agglutination mit den kombinierten Faktorenseren 6, 7, 8 (Gruppe C) oder 3, 10, 15 (Gruppe E) muß die Gruppenaufsplitterung mit den monofaktoriellen O-Seren erfolgen (Tab. 54).

b) H-Antigenbestimmung: Die endgültige Feststellung des Serovars erfolgt durch die Bestimmung der H-Antigene. Die H-Antigene (Phasen) sind hitze-, säure- und alkohollabile und in den Geißeln lokalisierte Proteine. Charakteristisch ist das Vorkommen zweier serologisch unterscheidbarer Phasen, nämlich der (spezifischen) Phase 1 und der (unspezifischen) Phase 2.

Die H-Antigene der Phase 1 wurden zunächst mit kleinen lateinischen Buchstaben bezeichnet (a–z), als die Buchstaben nicht mehr ausreichten, mit z_1, z_2 bis z_{57}. Die H-Antigene der Phase 2 werden mit den Ziffern 1–7 gekennzeichnet, die mit denen der O-Antigene nicht identisch sind, zum Teil mit kleinen Buchstaben, d. h., daß sich bestimmte in der Phase 1 vorkommende H-Antigene auch in der Phase 2 finden.

Ein Salmonellenstamm kann unter natürlichen Bedingungen in der Phase 1 vorliegen, d. h. es überwiegen Geißeln mit der Antigenstruktur der Phase 1 oder es überwiegt Phase 2 oder der Stamm hat beide Phasen etwa gleichstark ausgebildet. Phasenwechsel s. S. 180.

Bei der Durchführung der H-Antigenanalyse führt ein planvolles Aussuchen der Prüfseren unter Anlehnung an die Antigentabelle zu einer Zeit- und Materialersparnis, denn man wird zunächst die H-Seren benutzen, die die am häufigsten vorkommenden Salmonellen anzeigen. Ein beispielhafter Untersuchungsgang ist in der Tab. 54 aufgezeigt.

■ **Phase variation and swarming method of Sven Gard**

Difficulties can arise in the identification when one is dealing with a diphasic type which is present in only one phase.

Example: S. paratyphi B 1, 4, 5, 12 : b : 1.2
S. typhimurium 1, 4, 5, 12 : i : 1.2

If S. paratyphi B is present in the second phase (1, 4, 5, 12 :–: 1.2) then it cannot be differentiated from S. typhimurium without a change of phase induced in vitro. Procedure: 1–2 drops of H-1,2-serum are added to 1% semisolid agar at 45 °C. The medium is poured into a Petri dish, inoculated centrally and incubated with the inoculated surface uppermost. Bacteria which possess the H-antigen 1,2 are prevented from swarming, but those in phase 1 will swarm unhindered, to be picked off at the edge of the growth zone and agglutinated with an H-b-serum.

When a rapid diagnosis is required, the serological antigen analysis provides a useful and adequately reliable result. However, salmonellae of quite diffe-

■ **Phasenwechsel und Schwärmverfahren nach Sven Gard**

Schwierigkeiten können bei der Bestimmung entstehen, wenn es sich um einen diphasischen Typ handelt, der nur in einer Phase vorliegt.

Beispiel: S. paratyphi B: 1, 4, 5, 12 : b : 1,2
S. typhimurium: 1, 4, 5, 12 : i : 1,2

Liegt der S. paratyphi B-Stamm nur in der 2. Phase vor (1, 4, 5, 12 : – : 1,2), ist eine Unterscheidung von S. typhimurium ohne einen in vitro herbeigeführten Phasenwechsel nicht möglich. Durchführung: Einem halbflüssigen, 1%igen Agar werden bei 45 °C 1 bis 2 Tropfen H-1,2-Serum zugefügt. Nach Ausgießen des Nährbodens in eine Petrischale wird das Medium zentral beimpft und mit der beimpften Seite nach oben bebrütet. Die das H-Antigen 1,2 besitzenden Bakterien werden am Ausschwärmen gehindert, die in der Phase 1 vorliegenden Bakterien schwärmen ungehindert aus und können vom Rand der Wachstumszone abgeimpft und mit einem H-b-Serum agglutiniert werden.

Die serologische Antigenanalyse führt unter den

Table 55: Extract from the Kauffman-White system, showing the salmonellae of the greatest veterinary importance

Tabelle 55: Auszug aus dem Kauffmann-White-Schema mit den veterinärmedizinisch wichtigsten Salmonellen

Serovar	O-antigen	H-antigens Phase 1	Phase 2
Group A			
S. paratyphi A	1, 2, 12	a	(1, 5)
Group B			
S. abortusequi	4, 12	–	e, n, x
S. paratyphi B	1, 4 (5), 12	b	1, 2
S. abortusbovis	1, 4, 12, 27	b	e, n, x
S. abortusovis	4, 12	c	1, 6
S. saintpaul	1, 4 (5), 12	e, h	1, 2
S. reading	1, 4 (5), 12	e, h	1, 5
S. chester	1, 4 (5), 12	e, h	e, n, x
S. derby	1, 4 (5), 12	f, g	(1, 2)
S. agona	1, 4, 12	f, g, s	–
S. typhimurium	1, 4 (5), 12	i	1, 2
S. bredeney	1, 4, 12, 27	l, v	1, 7
S. brandenburg	1, 4, 12	l, v	e, n, z_{15}
S. heidelberg	1, 4 (5), 12	r	1, 2
Group C_1			
S. paratyphi C	6, 7 (Vi)	c	1, 5
S. choleraesuis	6, 7	(c)	1, 5
S. typhisuis	6, 7	c	1, 5
S. isangi	6, 7, 14	d	1, 5
S. livingstone	6, 7	d	l, 4
S. braenderup	6, 7, 14	e, h	e, n, z_{15}
S. montevideo	6, 7	g, m (p), s	–
S. thompson	6, 7, 14	k	1, 5
S. potsdam	6, 7	l, v	e, n, z_{15}
S. infantis	6, 7, 14	r	1, 5
S. bareilly	6, 7, 14	y	1, 5
S. tennessee	6, 7	z_{29}	–

Table 55: continued   Tabelle 55: Fortsetzung

Serovar	O-antigen	H-antigens Phase 1	Phase 2
Group C_2			
S. muenchen	6, 8	d	1, 2
S. newport	6, 8	e, h	1, 2
S. blockley	6, 8	k	1, 5
S. manchester	6, 8	l, v	1, 7
S. bovismorbificans	6, 8	r	1, 5
S. goldcoast	6, 8	r	l, w
Group C_4			
S. eimsbuettel	6, 7, 14	d	l, w
Group D_1			
S. typhi	9, 12 (Vi)	d	–
S. enteritidis	1, 9, 12	g, m	(1, 7)
S. dublin	1, 9, 12 (Vi)	g, p	–
S. panama	1, 9, 12	l, v	1, 5
S. gallinarum-pullorum	1, 9, 12	–	–
Group E_1			
S. anatum	3, 10	e, h	1, 6
S. meleagridis	3, 10	e, h	l, w
S. give	3, 10	l, v	1, 7
Group E_2			
S. newington	3, 15	e, h	1, 6
S. binza	3, 15	y	1, 5
Group E_3			
S. thomasville	3, 15, 34	y	1, 5
Group E_4			
S. senftenberg	1, 3, 19	g (s), t	–

( ) antigen factors or phases can be lacking

rent pathogenicity and epidemiology can possess the same antigenic formula and under such circumstances, the differentiation has to rely on biochemical tests (tab. 56).

Anforderungen einer schnellen Diagnose meistens zu einem verwertbaren und ausreichend sicheren Ergebnis. Es können aber auch nach Pathogenität und Epidemiologie unterschiedliche Salmonellen eine gleiche Antigenformel besitzen, ihre Differenzierung muß dann biochemisch erfolgen (Tab. 56).

Table 56: Differentiation of the pig-specific salmonella and S. paratyphi C (20)

Tabelle 56: Differenzierung von schweinespezifischen Salmonellen und S. paratyphi C (20)

antigen formula	S. paratyphi C 6, 7 (Vi) : c : 1, 5	S. typhisuis 6, 7 : c : 1, 5	S. choleraesuis 6, 7 : c : 1, 5	S. choleraesuis var. kunzendorf 6, 7 :– 1, 5
Dul	+	–	–	–
Man	+	–	+	+
Xyl	+	+	+	+
Tre	$+^{2-3\,d}$	$+^{1-2\,d}$	–	–
Ara	v^+	+	–	–
Rha	$+^{1-2\,d}$	+	+	+
H_2S	+	–	–	+

Bibliography / Literatur

1. BERGMANN, G., & U. GÖTZE (1965): Ein Beitrag zum Vorkommen von Salmonellen in Schlachthofabwässern und zur Frage einer Behandlung des Abwassers vor seiner Einleitung. Fleischwirtschaft **45**, 626–631.
2. BISPING, W., H. BERNS, E. JÄNECKE, I. B. ANDERSEN, B. SONNENSCHEIN & K. G. WAECHTER (1981): Salmonellen-Probleme in Tierkörperbeseitigungsanstalten 2. Untersuchungen über die Rekontamination von Tierkörpermehlen durch Salmonellen. Berl. Münch. tierärztl. Wschr. **94**, 195–197.
3. BECKER, H., & G. TERPLAN (1986): Salmonellen in Milch und Milchprodukten. Zbl. Vet. Med. B, **33**, 1–25.
4. BOCKEMÜHL, J., & H. P. R. SEELIGER (1985): Die Auswirkungen neuer taxonomischer Erkenntnisse auf die Nomenklatur von bakteriellen Seuchenerregern. Bundesgesundheitsbl. **28**, 61–69.
5. BOOS, G. (1981): Salmonellen in Fleisch unterschiedlicher Vermarktung. Fleischwirtsch. **61**, 261–265.
6. BULLING, E. (1968): Die Bedeutung und Bekämpfung der Salmonella-Infektionen bei Mensch, Tier und Lebensmitteln tierischer Herkunft. Bundesgesundheitsbl. **11**, 375–387.
7. BULLING, E. (1966): Salmonella-Infektionen bei Tieren und ihre Beziehungen zur menschlichen Gesundheit. Bundesgesundheitsbl. **9**, 240–245.
8. BULLING, E. (1962): Verbreitung und Bedeutung der Tiersalmonellosen in der Bundesrepublik. Ber. d. 5. Kongr. d. Dtsch. Vet. med. Ges. 216–225.
9. FEY, H., A. BÜRGI, A. MARGADANT & E. BOLLER (1978): An economic and rapid diagnostic procedure for the detection of Salmonella/Shigella using the polyvalent Salmonella phage 0–1. Zbl. Bakt. I. Orig. A **240**, 7–15.
10. HAZEM, A. S. (1978): Salmonella paratyphi bei Tieren und in der Umwelt. Dtsch. tierärztl. Wschr. **85**, 296–303.
11. HELLMANN, E. (1977): Latente Salmonella-Infektionen der Tiere und ihre Ursachen. Wiener tierärztl. Mschr. **64**, 173–180.
12. HESS, E., & C. BREER (1975): Salmonellenepidemiologie und Grünlanddüngung mit Klärschlamm. Zbl. Bakt. I. Orig. B **161**, 54–60.
13. HESS, E., G. LOTT & C. BREER (1974): Klärschlamm u. Freilandbiologie von Salmonellen. Zbl. Bakt. I. Orig. B **158**, 446–485.
14. JONAS, D., H. POLLMANN & G. BUGL (1986): Salmonella-Isolierungen aus Lebensmitteln tierischer Herkunft — Vergleichsuntersuchungen zur Leistungsfähigkeit des modifizierten Rappaportmediums (R10). Arch. Lebensmittelhyg. **37**, 65–66.
15. KAUFFMANN, F. (1966): The bacteriology of enterobacteriaceae. Copenhagen: Munksgaard.
16. KEMPF, G., & O. PIETZSCH (1981): Salmonellenprobleme in Tierkörperbeseitigungsanstalten. 1. Mittl.: Salmonellen in Tierkörpermehl. Berl. Münch. tierärztl. Wschr. **94**, 189–194.
17. KOTTER, L., H. SCHELS & G. TERPLAN (1964): Zum Vorkommen von Salmonellen in Fleisch- und Fleischerzeugnissen sowie anderen Lebensmitteln tierischer Herkunft. Arch. Lebensmittelhyg. **15**, Nr. 8, 20.
18. LE MINOR, L., M. VÉRON & M. POPOFF (1982): Taxonomie des Salmonella. Ann. Microbiol. (Inst. Pasteur) **133 b**, 223–243.
19. LE MINOR, L., M. VÉRON & M. PROPOFF (1982): Proposition pour une nomenclature des Salmonella. Ann. Microbiol. (Inst. Pasteur) **133 b**, 245–254.
20. SOJKA, W. J., & M. GITTER (1961): Salmonellosis in pigs with reference to its public health significance. Vet. Rev. Annot. **7**, 11.
21. SONTAG, M. (1962): Über den Salmonellenbefall pflanzlicher und tierischer Futtermittel unter besonderer Berücksichtigung von inländischem Knochenfuttermehl und Futterknochenschrot. Vet. med. Diss. Univers. Gießen.
22. STRAUCH, D. (1976): Verbreitung der Salmonellen über Abwasser und Abfälle. Fleischwirtschaft **56**, 917–925.
23. STRAUCH, D. (1964): Über das Vorkommen von Salmonellen in Futtermitteln, Abwasser, Wasser und Boden. Wiener tierärztl. Mschr. **51**, 757–767.
24. PIETZSCH, O. (1979): Verbreitung der Salmonella-Infektionen bei Tieren, tierischen Lebens- und Futtermitteln in der Bundesrepublik Deutschland einschl. Berlin (West). Bundesgesundheitsbl. **22**, 153–175.
25. PIETZSCH, O., & G. KEMPF (1984): Salmonellen in Futtermitteln. Zbl. Vet. Med. B **31**, 343–357.
26. PIETZSCH, O. (1981): Salmonella. In: H. BLOBEL & T. SCHLIESSER (Hrsg.): Handbuch der bakteriellen Infektionen bei Tieren. Bd. 3, S. 344–452. Jena: VEB Gustav Fischer.
27. PIETZSCH, O. (1978): Verbreitung der Salmonella-Infektionen bei Tieren, tierischen Lebens- und Futtermitteln in der Bundesrepublik Deutschland einschl. Berlin (West). Bundesgesundheitsbl. **21**, 389–411.
28. VASSILIADIS, P. (1983): The Rappaport-Vassiliadis (RV) enrichment medium for the isolation of salmonellas: An overview. J. appl. Bact. **54**, 69–76.
29. WEISS, R., K. G. DRÄGER, D. COBANOGLU & H. R. SCHÜTZE (1984): Zur Effizienz von modifiziertem Rappaportmedium, pH 7,0 zur Anreicherung von Salmonellen. Berl. Münch. tierärztl. Wschr. **97**, 206–208.

4.1.4 Genus: Shigella (Sh.)

Four species fall into this genus, and they differ in their geographical distribution:

Sh. dysenteriae — tropics and subtropics,
Sh. boydii — Near East and North Africa,
Sh. flexneri — world-wide,
Sh. sonnei — world-wide.

■ **Incidence and veterinary significance**
Under natural conditions, shigellae are responsible for dysentery only in man.

Infections of animals are rare, and then they affect mainly captive primates in which they cause gastro-enteritis and occasionally abortion and pneumonia (2, 3, 6, 8, 9).

In domestic animals infections are very rare and

4.1.4 Gattung: Shigella (Sh.)

Zu der Gattung zählen 4 Arten, die geographisch unterschiedliche Schwerpunkte besitzen:

Sh. dysenteriae — Tropen und Subtropen,
Sh. boydii — Vorderasien, Nordafrika,
Sh. flexneri — weltweit,
Sh. sonnei — weltweit.

■ **Vorkommen und medizinische Bedeutung**
Shigellen kommen als Erreger der bakteriellen Ruhr (Dysenterie) unter natürlichen Verhältnissen fast ausschließlich beim Menschen vor.

Infektionen bei Tieren sind selten. Sie betreffen besonders in Gefangenschaft gehaltene Primaten und verursachen Gastroenteritiden und vereinzelt Aborte und Pneumonien (2, 3, 6, 8, 9).

generally latent or they produce signs of enteritis. Shigella infections have been reported in, amongst others, dogs and cats (5, 7, 10, 12), cattle (4, 5, 13), pigs (1, 13), tigers (14) and guinea pigs. Most commonly these are *Sh. flexneri* infections.

However, although food materials of animal origin cannot be excluded altogether as a source of infection, this route is only of very marginal epidemiological significance (11).

■ Culture (figs. 132 and 133)

The primary isolation of shigellae is difficult. This is especially the case when examining food materials where, unlike clinical samples, only a few bacteria are likely to be present. In comparison with other *Enterobacteriaceae* the generation time of shigella is longer, so that they easily become overgrown in culture. Besides, no entirely satisfactory medium is available for their enrichment. The most likely is the selenite broth of Leifson. Tetrathionate media are unsuitable. Direct plating is therefore very important (11). MacConkey agar (without glucose) has been found effective and shigella grows as small colonies with an irregularly serrated edge. Other recommended media are: Salmonella-shigella (SS) agar, Sodium desoxycholate citrate agar, XLD agar.

■ Biochemical properties
See table 48.

■ Antigenic structure and serological differentiation

The agglutination test can be used for the recognition of shigella. However, the proof for identification of suspect colonies can be impeded by the O-inagglutinability or overlapping reactions with other genera.

Bei Haustieren sind Infektionen sehr selten und verlaufen meistens latent oder unter Erscheinungen einer Enteritis. Sie wurden u. a. gefunden beim Hund und bei der Katze (5, 7, 10, 12), beim Rind (4, 5, 13), beim Schwein (1, 13), beim Tiger (14) und bei Meerschweinchen. Meistens handelt es sich um Infektionen mit *Sh. flexneri*.

Infektionen durch Lebensmittel tierischer Herkunft können nicht völlig ausgeschlossen werden, ihnen kommt epidemiologisch nur eine Randbedeutung zu (11).

■ Kultur (Abb. 132 u. 133)

Die Anzüchtung von Shigellen aus Untersuchungsmaterial ist schwierig, besonders dann, wenn bei der Untersuchung von Lebensmitteln — im Gegensatz zu Infektionsfällen — nur mit wenigen Shigellen zu rechnen ist. Im Vergleich zu den anderen *Enterobacteriaceae* ist die Generationszeit der Shigellen länger, so daß sie leicht überwuchert werden, und ihre Tenazität ist gering. Zudem steht für die Anreicherung kein voll befriedigendes Medium zur Verfügung, am ehesten kommt die Selenitbrühe nach Leifson in Frage. Tetrathionatnährböden sind ungeeignet. Deswegen spielt die direkte Plattenkultur eine wichtige Rolle (11). Bewährt hat sich der MacConkey-Agar (ohne Glucose), auf dem die Shigellen in kleinen Kolonien mit einem unregelmäßig gezackten Rand wachsen. Weitere empfohlene Nährböden sind: Salmonella-Shigella-(SS-)Agar, Natriumdesoxycholatcitratagar, XLD-Agar.

■ Kulturell-biochemische Eigenschaften
Siehe Tab. 48.

■ Antigenstruktur und serologische Differenzierung

Für die Erkennung der Shigellen kann die Agglutination benutzt werden. Die Prüfung verdächtiger Kolonien kann aber durch eine O-Inagglutinabilität oder durch übergreifende Reaktionen zu anderen Gattungen gestört werden.

Bibliography / Literatur

1. BAKER, W. L. (1960): Shigella dysenteriae in swine. Vet. Med. **55**, 413–422.
2. CARPENTER, K. P. (1965): An attempt to find Shigellae in wild primates. J. Comp. Path. **75**, 201–204.
3. COOPER, J. E., & J. R. NEEDHAM (1976): An outbreak of shigellosis in laboratory marmosets and tamarins (Family: Callithricidae). J. Hyg. **76**, 415–424.
4. DEOM, J., & J. MORTELMANS (1954): A case of Shigella sonnei septicaemia in a calf. Nature **174**, 316.
5. DINOW, W. (1962): Isolierung von Shigella flexneri aus einem Hund und einer Kuh. Zbl. Bakt. I. Orig. **186**, 131–133.
6. FINCHAM, J. E., & J. V. SEIER (1981): Endemic enteric disease in vervet monkeys. J. S. Afr. Vet. Ass. **52**, 177–179.
7. FLOYD, T. M. (1955): Isolation of Shigella from dogs in Egypt. J. Bact. **70**, 621.
8. FOX, J. G. (1975): Transmissible drug resistance in Shigella and Salmonella isolated from pet monkeys and their owners. J. Med. Primat **4**, 165–171.
9. HARTLEY, E. G. (1975): The incidence and antibiotic sensitivity of Shigella bacteria isolated from newly imported macaque monkeys. Brit. Vet. J. **131**, 205–212.
10. KHAN, A. Q. (1968): Shigella infection in animals in the Sudan. Brit. Vet. J. **124**, 171–173.
11. REUSSE, U. (1984): Untersuchungen zur Isolierung von Shigellen aus Lebensmitteln tierischer Herkunft. Arch. Lebensmittelhyg. **35**, 138–141.

12. Shouman, M. T., F. F. Goda & S. M. El-Gibaly (1981): Preliminary investigation on stray dogs as carriers for pathogenic E. coli, Salmonella and Shigella. J. Egypt. Vet. Med. Ass. **39**, 59–65.
13. Ueda, S., S. Sasaki, M. Kabuto & W. Ninimiya (1963): Shigella organisms isolated from slaughtered cattle and hogs. Jap. J. Vet. Sci. **25**, 127–128.
14. Zaki, S., T. S. Nalini, M. S. Rao & B. S. Keshavamurtha (1980): Isolation of Shigella flexneri from two tiger cubs. Curr. Sci. **49**, 288.

4.1.5 Genus: Edwardsiella (Ed.)

The following species are recognized in this genus: *Ed. tarda*, *Ed. hoshinae* and *Ed. ictaluri*.

4.1.5.1 Edwardsiella tarda

This has been isolated from all classes of vertrebrates — fish, amphibia, reptiles, birds and mammals, as well as from mussels and crabs and from water, effluent and mud. Reptilian gut is believed to be the normal habitat of this organism (12, 16, 17), and presumably the bacterium gains access to water through faecal contamination. Thus it is fish, sealions and other animals in contact with surface water, which are the most likely animals to become infected. Frequently the infection is latent but it can also lead to disease.

Various lesions, including abscesses in muscles, liver and kidney, ecchymoses and petechiae in different regions of the body (including the fins), skin ulceration and others have been described in numerous species of fish, especially eel and catfish (EPDC = emphysematous putrefying disease of catfish) (1, 7, 10, 11, 18).

Tortoises are the most common reptiles to be affected and they mainly contract a latent intestinal infection (2, 8, 12, 16, 19, 21). Infections have occasionally been reported not only in seals, sealions and dolphins, but also in such mammals as pigs (4, 5, 13), cattle (3, 6), dogs and others (20). Generally the animals were clinically healthy, presenting only with diarrhoea.

Ed. tarda infections occur rarely also in birds and especially aquatic birds (2, 8).

Diseases caused by *Ed. tarda* are occasionally encountered in man, where they involve primarily the gastro-intestinal tract. Other forms are meningitis, abscess formation, septicaemia, urogenital infections, bronchopneumonia etc. (15).

Ed. tarda appears to have a world wide distribution; it is also found in Germany, though its primary location is Eastern Africa.

The biochemical characters are summarized in table 48. This is a motile, straight bacillus, 2–3 μm long. In 24 hours on simple media it will form colonies 0.5–1 mm in diameter at an optimum tem-

perature of 37 °C. It is haemolytic and lactose-negative.

4.1.5.2 Edwardsiella ictaluri

This bacterium was isolated by HAWKE (9) from river catfish which had developed a septicaemic disease, which he termed ESC (enteric septicaemia of catfish). The lesions consist of ulcers between the eyes, haemorrhages in the skin, the mouth and the neck region as well as at the base of the fins and other parts of the body. The muscles and internal organs also show haemorrhagic infiltrations (14).

Die kulturell-biochemischen Gattungsmerkmale sind in der Tab. 48 zusammengestellt. Es handelt sich um ein gerades, 2–3 µm langes, bewegliches Stäbchen. Es bildet auf einfachen Nährböden nach 24 h 0,5–1 mm große Kolonien, das Temperaturoptimum liegt bei 37 °C. Es wächst hämolytisch und ist lactosenegativ.

4.1.5.2 Edwardsiella ictaluri

Das Bakterium wurde von HAWKE (9) aus Flußwelsen isoliert, die eine septikämische Erkrankung aufwiesen, die vom Autor als ESC (enteric septicaemia of catfish) bezeichnet wurde. Das Krankheitsbild besteht in Ulcera zwischen den Augen, Blutungen in der Haut, im Maul- und Halsbereich sowie an der Flossenbasis und an anderen Körperstellen. Blutige Infiltrationen treten auch in der Muskulatur und in den inneren Organen auf (14).

Bibliography / Literatur

1. AMANDI, A., S. F. HIU, J. S. ROHOVEC & L. FRYER (1982): Isolation and characterization of Edwardsiella tarda from fall chinook salmon (Oncorhynchus tshawytscha). Appl. Environm. Microbiol. **43**, 1380–1394.
2. BAUWENS, L., P. DE MEURICHY, P. LEMMERN & J. VANDEPITTE (1983): Isolation of Plesiomonas shigelloides and Edwardsiella species in the Antwerp Zoo. Acta. Zool. Path. **77**, 61–73.
3. DAMME, L. R., & J. VANDEPITTE (1980): Frequent isolation of Edwardsiella tarda and Plesiomonas shigelloides from healthy Zairese freshwater fish: a possible source of sporadic diarrhoe in the tropics. Appl. Environm. Microbiol. **39**, 475–479.
4. DWIGHT, R. O., S. L. NELSON & J. B. ADDISON (1974): Isolation of Edwardsiella tarda from swine. Appl. Microbiol. **27**, 703–705.
5. ELAZHARY, M., A. TREMBLAY, A. LAGACE & R. S. ROY (1973): A preliminary study on the intestinal flora of cecum and colon of eight, ten and twelve week old swine. Can. J. Comp. Med. **37**, 369–374.
6. EWING, W. H., A. C. MCWHORTER, M. R. ESCOBAR & A. H. LUBIN (1965): Edwardsiella, a new genus of Enterobacteriaceae based on a new species, E. tarda. Int. Bull. Bact. Nomencl. Taxon. **15**, 33–38.
7. FUHRMANN, H., K. H. BÖHM & H. J. SCHLOTFELDT (1984): On the importance of enteric bacteria in the bacteriology of freshwater fish. Bull. Europ. Ass. Fish Path. **4**, 42–46.
8. GRIMONT, P. A., F. GRIMONT, C. RICHARD & R. SAKASAKI (1980): Edwardsiella hoshinae, a new species of Enterobacteriaceae. Curr. Microbiol. **4**, 347–351.
9. HAWKE, J. P. (1979): A bacterium associated with disease of pond cultured channel catfish, Ictalurus punctatus. J. Fish Res. Board Can. **36**, 1508–1512.
10. HOSHINA, T. (1962): On a new bacterium, Paracolobactrum anguillimortiferum n. sp. Bull. Jap. Soc. Sci. Fish **28**, 162–164.
11. MEYER, F. P., & G. L. BULLOCK (1973): Edwardsiella tarda, a new pathogen of channel catfish. Appl. Microbiol. **25**, 155–156.
12. MÜLLER, H. E. (1972): The aerobic faecal flora of reptiles with special reference to the enterobacteria of snakes. Zbl. Bakt. I. Orig. **222**, 487–495.
13. OWENS, D. R., S. L. NELSON & J. B. ADDISON (1974): Isolation of Edwardsiella tarda from swine. Appl. Microbiol. **27**, 703–705.
14. PLUMB, J. A., & T. E. SCHWEDLER (1982): Enteric septicemia of catfish (ESC): a new bacterial problem surfaces. Aquacult Mag. **8**, 26–27.
15. RENKEN-ZÜRNER, A. (1985): Vorkommen und veterinärmedizinische Bedeutung von Bakterien aus der Familie der Enterobacteriaceae mit Ausnahme der Gattungen Escherichia und Salmonella sowie der Spezies Yersinia pestis. Vet. Med. Diss. Hannover.
16. ROGGENDORF, M., & H. E. MÜLLER (1976): Enterobakterien bei Reptilien. Zbl. Bakt. I. Orig. A **236**, 22–35.
17. SAKAZAKI, R. (1967): Studies on the Asakusa group of Enterobacteriaceae (Edwardsiella tarda). Jap. J. Med. Sci. Biol. **20**, 205–212.
18. SAVIDIS, G. (1984): Qualitative Untersuchungen über das Vorkommen von Enterobacteriazeen aus dem Darm von Süßwasserfischen unter besonderer Berücksichtigung von Yersinia ruckeri, dem ätiologischen Agens von ERD. Vet. Med. Diss. Hannover.
19. SELBITZ, H. J., & W. E. ENGELMANN (1984): Die häufigsten bakteriellen Infektionen bei Reptilien. Mh. Vet. Med. **39**, 383–386.
20. TACAL, J. V., & C. F. MENEZ (1968): The isolation of Edwardsiella tarda from a dog. Philipp. J. Vet. Med. **7**, 143–145.
21. WYATT, L. E., R. NICKELSON & C. VANDERZANT (1979): Edwardsiella tarda in freshwater catfish and their environment. Appl. Environm. Microbiol. **38**, 710–714.

4.1.6 Genus: Klebsiella (K.)

The taxonomy of this genus has seen revision over the years but Bergey's manual (14) differentiates the following:
▷ *K. pneumoniae* with the subspecies
▷ *K. pneumoniae* subsp. *pneumoniae*, occurs normally in the digestive tract of animals and in their environment (soil, water, food stuffs etc.); it is a facultative pathogen,
K. pneumoniae subsp. *ozaenae* (syn.: *K. ozaenae* and
K. pneumoniae subsp. *rhinoscleromatis*) (syn.: *K. rhinoscleromatis,*) which is found in some chronic respiratory diseases of man;

4.1.6 Gattung: Klebsiella (K.)

Die Taxonomie der Gattung hat im Laufe der Zeit Wandlungen erfahren. Nach Bergey's manual (14) werden unterschieden:
▷ *K. pneumoniae* mit den Unterarten
▷ *K. pneumoniae* subsp. *pneumoniae*, die normalerweise im Darmtrakt der Tiere und ihrer Umwelt (Boden, Wasser, Futtermittel u. a.) vorkommt und fakultativ pathogen ist,
K. pneumoniae subsp. *ozaenae* (Syn.: *K. ozaenae*) und
K. pneumoniae subsp. *rhinoscleromatis* (Syn.: *K. rhinoscleromatis*), die bei chronischen Erkrankungen des Respirationstraktes des Menschen gefunden wird;

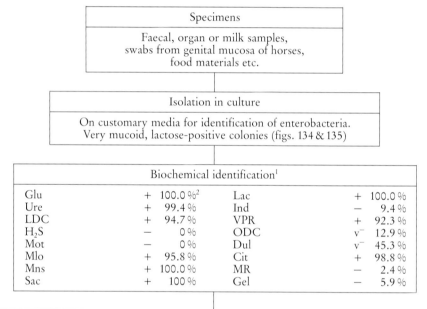

Specimens
Faecal, organ or milk samples, swabs from genital mucosa of horses, food materials etc.

Isolation in culture
On customary media for identification of enterobacteria. Very mucoid, lactose-positive colonies (figs. 134 & 135)

Biochemical identification[1]				
Glu	+ 100.0 %[2]	Lac	+	100.0 %
Ure	+ 99.4 %	Ind	−	9.4 %
LDC	+ 94.7 %	VPR	+	92.3 %
H_2S	− 0 %	ODC	v^-	12.9 %
Mot	− 0 %	Dul	v^-	45.3 %
Mlo	+ 95.8 %	Cit	+	98.8 %
Mns	+ 100.0 %	MR	−	2.4 %
Sac	+ 100 %	Gel	−	5.9 %

Differentiation of Klebsiella spp.								
Species	Gas from Glu	Acid from Lac	Dul	MR	VPR	Cit	Ure	Mlo	Ind
K. pneumoniae									
subsp. pneumoniae	+	+	v	−	+	+	+	+	−
subsp. ozaenae	v	(+)	−	+	−	v	v	−	−
subsp. rhinoscleromatis	−	−	−	+	−	−	−	+	−
K. oxytoca	+	+	v	−	+	+	+	v	+

Serological typing of K. pneumoniae subsp. pneumoniae
1. Identification of O-antigen without diagnostic significance
2. Identification of K-antigen provides real information about the virulence of the strain, can provide answers to epidemiological problems

[1] Strains from cattle, pigs, dogs, wild and captive animals (13); [2] Percentage of positive reactions

Fig. 136: Demonstration and identification of klebsiellae Abb. 136: Nachweis und Bestimmung von Klebsiellen

▷ *K. oxytoca*, an indole-positive type of klebsiella, which is also found in the intestinal tract and other organs of animals, as well as their environment and which may be isolated from pathological lesions;
▷ *K. terrigena* and
▷ *K. planticola* which occur mainly outside living creatures in the soil and water.

4.1.6.1 Klebsiella pneumoniae subsp. pneumoniae

■ **Incidence and veterinary significance**

K. pneumoniae is distributed not only in the environment of animals (soil, water, bedding, food materials, plants, sewage etc.) but it also settles in mucous membranes and particularly often in the gut. Under certain circumstances pathological conditions can develop, the most important of which are:
▷ In horses: inflammation of the genital mucosa and abortion, generalized infections of foals (6, 7, 8, 11, 17, 18, 19).
▷ In cattle: mastitis, generalized infections and enteritis of calves (1, 5, 9, 15, 20).
▷ In pigs: in the majority of instances the nasopharyngeal region and the digestive tract are infected without causing clinical signs. An aetiological role in piglet diarrhoea and the MMA syndrome has been attributed to *K. pneumoniae* (3, 4, 21).

Klebsiella infections can occasionally occur in other animals as well, especially in poultry.

■ **Morphology**
This is a non-motile, encapsulated rod, 0.3–1.5 × 0.6–6.0 µm, which arranged singly, in pairs or short chains.

■ **Culture** (figs. 134 and 135)
K. pneumoniae is culturally undemanding and will grow on all the usual media including those which are used for the demonstration of *Enterobacteriaceae*. The colonies are mucoid, but the degree of this depends on the strain and the medium, and it can be lost during passage.

■ **Biochemical properties**
The biochemical properties of *K. pneumoniae* and its three subspecies are summarized in figure 136. Its biochemical separation from *Enterobacter* strains which behave similarly is of importance from a differential diagnostic point of view (tab. 58). Since there is no single character which will differentiate the two genera, one has to con-

sider the whole range of reactions which are likely to separate them (18). Furthermore, there is a possibility of confusion with the mucoid strains of *E. coli* (fig. 125).

■ Antigenic structure

K. pneumoniae has O- and K-antigens. The O-antigens are of little importance in the differentiation, because they are difficult to demonstrate. They are masked by the capsule which is incompletely destroyed by heating to 100 °C for 2½ hours. Thus the klebsiellae cannot be agglutinated with O-antisera although eleven O-antigens have been identified.

More than 70 strains can be identified using the K-antigens. This is done with the capsular swelling reaction. The procedure is as follows: on a slide 1 drop of bacterial suspension is mixed with 1 drop of antiserum and a small amount of 10% methylene blue. Compared with the control, the bacteria in the positive test acquire an indistinct outline after 5 minutes, they are surrounded by a broad lighter zone which has a black border (precipitation) on the outside.

It is only possible to a limited degree to attribute certain capsular types to particular diseases or animal species. Many different types are found in bovine mastitis (5). The capsular types 1, 2 and 5 are, apparently, of greater pathogenic significance in genital infections of the mare, while type 7 is more frequently found in healthy stallions (2, 10, 17).

4.1.6.2 Klebsiella oxytoca

This bacterium is distinguished from *K. pneumoniae* by the fact that it forms indole (fig. 136). It is not known with certainty whether *K. oxytoca* is pathogenic to animals, although it has been isolated from disease conditions; from the genital tract of the horse for example. Its facultative pathogenicity appears to be less pronounced than that of *K. pneumoniae*.

■ Antigenstruktur

K. pneumoniae besitzt O- und K-Antigene. Die O-Antigene spielen bei der Differenzierung eine geringe Rolle, da sie schwer nachweisbar sind. Durch die Kapsel, die auch durch Erhitzung (2½ h/100 °C) ungenügend zerstört wird, werden die O-Antigene maskiert, so daß die Klebsiellen durch O-Antiseren inagglutinabel sind. Es sind 11 O-Antigene bekannt.

Durch den K-Antigennachweis lassen sich über 70 Serotypen nachweisen. Der Nachweis wird durch die Kapselquellreaktion geführt. Dabei wird auf einem Objektträger je ein Tropfen Bakteriensuspension und Antiserum mit einer geringen Menge einer 10%igen Methylenblaulösung vermischt. Im positiven Fall wird im Vergleich zu einer Kontrolle nach 5 min der Bakterienkörper unscharf und ist von einem breiten hellen Saum umgeben, der nach außen durch einen schwarzen Rand (Präzipitation) begrenzt wird.

Die Zuordnung einzelner Kapseltypen zu bestimmten Krankheitsbildern bzw. Tierarten ist nur begrenzt möglich. Bei der Rindermastitis finden sich zahlreiche verschiedene Typen (5). Für die Genitalinfektionen der Stuten haben offenbar die Kapseltypen 1, 2 und 5 eine größere pathogene Bedeutung, während der Typ 7 bevorzugt bei gesunden Hengsten gefunden wird (2, 10, 17).

4.1.6.2 Klebsiella oxytoca

Das Bakterium ist durch die Indolbildung von *K. pneumoniae* zu unterscheiden (Abb. 136). Über die Pathogenität für das Tier ist eine sichere Aussage noch nicht möglich, es wird jedoch aus pathologischen Prozessen isoliert, z. B. aus dem Genitaltrakt beim Pferd. Im Vergleich zu *K. pneumoniae* scheint die fakultative Pathogenität geringer zu sein.

Bibliography / Literatur

1. Amtsberg, G., & W. Fischer (1977): Untersuchungen zur pathogenen Bedeutung von Klebsiellen beim Kalb. Dtsch. tierärztl. Wschr. **84**, 296–300.
2. Atherton, J. G. (1975): The identification of equine genital strains of Klebsiella and Enterobacter species. Equ. Vet. J. **7**, 207–209.
3. Bertschinger, H. U., J. Pohlenz & J. Hemlep (1977): Untersuchungen über das Mastitis-Metritis-Agalaktie-Syndrom (Milchfieber) der Sau. II. Bakteriologische Befunde bei Spontanfällen. Schweiz. Arch. Tierhk. **119**, 223–233.
4. Bertschinger, H. U., J. Pohlenz & D. Middleton-Williams (1977): Untersuchungen über das Mastitis-Metritis-Agalaktie-Syndrom (Milchfieber) bei der Sau. III. Galaktogene Erzeugung von Klebsiellen-Mastitis. Schweiz. Arch. Tierhk. **119**, 265–275.
5. Braman, S. K., R. J. Eberhart, M. A. Asbury & G. J. Hermann (1973): Capsular types of Klebsiella pneumoniae associated with bovine mastitis. J. Am. Vet. Med. Assoc. **162**, 109–111.
6. Crouch, J. R. F., J. G. Atherton & H. Platt (1972): Venereal transmission of Klebsiella aerogenes in a thoroughbred stud from a persistently infected stallion. Vet. Rec. **90**, 21–24.
7. Floer, W. (1974): Zum Vorkommen von Klebsiellen in den Geschlechtsorganen und Feten von Vollblutpferden. Dtsch. tierärztl. Wschr. **81**, 20–22.

8. GREENWOOD, E. S., & D. R. ELLIS (1976): Klebsiella aerogenes in mares. Vet. Rec. **99**, 439.
9. GRUNERT, E., & U. WEIGT (1964): Beitrag zur Klebsiellen-Mastitis beim Rind. Berl. Münch. tierärztl. Wschr. **77**, 116–120.
10. HEUSER, H. (1974): Mikrobiologische und serologische Untersuchungen an equinen Klebsiellen. Vet. Med. Diss. Hannover.
11. MERKT, H., E. KLUG, K. H. BÖHM & R. WEISS (1974): Erfahrungen über Klebsiellen als Genitalinfektionserreger beim Pferd. Berl. Münch. tierärztl. Wschr. **87**, 405–409.
12. NEUMANN, P., & K. WENDT (1985): Zur Ätiopathogenese der Klebsiella-Mastitis. Mh. Vet. Med. **40**, 120–123.
13. NIAZI, Z. M., G. KIRPAL, G. AMTSBERG & M. REFAI (1977): Biochemie, Serologie, Mäusepathogenität und Antibiotikaresistenz von Klebsiellen verschiedener Tierarten. Berl. Münch. tierärztl. Wschr. **90**, 435–440.
14. ØRSKOV, I. (1984): Genus Klebsiella. In: Bergey's manual of determinative bacteriology. Vol. 1, S. 461–465. Baltimore: Williams & Wilkins.
15. RENK, W. (1962): Mastitiden bei Infektionen mit Escherichia coli, Aerobacter aerogenes und Klebsiella. Zbl. Vet. Med. **9**, 264–281.
16. WEBER, A., U. NEUMEIER & TH. SCHLIESSER (1975): Untersuchungen über das biochemische Verhalten und die Antibiotikaempfindlichkeit von Keimen der Gattung Klebsiella, isoliert aus Untersuchungsmaterial von Pferden. Berl. Münch. tierärztl. Wschr. **88**, 121–123.
17. WEISS, R., H. TILLMANN & K. G. DRÄGER (1985): Paarungsinfektionen bei Pferden durch Klebsiella pneumoniae, Kapseltyp 1. Prakt. Tierarzt **66**, 114–120.
18. WEISS, R., K. H. BÖHM, H. MERKT, E. KLUG & H. HEUSER (1976): Untersuchungen zur Besiedlung der Genital- und Nasenschleimhaut des Pferdes, insbesondere des Hengstes mit in der Pferdezucht bedeutsamen bakteriellen Infektionserregern, unter besonderer Berücksichtigung der Klebsiellen. II. Morphologische und biochemische Untersuchungen an Klebsiellen. Berl. Münch. tierärztl. Wschr. **89**, 152–156.
19. WEISS, R., K. H. BÖHM, H. MERKT & E. KLUG (1975): Untersuchungen zur Besiedlung der Genital- und Nasenschleimhaut des Pferdes, speziell des Hengstes mit in der Pferdezucht bedeutsamen bakteriellen Infektionserregern, unter besonderer Berücksichtigung der Klebsiellen. I. Epidemiologische Erhebungen. Berl. Münch. tierärztl. Wschr. **88**, 436–440, 445–449.
20. WHITE, F. (1967): An outbreak of mastitis in cattle and death of calves due to infection with an organism of the Friedländer group (Klebsiella). Vet. Rec. **22**, 566–568.
21. WILCOCK, B. P. (1979): Experimental Klebsiella and Salmonella infection in neonatal swine. Can. J. Comp. Med. **43**, 200–206.

4.1.7 Genus: Enterobacter (Eb.)

The genus contains the following: *Eb. cloacae*, *Eb. sakazakii*, *Eb. agglomerans*, *Eb. aerogenes*, *Eb. gergoviae*.

■ Incidence and veterinary significance

Members of this genus inhabit mainly the environment (water, soil, plants etc.) and they are also found in the digestive tract of animals. For the latter reason they are not infrequently isolated from specimens of animal origin. The most common are *Eb. cloacae* and *Eb. aerogenes*, but the other species are by no means uncommon.

The facultative pathogenicity of these bacteria must be rated as low, for in the majority of cases their isolation results from clinically unimportant colonization of the mucous membranes. Some aetiological significance has been attributed to *Enterobacter spp.* in the following conditions:
▷ Horse: abortion and infection of the genital tract leading to infertility. In stallions, the genital mucosa often carries the infection but without any clinical evidence (3, 8),
▷ Cattle: abortion, mastitis (4, 5, 9),
▷ Pigs: agalactia syndrome (1, 2).

No definite statement can be made at present as to whether in animals *Enterobacter* plays a similar causal part in urinary infection, delayed wound healing, pneumonia, enteritis and generalized infections as it does in man. Further reports of the occurrence of enterobacter in animals are reviewed by RENKEN/ZÜRNER (10).

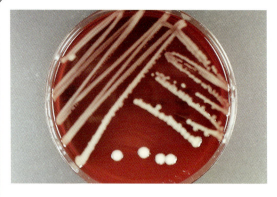
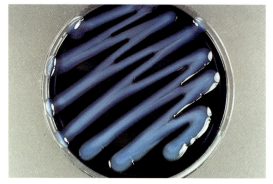
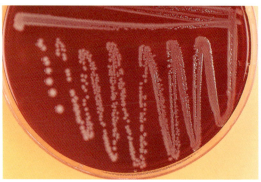
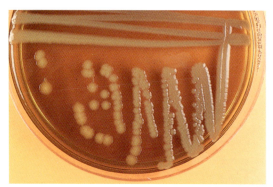

▲ Fig. 137: *Enterobacter aerogenes*, pure culture on blood agar, large moist, glistening colonies, 48 h, 37 °C. Magnification x 0.25
▼ Fig. 139: *Enterobacter cloacae*, pure culture on blood agar, large, moist colonies, 48 h, 37 °C. Magnification x 0.4

▲ Fig. 138: *Enterobacter aerogenes*, pure culture on Gassner agar, lactose-positive, mucoid colonies easily confused with Klebsiella (fig. 135) and mucoid growth of *E. coli* (fig. 125), 48 h, 37 °C. Magnification x 0.25
▼ Fig. 140: *Enterobacter cloacae*, pure culture on Gassner agar, large moist colonies, occasionally lactose-negative, 48 h, 37 °C. Magnification x 0.4

▲ Abb. 137: *Enterobacter aerogenes*, Reinkultur auf Blutagar, große feucht-schleimige Kolonien, 48 h, 37 °C, Abb.-M. 1 : 4
▼ Abb. 139: *Enterobacter cloacae*, Reinkultur auf Blutagar, große feuchte Kolonien, 48 h, 37 °C, Abb.-M. 1 : 2,5

▲ Abb. 138: *Enterobacter aerogenes*, Reinkultur auf Gaßner-Agar, lactosepositive Kolonien, schleimiges Wachstum, leichte Verwechselung mit Klebsiellen (Abb. 135) und schleimig wachsender *E. coli* (Abb. 125) 48 h, 37 °C, Abb.-M. 1 : 4
▼ Abb. 140: *Enterobacter cloacae*, Reinkultur auf Gaßner-Agar, große, feuchte Kolonien, ausnahmsweise lactosenegativ, 48 h, 37 °C, Abb.-M. 1 : 2,5

■ **Bacteriological properties** (figs. 137 to 140)
This is a motile rod which grows as colonies very similar to those of *E. coli* or klebsiellae; they can be very mucoid.

The identification of the genus (fig. 48) and the species (tab. 57) relies on the biochemical properties. Table 58 accents the characters which permit the differentiation from the genus *Klebsiella*.

■ **Bakteriologische Eigenschaften** (Abb. 137 bis 140)
Es handelt sich um bewegliche Stäbchen, die in der Kultur *E. coli* oder Klebsiellen sehr ähnlich sind, sie können in stark schleimigen Kolonien wachsen.

Die Bestimmung der Gattung (Tab. 48) und der Arten (Tab. 57) erfolgt anhand der biochemischen Eigenschaften. Merkmale, die eine Abgrenzung zur Gattung Klebsiella erlauben, enthält Tab. 58.

Table 57: Biochemical differentiation of the *Enterobacter* spp.

Tabelle 57: Kulturell-biochemische Unterscheidung der Enterobacterarten

Property	cloacae	sakasakii	Enterobacter gergoviae	aerogenes	agglomerans
Glu/Ga	+/+	+/+	+/+	+/+	+/v$^-$
LDC	−	−	v$^+$	+	−
ODC	+	+	+	+	−
H$_2$S	−	−	−	−	−
Ind	−	v$^-$	−	−	v$^-$
Ado	v$^-$	−	−	+	−
Lac	+	+	v$^-$	+	v
Ara	+	+	+	+	+
Sor	+	−	−	+	v$^-$
VPR	+	+	+	+	v$^+$
Dul	v$^-$	−	−	−	v$^-$
PAD	−	−	−	−	v$^-$
Ure	v$^+$	−	+	−	v$^-$
Cit	+	+	+	+	v$^+$

Bibliography / Literatur

1. ARMSTRONG, C. H., B. E. HOOPER & C. E. MARTIN (1968): Microflora associated with agalactia syndrome of sows. Am. J. Vet. Res. 29, 1401–1407.
2. BERTSCHINGER, H. U., J. POHLENZ & I. HEMLEP (1977): Untersuchungen über das Mastitis-Metritis-Agalaktie-Syndrom (Milchfieber) der Sau. II. Bakteriologische Befunde bei Spontanfällen. Schweiz. Arch. Tierk. 119, 223–233.
3. GIBSON, J. A., L. E. LEAVES & B. M. O'SULLIVAN (1982): Equine abortion associated with Enterobacter agglomerans. Equ. Vet. J. 14, 122–125.
4. JASPER, D. E., J. D. DELLINGER & R. B. BUSHNELL (1975): Herd studies on coliform mastitis. J. Am. Vet. Med. Ass. 166, 778–780.
5. MCDONALD, T. J., J. S. MCDONALD & D. L. ROSE (1970): Aerobic gram-negative rods isolated from bovine udder infections. Am J. Vet. Res. 31, 1937–1941.
6. NIAZI, Z. M., G. KIRPAL, G. AMTSBERG & M. REFAI (1977): Biochemie, Serologie. Mäusepathogenität und Antibiotikaresistenz von Klebsiellen verschiedener Tierarten. Berl. Münch. tierärztl. Wschr. 90, 435–440.
7. PITRE, J. (1966): La flore microbienne mise en évidence par la technique de l'écouvillonnage cerveal chez la jument. Rec. Med. Vet. 142, 591–606.
8. PLATT, H., J. ATHERTON & I. ØRSKOV (1976): Klebsiella and Enterobacter isolated from horses. J. Hyg. 77, 401–408.
9. RENK, W. (1962): Mastitiden bei Infektionen mit Escherichia coli, Aerobacter aerogenes und Klebsiella. Zbl. Vet. Med. 9, 264–281.
10. RENKEN-ZÜRNER, A. (1985): Vorkommen und veterinärmedizinische Bedeutung von Bakterien aus der Familie der Enterobacteriaceae mit Ausnahme der Gattungen Escherichia und Salmonella sowie der Species Yersinia pestis. Vet. Med. Diss. Hannover.

4.1.8 Genus: Hafnia (H.)

The genus contains bacteria which resemble *Eb. aerobacter* but do not liquefy gelatine. One species is recognized: *H. alvei* (syn.: *Enterobacter alvei, Enterobacter aerogenes subsp. hafniae*).

These are bacteria of the environment (soil, wa-

4.1.8 Gattung: Hafnia (H.)

Die Gattung enthält *Eb. aerogenes* ähnliche Bakterien, die Gelatine nicht verflüssigen. Es wird eine Art unterschieden: *H. alvei* (Syn.: *Enterobacter alvei, Enterobacter aerogenes subsp. hafniae*).

Das Bakterium kommt in der Umwelt (Erdbo-

Table 58: Biochemical distinction of the genera *Klebsiella* and *Enterobacter* on strains of animal origin (NIAZI et al., 6)

Tabelle 58: Biochemische Unterscheidung der Gattungen *Klebsiella* und *Enterobacter* anhand von Stämmen tierischer Herkunft (NIAZI et al., 6)

Genus	Lac	Ure	LDC	Gel	Mlo	ADH	ODC	Mot
Klebsiella	+ 100 %[1]	+ 99.4 %	+ 94.7 %	− 5.9 %	+ 95.9 %	− 6.4 %	v$^-$ 12.9 %	− 0 %
Enterobacter	v$^+$ 87.5 %	v$^-$ 28.6 %	v$^-$ 33.9 %	v$^+$ 69.6 %	v$^+$ 75 %	v$^+$ 76.8 %	+ 100 %	+ 100 %

[1] Percentage of positive reactions

[1] Prozentsatz positiver Reaktionen

ter, effluent and intestinal content). It is also identified in pathological specimens, but so far it has not been shown to cause disease although it has been isolated from:
▷ horses in cases of abortion (5),
▷ cows in mastitis (1),
other animals, including cold-blooded species (3, 4).

Biochemical properties of *H. alvei* are shown in tables 48 and 59, their comparison with the genera *Enterobacter* and *Serratia* will be found in table 60.

den, Wasser, Abwasser, Darminhalt) vor. Es wird auch in pathologischen Materialien nachgewiesen, ohne daß bisher eine ätiologische Bewertung möglich ist. Solche Isolierungen betreffen:
▷ Pferd: Abort, Endometritis (5),
▷ Rind: Mastitis (1)
und andere Tiere einschließlich Kaltblütler (3, 4).

Die kulturell-biochemischen Eigenschaften von *H. alvei* sind in den Tab. 48 und 59 und im Vergleich zu den Gattungen *Enterobacter* und *Serratia* in der Tab. 60 dargestellt.

Table 59: Biochemical characters of *Hafnia alvei*

Tabelle 59: Kulturell-biochemische Merkmale von *Hafnia alvei*

Ind		−	Gel	−	ODC	+
VPR	22 °C	+	Ure	−	Mlo	v
	35 °C	v	PAD	−	gas from Glu	+
Cit	22 °C	v	LDC	+	Mot	+
	35 °C	−	ADH	−	H_2S	−

Bibliography / Literatur

1. BINDE, M., & O. HERMANSEN (1982): Hafnia alvei in mastitis secretion, a case report. Nor. Veterinaertidsskr. **94**, 569–570.
2. KUME, T. (1962): A case of abortion possibly due to Hafnia organism. J. Hokkaido Vet. Ass. **6**, 1–4.
3. PITRE, J. (1966): La flore microbienne mise en évidence par la technique de l'écouvillonnage cerveal chez la jument. Rec. Méd. Vét. **142**, 591–610.
4. RENKEN-ZÜRNER, A. (1985): Vorkommen und veterinärmedizinische Bedeutung von Bakterien aus der Familie der Enterobacteriaceae mit Ausnahme der Gattungen Escherichia und Salmonella sowie der Spezies Yersinia pestis. Vet. Med. Diss. Hannover.
5. ROJAS, X., & O. ALONSO (1983): Isolation of Hafnia alvei from an aborted equine fetus. Arch. Med. Vet. Chile **15**, 90–91.

Table 60: Biochemical differentiation between the genera *Hafnia*, *Enterobacter* and *Serratia*

Tabelle 60: Kulturell-biochemische Unterscheidungsmerkmale zwischen den Gattungen *Hafnia*, *Enterobacter* und *Serratia*

Characters	Hafnia	Enterobacter	Serratia
Cit	−/(+)	+	+
Gel	−	v	+
LDC	+	v	v
ADH	−	v	−
Raf	−	+	v
Sac	−	+	v
Lac	−	v	v
D-Ado	−	v	v

4.1.9 Genus: Serratia (Sr.)

The following species are members of this genus: *Sr. marcescens* (Syn.: *Bacterium prodigiosum*),

4.1.9 Gattung: Serratia (Sr.)

Innerhalb der Gattung werden unterschieden: *Sr. marcescens* (Syn.: *Bacterium prodigiosum*),

Sr. rubidaea, Sr. liquefaciens, Sr. plymuthica, Sr. odorifera, Sr. ficaria.

The bacteria of this group occur naturally in the soil, in water and in food materials. As a consequence, they can be isolated as contaminants from specimens of animal origin. They are generally considered to be non-pathogenic, although they can occasionally participate in inflammatory conditions; this is particularly the case in *Sr. marcescens*.

Thus, they have been found in:
▷ horses in conjunctivitis, pneumonia, septicaemic diseases, particularly in foals, and in endometritis (1, 9).
▷ cattle in mastitis, where the greatest number of serratia infections are observed, and in abortion (4, 5, 6, 10).

Occasional infections have also been reported in dogs, cats, pigs and other animals. For a summary see (8).

■ Bacteriological properties

The identification of the genus (tab. 48) and of the species (tab. 61) relies on the biochemical characters. The species occurring most commonly in animals are, in descending order of frequency, *Sr. marcescens*, *Sr. rubidaea*, and *Sr. liquefaciens*. The first two are able to produce the red pigment prodigiosin (fig. 141). However, not all biotypes of *Sr. marcescens* have this capacity. The occurrence of the other species is confined mainly to the environment and no information is available about their veterinary significance.

Bibliography / Literatur

1. COLAHAN, P. T., L. C. PEYTON, M. R. CONNELLY & R. PETERSON (1984): Serratia spp. infection in 21 horses. J. Am. Vet. Med. Ass. **185**, 209–211.
2. DEOM, J., & J. MORTELMANS (1953): Etude d'une souche pathogène de Serratia marcescens. Rev. Immunol. **17**, 394–398.
3. FOX, J. G., C. M. BEAUCAGE, C. A. FOLTA & G. W. THORNTON (1981): Nosocomial transmission of Serratia marcescens in a veterinary hospital due to contamination by benzalkonium chloride. J. clin. Microbiol. **14**, 157–160.

Table 61: Biochemical differentiation of *Serratia spp.*

Property	marcescens	liquefaciens	rubidaea
Glu/Ga	+/+	+/v$^+$	+/v$^-$
LDC	+	v$^+$	v$^+$
ODC	+	+	−
H$_2$S	−	−	−
Ind	−	−	−
Ado	v	−	v$^+$
Lac	−	v$^-$	+
Ara	−	+	+
Sor	+	+	−
VPR	+	v	+
Dul	−	−	−
PAD	−	−	−
Ure	v$^-$	−	−
Cit	+	+	v$^+$

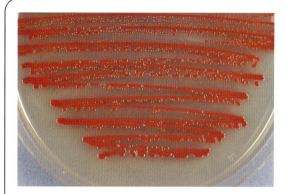
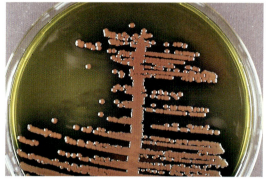
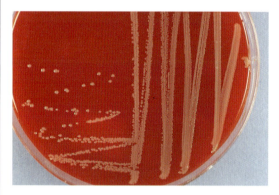
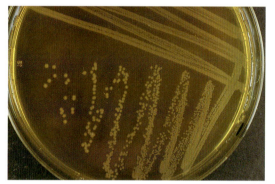

▲ Fig. 141: *Serratia marcescens,* pure culture on nutrient agar, formation of red prodigiosin, 48 h, 37 °C. Magnification x 0.4
▼ Fig. 143: *Serratia liquefaciens,* pure culture on blood agar, no pigmentation, 48 h, 37 °C. Magnification x 0.4

▲ Abb. 141: *Serratia marcescens,* Reinkultur auf Nähragar, Bildung von rotem Prodigiosin, 48 h, 37 °C, Abb.-M. 1 : 2,5
▼ Abb. 143: *Serratia liquefaciens,* Reinkultur auf Blutagar, keine Pigmentbildung, 48 h, 37 °C, Abb.-M. 1 : 2,5

▲ Fig. 142: *Serratia rubidea,* pure culture on Gassner agar, formation of red prodigiosin, lactose-positive colonies, 48 h, 37 °C. Magnification x 0.33
▼ Fig. 144: *Serratia liquefaciens,* pure culture on Gassner agar, lactose-negative colonies, no pigmentation, 48 h, 37 °C. Magnification x 0.4

▲ Abb. 142: *Serratia rubidea,* Reinkultur auf Gaßner-Agar, Bildung von rotem Prodigiosin, lactosepositive Kolonien, 48 h, 37 °C, Abb.-M. 1 : 3
▼ Abb. 144: *Serratia liquefaciens,* Reinkultur auf Gaßner-Agar, lactosenegative Kolonien, keine Pigmentbildung, 48 h, 37 °C, Abb.-M. 1 : 2,5

4. Isaksson, A., & O. Holmberg (1984): Serratia-mastitis in cows as a herd problem. Nord. Vet. Med. **36**, 354–360.
5. Kim, T. J., & B. H. Kim (1979): Biochemical and cultural characteristics and antimicrobial drug sensitivity of cultures of Serratia marcescens isolated from mastitis milk. Korean J. Vet. Publ. Health **3**, 15–21.
6. Nicholls, T. J., & M. G. Barton (1981): Serratia liquefaciens as a cause of mastitis in dairy cows. Vet. Rec. **109**, 288.
7. Pitre, J. (1966): La flore microbienne mise en évidence par la technique de l'écouvillonnage cervecal chez la jument. Rec. Med. Vet. **142**, 591–606.
8. Renken-Zürner, A. (1985): Vorkommen und veterinärmedizinische Bedeutung von Bakterien aus der Familie der Enterobacteriaceae mit Ausnahme der Gattungen Escherichia und Salmonella sowie der Spezies Yersinia pestis. Vet. Med. Diss. Hannover.
9. Shaftoe, S. (1984): Serratia marcescens septicaemia in a neonatal Arabian foal. Equ. Vet. J. **16**, 389–392.
10. Smith, R. E., & I. M. Reynolds (1970): Serratia marcescens associated with bovine abortion. J. Am. Vet. Med. Ass. **157**, 1200–1203.

Table 62: Gram-negative, pigment-producing bacteria which occur in animals

Tabelle 62: Bei Tieren vorkommende gramnegative, pigmentbildende Bakterien

Bacteria	Pigment	Chromopar[1]	Chromophor[2]	Oxi	Mot	Gel	Ind	Lac
Pseudomonas aeruginosa	pyocyanin, blue-green, chloroform-soluble fluorescin, yellow-green, water soluble	+ +	– –	+	+	+	–	–
Pseudomonas fluorescens	fluorescin, yellow-green, water soluble	+	–	+	+	+	–	–
Serratia marcescens	prodigiosin, red only produced at room temperature	–	+	–	+	–	–	–
Serratia rubidaea	prodigiosin red	–	+	–	+	–	–	+
Erwinia	yellow pigment	–	+	–	+	–	–	–
Flavobacterium	yellow pigment	–	+	+	v^+	+	(+)	v
Chromobacterium violaceum	blue-violet pigment	–	+	–	+	+ 7 d 20 °C	–	–

[1] Pigment diffuses into the medium;
[2] Pigment remains confined to colonies

[1] Pigment diffundiert in das Nährmedium;
[2] Pigment bleibt in den Kolonien

4.1.10 Genus: Proteus, Providencia, Morganella

The bacteria belonging to these genera have gone through numerous taxonomic changes. They are widely distributed in nature and participate to a large degree in the breakdown of organic substances. An important habitat is the intestinal tract of man and animals. Accordingly, they are frequently isolated from specimens of animal origin. However, their presence is most frequently merely the result of a clinically unimportant contamination and not of aetiological significance.

PENNER (15) differentiates the following genera:

4.1.10.1 Genus: Proteus (Pr.)

No distinction is usually made between these two species when they are isolated from pathological material, even though this could be done biochemically without much effort (tab. 63). Both bacteria undergo swarming (fig. 146), a phenomenon which

4.1.10 Gattungen: Proteus, Providencia, Morganella

Die Taxonomie der zu diesen Gattungen gehörenden Bakterien hat vielfachen Wandlungen unterlegen. Sie kommen weit verbreitet in der Natur vor, beteiligen sich vielfach am Abbau der organischen Substanz, und ein wichtiger Standort ist der Darm von Mensch und Tier. Dementsprechend werden sie häufig aus tierischen Untersuchungsstoffen isoliert. Ihr Nachweis ist meistens Folge einer klinisch bedeutungslosen Kontamination und selten von ursächlicher Bedeutung für ein Krankheitsgeschehen.

Nach PENNER (15) werden folgende Gattungen und Arten unterschieden:

4.1.10.1 Gattung: Proteus (Pr.)

Zwischen beiden Arten wird bei ihrer Isolierung aus pathologischem Material meistens nicht differenziert, auch wenn dies biochemisch ohne besonderen Aufwand möglich ist (Tab. 63). Bei beiden Bakterienarten handelt es sich um schwärmende Bakte-

Fig. 145–148 see page 198.

Abb. 145–148 siehe Seite 198.

is easily recognized in culture. *Pr. mirabilis* is found more often in animal specimens than *Pr. vulgaris*. They are both facultative pathogens and as such they are responsible for the same disease conditions:
▷ horses: endometritis, urogenital infections (4, 5, 21, 22),
▷ cattle: mastitis, endometritis (6, 7, 11, 14),
▷ calves: sepsis, gastro-enteritis, arthritis (3, 16),
▷ pigs: diarrhoea, MMA-complex, urinary tract infections (1, 2, 8),
▷ dogs and cats: urinary tract infections, cystitis, otitis externa, sepsis (12, 13, 18).

Apart from these, *Proteus spp.* can occasionally be isolated from disease conditions of other animals.

Latent infections of the bull's prepuce are very common, and *Proteus*, being a putrefying agent, is important in food hygiene; it can produce non-specific infections of food materials (19, 20).

■ **Culture** (fig. 146)
These bacteria are not fastidious and will grow on the usual media, a very characteristic feature is the swarming on the surface in the medium.

■ **Biochemical properties** (tab. 63)
A typical feature is the deamination of phenyl-alanine. Only *Pr. mirabilis* does not produce indole. On selective media, these organisms grow as lactose-negative colonies.

■ **Antigenic structure**
Numerous O- and H-antigens are differentiated in the various species, but they are of no importance in diagnosis.

4.1.10.2 Genus: Providencia (Prov.)

Contains the following species: *Prov. alcalifaciens*,

Table 63: Biochemical differentiation of *Pr. mirabilis*, *Pr. vulgaris*, *Providencia* and *Morganella*

Property	Proteus mirabilis	Proteus vulgaris	Providencia	Morganella
Swarming	+	+	−	−
PAD	+	+	+	+
Ind	−	+	+	+
H_2S	+	+	−	−
Gel	+	+	−	−
Cit	v	v⁻	+	−
ODC	+	−	−	+

Prov. stuartii (syn.: *Pr. stuartii*) and *Prov. rettgeri* (syn.: *Pr. rettgeri*).

These bacteria are occasionally isolated from animal material, but there is no conclusive evidence about their pathogenicity. They are similar to *Proteus*, but they do not swarm on solid media (figs. 147 and 148) and they can be distinguished by biochemical means (tab. 63).

4.1.10.3 Genus: Morganella (Mg.)

The species *Mg. morganii* (syn.: *Pr. morganii*), occurs in the faeces of animals and as facultative pathogen it may perhaps be implicated as a cause of enteritis. Biochemical properties are summarized in table 63.

(Syn.: *Pr. stuartii*) und *Prov. rettgeri* (Syn.: *Pr. rettgeri*).

Die Bakterien werden gelegentlich aus tierischen Untersuchungsmaterialien isoliert, sichere Erkenntnisse über ihre Pathogenität liegen nicht vor. Sie sind den *Proteus*-Bakterien ähnlich, zeigen jedoch auf der Kultur kein Ausschwärmen (Abb. 147 u. 148) und lassen sich kulturell-biochemisch abtrennen (Tab. 63).

4.1.10.3 Gattung: Morganella (Mg.)

Mit der Art *Mg. morganii* (Syn.: *Pr. morganii*), die im Kot von Tieren vorkommt und vielleicht als fakultativ pathogenes Bakterium ursächlich an Enteritiden beteiligt sein kann. Kulturell-biochemische Eigenschaften siehe Tab. 63.

Bibliography / Literatur

1. BERNER, H. (1981): Untersuchungen zum Vorkommen von Harnwegsinfektionen beim Schwein. Tierärztl. Umschau **36**, 162–171.
2. BERTSCHINGER, H. U., J. POHLENZ & I. HEMLEP (1977): Untersuchungen über das Mastitis-Metritis-Agalaktie-Syndrom der Sau. II. Bakteriologische Befunde bei Spontanfällen. Schweiz. Arch. Tierhk. **119**, 223–233.
3. BOTES, H. J. W. (1964): Proteus mirabilis as a cause of disease in calves. J. S. Afr. Vet. Med. Ass. **35**, 187–191.
4. COLLINS, S. M. (1961): A study of the incidence of cervical and uterine infection in thoroughbred mares in Ireland. Vet. Rec. **76**, 673–676.
5. DIVERS, T. J., T. D. BRYARS, O. MURCH & C. W. SIGEL (1981): Experimental induction of Proteus mirabilis cystitis in the pony and evaluation of therapy with trimethoprim-sulfadiazine. Am. J. Vet. Res. **42**, 1203–1205.
6. JASPER, D. E., J. D. DELLINGER & R. B. BUSHNELL (1975): Herd studies on coliform mastitis. J. Am. Vet. Med. Ass. **166**, 778–780.
7. KOLEFF, W. K., M. P. BOGDANOFF & S. A. WENEFF (1973): Vergleichende Untersuchungen über die Wirksamkeit verschiedener Antibiotika bei der Therapie von Endometritiden beim Rind. Tierärztl. Umschau **28**, 80–84.
8. LOVEDAY, R. K. (1964): Lactational failure in the sow. J. S. Afr. Vet. Med. Ass. **35**, 229–233.
9. LOVELL, R. (1929): The isolation of Bacterium morgani from the mammals, birds and reptiles in the zoological gardens. J. Path. Bact. **32**, 79–83.
10. MARONPOT, R. R., & L. G. PETERSON (1981): Spontaneous Proteus nephritis among male C3H/HeJ mice. Lab. Anim. Sci. **31**, 697–700.
11. McDONALD, T. J., J. S. McDONALD & D. L. ROSE (1970): Aerobic gramnegative rods isolated from bovine udder infections. Am. J. Vet. Res. **31**, 1937–1941.
12. MURDOCH, D. B., & J. R. BAKER (1977): Bacterial endocarditis in the dog. J. Small Anim. Pract. **18**, 687–699.
13. MORENE, G., C. FIGUEIREDO & C. A. M. LOPES (1975): Bacteriological findings in otitis in dogs. Arg. Inst. Biol. Sao Paulo **42**, 297–300.
14. NYAK, B., I. E. CRAIG & C. L. PADMORE (1981): Gangrenous mastitis in a sow. Mod. Vet. Pract. **62**, 543–544.
15. PENNER, J. L. (1984): Proteus, Morganella. In: Bergey's Manual of Systematic Bacteriology. Vol. 1, S. 491–498. Baltimore, London: Williams & Wilkins.
16. POHL, P. (1975): Présence de Protéus et échecs de l'antibiothérapie dans les diarrhées néonatales du veau. Ann. Méd. Vét. **119**, 435–442.
17. PÜSCHNER, J., & H. TOEPFER (1965): Die Bedeutung des Vorkommens von Proteus-Bakterien bei Schlachttieren. Fleischwirtschaft **45**, 41–47.
18. RIDGEWAY, R. L., J. P. HEGGERS, P. B. JENNINGS & W. J. HUNTER (1978): Hematogenous Bacteroides fragilis and Proteus mirabilis infection in a dog with lymphocytic lymphoma of the spleen. J. Am. Vet. Med. Ass. **172**, 711–713.
19. SEIDL, G. (1957): Über unspezifische Lebensmittelvergiftungen. Arch. Lebensmittelhyg. **8**, 219–220.
20. SZÁZADOS, I. (1980): Bewertung der Keime der Proteus-Gruppe im Rahmen der bakteriologischen Fleischuntersuchung. Fleischwirtschaft **60**, 2058–2062.
21. O'DRISCOLL, J. G., P. T. TROY & F. J. GEOGHEGAN (1977): An epidemic of venereal infection in thoroughbreds. Vet. Rec. **101**, 359–360.
22. O'DRISCOLL, J., J. GEOGHEGAN & P. TROY (1978): Bacillus proteus and CEM. Vet. Rec. **102**, 20.

4.1.11 Genus: Erwinia

This is a very heterogenous group of bacteria which occur mainly in plants and sometimes as plant pathogens. They possess the properties of *Enterobacteriaceae* and produce a yellow pigment on culture (figs. 149 and 150). They are isolated from specimens of animal origin with relative frequency,

4.1.11 Gattung: Erwinia

Es handelt sich um eine sehr heterogene Bakteriengruppe, die hauptsächlich bei Pflanzen und teilweise als Krankheitserreger bei diesen vorkommt. Die Bakterien besitzen die Eigenschaften der *Enterobacteriaceae* und bilden auf der Kultur gelbes Pigment (Abb. 149 u. 150). Sie werden relativ häufig aus

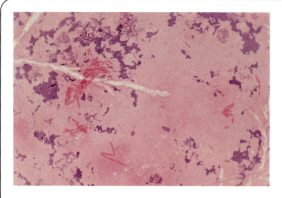
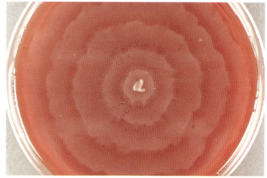
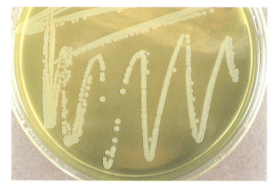
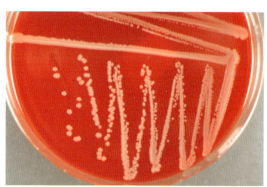

▲ Fig. 145: *Proteus sp.*, smear from urine sediment of a dog. Gram stain, about 10⁶ organisms per ml. Magnification x 1000
▼ Fig. 147: *Providencia (Proteus) rettgeri*, pure culture on Gassner agar, lactose-negative colonies without swarming, 48 h, 37 °C. Magnification x 0.4

▲ Fig. 146: *Proteus vulgaris*, pure culture on blood agar, central spot inoculation leading to wave-like swarming of the bacteria, 48 h, 37 °C. Magnification x 0.5
▼ Fig. 148: *Providencia (Proteus) stuartii*, pure culture on blood agar, no swarming, 48 h, 37 °C. Magnification x 0.4

▲ Abb. 145: *Proteus sp.*, Ausstrich eines Harnsedimentes vom Hund, Gram-Färbung, etwa 10⁶ Keime/ml Abb.-M. 1000:1
▼ Abb. 147: *Providencia (Proteus) rettgeri*, Reinkultur auf einer Gaßner-Platte, lactosenegative Kolonien, kein Ausschwärmen, 48 h, 37 °C, Abb.-M. 1:2,5

▲ Abb. 146: *Proteus vulgaris*, Reinkultur auf Blutagar, nach zentraler punktförmiger Beimpfung, wellenförmiges Ausschwärmen der Bakterien, 48 h, 37 °C, Abb.-M. 1:2
▼ Abb. 148: *Providencia (Proteus) stuartii*, Reinkultur auf Blutagar, kein Ausschwärmen 48 h, 37 °C, Abb.-M. 1:2,5

without there being any evidence about their pathogenicity. It is presumed that the strains isolated from animals, like those from human sources, belong to the *Erwinia herbicola* group, which had also been termed *Enterobacter agglomerans*. Their biochemical properties are listed in table 48.

To this day, the differentiation of this species from *Enterobacter agglomerans* is difficult, if not, in fact, impossible. Strains which are not infrequently isolated from uterine swabs from mares

tierischen Untersuchungsstoffen isoliert, ohne daß gesicherte Kenntnisse über ihre Pathogenität bestehen. Die aus Tieren isolierten Stämme gehören vermutlich ebenso wie die vom Menschen stammenden der *Erwinia herbicola*-Gruppe an, die auch als *Enterobacter agglomerans* bezeichnet wurde. Kulturell-biochemische Eigenschaften siehe Tab. 48.

Die Abgrenzung von *Enterobacter agglomerans* ist bis heute schwierig, wenn nicht unmöglich. Stämme, die aus Uterustupfern von Stuten häufig

Oxidase-negative and fermentative bacteria

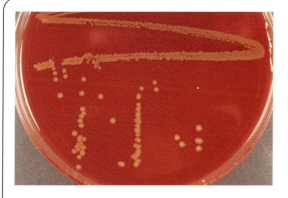
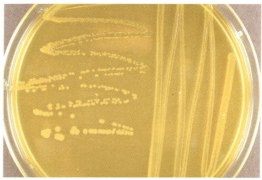
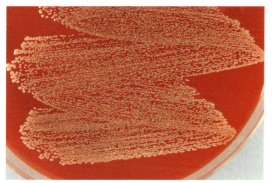
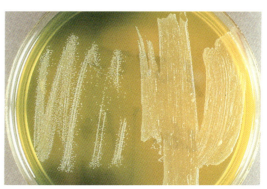

▲ Fig. 149: *Erwinia sp.*, pure culture on blood agar, formation of a yellowish-red pigment, 48 h, 37 °C. Magnification x 0.4
▼ Fig. 151: *Yersinia pseudotuberculosis*, direct culture on blood agar from the liver of a monkey, 48 h, 37 °C. Magnification x 0.4

▲ Fig. 150: *Erwinia sp.*, pure culture on Gassner agar, lactose-negative, yellowish colonies, 48 h, 37 °C. Magnification x 0.4
▼ Fig. 152: *Yersinia pseudotuberculosis*, direct culture on Gassner agar from the organs of a chinchilla, left = spleen, right = liver smear, lactose-negative colonies, 48 h, 37 °C. Magnification x 0.4

▲ Abb. 149: *Erwinia sp.*, Reinkultur auf Blutagar, Bildung eines gelbrötlichen Pigmentes, 48 h, 37 °C, Abb.-M. 1 : 2,5
▼ Abb. 151: *Yersinia pseudotuberculosis*, Direktkultur der Leber eines Affen auf Blutagar, 48 h, 37 °C, Abb.-M. 1 : 2,5

▲ Abb. 150: *Erwinia sp.*, Reinkultur auf einer Gaßner-Platte, lactosenegative Kolonien, Wachstum in gelblichen Kolonien, 48 h, 37 °C, Abb.-M. 1 : 2,5
▼ Abb. 152: *Yersinia pseudotuberculosis*, Direktkultur von Organen eines Chinchillas auf Gaßner-Agar, links Milz-, rechts Leberausstrich, lactosenegative Bakterien, 48 h, 37 °C, Abb.-M. 1 : 2,5

show the biochemical properties listed in table 64. It is doubtful, however, as to whether these characters are representative of all the strains that occur in animals.

zu isolieren sind, weisen die in der Tab. 64 dargestellten Eigenschaften auf. Es bleibt aber fraglich, ob diese Stämme für die insgesamt bei Tieren vorkommenden repräsentativ sind.

Bibliography / Literatur

1. STARR, M. P., & A. K. CHATTERJEE (1972): The genus Erwinia: Enterobacteria pathogenic to plants and animals. Ann. Rev. Microbiol. 26, 389–426.
2. GRAEVENITZ, A. VON (1977): The role of opportunistic bacteria in human disease. Ann. Rev. Microbiol. 31, 447–471.
3. STARR, M. P. (1981): The genus Erwinia. In: The Prokaryotes. Vol. 2, S. 1260–1271. Berlin, Heidelberg, New York: Springer.

Table 64: Biochemical behaviour of *Erwinia* or *Enterobacter agglomerans* strains obtained from cervical swabs of mares

Tabelle 64: Kulturell-biochemisches Verhalten von aus Zervixtupfern von Stuten stammenden *Erwinia* oder *Enterobacter agglomerans*-Stämmen

Glu	+	ODC	−	Sor	−
Glu/Ga	−	H_2S	−	VPR	v
Mot	+	Ind	−	Dul	−
LDC	−	Ado	−	PAD	−
Lac	−	Ure	−	Ara	v^+
Cit	−				

4.1.12 Genus: Yersinia (Y.)

The subclassification of this genus has undergone many changes in the last years. Recent findings, using the DNA hybridization tests have shown that there is a close relationship between *Y. pestis* (causal organism of human plague) and *Y. pseudotuberculosis*, so much so that it has been considered classing them as subspecies of the one species (1, 2).

Y. enterocolitica has for a long time included not only pathogens but also a number of non-pathogenic environmental bacteria (»*Y. enterocolitica*-like bacteria«). Taxonomic investigations have resulted in the exclusion of *Y. frederiksenii*, *Y. kristensenii*, *Y. intermedia* and *Y. aldovae*, all non-pathogenic bacteria of the environment. This means that only pathogenic organisms remain part of *Y. enterocolitica*.

The primary clinical significance in veterinary medicine is attributed to *Y. pseudotuberculosis* (41). The incidence of *Y. enterocolitica* is principally of epidemiological interest in respect of its transmissibility to man (serotypes 0 3, 0 9), because the bacterium produces disease only in chinchillas and hares (serotypes 0 2a, 0 2b, 0 3).

4.1.12.1 Yersinia pseudotuberculosis

■ **Incidence and veterinary significance**

Y. pseudotuberculosis is the cause of pseudotuberculosis or rodentiosis. The organism is more or less widely distributed among wild and domestic animals. Rodents are, however, especially prone and severe losses can occur among hares and wild rabbits (4, 7, 49). The infection is also found in many types of birds (summary 10, 19) and both wild and domestic birds are susceptible. In the latter, canaries and turkeys are primarily affected (12, 16, 21, 52). Isolated cases of disease and frequent latent intestinal infections occur in farm animals such as horses, cattle, pigs, sheep, goats etc. (6, 13, 22, 26, 27, 31, 32, 35, 46). Infections appear to be rare also in dogs, while they occur more frequently in cats (25, 34, 51).

The clinical picture is not uniform in animals and can vary from species to species. It ranges from the

acute form, a septicaemia with severe generalized symptoms, to a latent infection of the digestive tract and in particular of the tonsils. In the acute form the pathological changes are confined to enlargement of the spleen, and various lymph nodes as well as enteritis. In the subacute to chronic course, which is frequently observed in rodents, tuberculosis-like nodules develop in the liver, spleen, kidneys, lungs and lymph nodes. They are millet to hazel nut-sized with a dry caseous content.

Less common symptoms encountered in ruminants are abortion, mastitis, respiratory diseases, which have also been found in foals. Orchitis and epididymitis occur in sheep (15, 22, 27, 30, 43, 44).

In children and adolescents mesenteric lymphadenitis, acute terminal ileitis and appendicitis may develop and enteritis, rarely septicaemia, is seen in adults.

■ Morphology
Y. pseudotuberculosis is an ovoid or more elongated, pleomorphic bacillus, which measures 0.4–0.8 × 0.8–6.0 µm and is motile at 22 °C. Its bipolar staining reaction is inconsistent and without diagnostic value.

■ Culture (figs. 151 and 152)
Y. pseudotuberculosis is culturally not fastidious and will grow on blood agar and the usual media used for growing *Enterobacteriaceae*, such as Gassner plates. After 48 hours the colonies become greyish-white to greyish-yellow and opaque. On Gassner plates the bacterium is lactose-negative.

The most favourable incubation temperature is between 24 °C and 37 °C and most rapid growth occurs at 28–30 °C. Cold enrichment is possible at 2–4 °C.

An increasing proportion of R-forms is produced at temperatures above 30 °C; such colonies are dry and flat. Motile bacteria can be expected only in the smooth form, grown at temperatures up to 28 °C.

Difficulties can arise in the cultural isolation from material with mixed infection, because little is known so far about the most advantageous enrichment and selective media. WEBER et al. (46) were able to demonstrate *Y. pseudotuberculosis* with the Schiemann selective agar.

■ Biochemical properties
The various characters are shown in figure 153. It is

Specimens
Intestinal content, organ and milk samples etc.

Isolation on culture

1. Cold enrichment may be necessary,
   Phosphate buffered saline, pH 7.6,
   Incubation 3 weeks at 4 °C, weekly subculture onto media as in (2)
2. Direct culture on:
   Blood agar (fig. 151)
   Gassner agar, very delicate, lactose-negative colonies (fig. 152),
   Desoxycholate-citrate agar,
   Salmonella-shigella agar, and others.
   Yersinia selective medium of Schiemann (p. 204).
   Incubation temperature 37 °C and perhaps additionally 22 °C

Biochemical differentiation

1. Generic characters

Ara	+	Mal	+	MR	+
Dul	−	Raf	−	Cat	+
Gal	+	Cit	−	Oxi	−
Dex	+	Gel	−	PAD	−
Inu	−	Ure (72 h)	+	β-galactosidase	+
Lac	−	H_2S	−	ODC	−
Man	+	Nit	+	LDC	−

Motility at 22 °C + at 37 °C −

2. Differentiation between Y. pseudotuberculosis and Y. enterocolitica

	Y. pseudotuberculosis	Y. enterocolitica
Indole	−	v
Ornithine decarboxylase	−	+
Aesculin	+	−
Adonitol	+	−
Maltose	+	−
Rhamnose	+	−
Salicin	+	−
Saccharose	−	+
Sorbitol	−	+
Xylose	−	v

Antigenic pattern

O-group	O-subgroup	O-antigen	H-antigen	cross reaction with O-antigen
I	B	2, 3	a, c	−
	B	2, 4	a, c	−
II	A	5, 6	a, d	Salmonella of group B
	B	5, 7	a, d	(04, 027)
III	−	8	a	−
IV	A	9, 11	b, a, b	Salmonella of group D
	B	9, 12	a, b, d	(09, 046) and group H (014) E. coli 077, 017
V	A	10, 14	a, a, e (b)	
	B	10, 15	a	
VI		13	a	E. coli 055

Fig. 153: Isolation and identification of *Yersinia pseudotuberculosis*

Abb. 153: Nachweis und Differenzierung von *Yersinia pseudotuberculosis*

not possible to differentiate the serogroups by means of their biochemical properties.

■ **Antigenic structure**

Y. pseudotuberculosis possesses 15 O-antigens which can be utilized to differentiate 6 non-cross-reacting O-groups (I to VI). Four of these are further divided into two subgroups (A, B; fig. 153). The O-antigen 1 (»rough antigen«) occurs in all serotypes, and this results in cross reactions within the species *Y. pseudotuberculosis* and between it and *Y. pestis* (KNAPP & WEBER, 19; THAL and KNAPP, 42). Serogroup I occurs in 70–80 % of animal infections with *Y. pseudotuberculosis* and about 10–20 % involve serogroups II and III. Strains of serogroups IV and V are rare in Europe and serogroup VI does not occur there at all. There are no fundamental differences between the distribution of the serogroups in man and animals.

4.1.12.2 Yersinia enterocolitica
(Syn.: *Pasteurella enterocolitica, Pasteurella X*)

■ **Incidence and veterinary significance**

In the past this species included strains which differed considerably not only in their properties but also in their clinical significance. It is important, for bacteriological and epidemiological reasons, to separate from other members of this species strains with markedly divergent properties, which were previously identified as *Y. enterocolitica*-like or atypical. Based on DNA hybridization experiments they are designated as new species *(Y. frederiksenii, Y. kristensenii, Y. intermedia)* (p. 206).

Y. enterocolitica, in the strict sense, has been identified in many animal species over the years (pig, horse, ox, sheep, goat, dog, cat, rodents etc.) (for a survey see WINBLAD, 50). The occurrence in these species is usually not associated with any evidence of disease; they are invaders of the gut and clinically latent. Clinical manifestations therefore occur only in isolated animals and they have been reported in chinchillas, hares, monkeys, goats and sheep, where they produced either generalized infections or enteritis (18, 25, 28, 50).

In man, on the other hand, certain strains of characteristic biotype and antigenic structure produce clinical symptoms. These are in serogroups O3, O9 and O8 (after WINBLAD & WAUTERS, 50), which are members of biotypes 4, 2 and 1.

The presence in animals of these human pathogens is of special interest in demonstrating cross infections. They are found most frequently in pigs (up to about 10 %) and serotype O3 is more common than O9 (3, 11, 14, 23, 31, 47, 53). However, numerous other serotypes are also encountered be-

sides these, but they are probably of no pathogenic significance to man (18). Figure 154 presents an example of the most common serotypes.

Yersinias have been isolated repeatedly from foods of animal origin, including milk, but most of the isolates are not pathogenic to man (24, 40).

Infections of human infants can lead to gastroenteritis, in children and adolescents acute terminal ileitis, mesenteric lymphadenitis and pseudo-appendicitis are produced, while in adults the infection may induce acute enteritis. Possible complications are erythema nodosa, arthritis, acute glomerulonephritis, myocarditis and generalized infections (17, 18, 29, 50). The epidemiological connections between animal and human yersiniosis are still not entirely resolved, but it is possible that the different species are infected from a common source (sapronosis, 45).

■ Culture

Y. enterocolitica will grow on blood agar and the usual substrates used for the identification of salmonellae. However, growth is slower and 48 hours are required to produce colonies as large as those of *E. coli*. The optimum temperature is around 28 °C and, therefore, the colonies which develop in 24–36 hours at 37 °C are relatively small. Selective media are employed when attempting to isolate *Y. enterocolitica* from specimens. Some such media are obtainable commercially. The medium of Schiemann (fig. 154; 33, 46), which appears to be suitable also for the isolation of *Y. pseudotuberculosis*, has been found very effective. It is an established fact that the number of isolations increases when several selective media are used in parallel.

A preceding cold enrichment (phosphate buffered saline, pH 7.6, storage temperature +4 °C; fig. 154) can considerably improve the results of the cultural examination.

■ Biochemical properties

Are summarized in figure 154 and table 64.

■ Antigenic structure

57 O-factors, 6 K-antigens and 19 H-antigens have so far been identified, if the *Y.-enterocolitica*-like strains are included. The O-factors can be identified in agglutination test with autoclaved cultures. The human pathogenic strains have been biochemically and serologically defined with certainty and they

Infektionsbeziehungen von besonderem Interesse. Am häufigsten (bis zu etwa 10 %) werden sie beim Schwein gefunden, dabei ist der Serotyp 03 häufiger als der Serotyp 09 (3, 11, 14, 23, 31, 47, 53). Daneben kommen zahlreiche andere Serotypen vor, denen aber eine pathogene Bedeutung für den Menschen wahrscheinlich nicht zukommt (18). Über die schwerpunktmäßige Verteilung der Serotypen gibt die Abb. 154 ein Beispiel.

Yersinien sind wiederholt aus Lebensmitteln tierischer Herkunft einschließlich Milch isoliert worden, doch gehören die meisten Isolate nicht den humanpathogenen Typen an (24, 40).

Beim Menschen kann die Infektion bei Kleinkindern zu einer Gastroenteritis, bei Kindern und Jugendlichen zu akuter terminaler Ileitis, *Lymphadenitis mesenterialis,* Pseudoappendizitis und bei Erwachsenen zu *Enteritis acuta* führen. Mögliche Komplikationen sind *Erythema nodosum,* Arthritis, *Glomerulonephritis acuta,* Myokarditis, Allgemeininfektion (17, 18, 29, 50). Die epidemiologischen Zusammenhänge zwischen der Tier- und Menschenyersiniose sind noch weitgehend ungeklärt, möglicherweise bestehen gleiche Infektionsquellen (Sapronose; 45).

■ Kultur

Y. enterocolitica wächst auf Blutagar und auf den üblichen zum Salmonellennachweis benutzten Substraten. Das Wachstum ist jedoch langsamer, und erst nach 48 h sind die Kolonien etwa so groß wie die der Colibakterien. Das Temperaturoptimum liegt bei 28 °C, daher sind die innerhalb von 24–36 h bei 37 °C gebildeten Kolonien relativ klein. Für die gezielte Isolierung von *Y. enterocolitica* aus einem Untersuchungsmaterial werden jedoch bevorzugt Selektivmedien benutzt, die zum Teil im Handel erhältlich sind. Am besten bewährt hat sich das Medium nach Schiemann (Abb. 154; 33, 46), das offenbar auch für den Nachweis von *Y. pseudotuberculosis* geeignet ist. Grundsätzlich gilt, daß mit der Parallelverwendung mehrerer Selektivmedien die Zahl der Isolierungen steigt.

Das Ergebnis der kulturellen Untersuchung kann wesentlich durch die Vorschaltung einer Kälteanreicherung (phosphatgepufferte NaCl-Lösung, pH 7,6, Aufbewahrungstemperatur +4 °C; Abb. 154) verbessert werden.

■ Kulturell-biochemische Eigenschaften

Sind in der Abb. 154 und in der Tab. 64 zusammengestellt.

■ Antigenstruktur

Unter Einbeziehung von *Y. enterocolitica*-ähnlichen Stämmen sind bisher 57 O-Faktoren, 6 K-Antigene und 19 H-Antigene festgestellt worden. Die O-Faktoren lassen sich in der Agglutination mit autoklavierten Kulturen nachweisen. Biochemisch und serologisch sicher definiert sind in erster Linie die

belong to the biotypes 2, 3 and 4. KNAPP & THAL (20) have drawn up a simplified survey of the O-groups of the human pathogenic strains; these are depicted in figure 154 along with their properties. A similar classification was suggested by WINBLAD (50).

Distinct antigenic relationships exist between *Y. enterocolitica* (serotype 09) and brucellae (p. 256).

humanpathogenen Stämme, die den Biotypen 2, 3 und 4 angehören. In vereinfachter Übersicht haben KNAPP & THAL (20) für die humanpathogenen Stämme O-Gruppen aufgestellt, die mit ihren Eigenschaften aus der Abb. 154 ersichtlich sind. Eine ähnliche Einteilung wurde von WINBLAD (50) vorgeschlagen.

Deutliche antigene Beziehungen bestehen zwischen *Y. enterocolitica* (Serotyp 09) und Brucellen

---

Specimens
Homogenized tonsillar tissue, faecal samples intestinal content, food materials etc.

Isolation by culture

1. Enrichment:
   Cold enrichment in phosphate buffered saline for up to 3 weeks at +4 °C, weekly subculture to selective plates; modified Rappaport broth after Wauters (contains malachite green, carbenicillin and other inhibitors), for 2 days incubation at room temperature, then subculture on selective solid media.
2. Selective solid media:
   Either direct culture or subculture from enrichment broth, Selective media for enterobacteria are suitable e. g. Gassner agar, salmonella-shigella agar, Leifson agar, Sodium desoxycholate-citrate-mannitol agar, MacConkey agar. The medium of Schiemann has proved especially useful, it contains cefsulodin, irgasan, novobiocin (Oxoid supplement) for the suppression of contaminants. The colonies have a characteristic appearance: a dark red centre surrounded by a clear zone (fig. 157). On the medium of Wauters yersinia grow as colourless, shiny colonies (fig. 158). Incubation 24–48 hours at 37 °C.

Biochemical differentiation

1. Rapid differentiation of suspect colonies:
   Glucose fermentation without gas formation
   Motility at 22 °C but not at 37 °C
   Urease positiv
   With triple sugar iron agar a yellow colour develops on slope surface and butt
2. Generic properties are listed in figure 153.
3. Differentiation between Y. enterocolitica and Y. pseudotuberculosis is presented in fig. 153.

Characteristics of *Y. enterocolitica* serogroups pathogenic to man

	O-groups			
	3^1 $I^{2,3}$	9^1 $V^{2,4}$	8^1 $VI^{2,5}$	$5,27^1$ $IV^{2,6}$
Indole	−	−	+	(+)
Lecithinase	−	−	+	−
Ornithine decarboxylase	+	+	+	+
Urease	+	+	+	+
Xylose	−	+	+	+
Saccharose	+	+	+	+
Lactose	−	−	−	−
Rhamnose	−	−	−	−
Melibiose	−	−	−	−
Raffinose	−	−	−	−
Citrate (25 °C)	−	−	−	−

[1] After Winblad/Wauters; [2] After Knapp/Thal; [3] causes 60–75 % and; [4] 25–40 % of human infections in Europe; [5] occurs almost exclusively in the USA; [6] is very rare

Fig. 154: Demonstration and isolation of *Yersinia enterocolitica* (after KNAPP, 17; KNAPP & THAL, 20)

Abb. 154: Nachweis und Differenzierung von *Yersinia enterocolitica* (nach KNAPP, 17; KNAPP & THAL, 20)

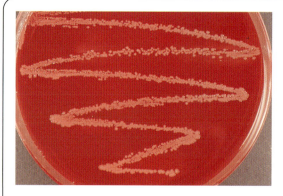
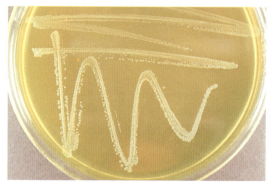
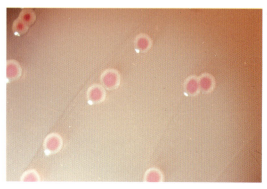
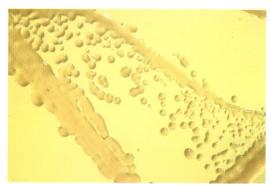

▲ Fig. 155: *Yersinia enterocolitica*, pure culture on blood agar, 48 h, 37 °C. Magnification x 0.4
▼ Fig. 157: *Yersinia enterocolitica*, pure culture on Schiemann selective medium (Oxoid), containing sodium desoxycholate and antibiotics to inhibit contaminants, red colonies with surrounding clear area, 48 h, 32 °C. Magnification x 2

▲ Abb. 155: *Yersinia enterocolitica*, Reinkultur auf Blutagar, 48 h, 32 °C, Abb.-M. 1 : 2,5
▼ Abb. 157: *Yersinia enterocolitica*, Reinkultur auf der Selektivplatte nach Schiemann (Oxoid), enthält Na-Desoxycholat, und Antibiotika zur Hemmung der Begleitflora, rote Kolonien mit einem klaren Hof, 48 h, 32 °C, Abb.-M. 2 : 1

▲ Fig. 156: *Yersinia enterocolitica*, pure culture on Gassner medium, lactose-negative colonies, 48 h, 32 °C. Magnification x 0.4
▼ Fig. 158: *Yersinia enterocolitica*, pure culture on Wauters selective medium (Merck), contains sodium desoxycholate, ox bile, brilliant green and a high citrate concentration for inhibition of contaminant inhibition, 48 h, 32 °C. Magnification x 2.6

▲ Abb. 156: *Yersinia enterocolitica*, Reinkultur auf einer Gaßner-Platte, lactosenegative Kolonien, 48 h, 32 °C, Abb.-M. 1 : 2,5
▼ Abb. 158: *Yersinia enterocolitica*, Reinkultur auf der Selektivplatte nach Wauters (Merck), enthält Na-Desoxycholat, Ochsengalle, Brillantgrün und hohe Citratkonzentration zur Hemmung der Begleitflora, 48 h, 32 °C, Abb.-M. 2,6 : 1

There are further antigenic associations with *Salmonella urbana* (O30) and *Morganella morganii*.

4.1.12.3 Y. frederiksenii, Y. intermedia, Y. kristensenii

These species include strains which differ fundamentally in their biochemical properties from *Y. en-*

(S. 256). Weitere Antigengemeinschaften bestehen mit *Salmonella urbana* (O30) und *Morganella morganii*.

4.1.12.3 Yersinia frederiksenii, Y. intermedia, Y. kristensenii

Unter diesen Artbezeichnungen werden Stämme zusammengefaßt, die sich von *Yersinia enterocoliti-*

Table 65: Biochemical differentiation between *Yersinia enterocolitica, frederiksenii, intermedia* and *kristensenii* (40)

Properties[1]	enterocolitica biotypes 1–4	5	frederiksenii	intermedia	kristensenii
Nit	+	−	+	+	+
VPR	+	+	+	+	−
Cel	+	+	+	+	+
Sac	+	+	+	+	−
Tre	+	+	+	+	+
Rha	−	+	+	+	−
Mel	−	−	−	+	−
Methyl glucoside	−	−	−	+	−
ODC	+	+	+	+	+
Ind	v	+	+	+	+
Sbs	+	+	+	+	+
Sor	+	+	+	+	+
Raf	−	−	−	+	−
Cit	−	v	v	+	−
Mal	+	+	+	+	+

[1] Assessment of reaction after 72 hours

terocolitica. In the literature they are also referred to as *Y. enterocolitica*-like or atypical strains. Apart from the above-named species there are other groups which fall into this category, but which have not been conclusively defined. They occur in many animal species, in their surroundings, in surface water and effluent. Most of the strains isolated from food materials, including milk, belong to this group. If they are of any medical importance at all, they are merely opportunists. Their clinical veterinary significance is largely unknown.

For biochemical properties see table 64. Rhamnose-positive strains are often isolated (18, 40, 50).

4.1.12.4 Yersinia ruckeri

This bacterium is the cause of enteric red mouth disease in trout and other salmonids (38). The course of this condition can vary from acute to chronic and the main signs are inflammation in the mouth region, enteritis and haemorrhages into the intestinal wall, haemorrhagic and ulcerative dermatitis and petechial haemorrhages at the base of the fins (9, 37, 39). In the Federal Republic of Germany the disease was first encountered by FUHRMANN (9) in trout, carp and eels.

Y. ruckeri can be grown on blood agar and the media normally used for demonstrating Enterobacteriaceae (e.g. Gassner plates). They are incubated at 25 °C to 28 °C (figs. 159 and 160). The biochemical properties (8, 9, 30) are shown in table 66.

Table 66: Biochemical properties of *Yersinia ruckeri* at incubation temperature of 25 °C for 48 h (9)

Tabelle 66: Kulturell-biochemische Eigenschaften von *Yersinia ruckeri* bei einer Bebrütungstemperatur von 25 °C/48 h (9)

Oxi	−	Nit	+
O/F (Glu)	+/+	VPR	+ 37 °C/48 h
Cat	+	MR	+
H₂S	−	Glu/Ga	+/v
Gel	+	Lac	−
Ure	v	Sac	−
LDC	+ 37 °C/48 h	Ara	−
ODC	+ 37 °C/48 h	Mal	v
PAD	−	Rha	−
Cit	+ 7 d	Tre	−
Ind	−		

Bibliography / Literatur

1. BERCOVIER, H., H. H. MOLLARET, J. M. ALONSO, J. BRAULT, G. R. FANNING, A. G. STEIGERWALT & D. J. BRENNER (1980): Intra- and interspecies relatedness of Yersinia pestis by DNA hybridization and its relationship to Yersinia pseudotuberculosis. Curr. Microbiol. **4**, 225–229.
2. BOCKEMÜHL, J., & H. P. R. SEELIGER (1985): Die Auswirkungen neuer taxonomischer Erkenntnisse auf die Nomenklatur von bakteriellen Seuchenerregern. Bundesgesundheitsbl. **28**, 65–69.
3. BOCKEMÜHL, J., H. SCHMITT, J. ROTH & E. SAUPE (1979): Die jahreszeitliche Häufigkeit der Ausscheidung von Yersinia enterocolitica im Kot gesunder Schweine. Zbl. Bakt. I. Orig. A **244**, 494–505.
4. BRÖMEL, J., & K. ZETTL (1976): Ergebnisse mehrjähriger Wilduntersuchungen im nordhessischen Raum. Prakt. Tierarzt **57**, 246–249.
5. CHRISTENSEN, S. G. (1981): Isolation and identification of Yersinia enterocolitica. Nord. Vet. Med. **33**, 210–217.
6. DEE, W. (1985): Yersinia pseudotuberculosis — Aborterreger beim Rind. Mh. Vet. Med. **40**, 721–722.
7. DINGELDEIN, W., & W. A. VALDER (1978): Infektionskrankheiten bei Hase und Wildkaninchen. Prakt. Tierarzt **59**, 347–352.
8. EWING, W. H., A. J. ROSS, D. J. BRENNER & G. R. FANNING (1978): Yersinia ruckeri sp. now., the redmouth bacterium. Int. J. Syst. Bact. **28**, 37–44.
9. FUHRMANN, H., K. H. BÖHM & H. J. SCHLOTFELD (1983): An outbreak of enteric redmouth disease in West Germany. J. Fish Dis. **6**, 309–311.
10. GLÜNDER, G., K. H. HINZ & A. WEBER (1986): Zum Vorkommen von Yersinien in Vögeln. Dtsch. tierärztl. Wschr. **93**, 27–29.
11. HAWARI, A. D., G. AMTSBERG & G. KIRPAL (1981): Kulturelle und serologische Untersuchungen zum Vorkommen von Yersinia-enterocolitica-Infektionen bei Schweinen und Rindern. Berl. Münch. tierärztl. Wschr. **94**, 404–409.
12. HINZ, K. H., E. F. KALETA, B. STIBUREK, G. GLÜNDER & K. GESSLER (1981): Eine durch Yersinia pseudotuberculosis bei Mastputen verursachte Myopathie. Dtsch. tierärztl. Wschr. **88**, 352–354.
13. HODGES, R. T., & M. G. CARMAN (1985): Recovery of Yersinia pseudotuberculosis from the faeces of healthy cattle. N.Z. Vet. J. **33**, 175–176.
14. HUNTER, D., S. HUGHES & E. FOX (1983): Isolation of Yersinia enterocolitica from pigs in the United Kingdom. Vet. Rec. **112**, 322–323.
15. JAMIESON, S., & M. A. SOLTYS (1947): Infectious epididymo-orchitis of rams associated with Pasteurella pseudotuberculosis. Vet. Rec. **59**, 351–353.
16. KILIAN, J. G., R. YAMAMOTO, W. E. BABCOCK & E. M. DICKINSON (1962): An unusual aspect of Pasteurella pseudotuberculosis in turkeys. Avian Dis. **6**, 403–405.
17. KNAPP, W. (1984): Die Gattung Yersinia — Yersiniosen. In: H. BRANDIS & H. J. OTTE (Hrsg.): Lehrbuch der medizinischen Mikrobiologie. 5. Aufl., S. 304–317. Stuttgart: Gustav Fischer.
18. KNAPP, W. (1983): Yersinia enterocolitica. Bundesgesundheitsbl. **26**, 381–389.
19. KNAPP, W., & A. WEBER (1982): Yersinia pseudotuberculosis. In: H. BLOBEL & TH. SCHLIESSER (Hrsg.): Handbuch der bakteriellen Infektionen bei Tieren. Bd. IV, S. 466–518. Jena: VEB Gustav Fischer.
20. KNAPP, W., & E. THAL (1973): Die biochemische Charakterisierung von Yersinia enterocolitica (syn.: Pasteurella X) als Grundlage eines vereinfachten O-Antigenschemas. Zbl. Bakt. I. Orig. A **223**, 88–105.
21. KRAUSS, H., & L. HENSEL (1961): Pseudotuberkulose bei Enten. Dtsch. tierärztl. Wschr. **68**, 144–146.
22. LANGFORD, E. V. (1969): Pasteurella pseudotuberculosis associated with abortion and pneumonia in the bovine. Can. Vet. J. **10**, 208–211.
23. LEEMANN, R. (1979): Nachweis von Yersinia enterocolitica in Kotproben von Schlachtschweinen. Zbl. Vet. Med. B, **26**, 214–221.
24. LEISTNER, L. (1975): Nachweis von Yersinia enterocolitica in Faeces und Fleisch von Schweinen, Rindern und Geflügel. Fleischwirtschaft **55**, 1599–1602.
25. LOTT-SCHOLZ, G. (1979): Yersiniose bei Heimtieren. Kleintierpraxis **26**, 97–99.
26. MAIR, N. S., & G. S. ZIFFO (1974): Isolation of Y. pseudotuberculosis from a foal. Vet. Rec. **94**, 152–153.
27. MAIR, N. S., & J. F. HARBOURNE (1963): The isolation of Pasteurella pseudotuberculosis from a bovine fetus. Vet. Rec. **75**, 559–561.
28. MCSPORRAN, K. D., L. M. HANSEM, B. W. SAUNDERS & A. DAMSTEEGT (1984): An outbreak of diarrhoea in hoggets associated with infection by Yersinia enterocolitica. N.Z. Vet. J. **32**, 38–39.
29. MASSHOFF, W. (1962): Die Pseudotuberkulose des Menschen. Dtsch. tierärztl. Wschr. **87**, 915–920.
30. MESSERLI, J. (1972): Yersinia pseudotuberculosis, Erreger einer Mastitis beim Rind. Zbl. Bakt. I. Orig. A **222**, 280–282.
31. NARUCKA, K., & J. F. WESTERDOORP (1977): Een onderzek naar het voorkomen van Yersinia enterocolitica en Yersinia pseudotuberculosis bij klinisch normale varkens. Tijdschr. Diergeneesk. **102**, 299–303.
32. NATTERMANN, H., F. HORSCH, M. SEEGER, W. DEE, C. SCHLINGMANN & H. SCHLINGMANN (1985): Epizootologie der Yersinia-enterocolitica-Infektion in einem Schweinebestand. Mh. Vet. Med. **40**, 366–370.
33. PRIMAVESI, C. A., & A. LORRA-EBERTS (1983): Erfahrungen mit einem neu entwickelten Selektiv-Agar nach Schiemann zum Nachweis von Yersinia enterocolitica. Lab. med. **7**, 59–61.

34. Rahko, T., & H. Saloniemi (1969): Beobachtungen über die Pathologie der natürlichen Yersinia pseudotuberculosis Infektion bei der Katze. Dtsch. tierärztl. Wschr. 76, 611–613.
35. Reuss, U. (1962): Enzootisches Auftreten der Rodentiose in einem Schweinebestand. Berl. Münch. tierärztl. Wschr. 75, 203–204.
36. Ross, A. J., & R. R. Rucker (1966): Description of a bacterium associated with redmouth disease of rainbow trout. Can. J. Microbiol. 12, 763–770.
37. Rübsamen, S., & J. Weis (1985): Nachweis von Enteric Redmouth Disease bei Regenbogenforellen, Salmo gairdneri Richardson, in Südbaden. Tierärztl. Umschau 40, 995–998.
38. Rucker, R. R. (1966): Redmouth Disease of rainbow trout. Bull. Off. Int. Epizoot. 65, 825–830.
39. Schlotfeld, H. J., K. H. Böhm, F. Pfortmüller & K. Pfortmüller (1985): »Rotmaulseuche«/ERM (Enteric Redmouth Disease) der Forelle und anderer Nutzfische in Nordwestdeutschland. Vorkommen, Therapie, Vakzinierungsergebnisse. Tierärztl. Umschau 40, 985–995.
40. Stengel, E. (1984): Vorkommen von Yersinia enterocolitica in Milch und Milchprodukten. Arch. Lebensmittelhyg. 35, 91–95.
41. Thal, E. (1974): Genus Yersinia — Veterinärmedizinische Bedeutung und bakteriologische Diagnostik. Berl. Münch. tierärztl. Wschr. 87, 212–214.
42. Thal, E., & W. Knapp (1971): A revised antigenic scheme of Yersinia pseudotuberculosis. Symp. Ser. immunbiol. Stand. 15, 219–222.
43. Ulsen, F. W. van (1960): Abortus beim Rind durch Salmonella und Listeria. Dtsch. tierärztl. Wschr. 67, 425–429.
44. Watson, W. A., & D. Hunter (1960): The isolation of Pasteurella pseudotuberculosis from an ovine fetus. Vet. Rec. 72, 770–777.
45. Weber, A. (1983): Welche Rollen spielen Heimtiere im Zusammenhang mit enteralen Yersiniosen beim Menschen? Prakt. Tierarzt 64, 666–672.
46. Weber, A., C. Lembke & R. Schäfer (1983): Vergleichende Anwendung von zwei im Handel erhältlichen Selektivnährböden zur Isolierung von Yersinia enterocolitica aus Tonsillen von Schlachtschweinen. Zbl. Vet. Med. B, 30, 532–536.
47. Weber, A., & W. Knapp (1981): Nachweis von Yersinia enterocolitica und Yersinia pseudotuberculosis in Kotproben gesunder Schlachtschweine in Abhängigkeit von der Jahreszeit. Zbl. Vet. Med. B, 28, 407–413.
48. Weber, A., & C. Lembke (1981): Vergleichende Anwendung von zwei Anreicherungsverfahren und fünf Selektivnährböden zur Isolierung von Yersinia enterocolitica aus Tonsillen von Schlachtschweinen. Zbl. Bakt. I. Orig. A, 250, 72–77.
49. Weidenmüller, H. (1959): Zur Rodentiose bei Tier und Mensch. Tierärztl. Umschau 14, 256–259.
50. Winblad, S. (1982): Yersinia enterocolitica. In: H. Blobel & Th. Schliesser (Hrsg.): Handbuch der bakteriellen Infektionen bei Tieren. Bd. 4, S. 519–535. Jena: VEB Gustav Fischer.
51. Winkenwerder, W. (1968): Zur Epizootiologie der Pseudotuberkulose bei einigen Haus- und Zootieren. Int. Symp. Pseudotuberk., Paris 1967, Symp. Ser. Immunbiol. Standard. 9, 69–74.
52. Wise, D. R., & P. K. Uppal (1972): Osteomyelitis in turkeys caused by Yersinia pseudotuberculosis. J. Med. Microbiol. 5, 128–130.
53. Wuthe, H. H., G. Schulz-Lell, I. Böhlck & S. Aleksśić (1982): Ergebnisse von kulturellen Untersuchungen auf Yersinia enterocolitica in Proben von Menschen und Schweinen in Schleswig-Holstein. Berl. Münch. tierärztl. Wschr. 95, 288–292.

5 Oxidase-negative and oxidative or glucose-inactive bacteria

(reaction type II b and II c)

5.1 Genus: Acinetobacter (A.)

This genus falls within the family Neisseriaceae (tab. 46).
These bacteria are widely distributed in the environment, in soil and in water. Therefore the members are isolated with relative frequency from specimens of animal origin. So far, little is known about their pathogenicity for animals. In the majority of cases the isolates are of no aetiological significance. But the following disease conditions have been associated with *Acinetobacter* as the cause:
Myositis, septicaemia and haematuria in the horse (10), bronchopneumonia in mink and rabbits (7, 9), septicaemic diseases of dogs (3) and pigs (3), as well as abortion in horses, cattle, buffalo and pigs (3, 5, 11) and infertility of mares (1).
A. calcoaceticus is the only species within this genus.

5 Oxidasenegative und oxidative oder glucoseinaktive Bakterien

(Reaktionstypen II b und II c)

5.1 Gattung: Acinetobacter (A.)

Taxonomisch gehört die Gattung zur Familie der Neisseriaceae (Tab. 46). Es handelt sich um Bakterien, die in der Umwelt, im Erdboden und im Wasser verbreitet vorkommen. Daher können sie relativ häufig in tierischen Untersuchungsstoffen nachgewiesen werden. Über ihre Pathogenität für Tiere ist bisher wenig bekannt. Überwiegend haben die Funde bei Tieren keine ätiologische Bedeutung. Bisher sind folgende Krankheitsprozesse mit Acinetobacter in ursächlichen Zusammenhang gebracht worden:
Myositis, Septikämie, Hämaturie bei Pferden (10), Bronchopneumonien bei Nerzen und Kaninchen (7, 9), septikämische Erkrankungen bei Hunden (3) und Schweinen (3) sowie Aborte bei Pferden, Rindern, Büffeln und Schweinen (3, 5, 11) und Unfruchtbarkeit der Stuten (1).
A. calcoaceticus ist die einzige Art der Gattung.

210 Gram-negative, aerobic or microaerophilic or facultatively anaerobic rods, with simple cultural requirements

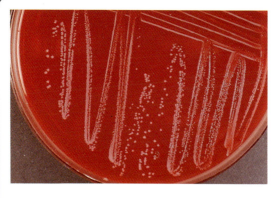
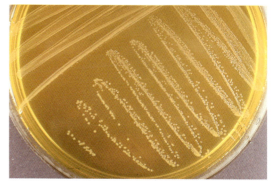
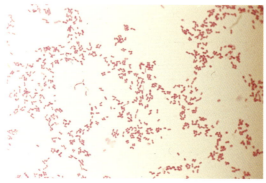
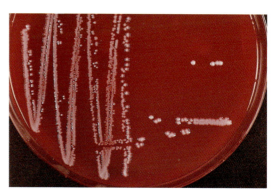

▲ Fig. 159: *Yersinia ruckeri*, pure culture on blood agar, 48 h, 25 °C. Magnification x 0.4
▼ Fig. 161: *Acinetobacter calcoaceticus*, culture smear, Gram stain, Gram-negative bacteria, some of which take on the characteristic diploid form. Magnification x 1000

▲ Abb. 159: *Yersinia ruckeri*, Reinkultur auf Blutagar, 48 h, 25 °C, Abb.-M. 1 : 2,5
▼ Abb. 161: *Acinetobacter calcoaceticus*, Kulturausstrich, Gram-Färbung, gramnegative, teilweise in charakteristischer Diploform gelagerte Bakterien, Abb.-M. 1000 : 1

▲ Fig. 160: *Yersinia ruckeri*, pure culture on Gassner medium. Lactose-negative colonies, 48 h, 25 °C. Magnification x 0.4
▼ Fig. 162: *Acinetobacter calcoaceticus*, pure culture on blood agar, 48 h, 37 °C. Magnification x 0.4

▲ Abb. 160: *Yersinia ruckeri*, Reinkultur auf Gaßner-Agar, lactosenegative Bakterien, 48 h, 25 °C, Abb.-M. 1 : 2,5
▼ Abb. 162: *Acinetobacter calcoaceticus*, Reinkultur auf Blutagar, 48 h, 37 °C, Abb.-M. 1 : 2,5

■ **Morphology** (fig. 161)
This a Gram-negative, non-motile rod, 0.9–1.6 × 1.5–2.5 µm which in the later phases of growth may be coccoid and partly encapsulated. Most are diplobacteria and less frequently they occur in short chains.

■ **Culture** (fig. 162)
A. calcoaceticus grows under aerobic conditions on

■ **Morphologie** (Abb. 161)
Es handelt sich um gramnegative, unbewegliche, 0,9–1,6 × 1,5–2,5 µm große, in späten Wachstumsphasen oft kokkenähnliche, teilweise bekapselte Stäbchen, die meistens als Diplobakterien und seltener in kurzen Ketten vorliegen.

■ **Kultur** (Abb. 162)
A. calcoaceticus wächst unter aeroben Bedingungen

Table 67: Biochemical properties of *Acinetobacter calcoaceticus*

Tabelle 67: Kulturell-biochemische Eigenschaften von *Acinetobacter calcoaceticus*

1. Species characters

Oxi	−	Hae	v	LDC	−	Gas from	
Mot	−	Gel	v	ADC	−	Glu	v
Cat	+	Ure	v	Cit	v	Ara	v
Ind	−	Nit	−			Xyl	v
H$_2$S	−	PAD	−			Lac	v

2. Differentiation of biotypes

Properties	anitratus	haemolyticus	alcaligenes	lwoffi
Glu	+	+	−	−
β-Hae	−	+	+	−
growth on SS and Gassner agar	−	+	+	−
Gel	−	+	+	−

simple media, forming non-pigmented colonies within 24–48 hours. The encapsulated forms produce mucoid colonies.

■ **Biochemical properties** (tab. 67)

Various phenotypes can be differentiated on the basis of their biochemical reactions (production of acid from glucose and other carbohydrates, utilization of various substances as sources of carbon). The following were classified in the older literature by the acid production from glucose: *var. glucidolyticus* (syn.: *Bact. anitratum, Acinetobacter anitratus, Herellea vaginicola* etc.). These variants were found more frequently in association with disease processes, at least in man.

Var. aglucidolyticus (syn.: *Mima polymorpha Acinetobacter lwoffi*). The four biotypes, listed in table 67 can be differentiated by using further characters (gelatinolysis, β-haemolysis, growth on SS agar). Other systems of biotyping have been drawn up by BAUMANN et al. (2) and JUNI (8) and they list up to 7 such biotypes. Aglucocidolytic strains, which are β-haemolytic, predominate among those isolated from animal materials. Thus, they are clearly differentiated from the oxidase-negative *Enterobacteriaceae* (1).

auf einfachem Nährboden und bildet in 24–48 h pigmentlose Kolonien. Die bekapselten Formen wachsen in schleimigen Kolonien.

■ **Kulturell-biochemische Eigenschaften** (Tab. 67)

Aufgrund biochemischer Reaktionen (Säurebildung aus Glucose und anderen Kohlenhydraten, Gelatinasebildung, Ausnutzung verschiedener Substanzen als C-Quelle) lassen sich verschiedene Phänotypen unterscheiden. Nach der Säurebildung aus Glucose werden in älteren Publikationen unterschieden:

var. glucidolyticus (Syn.: *Bact. anitratum, Acinetobacter anitratus, Herellea vaginicola* u. a.), diese Variante wird, zumindest beim Menschen, häufiger in Verbindung mit Krankheitsprozessen gefunden; *var. aglucidolyticus* (Syn.: *Mima polymorpha, Acinetobacter lwoffi*). Unter Heranziehung weiterer Merkmale (Gelatinolyse, β-Hämolyse, Wachstum auf SS-Agar) lassen sich die in der Tab. 67 aufgeführten 4 Biotypen unterscheiden. Weitere Biotypisierungsschemata sind von BAUMANN et al. (2) sowie JUNI (8) aufgestellt worden und unterscheiden bis zu 7 Biotypen. Bei den Isolierungen aus tierischen Untersuchungsstoffen überwiegen aglucidolytische Stämme, die sich dadurch von den auch oxidasenegativen *Enterobacteriaceae* deutlich abheben und keine β-Hämolyse bilden (1).

Bibliography / Literatur

1. ALBERTA, R. (1986): Untersuchungen zum Vorkommen Glukose nichtfermentierender gramnegativer Bakterien in den Geschlechtsorganen von Pferden mit einem Beitrag zu ihrer bakteriologischen Differenzierung. Vet. Med. Diss. Hannover.
2. BAUMANN, P., M. DOUDOROFF & R. Y. STANIER (1968): A study of the Moraxella group II. Oxydative-negative species (Genus Acinetobacter). J. Bact. **95**, 1520–1541.
3. CARTER, G. R., T. I. ISOUN & K. K. KEAHEY (1970): Occurrence of Mima and Herellea species in clinical specimens from various animals. J. Am. Vet. Med. Ass. **156**, 1313–1318.

4. DAS, A. M., & V. L. PARANJAPE (1986): Acinetobacter calcoaceticus in three cases of late abortion in water buffaloes. Vet. Rec. **118**, 214.
5. GIBSON, J. A., & L. E. EAVES (1981): Isolation of Acinetobacter calcoaceticus from an aborted equine foetus. Austr. Vet. J. **57**, 529–531.
6. GOTTSCHALK, M. G., M. I. PASINI & A. G. LIANOS (1984): Acinetobacter lwoffi and Moraxella sp. from mares with reproductive disorders. Vet. Argent. **1**, 488–491.
7. GRABELL, I., & K. G. NYSTRÖM (1961): Haemorrhagic pneumonia in mink caused by Herellea. Acta vet. scand. **2**, 281–299.
8. JUNI, E. (1978): Genetics and physiology of Acinetobacter. Ann. Rev. Microbiol. **32**, 349–371.
9. KUNSTYR, I., & H. HANSEN (1978): Acinetobacter als mögliche Ursache von Bronchopneumonie bei einem Kaninchen. Dtsch. tierärztl. Wschr. **85**, 293–295.
10. RAJASEKHAR, M., L. MUNIYAPPA & B. MURTHY (1978): Chronic haematuria caused by Acinetobacter calcoaceticus in a race horse. Vet. Rec. **102**, 557.
11. ROSS, H. M. (1968): The isolation of Bacterium anitratum (Acinetobacter anitratus) and Mima polymorpha (Acinetobacter lwoffii) from animals in Uganda. Vet. Rec. **83**, 483–486.

6 Further Gram-negative, oxidase-negative and rarely encountered bacteria

6.1 Genus: Francisella (Fr.)
6.1.1 Francisella tularensis

■ **Incidence and veterinary significance**

Fr. tularensis is the cause of tularaemia. Two variants of the bacterium can be differentiated by their geographic distribution:
▷ *var. palaearctica:* USSR, North America, Northern and Eastern Europe, Iran, Israel, Turkey;
▷ *var. tularensis:* North America.

The disease occurred in Germany in 1950/51, 1958, and 1968 and was particularly prominent on the peninsula Eiderstedt. The frequent occurrence of the disease in winter is associated with the hunting season, when there tends to be a concentration of hares resulting from drives.

Fr. tularensis affects primarily rodents (hares, rats, mice, hamsters etc.). The clinical picture can vary from that of a latent infection to a generalized septicaemia. In protracted cases there are swelling and caseation of the lymph nodes and the development of necrotic lesions in the internal organs. The disease can become epidemic leading to widespread deaths.

Fatal septicaemic diseases due to *Fr. tularensis* are rare in domestic animals, but they have been observed in sheep (lambs being particularly susceptible), in pigs, cattle, dogs, cats and poultry. The infection can be transmitted to man through contact with an infected animal, through arthropods or, in very rare instances, through food materials. The site of entry of the infection determines whether the external (e. g. cutaneo-glandular) or the internal (e. g. pulmonary) form of the disease supervenes.

■ **Morphology**

Fr. tularensis is a Gram-negative, non-motile rod which, especially in old cultures, appears coccoid. It is best stained with carbol fuchsin, gentian violet

or by Giemsa's method. The latter method shows up the bipolar staining particularly well.

■ **Culture and biochemical properties**
This bacterium, when first isolated, demands special media and the blood glucose cystine agar of FRANCIS (cystine heart agar, Difco with 10% rabbit blood) has been found useful after the addition of each: 100 IU or µg/ml of penicillin, polymyxin B sulphate and nystatin. Round, moist, milky white colonies about 1 mm in diameter develop after 48 hours aerobic incubation at 37 °C. Culture is also successful on the egg yolk medium of McCOY and CHAPLIN (60% egg yolk and 40% NaCl solution are mixed, filled into tubes and coagulated for 2 days at 72 °C in a steamer). The agglutination test, using specific serum, and the biochemical characters are used to identify the organism. Certain carbohydrates or alcohols are fermented without gas production: Glu +, Sac (+), Man +, Mal +, Lac −, Gel −, Ind −, Ure −. The bacterium is oxidase-negative and weakly catalase-positive.

■ **Animal inoculation**
Guinea pigs and mice are suitable for inoculation experiments. Rabbits are resistant to *var. palaearctica*. The inoculated animals die after 4 to 7 days and the organism can be cultured from the organs.

6.1.2 Francisella novicida

Fr. novicida was isolated from tularaemia-like changes in mice, guinea pigs and hamsters.

Bibliography / Literatur
1. KNOTHE, H. (1969): Tularämie. In: A. GRUMBACH & O. BONIN (Hrsg.): Die Infektionskrankheiten des Menschen und ihre Erreger, 2. Aufl., Band II, S. 1016–1022. Stuttgart: Georg Thieme.
2. LEMBKE, U. (1969): Zur Epidemiologie der Tularämie in Deutschland unter besonderer Berücksichtigung der Jahre 1956–1968. Bundesgesundheitsb. **12**, 377–379.

6.2 Genus: Streptobacillus
Streptobacillus moniliformis
(syn.: *Actinobacillus muris*)

■ **Incidence and veterinary significance**
The bacterium inhabits the nasopharynx of rats and is the cause of rat-bite fever. Arthritis of turkeys, and rarely in other animals, has been attributed to this (1, 2, 3).

■ **Morphology** (fig. 194)
A Gram-negative, pleomorphic, non-motile bac-

fuchsin, Gentianaviolett oder nach Giemsa zu färben. Besonders bei der letzteren kann es eine Bipolarität zeigen.

■ **Kultur und kulturell-biochemische Eigenschaften**
Das Bakterium stellt bei der Isolierung hohe Nährbodenansprüche. Bewährt hat sich der Blut-Glucose-Cystin-Agar nach Francis (cystin-heart-agar, Difco, mit 10% Kaninchenblut) mit Zusatz von je 100 IE bzw. µg/ml Penicillin, Polymyxin-B-Sulfat und Nystatin. Bebrütung aerob bei 37 °C. Nach 48 h bilden sich runde, feuchte, milchigweiße, etwa 1 mm große Kolonien. Die Kultur gelingt auch auf dem Eidotter-Nährboden nach McCoy und Chapin (60% Eigelb und 40% NaCl-Lösung mischen, in Röhrchen abfüllen und an 2 d bei 72 °C im Dampftopf koagulieren). Die Identifizierung des Erregers erfolgt durch Agglutination mit spezifischem Serum und durch biochemische Reaktionen (Kohlenhydrate bzw. Alkohole ohne Gasbildung: Glu +, Sac [+], Man +, Mal +, Lact −, Gel −, Ind −, Ure −). Das Bakterium ist oxidasenegativ und schwach katalasepositiv.

■ **Tierversuch**
Geeignet für den diagnostischen Tierversuch sind Meerschweinchen und Mäuse. Kaninchen sind gegen die *var. palaearctica* resistent. Die Versuchstiere sterben nach 4–7 d oder später, und der Erreger kann aus den Organen kulturell isoliert werden.

6.1.2 Francisella novicida

Fr. novicida wurde aus tularämieähnlichen Veränderungen bei Mäusen, Meerschweinchen und Hamstern isoliert.

6.2 Gattung: Streptobacillus
Streptobacillus moniliformis
(Syn.: *Actinobacillus muris*)

■ **Vorkommen und medizinische Bedeutung**
Das Bakterium kommt im Nasopharynx von Ratten vor und gilt als Ursache des Rattenbißfiebers des Menschen. Gelenkserkrankungen sind bei Puten und selten bei anderen Tierarten beschrieben worden (1, 2, 3).

■ **Morphologie** (Abb. 194)
Es handelt sich um gramnegative, polymorphe, un-

terium. Apart from coccoid forms, filaments may occur which have spindle-shaped or round enlargements (fig. 194). The length of the rods varies between 1 µm and 5 µm and the enlargement can reach a diameter of 1 µm to 3 µm.

■ **Culture** (fig. 195)
Streptobacillus moniliformis grows under microaerophilic conditions on protein-containing media (blood agar, serum broth). On blood agar they form small (ca. 0.3–0.5 mm), grey, non-haemolytic colonies within 48 to 72 hours (fig. 195).

■ **Biochemical properties**
Oxi −, Cat −, Ure −, Ind −, H_2S v^+, Nit −, Gel −, Glu +, Lac −, Mal v, Sac v, Ara v, Tre v^-, Dul −, Sor v^-, Sal v. 20 % serum must be added to the test media.

■ **Animal inoculation**
Inoculated mice succumb either to a rapidly fatal generalized infection or a chronic arthritis with joint swelling. This sign can also be induced in turkeys.

■ **Kultur** (Abb. 195)
Das Bakterium wächst unter mikroaerophilen oder anaeroben Bedingungen auf eiweißhaltigen Nährböden (Blutagar, Serumbouillon). Auf Blutagar bilden sich nach 48 bis 72 Stunden kleine, etwa 0,3–0,5 mm große, graue, nichthämolysierende Kolonien (s. Abb. 195).

■ **Kulturell-biochemische Eigenschaften**
Oxi −, Kat −, Ure −, Ind −, H_2S v^+, Nit −, Gel −, Glu +, Lact −, Mal v, Sac v, Ara v, Tre v^-, Dul −, Sor v^-, Sal v. Die Testmedien müssen einen Zusatz von 20 % Serum enthalten.

■ **Tierversuch**
Die Infektion von Mäusen führt entweder zu einer rasch tödlich verlaufenden Allgemeininfektion oder zu chronischen Gelenkserkrankungen mit Anschwellungen. Das Krankheitsbild läßt sich auch bei Puten erzeugen.

Bibliography / Literatur

1. GLÜNDER, K., K. H. HINZ & B. STIBUREK (1982): Eine durch Streptobacillus moniliformis bedingte Gelenkserkrankung. Dtsch. tierärztl. Wschr. **89**, 367–370.
2. MOHAMED, Y. S., P. D. MOORHEAD & E. H. BOHL (1969): Natural Streptobacillus moniliformis infection of turkeys, sheep and pigs. Avian Dis. **13**, 379–385.
3. YAMAMOTO, R., & G. T. CLARK (1966): Streptobacillus moniliformis infection in turkeys. Vet. Rec. **79**, 95–100.

Gram-negative, comma-shaped or spiral bacteria (Family: Spirillaceae)

Gramnegative, komma- bis spiralförmige Bakterien (Familie: Spirillaceae)

1   Genus: Spirillum

This is a bacterium that is twisted like a cork-screw and occurs mainly in water and effluent. Its motility is due to 5 to 20 flagella which are usually present on both poles. The various species are non-pathogenic, with the exception of *Spirillum minus* which causes rat-bite fever in man. This organism occurs in the blood of rats and mice and can be transmitted to man through a bite. The disease is very rare in Germany. It is doubtful whether this species actually belongs to the genus *Spirillum*.

Among the non-pathogens there is *Spirillum volutans*, one of the largest bacteria, measuring up to 60 µm, which is striking because of the volutin bodies inside the cell.

2   Genus: Campylobacter (C.)

A Gram-negative, non-spore forming rod, that measures 0.2–0.8 × 0.5–5 (8) µm and is twisted into a spiral of up to several coils. Coccoid forms can occur in culture. They are motile due to monotrichous flagellation at one or both ends of the bacterium. It is oxidase-positive, and neither ferments nor oxidizes carbohydrates. MR and VPR are negative. Its growth is anaerobic or micro-aerophilic.

The species belonging to this genus are listed in table 68.

A distinction is being made in the following description between campylobacter infection of the reproductive organs and of the gut. This grouping, which is related to the primary site of the infection

1   Gattung: Spirillum

Es handelt sich um korkenzieherartig gewundene Bakterien, die vorwiegend in Gewässern und Abwässern vorkommen. Ihre Beweglichkeit beruht auf dem Vorhandensein von 5 bis 20 Geißeln, meistens an beiden Polen des Bakteriums. Die verschiedenen Arten sind apathogen mit Ausnahme von *Spirillum minus,* das das Rattenbißfieber beim Menschen verursacht. Dieser Erreger kommt im Blut von Ratten und Mäusen vor und kann durch Biß auf den Menschen übertragen werden. In Deutschland ist die Erkrankung sehr selten. Die Zugehörigkeit dieses Erregers zur Gattung Spirillum ist fraglich.

Unter den apathogenen Vertretern ist *Spirillum volutans* eines der größten Bakterien (bis 60 µm) mit auffallenden Volutinkörperchen im Zellinnern.

2   Gattung: Campylobacter (C.)

Es handelt sich um gramnegative, sporenlose, ein- bis mehrfach spiralförmig gewundene, 0,2–0,8 × 0,5–5 (8) µm große Stäbchen. In der Kultur können auch kokkoide Formen auftreten. Die Beweglichkeit beruht auf einer monotrichen Begeißelung an einem oder beiden Enden des Bakteriums. Oxidase-positiv, Kohlenhydrate werden weder fermentiert noch oxidiert, MR und VPR negativ. Mikroaerophiles bis anaerobes Wachstum.

Die zu der Gattung gehörenden Arten sind in der Tab. 68 zusammengestellt.

In der folgenden Beschreibung wird zwischen Infektionen der Geschlechtsorgane und des Darmes durch Campylobacterarten unterschieden. Von die-

Table 68: Nomenclature, incidence and aetiological significance of *Campylobacter* in man and animals
Tabelle 68: Nomenklatur, Vorkommen und ätiologische Bedeutung von *Campylobacter* bei Mensch und Tier

Species/Name	Synonyms	Occurrence in the gut	Animals	Clinical picture man
Campylobacter fetus subsp. venerealis	Campylobacter fetus subsp. fetus, Vibrio fetus subsp. venerealis		cattle: enzootic sterility, abortion sheep: abortion	generalized infection
Campylobacter fetus subsp. fetus	Campylobacter fetus subsp. intestinalis, Vibrio fetus subsp. intestinalis	Cattle, sheep, pigs, birds	cattle: sporadic abortion sheep, pig: enzootic abortion	enteritis
Campylobacter jejuni	Campylobacter fetus subsp. jejuni (C. jejuni and C. coli were not separated)	numerous species	ox, dog etc.: enteritis cow: mastitis, sheep: abortion birds: infectious hepatitis	enteritis (?)
Campylobacter coli	Vibrio jejuni/coli related vibrios	Primarily pig, less often other species	pig: enteritis (?)	enteritis (?)
Campylobacter laridis	NARTC = nalidixic acid-resistant thermophile Campylobacter	Birds and other species of animals	latent intestinal infection	enteritis (?)
Campylobacter sputorum subsp. sputorum				mouth cavity
Campylobacter sputorum subsp. mucosalis		Pig	intestinal adenomatosis, necrotizing enteritis, regional ileitis, proliferative haemorrhagic enteropathy	
Campylobacter sputorum subsp. bubulus		Numerous animal species	frequent, clinically latent infection of bull's prepuce	
Campylobacter fecalis		ox, sheep	cattle: enteritis (?)	
aerotolerant Campylobacter			pig: abortions (?), cattle: mastitis, infection of prepuce, abortions (?)	

or of disease development, has certain exceptions. Thus, *C. fetus subsp. fetus* and *C. sputorum subsp. bubulus* are classed as genital campylobacters, but both also occur in the gut.

2.1 Campylobacter infections of the reproductive organs

These species occur mainly in cattle and sheep, less often in pigs. They are listed in table 68 along with their synonymous designations and their clinical significance.

2.1.1 Campylobacter fetus subsp. venerealis

Is the cause of a notifiable (in Germany) venereal disease of cattle, which is characterized by failure of conception, prolonged periods between oestrus and abortion. In bulls there is usually an asymptomatic invasion of the preputial mucosa without tendency towards an ascending spread of the infection (21, 32, 56, 67, 68, 86, 104).

■ **Culture** (fig. 165)
The bacterium grows best under micro-aerophilic conditions on a thioglycollate plate with additional 10% bovine blood, where it produces small (0.5–1 mm), shiny, slightly cloudy and often pink coloured colonies that have a tendency to spread over the surface of the medium. The routine for cultural investigation is shown in figure 163.

In thioglycollate broth *Campylobacter* grows in a layer immediately below the surface (fig. 167).

■ **Biochemical properties**
See figure 163 and section 2.1.4.2.

■ **Antigenic structure**
The subspecies possess a common O-antigen which was designated O1-antigen by MITSCHERLICH & LIESS (6). Further antigen identification are given by GARCIA et al. (32). For serological differentiation see section 2.1.4.3.

2.1.2 Campylobacter fetus subsp. fetus

This subspecies is found mainly in cattle and sheep (tab. 68). Sporadic abortion is seen in cattle on occasion, but apart from that no fertility problems are caused, even though this bacterium is occasionally isolated from the vaginal and preputial mucosae

(7, 17, 22, 112, 117). In the sheep *C. fetus subsp. fetus* is responsible for epidemic abortion.

In cattle and sheep the natural habitat of the organism is the intestinal tract and the infection is transmitted by mouth; venereal transmission is without significance. It remains questionable as to whether this subspecies is capable of inducing intestinal disease, but AL-MASHAT & TAYLOR (2) report such observations.

■ **Culture**
Subsp. fetus behaves in culture similar to *subsp. venerealis* (see section 2.1.1).

■ **Biochemical properties**
See figure 163 and section 2.1.4.2.

■ **Antigenic structure**
This subspecies contains the serotypes O1, O2, O7 and O13 (MITSCHERLICH, 68; MITSCHERLICH & LIESS, 69), which are the causes of sheep abortion and occur with varying regional frequency. The serological differentiation is discussed in section 2.1.4.3.

2.1.3 Campylobacter sputorum subsp. bubulus

This subspecies occurs very frequently on the preputial mucosa of the bull; LEIN et al. (61) were able to isolate it in 86% of animals examined. It is considered to be non-pathogenic. Other isolations were made from the vaginal mucosa (50), aborted calf foetuses (119) and from intestinal content (112).

■ **Morphology**
They are relatively small organisms (0.3–0.6 × 2.4 μm) when compared with *C. fetus*, and they exhibit exceptionally lively behaviour in an unstained smear, when taken from a broth culture (»swarming midge movement«).

■ **Culture** (fig. 166)
Subsp. bubulus forms greenish-brown colonies on thioglycollate blood agar.

■ **Biochemical properties**
Are summarized in figure 163 and section 2.1.4.2.

■ **Antigenic structure**
According to the classification of MITSCHERLICH & LIESS (69) one can at least differentiate the O-antigens 3, 4 and 5.

---

ginal- oder Präputialschleimhaut isoliert werden kann (7, 17, 22, 112, 117). Beim Schaf ist *C. fetus subsp. fetus* Ursache eines seuchenhaften Verlammens.

Der natürliche Standort des Erregers ist bei Rind und Schaf der Darmkanal, die Infektion wird oral übertragen, die venerische Verbreitung ist ohne größere Bedeutung. Ob die Subspezies fetus Darmerkrankungen verursachen kann, bleibt fraglich, über entsprechende Beobachtungen ist von AL-MASHAT & TAYLOR (2) berichtet worden.

■ **Kultur**
In der Kultur verhält sich *subsp. fetus* ähnlich wie *subsp. venerealis* (s. Kapitel 2.1.1).

■ **Kulturell-biochemische Eigenschaften**
Siehe Abb. 163 und Kapitel 2.1.4.2.

■ **Antigenstruktur**
Innerhalb der Subspezies gibt es die Serotypen 01, 02, 07 und 013 (MITSCHERLICH, 68; MITSCHERLICH & LIESS, 69), die namentlich als Schafaborterreger regional unterschiedlich häufig vorkommen. Serologische Differenzierung s. Kapitel 2.1.4.3.

2.1.3 Campylobacter sputorum subsp. bubulus

Die Subspezies kommt sehr häufig auf der Präputialschleimhaut des Bullen vor, so konnten z. B. LEIN et al. (61) sie in 86% der untersuchten Tiere isolieren. Sie gilt als apathogen. Weitere Isolierungen stammen von der Vaginalschleimhaut (50), abortierten Rinderfeten (119) und aus dem Darminhalt (112).

■ **Morphologie**
Im Vergleich zu *C. fetus* relativ kleine *Campylobacter* (0,3–0,6 × 2–4 μm), die im Nativpräparat aus einer Bouillon eine besonders lebhafte Bewegung (Mückenschwarmbewegung) zeigen.

■ **Kultur** (Abb. 166)
Auf der Thioglykolat-Blutplatte wächst *subsp. bubulus* in grün-braunen Kolonien.

■ **Kulturell-biochemische Eigenschaften**
Siehe Abb. 163 und Kapitel 2.1.4.2.

■ **Antigenstruktur**
Entsprechend der Einteilung nach MITSCHERLICH & LIESS (69) können mindestens die O-Antigene 3, 4 und 5 unterschieden werden.

```
                          ┌─────────────────────────────────────────────────┐
                          │                   Specimens                      │
                          ├─────────────────────────────────────────────────┤
                          │ Placenta, abomasal content from aborted foetuses,│
                          │ vaginal and preputial rinses, and from inside the│
                          │   artificial vagina after taking semen sample    │
                          └─────────────────────────────────────────────────┘
```

┌──┐
│   Examination by culture   │
├──┤
│ 1. Treatment of test material and inoculation of media: │
│ 1a. Placenta, abomasal content: direct culture on selective media   │
│ 1b. Rinsing samples: │
│   Filtration method: centrifuge 3–5 minutes, expel supernatant through filter with pore size 0.65 µm. |
| Spread a few drops onto a thioglycollate blood plate;   │
│   Selective method: centrifuge ca. 20 minutes, inoculate sediment onto blood agar plate which contains |
| antibiotics as a selective agent, e. g. supplement of Skirrow [each 500 ml medium contains 5 mg |
| vancomycin, 1250 IU polymyxin B, 2.5 mg trimethroprim lactate (Oxoid)]   │
│ 2. Microaerophilic incubation: │
│   Anaerobic flask is evacuated to a negative pressure of 0.9 atm. and filled with a mixture of 95 % N_2 and |
| 5 % CO_2 to a negative pressure of 0.2 atm. Commercial gas generators are available. Incubation time |
| 4–6 days.   │
│ 3. Assessment of cultures: │
│   Suspicious colonies examined under phase contrast for the presence of campylobacter and motility in |
| a fresh preparation. Oxidase test if required. Pure cultures are prepared on a thioglycollate-blood |
| plates or in liver broth.   │
└──┘

Biochemical differentiation								
	Catalase	H_2S^1	H_2S^2	3,5 % NaCl	1 % Glycine	0.1 % Selenite	25 °C	43 °C
Campylobacter fetus								
subsp. venerealis	+	–	v	–	v	–	+	–
subsp. fetus	+	–	+	v	+	+	+	–
Campylobacter jejuni	+	v^3	+	–	+	+	–	+
Campylobacter sputorum								
subsp. bubulus	–	+	+	+	+	v	+	+

[1] insensitive test, demonstration in liver broth with strip of lead acetate paper suspended in it (fig. 167) or in 2-sugar-iron agar after Kligler;
[2] sensitive test, demonstration in nutrient broth containing 0.025 % cysteine and a suspended strip of lead acetate paper;
[3] Biotype 1 – negative, biotype 2 – positive

Fig. 163: Cultural isolation and differentiation of *Campylobacter species* of the genital tract

2.1.4 Diagnosis of the genital Campylobacter infection

The diagnostic methods used for the demonstration of the listed *Campylobacter* species in clinical material are the same in principle as those used to differentiate the species; they are therefore discussed together.

2.1.4.1 Identification of causal agent

The most reliable method of identifying the organism is by means of culture, because only when the bacteria have been isolated is it possible to differen-

tiate between the various *Campylobacter spp.* occurring in the genital organs.

It is possible to demonstrate the agent by fluorescence microscopy as a rapid method (9, 10, 14, 25, 65, 76, 77, 115), but its specificity is limited because the O-antigen 1 which is typical for *subspecies venerealis*, also occurs in strains of *subsp. fetus;* thus there is antigen identity. Furthermore, there is partial antigen uniformity between the *subspecies venerealis* and *fetus*, because the former bears not only the O1-antigen, but it can also possess small amounts of O2-antigen and *vice versa*, so that cross reactions can occur. They can only be avoided by serum absorption (90).

The materials and methods which can be used for the cultural investigation are summarized in figure 163. Instead of rinsing the prepuce and sampling the rinsing fluid it has been found just as effective and much easier to rinse out the inside of the artificial vagina, immediately after taking semen (15). Thioglycollate broth without the addition of agar can be used as rinsing fluid.

The cultures must be set up on the day the sample is taken (if possible within 6 hours). Otherwise it is likely that the campylobacters would die. Various transport media have been devised which would ensure a prolonged survival time. The specimens should not be sent in cool boxes (20, 33, 60, 114).

Contaminants are often very numerous, especially in preputial rinses, and in order to control these the sample is either filtered before culture or it is spread on selective media which contain antibiotics (fig. 163; 8, 15, 26, 52, 76, 79, 92, 100, 116). Both methods have their advantages and disadvantages, but on the whole the direct culture on antibiotic-containing media appears to demonstrate more campylobacters than does the filtration method, because many bacteria seem not to pass the filters (15, 115, 116). In actual fact, it is advisable to do both methods in parallel for the best results. Even so, a single test on an individual animal is no guarantee. The test should be repeated at least three times in order to be sure.

2.1.4.2 Biochemical differentiation

The characters of *C. fetus* are summarized in figure 163. The following methods of investigation have proved successful:
▷ Catalase production: Broth culture is mixed with an equal volume of 3% hydrogen peroxide solution: oxygen is formed immediately.

in den Genitalorganen vorkommenden *Campylobacter*-Arten möglich ist.

Die fluoreszenzmikroskopische Untersuchung zum Erregernachweis ist als eine diagnostische Schnellmethode im Prinzip möglich (9, 10, 14, 25, 65, 76, 77, 115), ihre Spezifität ist jedoch begrenzt, da das für die *subsp. venerealis* typische O-Antigen 1 auch bei Stämmen der *subsp. fetus* vorkommt, so daß eine Antigenidentität vorliegt. Darüber hinaus bestehen zwischen den *subsp. venerealis* und *fetus* teilweise Antigenübereinstimmungen, da *venerealis* neben dem O1- auch geringe Mengen O2-Antigen enthalten kann und umgekehrt, so daß Kreuzreaktionen auftreten, die nur durch Serumabsorptionen zu vermeiden sind (90).

Die für die kulturelle Untersuchung in Frage kommenden Materialien und Methoden sind in der Abb. 163 zusammengestellt. An Stelle der Präputialspülprobe hat sich die sehr viel leichter durchzuführende Spülung der Innenwand der künstlichen Scheide bewährt, die unmittelbar nach der Samenentnahme vorgenommen wird (15). Als Spülflüssigkeit kann Thioglykolatbouillon ohne Agarzusatz benutzt werden.

Das Untersuchungsmaterial muß am Tag der Entnahme bakteriologisch angelegt werden (möglichst innerhalb von 6 h), da sonst mit dem Absterben von Campylobacter zu rechnen ist. Für eine verlängerte Überlebenszeit sind verschiedene Transportmedien beschrieben worden. Das Material soll nicht gekühlt versendet werden (20, 33, 60, 114).

Für die Ausschaltung der besonders in Präputialspülproben sehr starken Begleitflora kann das Material entweder vorher filtriert oder auf antibiotikahaltige Selektivplatten ausgestrichen werden (Abb. 163) (8, 15, 25, 26, 52, 76, 78, 79, 92, 100, 116). Beide Methoden weisen Vor- und Nachteile auf. Im allgemeinen scheint die Direktkultur auf antibiotikahaltigen Platten häufiger zum Campylobacternachweis zu führen als die Filtrationsmethode, bei der offenbar viele Bakterien den Filter nicht passieren (15, 115, 116). Empfehlenswert ist es, beide Methoden parallel zu benutzen, da damit die größte Ausbeute zu erzielen ist. Dennoch besitzt eine einmalige Untersuchung eines Tieres keine ausreichende Sicherheit, die Untersuchung sollte mindestens dreimal wiederholt werden.

2.1.4.2 Kulturell-biochemische Identifizierung

Die Merkmale von *C. fetus* sind in der Abb. 163 zusammengestellt. Folgende Untersuchungsmethoden haben sich bewährt:
▷ Katalasebildung: 3%ige Wasserstoffperoxidlösung und Bouillonkultur werden im gleichen Verhältnis gemischt, unmittelbar danach kommt es zur Bildung von Sauerstoff.

▷ Insensitive H_2S test: A strip of lead acetate paper is suspended in a tube of liver broth. Incubation at 37 °C and normal atmosphere for 3 days (fig. 167). The test can also be performed with the double sugar iron agar of KLIGLER.
▷ Sensitive H_2S test: A strip of lead acetate paper is suspended in 0.025 % cysteine broth. Incubation for 4 days at 37 °C under normal atmospheric conditions.
▷ Salt tolerance: Sodium thioglycollate broth containing 3.5 % NaCl and 0.1 % agar is heavily inoculated and incubated for 4 days at 37 °C under normal atmospheric conditions. Growth is indicated by a layer of growth immediately below the surface. Microscopic examination under phase contrast shows the motile bacteria.
▷ Glycine tolerance: Follows the same principle as the salt tolerance test. One should aim at testing concentrations of 0.8, 1.0 and 1.2 % (BISPING, 15).
▷ Nalidixic acid (NA) and triphenyl tetrazolium chloride (TTC) tolerance: Can be tested on blood agar to which 40 mg NA or 1 g TTC has been added per l.
▷ Hippurate hydrolysis: See page 31.
▷ Sodium selenite reduction: 0.1 sodium selenite broth, without added agar is heavily inoculated and incubated micro-aerophilically for 4 days. The sodium selenite must not be added to the broth until after autoclaving. A red colour indicates a positive reaction.
▷ Testing growth at 25 °C and 37 °C: This is done in liver broth.

The majority of strains can be identified with relative certainty by the results of these biochemical tests (fig. 163). However, there may be certain strains which give aberrant reactions; these cannot be classified with absolute reliability.

The differentiation between *C. fetus subsp. venerealis* and *C. fetus subsp. fetus* is essentially based on:
▷ H_2S production which in *subsp. venerealis* is negative even in the sensitive test (deviant reactions are possible);
▷ The glycine tolerance in *subsp. venerealis* extends to 0.8 %, rarely even to 1 % (according to DEDIÉ et al. [22], to 1.1 %), while in *subsp. fetus* at least 1.4 % is tolerated; sodium selenite reduction is positive in *subsp. fetus* and is considered to be a particularly reliable indication (17).

C. sputorum subsp. bubulus is easy to identify among the genital *Campylobacter spp.*, because it produces no catalase, is distinctly H_2S-positive and will grow in 3.5 % NaCl broth.

▷ Unempfindlicher H_2S-Test: In ein Leberbouillonröhrchen wird ein Bleiacetatstreifen eingehängt. Bebrütungsdauer 4 d bei 37 °C unter normalen atmosphärischen Bedingungen (Abb. 167). Der Test kann auch mit 2-Zucker-Eisen-Agar nach Kligler durchgeführt werden.
▷ Empfindlicher H_2S-Test: In eine 0,025 %ige Cystein-Nährbouillon wird ein Bleiacetatstreifen eingehängt. Bebrütungsdauer 4 d bei 37 °C unter normalen atmosphärischen Bedingungen.
▷ Kochsalztoleranz: Na-Thioglykolatbouillon mit 3,5 % NaCl und 0,1 % Agar wird kräftig beimpft und 4 d bei 37 °C unter normalen atmosphärischen Bedingungen bebrütet. Das Wachstum zeigt sich durch ringförmige Trübung dicht unter der Oberfläche. Bei der mikroskopischen Kontrolle (Phasenkontrast) sind bewegliche Bakterien vorhanden.
▷ Glycintoleranz: Erfolgt nach prinzipiell gleichem Versuchsansatz wie die Prüfung der Kochsalztoleranz. Es sollten möglichst die Konzentrationen 0,8, 1,0 und 1,2 % (BISPING et al., 15) geprüft werden.
▷ Nalidixinsäure- (NA) und Triphenyltetrazoliumchloridtoleranz (TTC): Kann auf Blutagar mit Zusatz von 40 mg NA oder 1 g TTC je l geprüft werden.
▷ Hippuratspaltung: s. S. 31.
▷ Natriumselenitreduktion: Eine 0,1 %ige Na-Selenitbouillon ohne Agarzusatz wird kräftig beimpft und unter mikroaerophilen Bedingungen 4 d bebrütet. Das Na-Selenit darf der Bouillon erst nach dem Autoklavieren zugesetzt werden. Positive Reaktion: Rotfärbung des Mediums.
▷ Prüfung des Wachstums bei 25 und 37 °C: Leberbouillon.

Der Ausfall dieser kulturell biochemischen Reaktionen (Abb. 163) erlaubt bei der Mehrzahl der Stämme eine relativ sichere Bestimmung. In Einzelfällen kann es Stämme geben, die durch abweichende Reaktionen nicht sicher einzuordnen sind.

Die Unterscheidung von *C. fetus subsp. venerealis* von *C. fetus subsp. fetus* erfolgt im wesentlichen durch:
▷ H_2S-Bildung, die bei der *subsp. venerealis* auch im empfindlichen Test negativ ausfällt (abweichende Reaktionen möglich);
▷ Glycintoleranz, die bei der *subsp. venerealis* meistens bis 0,8 % und selten bis 1 % (nach DEDIÉ et al. [22] bis 1,1 %) reicht, bei der *subsp. fetus* mindestens 1,4 % beträgt; Na-Selenitreduktion, die bei *subsp. fetus* positiv ist und als besonders sicheres Kennzeichen gilt (17).

Von den genitalen *Campylobacter*-Arten ist *C. sputorum subsp. bubulus* leicht zu identifizieren, da er keine Katalase bildet, deutlich H_2S-positiv ist und in einer 3,5%igen NaCl-Bouillon wächst.

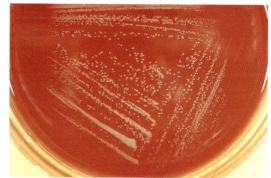
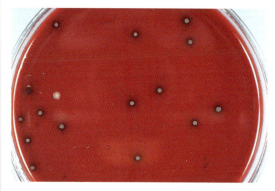
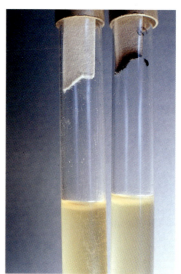

▲ Fig. 164: *Campylobacter fetus subsp. venerealis*, fresh preparation from a culture, phase contrast. Magnification x 1000
▼ Fig. 166: *Campylobacter sputorum subsp. bubulus*, direct culture from a bull's preputial rinse on thioglycollate blood agar, mixed culture: the campylobacter colonies are surrounded by a dark zone, 4 d micro-aerophilic incubation at 37°C. Magnification x 0.33

▲ Abb. 164: *Campylobacter fetus subsp. venerealis*, Nativpräparat von einer Kultur, Phasenkontrast, Abb.-M. 1000 : 1
▼ Abb. 166: *Campylobacter sputorum subsp. bubulus*, Direktkultur der Präputialspülprobe eines Bullen auf Thioglykolat-Blutagar, Mischkultur, die Campylobacter-Kolonien sind von einem dunklen Hof umgeben, 4 d, mikroaerophil bei 37°C, Abb.-M. 1 : 3

▲ Fig. 165: *Campylobacter fetus subsp. venerealis*, culture on thioglycollate blood agar, 4 d micro-aerophilic incubation at 37°C. Magnification x 0.4
▼ Fig. 167: *Campylobacter* cultures in liver broth: right *C. sputorum subsp. bubulus*, H_2S-positive, left *C. fetus subsp. venerealis* H_2S-negative. Formation of H_2S demonstrated with strip of lead acetate. The bacteria grow in the form of a ring immediately below the surface. Magnification x 0.5

▲ Abb. 165: *Campylobacter fetus subsp. venerealis*, Kultur auf Thioglykolat-Blutagar, 4 d, mikroaerophil bebrütet bei 37°C, Abb.-M. 1 : 2,5
▼ Abb. 167: *Campylobacter*-Kulturen in Leberbouillon, rechts: *C. sputorum subsp. bubulus*, H_2S-positiv, links: *C. fetus subsp. venerealis*, H_2S-negativ, Nachweis der H_2S-Bildung mittels Bleiacetatstreifen. Wachstum der Bakterien in Form eines Ringes dicht unter der Oberfläche, Abb.-M. 1 : 2

2.1.4.3 Serological identification

C. fetus subsp. *venerealis* and subsp. *fetus* possess characteristic O-antigens (pp. 217, 218), which can be demonstrated with the agglutination test and more clearly with the complement fixation test. They can be used for the serological differentiation of the two subspecies (13, 69, 97). MITSCHERLICH & LIESS (69) described the serological differentiation by means of the complement fixation test and the method of obtaining the antigen (phenolic extracts).

The reliability of the serological antigen determination is lessened by the observation that there are strains with O-antigen 1 which behave biochemically like subsp. *fetus* (glycine tolerance, positive selenite reduction), without causing epidemic venereal disease (13, 15, 22, 64). Also, there are strains in which O-antigen 1 predominates while small amounts of O-antigen 2 are also present, and there are other strains where the situation is reversed. MITSCHERLICH & HEIDER (66) have encountered isolated strains which initially possessed the O-antigen 1, but lost it during culture passages while they formed O-antigen 2. The converse has not been observed.

For these reasons the identification of *C. fetus* subsp. *venerealis* is based primarily on biochemical tests, although in special cases the complement fixation test can be used as an additional aid.

2.1.5 Aerotolerant Campylobacter (Campylobacter cryaerophilia)

In recent years several authors have isolated aerotolerant strains of campylobacter, which were implicated as a cause of abortion, especially in pigs. However, they have also been demonstrated in the foetuses of other species (cattle, horses, sheep) (27, 28, 43, 46, 70, 72). Other strains originate from the prepuce or from cases of mastitis (62).

They differ fundamentally from other species of campylobacter in that they are aerotolerant and by the fact that they do not grow in primary culture on the ordinary solid media, but require semi-solid media. The semi-solid EMJH leptospira medium (p. 280) with the addition of 5-fluorouracil (100 mg/ml) has been found useful. Subcultures can then be made onto solid media containing blood (and 125 μg carbenicillin/ml). On this medium the strains will

Table 69: Biochemical properties of aerotolerant strains of *Campylobacter* (46, 71, 72)

Growth at 25 °C	+
Growth at 43 °C	−
Growth with 1 % glycine	v
Cat	+
H_2S (without cysteine)	−
H_2S (with 0.02 % cysteine)	v^-
TTC resistance	−
NA resistance	v^-
Sel	v^-

grow aerobically but a better growth is produced in reduced O₂ tension. The optimum incubation temperature is 30 °C (70).

Biochemical properties see tab. 69.

2.2 Campylobacter infections of the gut

The species falling into this category are summarized in table 68.

2.2.1 Campylobacter jejuni

This is present in the intestine of many animal species and has been isolated, for instance, from cattle, sheep, goats, pigs, dogs, cats, poultry, rabbits, guinea pigs, rats and mice (19, 31, 47, 48, 73, 80, 85, 102, 108, 111, 120 and many others).

In the majority of cases the isolation of *C. jejuni* merely indicates an asymptomatic presence in the gut, although it can also be associated with enteritis. The first report of a *C. jejuni* enteritis was that of JONES & LITTLE (1931) but it is not certain whether this was the same bacterium which is recognized today by that name. Other reports as a cause of enteritis pertain mainly to cattle, sheep and dogs and were made by VANDENBERGHE et al., 103; RÜBSAMEN et al., 89; FIREHAMMER & MYERS, 30; AL-MASHAT & TAYLOR, 2; HOSIE et al., 45. Sheep can abort after an initial intestinal infection.

C. jejuni is also widely distributed among birds and they can have either a latent infection of the gut, and this has been found in a large variety of birds (1, 23, 35, 40, 84, 110 etc.), or they can be affected with infectious campylobacter hepatitis (»vibrio hepatitis«), a disease primarily of fowls. It is a subacute to chronic hepatitis with swelling of the liver with necroses, haemorrhages and haematomata (11, 16, 37, 44, 51, 76, 91, and others).

C. jejuni, the causal organism of infectious hepatitis, has occasionally been confused in the literature with *V. metschnikovi* (p. 139). The two species can be differentiated, however, by the fact that *V. metschnikovi* grows under aerobic conditions, ferments carbohydrates, forms indole and remains alive for 10 months in broth cultures at room temperature (58).

C. jejuni is being identified with increasing frequency as the cause of enteritis in man. It is said that contact with animals (especially poultry, cattle, sheep, pigs and dogs) or with food materials of animal origin (meat, including poultry, milk) play an important epidemiological role (12, 93).

Morphology and culture
C. jejuni is very similar in its morphology and cultural behaviour to C. fetus and the routine for cultural examination is shown in figure 168.

Biochemical properties
See figure 168 and section 2.2.

Antigenic structure
The antigenic structure of C. jejuni is very heterogenous. A number of serotypes were established with the aid of serological methods such as agglutination, passive haemagglutination, complement fixation and ELISA so that the establishment

erreger beim Menschen festgestellt worden. Dabei soll der Kontakt zu Tieren (insbesondere Geflügel, Rinder, Schafe, Schweine, Hunde) oder zu Lebensmitteln tierischer Herkunft (Fleisch einschließlich Geflügelfleisch, Milch) eine wichtige epidemiologische Rolle spielen (9, 12, 93).

Morphologie und Kultur
Im morphologischen und kulturellen Verhalten ähnelt C. jejuni weitgehend C. fetus. Die kulturelle Untersuchung ist in der Abb. 168 zusammengestellt.

Kulturell-biochemische Eigenschaften
Siehe Abb. 168 und Kapitel 2.2.

Antigenstruktur
C. jejuni ist in seiner Antigenstruktur sehr heterogen. Mit verschiedenen serologischen Methoden (Agglutination, passive Hämagglutination, KBR, ELISA) konnten zahlreiche Serotypen ermittelt werden, die eine Aufstellung eines Serotypisie-

Specimens
Faecal samples, intestinal content, food samples etc.

Examination by culture
1. Direct culture on selective media e. g. Thioglycollate blood plates with Butzler's supplement [bacitracin, cycloheximide, colistin, cephazolin, novobiocin (Oxoid)] (107); 2. 1 g test material in 10 ml saline, briefly centrifuged, then filtered and inoculated onto a thioglycollate blood or selective plate; 3. It may be necessary to precede with an enrichment broth, e. g. Rosef (85) which contains rezasurin, vancomycin, trimethoprim, polymyxin B. 24–48 h incubation at 43 °C, then subculture on selective plate as in 1. 4. Micro-aerophilic incubation at 43 °C, for 3–4 d in an atmosphere e. g. anaerobic jar of Oxoid with a Campylobacter gas generating kit without catalyst.

Biochemical identification of pure culture				
Properties	C. jejuni	C. coli	C. laridis (NARTC)[1]	C. fecalis
Morphology	spiral, later coccoid	spiral, partly coccoid	spiral, later coccoid	spiral
Catalase	+	+	+	−
Nitrate	+	+	+	+
Oxidase	+	+	+	+
1 % Glycine	+	+	+	+
Hippurate	+	−	−	−
H_2S insensitive test[2]	−	−	−	+
H_2 sensitive test[3]	+	+	+	+
NA resistance (30 µg)	−	−	+	+
Cephalothin resistance (30 µg)	−	−	−	+
25 °C	−	−	−	(+)
43 °C	+	+	+	(+)

[1] Nalidixic acid resistant, thermophile campylobacter; [2] Lead acetate strip in liver broth or Kligler medium;
[3] Lead acetate strip in broth containing 0.025 % cysteine

Fig. 168: Demonstration and identification of intestinal *Campylobacter species*

Abb. 168: Nachweis und Bestimmung im Darm vorkommender *Campylobacter*

of a serotyping system is made all the more difficult (54, 55, 59, 69, 113). But the serological typing does permit the demonstration of a probable epidemiological association between human infections and the presence of certain organisms in animal materials (e.g. milk) (32, 49, 59, 101).

2.2.2 Campylobacter coli

C. coli occurs in animals under similar circumstances as C. jejuni. The pig is the most important link in the spread of this organism. In this instance too, as with C. jejuni, the intestine appears to be the site of settlement without any clinical consequences. Starting with the observations of DOYLE (24), C. coli has for a long time been considered to be the cause of swine dysentery (»vibrio dysentery«), but this view has been dropped and treponemas are now believed to be responsible (p. 286). Nevertheless, it is still possible, as infection experiments have shown, that C. coli may have a synergistic effect in supporting the treponemas in their pathogenicity (29). Also, it remains likely that C. coli can induce an enteritis in piglets (74, 101). This campylobacter plays a lesser role in inducing enteritis in man than does C. jejuni.

■ **Morphology**
C. coli usually occur as slender forms which have pointed ends. They measure 0.2–0.4 × 1.5–3.5 µm. Flagella are generally present on both ends.

■ **Biochemical properties**
See figure 168 and section 2.2.

■ **Antigenic structure**
It is very probable that C. coli possesses numerous O-antigens, so that the position is similar to that of C. jejuni. It is usually possible to differentiate between these two campylobacters by means of the complement fixation and the passive haemagglutination tests (55, 68).

2.2.3 Campylobacter laridis

Is a species which has been identified in sea gulls and may be of significance as a cause of enteritis in man. The bacterium is very similar to C. jejuni and C. coli, but it is resistant to nalidixic acid (30 to 40 µg) (NARTC strains = nalidixic acid resistant thermophile campylobacter) and does not hydrolyse sodium hippurate. It is not yet clear whether there are other clinical or epidemiological peculiarities.

2.2.4 Diagnosis of infections by C. jejuni and C. coli

Both bacteria are resident in the gut and they share many bacteriological properties, so that they are detected by the same methods. The diagnostic routine is shown in figure 168, and the cultural investigation is the most important. Storing the broth cultures presents some difficulty, because the organisms die off after a few days. Therefore, they must be lyophilized immediately or they can be maintained for months in liver broth or as a bacterial suspension in a glycerol-skimmed milk mixture at $-70\,°C$.

The biochemical properties are shown in figure 168. Growth at 43 °C (»thermophile *Campylobacter*«) or the lack of growth at 25 °C and the sensitivity to nalidixic acid are important in the differentiation between *C. coli* and *C. jejuni* on the one hand and *C. fetus* on the other (38, 41, 42, 83, 95). The distinction between *C. jejuni* and *C. coli* (see fig. 168) relies on the hydrolysis of hippurate and the absence of or retarded growth of *C. jejuni* on triphenyl tetrazolium chloride blood agar (*C. coli* grow after 3 days, *C. jejuni* after 1 week or not at all; 5, 42, 105). SKIRROW & BENJAMIN (96) described thermophile strains which are also nalidixic acid resistant (NARTC) (fig. 168).

Table 70: Biochemical properties of the subspecies of *C. sputorum* (58)

Characters	sputorum	bubulus	mucosalis
Cat	−	−	−
Oxi	(+)	+	(+)
H_2S^1	v⁻	+	+
H_2S^2	+	+	+
1 % glycine	+	+	−
1.5 % glycine	v⁺	+	−
1.5 % NaCl	v⁺	+	+
2 % NaCl	−	+	−
3 % NaCl	−	+	−

[1] Demonstration with triple sugar iron agar;
[2] Medium containing 0.05 % cysteine hydrochloride

Table 71: Biochemical properties of *Campylobacter hyointestinalis* (53)

Character	Reaction	Character		Reaction
Cat	+	Growth	TTC[1]	+
aerobic growth	−	inhibition	1 % glycine	v
OF-Glu	−		30 µg cephalotin	+
Mot	+		30 µg nalidixic acid	−
Growth at 25 °C	−	H$_2$S production	Pb acetate strip	
Growth at 43 °C	−		over blood agar[2]	+
Nit	+		Pb acetate strip	
			over blood agar	
			with 0.02 % cysteine	+
Hippurate	−		triple sugar iron agar	+

[1] Triphenyl tetrazolium chloride; [2] Sheep blood agar, incubated in 6 % O$_2$, 10 % CO$_2$, 84 % H$_2$

2.2.5 Campylobacter sputorum subsp. mucosalis

The causal agency of intestinal adenomatosis is attributed to this campylobacter. It occurs in weaning piglets and affects the lower part of the ileum and the caecum where it produces a substantial proliferation of the intestinal mucosa. The organism can be demonstrated within the cells in these lesions. As a rule the adenomatosis subsides but it can proceed to a necrotizing enteritis or regional ileitis. The bacterium may also reside in the oral cavity of pigs (81, 82, 87, 88, 106).

■ **Biochemical properties**
See table 70 (57, 58, 63).

2.2.6 Campylobacter hyointestinalis

A species that has not until now been finally classified. GEBHART et al. (34) isolated it from proliferative ileitis of the pig.

■ **Biochemical properties**
See table 71.

2.2.7 Campylobacter fecalis

C. fecalis is mainly apathogenic and can be isolated from the intestinal tract of cattle and sheep and from the preputial and vaginal mucosa of these animals. AL-MASHAT & TAYLOR (4) were able to induce an experimental enteritis in calves with this bacterium.

■ **Biochemical properties**
See figure 168.

Bibliography / Literatur

1. ABDALLAH, I. S., & W. WINKENWERDER (1965): Haussperlinge (Passer domesticus L.) als Überträger von Vibrionen. Zbl. Vet. med. 13, 338–344.
2. AL-MASHAT, R. R., & D. J. TAYLOR (1983): Production of enteritis of calves by the oral inoculation of pure cultures of Campylobacter fetus subsp. intestinalis. Vet. Rec. 112, 54–58.
3. AL-MASHAT, R. R., & D. J. TAYLOR (1983): In vitro sensitivity of 28 bovine isolates of campylobacter to some commonly used antimicrobials. Vet. Rec. 113, 89.
4. AL-MASHAT, R. R., & D. J. TAYLOR (1981): Production of enteritis in calves by the oral inoculation of pure cultures of Campylobacter fecalis. Vet. Rec. 109, 97–101.
5. AL-MASHAT, R. R., & D. J. TAYLOR (1980): Campylobacter spp. in enteric lesions in cattle. Vet. Rec. 107, 31–34.
6. AL-MASHAT, R. R., & D. J. TAYLOR (1980): Production of diarrhoe and dysentery in experimental calves by feeding pure cultures of Campylobacter fetus subsp. jejuni. Vet. Rec. 107, 459–464.
7. AGUMBAH, J. O., & J. S. OGAA (1979): Genital tropism and coital transmission of Campylobacter fetus subsp. intestinalis. Brit. Vet. J. 135, 83–91.
8. ANDREWS, PH. J., & F. W. FRANK (1974): Comparison of four diagnostic tests for detection of bovine genital vibriosis. J. Am. Vet. Med. Ass. 165, 695–697.
9. ARDEY, W. B., P. ARMSTRONG, W. A. MEINERSHAGEN & F. W. FRANK (1972): Diagnosis of ovine vibriosis and enzootic abortion of ewes by immunfluorescence technique. Am. J. Vet. Res. 33, 2535–2538.
10. BARNARD, B. J. H. (1969): The diagnosis of vibriosis by the fluorescent antibody technique. J. S. Afr. Vet. Med. Ass. 40, 407–409.
11. BAUDITZ, R. (1966): Die infektiöse Hepatitis des Huhnes. Vet. med. Nachr. 118–132.
12. BEHRENS, R., M. KIST & H. HELWIG (1983): Campylobacterinfektionen bei Kindern. Immun. Infekt. 11, 55–60.
13. BERG, R. L., J. W. JUTILA & B. D. FIREHAMMER (1971): A revised classification of Vibrio fetus. Am. J. Vet. Res. 32, 11–22.
14. BINGÖL, R., & H. BLOBEL (1970): Immunfluoreszenz- und Agglutinationsreaktionen von Vibrio fetus. Zbl. Bakt. I. Orig. 215, 316–319.
15. BISPING, W., G. KIRPAL & B. SONNENSCHEIN (1981): Die Diagnose und Bekämpfung der Campylobacter fetus subsp. fetus-Infektion beim Besamungsbullen. Tierärztl. Umschau 36, 667–674.
16. BISPING, W., U. FREYTAG & H. KRAUSS (1963): Feststellung der Vibrionenhepatitis der Hühner in Nordwestdeutschland. Berl. Münch. tierärztl. Wschr. 76, 456–461.
17. BLUMENSCHEIN, W. (1980): Untersuchungen über das Vorkommen von Campylobacter fetus in Darm und Galle bei Rindern und Kälbern unter besonderer Berücksichtigung der Biotypen intestinalis und venerealis in Baden-Württemberg. Vet. Med. Diss. München.
18. BORKENHAGEN, M., & W. LETZ (1974): Vibrio fetus Typ 1 als Ursache seuchenhaften Verlammens bei Schafen. Mh. Vet. Med. 29, 250–252.
19. BRUCE, D., W. ZOCHOWSKI & G. A. FLEMING (1980): Campylobacter infections in cats and dogs. Vet. Rec. 107, 200–201.
20. CLARK, B. L., J. H. DUFTY & M. J. MONSBOURGH (1972): A method for maintaining the viability of Vibrio fetus var. venerealis in samples of preputial secretions collected from carrier bulls. Aust. Vet. J. 48, 462–464.
21. DEDIÉ, K., R. POHL, H. ROMER, F. WAGENSEIL, E. ALBRECHT & G. HÜHNERMUND (1982): Zur Verbreitung, Ermittlung und Bekämpfung der venerischen Campylobacteriosis (Vibriosis genitalis) beim Rind in Beständen mit Bullenhaltung. Tierärztl. Umschau 37, 80–96.
22. DEDIÉ, K., R. POHL & K. REISSHAUER (1977): Vorkommen und Pathogenität glycin-positiver Stämme des Campylobacter (Vibrio) fetus Serotyp O1. Zbl. Vet. Med. B, 24, 767–770.
23. DEVRIESE, L., & A. DAVOS (1971): Vibrio spp. bij pluimvee: isolatie, identficatie en experimentele infectie. Tijdschr. Diergeneesk. 96, 193–201.
24. DOYLE, L. P. (1948): The etiology of swine dysentery. Amer. J. Vet. Res. 9, 50–51.
25. DUFTY, J. H. (1967): Diagnosis of vibriosis in the bull. Austr. Vet. J. 43, 433–437.
26. DUNN, H. O., K. BURDA, W. C. WAGNER & H. L. GIMAN (1965): Isolation of Vibrio fetus from bovine semen. Cornell Vet. 55, 220–229.
27. ELLIS, W. A., S. D. NEIL, J. J. O'BRIEN & J. HANNA (1978): Isolation of Spirillum-like organism from pig fetuses. Vet. Rec. 102, 106.
28. ELLIS, W. A., S. D. NEIL, J. J. O'BRIEN, H. W. FERGUSON & J. HANNA (1977): Isolation of Spirillum/Vibrio-like organism from bovine fetuses. Vet. Rec. 100, 451–452.
29. FERNIE, D. S., R. M. GRIFFIN & R. W. A. PARK (1975): The possibility that Campylobacter (Vibrio) coli and Treponema hyodysenteriae are both involved in swine dysentery. Brit. Vet. J. 131, 335–338.
30. FIREHAMMER, B. D., & L. L. MYERS (1981): Campylobacter fetus subsp. jejuni: Its possible significance in enteric disease of calves and lambs. Am. J. Vet. Res. 42, 918–922.
31. FLEMING, M. P. (1980): Incidence of campylobacter infection in dogs. Vet. Rec. 107, 202.
32. GARCIA, M. M., M. D. EAGLESOME & C. RIGBY (1983): Campylobacters important in veterinary medicine. Vet. Bull. 53, 793–818.
33. GARCIA, M. M., R. B. STEWART & G. M. RUCKERBAUER (1984): Quantitative evaluation of a transport enrichment medium for Campylobacter fetus. Vet. Rec. 115, 434–436.
34. GEBHART, C. J., G. E. WARD, K. CHANG & H. J. KURTZ (1983): Campylobacter hyointestinalis (new species) isolated from swine with lesions of proliferative ileitis. Am. J. Vet. Res. 44, 361–367.
35. GOREN, E., & A. DE JONG (1980): Campylobacter fetus subsp. jejuni bij pluimvee. Tijdschr. Diergeneesk. 105, 724–726.
36. GÖRGEN, M., G. KIRPAL & W. BISPING (1983): Untersuchungen zum Vorkommen von Keimen der Gattung Campylobacter beim Schwein. I. Kulturelle Untersuchungen von Kot, Darminhalt und Gallenblasen sowie Infektionsversuche. Berl. Münch. tierärztl. Wschr. 96, 86–89.
37. GRÜNBERG, W., & E. OTTE (1963): Vibrionen-Hepatitis bei Trappenküken. Wiener tierärztl. Mschr. 50, 862–870.
38. HÄNNINEN, M. (1980): Characterization of Campylobacter jejuni/coli isolated from different sources. Acta vet. scand. 23, 88–98.
39. HARVEY, S. M. (1980): Hippurate hydrolysis by Campylobacter fetus. J. clin. Microbiol. 11, 435–437.
40. HARTOG, B. J., G. J. A. DE WILDE & E. DE BOER (1983): Poultry as a source of Campylobacter jejuni. Arch. Lebensmittelhyg. 34, 116–122.
41. HASSELBACH, P., G. KIRPAL, M. GÖRGEN & W. BISPING (1984): Untersuchungen zum Vorkommen von Keimen der Gattung Campylobacter beim Schwein. Teil II: Kulturelles Verhalten, Differenzierung und Resistenzprüfung der isolierten Campylobacterstämme. Berl. Münch. tierärztl. Wschr. 97, 113–119.
42. HASSELBACH, P. (1983): Untersuchungen über die kulturell-biochemische Differenzierung tierischer Campylobacterstämme. Vet. Med. Diss. Hannover.
43. HIGGINS, R., & R. DEGRE (1979): Isolation of Spirillum-like organisms from pig and bovine fetuses. Vet. Rec. 104, 262–263.

44. Hofstad, M. S., E. H. McGehee & P. C. Bennett (1958): Avian infectious hepatitis. Avian Dis. **2**, 358–364.
45. Hosie, B. D., T. B. Nicolson & D. B. Henderson (1979): Campylobacter infections in normal and diarrhoeic dogs. Vet. Rec. **105**, 80.
46. Jahn, B. (1983): Campylobacter im Genitaltrakt des Schweines. Vet. Med. Diss. Hannover.
47. Jørgensen, K. (1981): Forekomst af Campylobacter fetus ssp. jejuni hos danske hunde. Nord. Vet. Med. **33**, 42–48.
48. Jørgensen, K. (1979): The occurrence of Campylobacter in swine. Nord. Vet. Med. **31**, 534.
49. Jones, D. M., J. D. Abbott, M. J. Painter & E. M. Sutcliffe (1984): A comparison of biotypes and serotypes of Campylobacter sp. isolated from patients with enteritis and from animal and environmental sources. J. Infect. **9**, 51–58.
50. Kamel, M. M. (1960): Isolierung und Differenzierung der beim Rind vorkommenden Vibrionen. Vet. med. Diss. Hannover.
51. Kölbl, O. (1964): Nachweis der Vibrionenhepatitis bei Hühnern in Österreich. Wiener tierärztl. Wschr. **51**, 165–170.
52. Kötsche, W. (1980): Untersuchungen zur Eignung von Membranfiltern für die Selektivzüchtung von Campylobacteriaceae und die gleichzeitige Eliminierung von Bacterium proteus aus Präputialspülproben von Bullen. Mh. Vet. Med. **35**, 452–456.
53. Lambert, M., J. M. W. Jones & S. A. Lister (1984): Isolation of Campylobacter hyointestinalis from pigs in the United Kingdom. Vet. Rec. **115**, 128–129.
54. Lauwers, S., L. Vlaes & J. P. Butzler (1981): Campylobacter serotyping and epidemiology. Lancet I, 158–159.
55. Lauwers, S., & J. L. Penner (1984): Serotyping Camplyobacter and Campylobacter coli on the basis thermostable antigens. In: J. P. Butzler: Campylobacter infection in man and animals. S. 51–59. Boca Raton, Florida: CRC Press.
56. Laing, J. A. (1960): Vibrio fetus infection of cattle. FAO Agricultural studies 51.
57. Lawson, G. H. K., J. L. Leaver, G. W. Pettigrew & A. C. Rowland (1981): Some features of Campylobacter sputorum subsp. mucosalis nov., nom. rev. and their taxonomic significance. Int. J. System. Bact. **31**, 385–391.
58. Lawson, G. H. K., A. C. Rowland & P. Wooding (1975): The characterization of Campylobacter sputorum subspecies mucosalis isolated from pigs. Res. Vet. Sci. **18**, 121–126.
59. Lior, H., L. Woodward, J. A. Edgar, L. J. Laroche & P. Gill (1982): Serotyping of Campylobacter jejuni by slide agglutination based on heat-labile antigenic factors. J. clin. Microbiol. **15**, 761–768.
60. Lisle, G. W. de, D. J. Stephens & M. M. E. Bird (1982): Transport media for Campylobacter fetus venerealis. N.Z. Vet. J. **30**, 31–32.
61. Lein, D., J. Erickson, A. Winter & K. McEntee (1968): Diagnosis, treatment and control of vibriosis in an artifical insemination center. J. Am. Vet. Med. Ass. **153**, 1574–1580.
62. Logan, E. F., S. D. Neill & D. P. Mackie (1982): Mastitis in dairy cows associated with an aerotolerant campylobacter. Vet. Rec. **110**, 229–230.
63. Love, D. N., R. J. Love & M. Bailey (1977): Comparison of Campylobacter sputorum subsp. mucosalis strains in PIA and PHE. Vet. Rec. **101**, 407.
64. Mehle, J. (1971): Vibrio fetus, Typ 1, im Verdauungstrakt der Rinder. Der Wert der serologischen KBR-Methode für die Diagnostik der Genitalvibriose der Färsen. Veterin. Glasnik **15**, 165–169.
65. Mellick, P. W., A. J. Winter & K. McEntee (1965): Diagnosis of Vibriosis in the bull by use of the fluorescent antibody technic. Cornell Vet. **55**, 280–294.
66. Mitscherlich, E., & R. Heider (1968): Formenwechsel der O-Antigene bei Vibrio fetus. Zbl. Vet. Med. B **15**, 486–493.
67. Mischerlich, E., & H. Prange (1959): Die Vibriosis genitalis des Rindes. Dtsch. tierärztl. Wschr. **66**, 521–526, 559–564.
68. Mitscherlich, E. (1981): Campylobacter und Vibrio. In: H. Blobel & T. Schliesser (Hrsg.): Handbuch der bakteriellen Infektionen bei Tieren, Bd. III, S. 1–74. Jena: VEB Gustav Fischer.
69. Mitscherlich, E., & B. Liess (1958): Die serologische Differenzierung von Vibrio fetus-Stämmen. Dtsch. tierärztl. Wschr. **65**, 2–5, 36–39.
70. Neill, S. D., J. J. O'Brien & W. A. Ellis (1980): The isolation of aerotolerant campylobacter. Vet. Rec. **106**, 152–153.
71. Neill, S. D., W. A. Ellis & J. J. O'Brien (1978): The biochemical characteristics of Campylobacter-like organisms from cattle and pigs. Res. Vet. Sci. **25**, 368–372.
72. Neill, S. D., W. A. Ellis & J. J. O'Brien (1979): Designation of aerotolerant Campylobacter-like organism from porcine and bovine abortions to the genus of Campylobacter. Res. Vet. Sci. **27**, 180–186.
73. Oosterom, J. (1980): Het voorkomen van Campylobacter fetus subsp. jejuni bij normale slachtvarkens. Tijdschr. Diergenessk. **105**, 49–50.
74. Olubunmi, P. A., & D. J. Taylor (1982): Production of enteritis in pigs by the oral inoculation of pure cultures of Campylobacter coli. Vet. Rec. **111**, 197–202.
75. Peckham, M. C. (1958): Avian vibrionic hepatitis. Avian Dis. **2**, 348–358.
76. Philpott, M. (1968): Diagnosis of Vibrio fetus infection in the bull. Vet. Rec. **82**, 458–463.
77. Philpott, M. (1966): The detection of Vibrio fetus in the bull. Vet. Rec. **79**, 811–812.
78. Plastridge, W. N., M. E. Koths & L. F. Williams (1961): Antibiotic mediums for the isolation of vibrios from bull semen. Am. J. Vet. Res. **22**, 867–870.
79. Plumer, G. J., W. C. Duvall & V. M. Shepler (1962): A preliminary report on a new technic for isolation of Vibrio fetus from carrier bulls. Cornell Vet. **52**, 110–122.
80. Prescott, J. F., & C. W. Bruin-Mosch (1981): Carriage of Campylobacter jejuni in healthy and diarrheic animals. Am. J. Vet. Res. **42**, 164–165.
81. Roberts, L. (1981): Natural infection of the oral cavity of young piglets with Campylobacter sputorum subsp. mucosalis. Vet. Rec. **109**, 17.
82. Roberts, L., G. H. K. Lawson & A. C. Rowland (1980): Experimental infection of neonatal pigs with Campylobacter sputorum subsp. mucosalis with special reference to the oral cavity. Vet. Microbiol. **5**, 249–255.
83. Rosef, O., & M. Yndestad (1982): Some characteristics of Campylobacter fetus subsp. jejuni isolated from pigs, birds and man. Acta vet. scand. **23**, 9–15.
84. Rosef, O. (1981): Forekomsten av Campylobacter fetus subsp. jejuni og salmoneller-bacterier hos noen viltlevende fugler. Nord. Vet. Med. **33**, 539–543.
85. Rosef, O. (1981): Isolation of Campylobacter fetus subsp. jejuni from the gallbladder of normal and slaughter pigs using an enrichment procedure. Act. vet. scand. **22**, 149–151.
86. Roslanowski, K., T. Losinski & J. Wyszanowski (1972): Vibriose bei Zuchtbullen. Med. veter. Warszawa **28**, 104–107.
87. Rowland, A. C., & G. H. K. Lawson (1975): Intestinal adenomatosis. A possible relationship with necrotic enteritis, regional ileitis and proliferative hemorrhagic enteropathy. Vet. Rec. **97**, 178–181.
88. Rowland, A. C., G. H. K. Lawson & A. Maxwell (1973): Intestinal adenomatosis in the pig: Occurrence of a bacterium in affected cells. Nature **243**, 417.
89. Rübsamen, S., K. Danner & R. Weiss (1982): Zur ätiologischen Bedeutung von Campylobacter fetus subsp. jejuni und Parvovirus für akute Enteritiden des Hundes. Zbl. Vet. Med. B, **29**, 521–531.

90. Schimmelpfennig, H., & E. Mitscherlich (1964): Zur Anwendung der Fluoreszenzserologie in der bakteriologischen Diagnostik. 1. Mitt.: Differenzierung von Vibrio fetus- und Vibrio El Tor-Stämmen mittels fluoreszierender Antikörper. Zbl. Vet. Med. B, **11**, 393–406.

91. Sevoian, M., R. W. Winterfield & C. L. Goldman (1958): Avian infectious hepatatis. 1. Clinical and pathological manifestations. 2. Some characteristics of the etiologic agent. Effect of various drugs on the course of the disease. Avian Dis. **2**, 3–18, 19–39.

92. Shepler, V. M., G. J. Plumer & J. E. Faber (1963): Isolation of Vibrio fetus from bovine preputial fluid, using millipore filters and an antibiotic medium. Amer. J. Vet. Res. **24**, 749–755.

93. Skirrow, M. B. (1982): Campylobacter enteritis — the first five years. J. Hyg. **89**, 175–184.

94. Skirrow, M. B. (1981): Campylobacter enteritis in dogs and cats: a new zoonosis. Vet. Res. Comm. **5**, 13–19.

95. Skirrow, M. B., & J. Benjamin (1980): Differentiation of enteropathogenic campylobacter. J. clin. Path. **33**, 1122.

96. Skirrow, M. B., & J. Benjamin (1980): "1001" Campylobacters: cultural characteristics of intestinal campylobacters from man and animals. J. Hyg. **85**, 427–442.

97. Söderlind, O. (1961): Serologische Differenzierung von Vibrio-fetus-Stämmen. Mh. Tierhk. **13**, 42–47.

98. Speck, J. (1969): Antigene Eigenschaften isolierter Hühnervibrionenstämme. Zbl. Vet. med. B, **16**, 579–587.

99. Speck, J. (1965): Die serologische Differenzierung von Hühnervibrionen mittels der Komplementbindungsreaktion. Zbl. Vet. Med. Reihe B, **12**, 541–546.

100. Stadtfeld, H., E. Nitzschke, W. Hahn & A. Konz (1982): Zum kulturellen Nachweis von Campylobacter fetus subspecies fetus in Präputialspülproben von Besamungs- und Deckbullen. Berl. Münch. tierärztl. Wschr. **95**, 393–397.

101. Taylor, O. J., & P. A. Olubunmi (1981): A reexamination of the role of Campylobacter fetus subsp. coli in enteric disease of the pig. Vet. Rec. **109**, 112–115.

102. Teufel, P. (1982): Campylobacter fetus ss. jejuni — Ausscheidungsraten beim Schwein und Überleben in Leitungswasser. Fleischwirtsch. **62**, 1344–1345.

103. Vandenberghe, J., S. Lauwers, P. Plehier & J. Hoorens (1982): Campylobacter jejuni related with diarrhoea in dogs. Brit. Vet. J. **138**, 356–361.

104. Vandeplassche, M. (1959): Die Epidemiologie und die Bekämpfung der Vibriosis genitalis bovis. Zuchthygiene **3**, 1–15.

105. Véron, M., & R. Chatelain (1973): Taxonomic study of genus Campylobacter Sebald and Véron and designation of the neotype strain for the type species Campylobacter fetus (Smith and Taylor) Sebald and Véron. Int. J. System. Bact. **23**, 122–134.

106. Waldmann, K. H. (1985): Campylobacter als Enteropathieursache beim Schwein. Prakt. Tierarzt **66**, 989–994.

107. Weber, A., C. Lemke, R. Schäfer & I. Bergmann (1983): Vergleichende Anwendung von zwei Selektivnährböden zur Isolierung von Campylobacter jejuni aus Kotproben von Tieren. Zbl. Vet. Med. B, **30**, 175–179.

108. Weber, A., C. Lemke, R. Schäfer, U. Seifert & H. Berg (1983): Nachweis von Campylobacter jejuni in Kotproben von Hunden. Berl. Münch. tierärztl. Wschr. **96**, 232–234.

109. Weber, A., C. Lembke & R. Schäfer (1982): Untersuchungen zum Vorkommen von Campylobacter jejuni bei Kaninchen, Meerschweinchen, Ratten und Mäusen in der Versuchstierhaltung. Berl. Münch. tierärztl. Wschr. **95**, 488–489.

110. Weber, A., C. Lembke & A. Kettner (1981): Nachweis von Campylobacter jejuni in Kotproben von klinisch gesunden Brieftauben. Berl. Münch. tierärztl. Wschr. **94**, 449–451.

111. Weisser, W. (1983): Erfahrungen mit der Isolierung und Klassifizierung von Campylobacter aus Fäzes von fleischfressenden Haustieren. Tierärztl. Umschau **38**, 717–721.

112. Winkenwerder, W., & T. Maciak (1965): Das Vorkommen von Vibrionen bei Rindern in Nordwestdeutschland. Berl. Münch. tierärztl. Wschr. **78**, 161–166.

113. Winkenwerder, W., & W. Bisping (1964): Kulturelle, serologische und tierexperimentelle Untersuchungen mit von Hühnern und Rindern isolierten Vibrionen. Zbl. Vet. Med. B, **11**, 603–616.

114. Winter, A. J., & A. T. Caveney (1978): Evaluation of a transport medium for Campylobacter (Vibrio) fetus. J. Am. Med. Ass. **173**, 472–474.

115. Winter, A. J., J. D. Samuelson & M. Elkana (1967): A comparison of immunfluorescence and cultural techniques for demonstration of Vibrio fetus. J. Amer. vet. med. Ass. **150**, 499–502.

116. Winter, A. J., W. Burda & H. O. Dunn (1965): An evaluation of cultural technics for the detection of Vibrio fetus in bovine semen. Cornell Vet. **55**, 431–444.

117. Witte, K. (1962): Zur Zuverlässigkeit des Kulturverfahrens, der Scheidenschleimagglutination und der Blutserumkomplementbindungsreaktion für den Nachweis der Vibrio fetus-Infektion bei weiblichen Rindern in akut und chronisch verseuchten Beständen. Dtsch. tierärztl. Wschr. **69**, 394–400, 421–424.

118. Wolfers, I. (1981): Untersuchungen zum Vorkommen von Campylobacter im Hundedarm mit einem Beitrag zu ihrer Isolierung und Differenzierung. Vet. Med. Diss. Hannover.

119. Wormstrand, A. (1968): The occurrence of Vibrio bubulus and its importance as a possible cause of abortion. Nord. Vet. Med. **20**, 634–637.

120. Wright, E. P. (1982): The occurrence of Campylobacter jejuni in dog faeces from a public park. J. Hyg. **89**, 191–194.

Haemophilic bacteria
Hämophile Bakterien

1 Genus: Haemophilus (H.)

Gram-negative coccoid to rod shaped bacteria which rarely form into filaments, are haemophilic but non-motile. Their growth is dependent on growth factors. The bacteria can form capsules which determine the colony form (tab. 73). Size: 0.2–0.3 × 0.5–2 µm.

■ **Incidence and veterinary significance**
Incidence and significance in animals see table 72. *Haemophilus species* probably occur in all types of animal. They can form part of the normal bacterial flora or, on the other hand, they can produce disease conditions. Some species have not been classified, or at least only incompletely characterized. In the following only those species will be discussed in detail which have definitely been described and/or which are of known clinical importance.

■ **Culture**
▷ Growth factor V: NAD (nicotinamide adenine dinucleotide) is thermolabile and participates in the oxidation-reduction processes of the growing bacterial cell. The factor occurs naturally in animal and plant cells and is produced by some bacteria, such as staphylococci (satellite phenomenon).
▷ Growth factor X: Haemin is a complex of protoporphyrin and an essential component of the bacterial respiratory enzymes.
The various species require for growth either both these factors or one and this fact is utilized in taxonomy (fig. 169).

In view of the growth factor requirements the bacteria can be grown on the following media: chocolate agar, contains X and V factors; blood agar, contains only X factor in accessible and sufficient amounts. It is therefore necessary to supply another strain of bacteria which can synthesize the

1 Gattung: Haemophilus (H.)

Gramnegative, pleomorphe, kokkoide bis stäbchenförmige, seltener Fäden bildende, unbewegliche, hämophile Bakterien, deren Wachstum von Wachstumsfaktoren abhängig ist. Die Bakterien können eine Kapsel ausbilden, die die Kolonieform bestimmt (s. Tab. 73). Größe: 0,2–0,3 × 0,5–2 µm.

■ **Vorkommen und medizinische Bedeutung**
Vorkommen und Bedeutung bei Tieren zeigt Tab. 72. *Haemophilus*-Arten dürften bei praktisch allen Tierarten vorkommen. Sie gehören einerseits zur normalen Keimflora, andererseits können sie teilweise Krankheitsprozesse verursachen. Einige Arten sind bisher nicht oder nur unvollständig identifiziert worden. Nachfolgend werden insbesondere die Arten genannt, die sicher beschrieben und (oder) von bekannter klinischer Bedeutung sind.

■ **Kultur**
▷ Wachstumsfaktor V: NAD (Nikotinamid-adenin-dinukleotid), thermolabil, beteiligt an Oxidoreduktionsprozessen der wachsenden Bakterienzelle. Der Faktor kommt natürlicherweise in tierischen und pflanzlichen Zellen vor und wird von einigen Bakterien produziert, z. B. von Staphylokokken (Ammen- und Satellitenphänomen).
▷ Wachstumsfaktor X: Hämin, Komplex aus Protoporphyrin und einem essentiellen Bestandteil der bakteriellen Atmungsenzyme.
Die einzelnen Arten brauchen zum Wachstum entweder beide oder einen der Wachstumsfaktoren, dies wird als taxonomisches Merkmal genutzt (Abb. 169).

Unter Berücksichtigung des Bedarfes an den Wachstumsfaktoren lassen sich die Bakterien auf folgenden Nährboden züchten: Kochblutagar, enthält X und V-Faktor; Blutagar, enthält nur den X-

Table 72: *Haemophilus species* of veterinary importance

Tabelle 72: Veterinärmedizinisch wichtige *Haemophilus*-Arten

Animal species	Haemophilus species	Clinical picture
Pig	parasuis	Glässer's disease, polyserositis and arthritis, secondary infections in cases of pneumonia, part of the normal bacterial flora of the nasal cavity (3, 24, 58, 81)
	pleuropneumoniae, syn.: parahaemolyticus	infectious pleuropneumonia, characterized by haemorrhagic necrotizing pneumonia, usually acute or peracute, rarely chronic, adhesive pleurisy, first seen in Germany in 1980; highly contagious, aerogenous contact infection, primary cause (17, 46, 53, 56)
Poultry	paragallinarum	contagious coryza of fowls, catarrhal and fibrinous pleurisy, sinusitis, conjunctivitis (27, 53) latent infections, virulence of strains differs
	avium	apathogenic or slightly virulent inhabitants of the respiratory organs (2, 28)
Dog	haemoglobinophilus syn.: canis	apathogenic inhabitant of the prepuce; haemophilus species have also been isolated from vaginitis and respiratory diseases
Ox	somnus[1]	(1) infectious, septicaemic thrombosing meningo-encephalitis (ISTME), sleeper syndrome (18, 35, 61, 71) (2) respiratory diseases, pneumonia, laryngitis, tracheitis (frequently mixed infections with other bacteria), pleurisy (13, 42) (3) arthritis, tenovaginitis (4) diseases and infections of the genital organs, endometritis with sterility, abortion (19, 48), occurs in semen and genital tract of bulls (11, 30, 40, 42, 62) (5) weak calf syndrome, weakly calves following infection at birth (79)
Horse	equigenitalis[1]	infection of the genital organs, endometritis, cervicitis, vaginitis, latent infections in mares and stallions (7, 9, 13, 70)
Sheep	ovis[1] agni[1]	bronchopneumonia (41) septicaemia, pneumonia, arthritis of lambs
Fish	piscium[1]	Ulcer disease of trout, ulcerating inflammation of gills and mouth

[1] membership of the genus *Haemophilus* doubtful or not proven

[1] Zugehörigkeit zur Gattung *Haemophilus* fraglich oder nicht gegeben

V factor (satellitism, fig. 173). For this purpose the strain to be examined is spread in parallel streaks onto blood agar and the satellite bacterium is inoculated in a single line at right angles to the others. After incubation the *Haemophilus* colonies exhibit a distinct growth stimulation in the region of the satellite bacteria. Other organisms, such as streptococci, can also exhibit the satellite phenomenon and the Gram stain is used to differentiate.

Levinthal agar or broth: These media contain the following blood extracts: nutrient broth (e. g. brain heart infusion) with 10 % horse blood is briefly boiled and the supernatant is filtered (first with filter paper then through Seitz filters). This »stock solution« is mixed either with agar (50 °C) or with broth at a ratio of 1 : 1.

NAD-haemin medium has growth factors added to the basic constituents at a final concentration of 1 to 10 µg/ml.

Faktor in ausreichend verfügbarer Menge, so daß die Mitführung eines den V-Faktor synthetisierenden Bakterienstammes notwendig ist (Ammenphänomen, s. Abb. 173). Dazu wird bei der Isolierung das zu untersuchende Material in parallelen Strichen auf die Blutplatte geimpft und senkrecht dazu in einem Einzelstrich der Ammenkeim aufgebracht. Nach Bebrütung zeigen die *Haemophilus*-Kolonien im Bereich des Ammenstriches eine deutliche Wachstumsförderung (auch andere Bakterien, z. B. Streptokokken, können ein Ammenphänomen zeigen, Kontrolle durch Gram-Färbung).

Levinthal-Agar oder -Bouillon: Diese Medien enthalten folgenden Blutextrakt: Nährbouillon (z. B. brain-heart-infusion) mit 10 % Pferdeblut wird kurz aufgekocht, und der Überstand wird filtriert (erst Papier-, dann Seitzfilter). Diese »Stammlösung« wird entweder mit Agar (50 °C) oder Bouillon im Verhältnis 1 : 1 gemischt.

```
┌─────────────────────────────┐
│         Specimens           │
└─────────────┬───────────────┘
              │
┌─────────────┴───────────────┐
│   Microscopic examination   │
├─────────────────────────────┤
│ Gram-negative coccoid rods, │
│ non-motile, rarely forming  │
│ filaments                   │
└─────────────────────────────┘
```

Examination by culture

1. Carried out under consideration of the dependence on X- and/or V-factors:
   Blood agar with Staphylococcus epidermidis to demonstrate satellitism
   Chocolate agar,
   Levinthal agar,
   Selective media (p. 235)
   Commercial haemophilus agar,
2. Incubation at 37 °C either aerobic or, in the case of micro-aerophilic species (see below) in 10 % CO_2 atmosphere

Biochemical identification

1. Assessment of dependence on X- and/or V-factors
   Disc test (other methods e. g. porphyrin test see page 235):

Growth around the discs			indicates:
X and V	V	X	
+	+	−	V dependence
+	−	−	X and V dependence
+	−	+	X dependence

2. Identification of biochemical properties[2]

Host	Haemophilus	X	V	CO_2	Oxi	Cat	Hae	Ind	Ure	Dex	Sac	Lac	Xyl	Man
Pig	parasuis	−	+	−	−	+	−	−	−	+	+	−	−	−
	pleuropneumoniae	−	+	+	v	v	+	−	+	+	+	v	+	+
	sp.[3]	−	+	−	+	+	v	−	+	+	+	+	−	−
Poultry	paragallinarum	−	+	+	−	−	−	−	−	+	+	v	v	+
	avium	−	+	−	+	−	−	−	−	+	+	v	v	+
Horse	equigenitalis[1]	−	−	+	+	+	−	−	−	−	−	?	?	?
Ox	somnus[1]	−	−	+	+	−	(+/−)	v	−	+	−	−	+	v
Sheep	ovis[1]	+?	−	−	?	?	−	−	?	+	+	v	v	+
	agni[1]	+?	−	?	?	?	?	−	?	(+)	v⁻	−	(+)	(+)
Dog	haemoglobinophilus	+	−	−	+	+	−	+	−	+	+	−	+	+
Fish	piscium[1]	−	−	−	+	−	−	−	−	+	+	−	−	−

```
┌────────────────────────────────────────────────┐
│ Serological determination of capsular antigens │
├────────────────────────────────────────────────┤
│ especially with H. parasuis, H. pleuropneumoniae, │
│ H. paragallinarum[4]                           │
└────────────────────────────────────────────────┘
```

[1] Membership of genus haemophilus is doubtful or not proven; [2] after Nicolet, 53; [3] minor group see p. 238;
[4] Review of methods, see Nicolet, 53

Fig. 169: Demonstration and identification of *Haemophilus species* of veterinary importance

Abb. 169: Nachweis und Identifizierung veterinärmedizinisch wichtiger *Haemophilus-Arten*

Selective media which incorporate inhibitors for the suppression of contaminants. Crystal violet (1 : 25,000) and 1.6 IU/ml bacitracin were recommended for the isolation of haemophilus in the pig (41). Incubation temperature 37 °C. Most species require an atmosphere of 10 % CO_2 for primary culture (fig. 169).

■ Biochemical properties

▷ Identification of dependence on X or V factors. In routine diagnosis the disc test is very popular. Filter paper discs impregnated with the appropriate factors are commercially available. The test procedure is similar to that of antibiotic sensitivity tests: the surface of an agar plate is evenly inoculated and the discs are deposited on top. Following incubation for 24—48 hours the growth is assessed in the diffusion zone around the discs (fig. 171).

Another method is to add NAD and/or haemin as pure substances to the medium (proteose peptone agar) (82).

The porphyrin test has been developed because the demonstration of X factor dependence can present difficulty. This test is based on the observation that strains which are not dependent on X factor synthesize porphyrins from δ-aminolaevulinic acid. The haemin dependence can thus be demonstrated indirectly if there is no such synthesis of porphyrin. The test medium consists of δ-aminolaevulinic acid (2.0 mM), Mg/SO$_4$ (0.8 mM) and a phosphate buffer (0.1 M, pH 6.9). The solution is tubed in 0.5 ml lots and inoculated with a loop of bacteria from a chocolate agar culture that had been incubated for 24 hours. This in turn is incubated for 24 or 48 hours at 37 °C. The precursor of porphyrin is demonstrated by adding a drop of Kovacs regent. A pink to red colour develops if the test is positive (36, 44).

NAD-Hämin-Medien, die neben dem Grundmedium Zusätze der Wachstumsfaktoren enthalten, Endkonzentrationen 1 bis 10 µg/ml.

Selektivmedien, die Hemmstoffe zur Unterdrückung der Begleitflora enthalten. Für die Isolierung von *Haemophilus* beim Schwein wurden Kristallviolett (1 : 25 000) und 1,6 IE/ml Bacitracin empfohlen (41). Bebrütungstemperatur 37 °C. Die meisten Arten erfordern für die Anzucht eine 10%ige CO_2-Atmosphäre (Abb. 169).

■ Kulturell-biochemische Eigenschaften

▷ Bestimmung der Abhängigkeit von X- und V-Faktor: Für die Routinediagnostik wird insbesondere der Blättchentest benutzt. Die mit den entsprechenden Faktoren getränkten Filterpapierscheiben sind im Handel erhältlich. Der Nachweis wird nach Art des Resistenztestes geführt, indem die Oberfläche eines Agarnährbodens gleichmäßig beimpft und anschließend die Blättchen aufgelegt werden. Nach der Bebrütung (24–48 h) wird das Wachstum im Bereich der Diffusionszone um die Blättchen herum beurteilt (Abb. 171).

Eine weitere Möglichkeit besteht darin, Nährböden (Proteose-Peptonagar) NAD und (oder) Hämin als Reinsubstanz zuzusetzen (82).

Da der Nachweis der X-Abhängigkeit schwierig sein kann, ist der Porphyrintest entwickelt worden. Er beruht auf der Beobachtung, daß X unabhängige Stämme aus δ-Aminolävulinsäure Porphyrine synthetisieren. Durch die ausbleibende Synthese kann indirekt die Häminabhängigkeit nachgewiesen werden. Das Testmedium besteht aus δ-Aminolävulinsäure (2,0 mM), MgSO$_4$ (0,8 mM) und einem Phosphatpuffer (0,1 M, pH 6,9). Die Lösung wird in Mengen von 0,5 ml abgefüllt, mit einer Öse Bakterienmaterial einer 24 h bebrüteten Kochblutkultur beimpft und 24 bzw. 48 h bei 37 °C bebrütet. Der Nachweis von Porphyrin (Vorstufe) geschieht durch Zusatz von einem Tropfen Kovacs-Reagens, im positiven Fall tritt eine Rosa- bis Rotverfärbung auf (36, 44).

Table 73: Colony variation in *Haemophilus pleuropneumoniae*, *paragallinarum* and *parasuis*

Tabelle 73: Kolonievariabilität bei *Haemophilus pleuropneumoniae*, *paragallinarum* und *parasuis*

Colony form	Appearance of colony	Capsule present	Direction of dissociation
M	Large, mucoid, confluent colonies, shiny surface, in oblique iridescent light	+	↑ [1]
S	Small, smooth, transparent colonies, no confluence nor iridescence	negative, except: H. pleuropneumoniae	
R	large colonies with crumpled surface and serrated edge	−	↓

[1] Reversible through animal passage

▷ Fermentation of Carbohydrates: This follows the usual technique. It may be necessary to add NAD and haemin to the media. BIBERSTEIN et al. (5) recommend a rapid method: The phenol red carbohydrate (0.5%) medium is put up in lots of 1 ml, heavily inoculated and, after 4 to 6 and 24 hours incubation at 37 °C it is checked for the production of acid.

▷ Haemolysis: This is tested on blood agar (5% defibrinated ox or sheep blood) using a non-haemolytic strain of *Staphylococcus epidermidis* as satellite.

CAMP test: The *Haemophilus* strain is inoculated onto a blood agar plate right up to the point where the zone of β-haemolysin of a previously inoculated *Staphylococcus aureus* is expected to extend, without actually touching it.

Methods for the demonstration of oxidase, catalase, urease, indole and nitrate reduction (26).

1.1 Haemophilus infections in pigs
1.1.1 Haemophilus suis

This bacterium is extremely sensitive and difficult to culture, being dependent on both V and X factors. It is not known, therefore, how widely it is distributed but apparently it is rare and, according to NICOLET (53), it merely remains of historical interest.

H. suis, like *H. parasuis*, is implicated as a cause of Glässer's disease and it occurs as a normal resident in the respiratory mucosa of healthy pigs.

Biochemical properties, see figure 169.

1.1.2 Haemophilus parasuis

See figs. 170 and 171. Veterinary significance, see table 72. Biochemical properties see figure 169.

Serogroups A–D have been identified, in correlation with the capsular antigens; Serotype C appears to be the most common.

1.1.3 Haemophilus pleuropneumoniae
(Syn.: *H. parahaemolyticus*)

The classification of *H. pleuropneumoniae* is uncertain despite its predominant V factor dependence. POHL et al. (60) and KIELSTEIN et al. (38) class it in the genus *Actinobacillus* (*Act. pleuropneumoniae*), because of the structure of its DNA bases.

■ Incidence and veterinary significance
See table 72.

Genus: Haemophilus (H.)

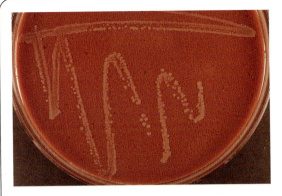
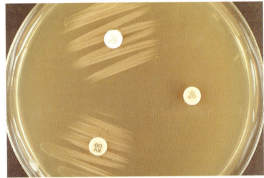
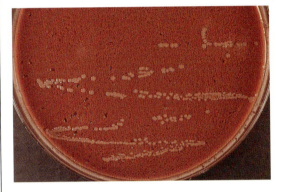
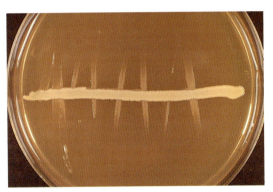

▲ Fig. 170: *Haemophilus parasuis*, pure culture on chocolate agar, 48 h, 37 °C. Magnification x 0.4
▼ Fig. 172: *Haemophilus pleuropneumoniae*, pure culture on chocolate agar, 48 h, 37 °C, incubated in 10 % CO_2 atmosphere. Magnification x 0.4

▲ Fig. 171: *Haemophilus parasuis*, pure culture on tryptose agar, demonstrating V-factor growth dependence in the disc test, 48 h, 37 °C. Magnification x 0.4
▼ Fig. 173: *Haemophilus pleuropneumoniae*, pure culture on tryptose agar, satellitism phenomenon, growth on either side of the *Staphylococcus epidermidis* inoculation streak, 48 h, 37 °C. Magnification x 0.4

▲ Abb. 170: *Haemophilus parasuis*, Reinkultur auf Kochblutplatte, 48 h, 37 °C, Abb.-M. 1 : 2,5
▼ Abb. 172: *Haemophilus pleuropneumoniae*, Reinkultur auf Kochblutplatte, 48 h, 37 °C, bebrütet in 10 %iger CO_2-Atmosphäre, Abb.-M. 1 : 2,5

▲ Abb. 171: *Haemophilus parasuis*, Reinkultur auf Tryptose-Agar, Nachweis der Wachstumsabhängigkeit vom V-Faktor im Blättchentest, 48 h, 37 °C, Abb.-M. 1 : 2,5
▼ Abb. 173: *Haemophilus pleuropneumoniae*, Reinkultur auf Tryptose-Agar, Ammenphänomen, Wachstum beiderseits des Impfstriches von *Staphylococcus epidermidis*, 48 h, 37 °C, Abb.-M. 1 : 2,5

■ **Morphology**
This is a coccoid or short rod, which may even form filaments after 48 hours.

■ **Culture** (figs. 172 and 173)
The cultural demonstration is carried out on blood agar with satellite and this permits a more easy recognition than on chocolate agar, because of the haemolysis. Two distinct colony forms are possible, one compact, waxy the other soft (tab. 73).

■ **Morphologie**
Es handelt sich um ein kokkoides bis kurzes Stäbchen, das nach 48 h auch Fäden ausbilden kann.

■ **Kultur** (Abb. 172 u. 173)
Der kulturelle Erregernachweis erfolgt auf Blutagar mit Amme, der aufgrund der Hämolyse eine leichtere Identifizierung erlaubt als Kochblutagar. Es können zwei verschiedene Kolonieformen auftreten, entweder eine kompakte, wachsartige oder eine visköse (Tab. 73).

■ **Biochemical properties**
See figure 169.

Most strains are NAD-dependent, but there is also a NAD-independent variant (»Pasteurella-like organism«). Very characteristic for their recognition is haemolysis of bovine or sheep blood and a positive CAMP test.

■ **Antigenic structure**
At least 10 serotypes of more or less distinct geographical distribution can be differentiated on the basis of the capsular antigens (25, 37, 49, 54, 65). Serotype 2 appears to be particularly common in Europe, but other serotypes (3, 7, 9) occur also. Type 5 predominates in Canada and the USA. Their differentiation is important for making vaccines and for serological diagnosis and it is facilitated by various serological methods (slide agglutination, precipitation tests).

■ **Serological diagnosis**
Antibodies can be demonstrated in infected animals by means of the complement fixation reaction; a titre of 1 : 10 is considered specific (54), there are no cross reactions between the serotypes (57).

■ **Further Haemophilus species**
There are certain to be more *Haemophilus* species in pigs as, for instance, the »minor group« of species (fig. 169). Our understanding of their pathogenic significance (as cause of pneumonia) is still incomplete (37).

1.2 Haemophilus infections in poultry
1.2.1 Haemophilus paragallinarum

Veterinary significance, see table 72. Biochemical properties, see figure 169.

1.2.2 Haemophilus avium

Is similar in distribution to *H. paragallinarum*, but it is considered to be mainly non-pathogenic. Biochemical properties, see figure 169.

H. avium is differentiated from *H. paragallinarum* mainly by the following biochemical reactions: Cat −, Gal +, Tre +, aerobic growth, no growth stimulation by fowl serum, production of a yellow pigment (2, 28). Recent taxonomic research has included *H. avium* in the genus *Pasteurella* (p. 125 and tab. 34).

1.3 Haemophilus haemoglobinophilus
(Syn.: *H. canis*)

A non-pathogen that occurs in the prepuce. Other species have been isolated from the oral cavity and the respiratory organs (53).

1.4 Haemophilus somnus

Veterinary significance, see table 72. Summarizing description of *H. somnus* in HUMPHREY & STEPHENS (30).

■ **Morphology**
Haemophilus somnus is a pleomorphic coccoid to filamentous rod. The coccoid forms may exhibit bipolar staining (CORBOZ & NICOLET, 10).

■ **Culture** (fig. 175)
Anaerobic or micro-aerophilic incubation produces colonies that are just visible after 24 hours and 0.5 to 1.5 mm in diameter after 48. Growth is indepen-

Specimens
Central nervous tissue, secretions from lungs, vagina, cervix, uterus, preputial rinses and semen samples

Microscopic examination
Gram-negative, coccoid or filamentous, pleomorphic bacteris, often difficult to stain and recognize as Gram-negative rods

Examination by culture
1. Medium: chocolate agar,   2. Incubation anaerobic or micro-aerophilic (5–10% CO_2), growth as delicate colonies, just visible after 24–48 h. All colonies are pigmented light- to lemon-yellow, haemolysis with viridans effect visible with varying distinctness below the colony; aerobic incubation: very slow growth, colonies visible after 3–4 days,   3. Incubation temperature 37 °C

Biochemical differentiation			
Dependence X-factor	−	Adonitol	v^-
Dependence V-factor	−	Salicin	v^-
Oxidase	+	Inositol	v^-
Lysine carboxylase	+	Saccharose	v^-
Aesculin	+	Catalase	v^-
Glucose	v^+	Indole	−
Mannitol	v^+	Citrate	−
Nitrate	v^+	Voges-Proskauer reaction	−
Lactose	v^-	Methyl red reaction	−
Dulcitol	v^-	Urease	−

Fig. 174: Isolation and characterization of *Haemophilus somnus* from the ox (10, 23, 37)

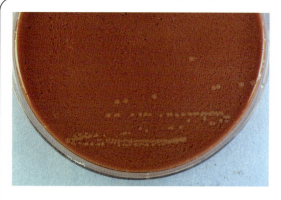
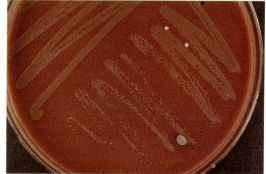
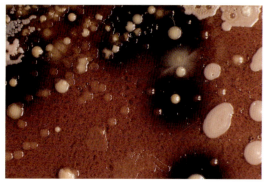
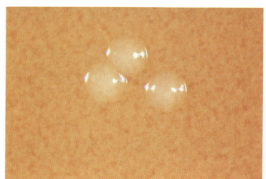

▲ Fig. 175: *Haemophilus somnus*, pure culture on chocolate agar, 48 h, 37 °C, incubated in a 10 % CO_2 atmosphere. Magnification x 0.4
▼ Fig. 177: *Haemophilus equigenitalis*, mixed culture from a swab from a mare, chocolate agar, 72 h, 37 °C, incubated in an atmosphere of 95 % N_2 and 5 % CO_2. Magnification x 0.67

▲ Fig. 176: *Haemophilus equigenitalis*, culture on chocolate agar, contaminated with *Staphylococcus epidermidis* and bacilli, 4 d, 37 °C, incubated in an atmosphere of 95 % N_2 and 5 % CO_2. Magnification x 0.4
▼ Fig. 178: *Haemophilus equigenitalis*, pure culture on chocolate agar, 4 d, 37 °C, incubated in an atmosphere of 95 % N_2 and 5 % CO_2. Magnification x 10

▲ Abb. 175: *Haemophilus somnus*, Reinkultur auf Kochblutplatte, 48 h, 37 °C, bebrütet in 10%iger CO_2-Atmosphäre, Abb.-M. 1 : 2,5
▼ Abb. 177: *Haemophilus equigenitalis*, Mischkultur aus einem Stutentupfer, Kochblutplatte, 72 h, 37 °C, bebrütet in 95%iger N_2- und 5%iger CO_2-Atmosphäre, Abb.-M. 1 : 1,5

▲ Abb. 176: *Haemophilus equigenitalis*, Kultur auf Kochblutplatte, verunreinigt mit *Staphylococcus epidermidis* und Bazillen, 4 d, 37 °C, bebrütet in 95%iger N_2- und 5%iger CO_2-Atmosphäre, Abb.-M. 1 : 2,5
▼ Abb. 178: *Haemophilus equigenitalis*, Reinkultur auf Kochblutplatte, 4 d, 37 °C, bebrütet in 95%iger N_2- und 5%iger CO_2-Atmosphäre, Abb.-M. 10 : 1

dent of a staphylococcal satellite. The colonies produce a yellow pigment, especially the older ones. A weak haemolysis can develop. A selective medium has been described by SLEE & STEPHENS (69).

Biochemical properties, see figure 174.

Das Wachstum ist nicht von einer Staphylokokkenamme abhängig. Die Stämme zeigen besonders in älteren Kulturen eine gelbe Pigmentierung. Es kann eine schwache Hämolyse auftreten. Ein Selektivmedium ist von SLEE & STEPHENS (69) beschrieben worden.

Kulturell-biochemische Eigenschaften siehe Abb. 174.

1.5 Haemophilus (Taylorella) equigenitalis
(Syn.: contagious equine metritis organism = CEMO)

The cause of contagious equine metritis (CEM) is a bacterium which was first describe by PLATT et al. (59) and provisionally termed *H. equigenitalis* by TAYLOR et al. (76) even though it is independent in its growth of either X or V factors and so does not fulfil the criterion of the genus *Haemophilus*.

■ Incidence and veterinary significance
CEM was first described in Great Britain (13, 15) but is apparently distributed throughout the world. Its occurrence in the Federal German Republic up to 1982 is reviewed by ECKSTEIN (20). Its occurrence in Germany has also been dealt with by BLOBEL et al. (7, 8), MUMME & AHLSWEDE (50) as well as KIRPAL & BISPING (39). The clinical signs in the mare are those of endometritis and, depending on the severity, a sero-mucinous or muco-purulent

Specimens
Mare: Smear from the fossa glandis (middle sinus) or as a second choice the fossa praeputialis; cervical swab: smear from inside the cervix including the internal cervical orifice and the inside of the body of the uterus[1];   Stallion: swab from the urethra, smear from fossa glandis, fore-secretion. Before taking the sample, the swabs must be moistened in the transport medium.

Shipment of the specimens
Immediately after taking the sample the swabs must be placed in transport medium (after Stuart or Amies, 21, 51, 66).

Isolation by culture
Chocolate agar: to exclude non-specific contaminants the material is split before being spread and/or selective media are used which contain, for example, 200 µg streptomycin sulphate, 5 µg amphotericin B or 5 µg clindamycin, 1 µg trimethoprim, 5 µg amphotericin B per ml. It is advisable to use two different media, one of which must not contain streptomycin, because some of the strains are streptomycin-resistant. Micro-aerophilic incubation (95% N_2, 5% CO_2) for at least 4 days at 37 °C. Prolonged incubation can increase the yield (1, 34, 77).

Identification of suspect bacteria
1. Gram-negative coccoid rods,   2. Growth exclusively under micro-aerophil conditions, after 3–4 days the colonies are recognizable and about 1 mm in size,   3. Biochemical properties: oxidase +, catalase +, phosphatase +; it is largely inactive where carbohydrate fermentation is concerned,   4. Slide agglutination tests with specific antiserum are positive (weak spontaneous agglutination often occurs in saline controls).

[1] See MERKT et al. (47) for taking the test samples

Fig. 179: Demonstration and identification of *Haemophilus equigenitalis* (CEMO)

secretion. Additionally, there may be vaginitis and cervicitis, and this may be the only sign in mild cases. The infection results in decreased fertility. The bacterium has also been isolated from cases of abortion (52). In some instances the infection may remain latent.

A clinically asymptomatic infection of the penis, the urethral mucosa and the fossa glandis can occur in stallions.

A summary of the disease will be found in BREWER (9) and in BLOBEL & BRÜCKLER (6).

■ **Morphology**
Gram-negative coccoid, pleomorphic, non-motile rod, measuring 0.3–0.6 × 1–2 µm.

■ **Culture** (figs. 176 to 178)
The examination routine is presented in figure 179. Chocolate agar is specially suitable for the primary isolation (33, 59, 63, 77). Growth is independent of X or V factors, although the X factor can enhance growth (68).

Incubation must be micro-aerobic (5–10% CO_2) and a gas mixture of 95% N_2 and 5% CO_2 also stimulates growth (70). KAMADA et al. (34) obtained the best growth by incubating in an atmosphere of 10% CO_2 and 75% N_2.

■ **Biochemical properties**
See figure 179 (75).

■ **Antigenic structure and serological identification**
Little is known so far about the complex antigenic structure. But the bacterium can be identified in the slide agglutination test using specific antisera produced in the rabbit (64, 75). The agglutination can be accentuated if the antibodies were linked beforehand to Protein-A-positive staphylococci (6).

■ **Serological diagnosis**
The indirect identification of infection has been attempted with various serological methods, but none has achieved any special clinical significance. The serum agglutination test and the antiglobulin tests can be used in acute infections, but the CFT is better in chronic infections, because the antibodies persist for longer periods (4, 14, 16, 22, 45).

2 Genus: Histophilus
2.1 Histophilus ovis

The bacterium is similar to *Haemophilus* species and has been isolated in Australia and New Zealand

Table 74: Biochemical properties of *Histophilus ovis*

Tabelle 74: Kulturell-biochemische Eigenschaften von *Histophilus ovis*

Cat	−	Ind	v	Man	+	Raf	−
Oxi	+	Nit	−	Sor	+	Sac	−
Mot	−	Glu	+[1]	Dul	−	H_2S	−
Hae	−	Mal	v	Lac	−		

[1] only acid production from carbohydrate fermentation

but also in Europe from sheep affected with the following conditions: epididymitis, abortion, polyarthritis, mastitis, synovitis, vaginitis.

This is a Gram-negative coccoid, non-motile rod. On blood agar it will produce shiny, non-haemolytic colonies 0.5 to 1 mm in diameter within 48 hours of micro-aerophilic incubation (10 % CO_2). On further incubation the colonies produce a yellow pigment. Weak aerobic growth is possible. It has been assumed that such a close relationship exists between *Histophilus ovis*, *Haemophilus somnus* and *Haemophilus agni* (»H-H-group«) that they can be grouped together in a new genus (11, 43, 72).

Europa von Schafen und Rindern im Zusammenhang mit folgenden Krankheitsbildern isoliert: Epididymitis, Abort, Polyarthritis, Mastitis, Synovitis, Vaginitis.

Es handelt sich um ein gramnegatives, kokkoides, unbewegliches Stäbchen, das unter mikroaerophilen Bedingungen (10 % CO_2) auf Blutagar innerhalb von 48 h 0,5 bis 1,0 mm große, glänzende, nichthämolytische Kolonien bildet. Bei weiterer Bebrütung bildet sich ein gelbes Pigment. Ein schwaches aerobes Wachstum ist möglich. Es ist angenommen worden, daß zwischen *Histophilus ovis* und *Haemophilus somnus* und *Haemophilus agni* eine so enge Verwandtschaft besteht (»H-H-group«), daß diese Bakterien deswegen in einer neuen Gattung zusammengefaßt werden können (11, 43, 72).

Bibliography / Literatur

1. ATHERTON, J. G. (1983): Evaluation of selective supplements used in media for the isolation of the causative of contagious equine metritis. Vet. Rec. 113, 299–300.
2. BLACKALL, P. J., & G. G. REID (1982): Further characterization of Haemophilus paragallinarum and Haemophilus avium. Vet. Microbiol. 7, 359–367.
3. BAEHLER, J. F., H. BURGISSER, P. A. DE MEURON & J. NICOLET (1974): Infection à Haemophilus parasuis chez le porc. Schweiz. Arch. Tierhk. 116, 183–188.
4. BENSON, J. A., F. L. M. DANSON, D. S. DURRANT, P. T. EDWARDS & D. G. POWELL (1978): Serological response in mares affected by contagious equine metritis 1977. Vet. Rec. 102, 277–280.
5. BIBERSTEIN, E. L., A. GUNNARSSON & B. HURVELL (1977): Cultural and biochemical criteria for the identification of Haemophilus spp. from swine. Am. J. Vet. Res. 38, 7–11.
6. BLOBEL, H., & J. BRÜCKLER (1981): Contagious equine metritis. In: H. BLOBEL & T. SCHLIESSER (Hrsg.): Handbuch der bakteriellen Infektionen bei Tieren, Bd. III, S. 545–556. Jena: VEB Gustav Fischer.
7. BLOBEL, H., J. BRÜCKLER, D. KITZROW & K. BLOBEL (1979): "Contagious equine metritis" (CEM). Prakt. Tierarzt 61, 41–47.
8. BLOBEL, H., D. KITZROW & K. BLOBEL (1978): Contagious equine metritis. Tierärztl. Umschau 33, 523–534.
9. BREWER, R. A. (1983): Contagious equine metritis: A. review. Vet. Bull. 53, 881–891.
10. CORBOZ, L., & J. NICOLET (1975): Infektionen mit sogenannten »Haemophilus somnus« beim Rind: Isolierung und Charakterisierung von Stämmen aus Respirations- und Geschlechtsorganen. Schweiz. Arch. Tierhk. 117, 493–502.
11. CORBEL, M. J., R. A. BREWER & R. SMITH (1986): Isolation of bacteria of the Haemophilus-Histophilus-group from the genital tracts of cattle. Vet. Rec. 118, 695–696.
12. CORSTVET, R. E., R. J. PANSIERA, H. B. RINKER, B. L. STARKS & C. HOWARD (1973): Survey of tracheas of feedlot cattle for Haemophilus somnus and other selected bacteria. J. Am. Vet. Med. Ass. 163, 870–873.
13. CROWHURST, R. S. (1977): Genital infection in mares. Vet. Rec. 100, 476.
14. CROXTON-SMITH, P., J. A. BENSON, F. L. M. DAWSON & D. G. POWELL (1978): A complement fixation test for antibody to the contagious equine metritis organism. Vet. Rec. 103, 275–278.
15. DAVID, J. S. E., C. J. FRANK & D. G. POWELL (1977): Contagious metritis 1977. Vet. Rec. 101, 189–190.
16. DAWSON, F. L. M., J. A. BENSON & P. CROXTON-SMITH (1978): The course of serum antibody development in two ponies experimentally infected with contagious metritis. Equine vet. J. 10, 145–147.
17. DIDIER, P. J., L. PERINO & J. URBANCE (1984): Porcine Haemophilus pleuropneumonia: microbiological and pathological findings. J. Am. Vet. Med. Ass. 184, 716–719.
18. DIRKSEN, G., E. KAISER & H. SCHELS (1978): Erstes Auftreten der infektiösen septikämisch-thrombosierenden Meningoenzephalitis (ISTME) bei Mastrindern in Süddeutschland. Prakt. Tierarzt 59, 766–775.
19. DREUMEL, A. A., & M. VAN KIERSTEAD (1975): Abortion associated with Haemophilus somnus infection in a bovine fetus. Canad. Vet. J. 16, 367–370.
20. ECKSTEIN, K. (1983): Verbreitung und Bedeutung der ansteckenden Gebärmutterentzündung der Pferde (CEM 77) in der Bundesrepublik Deutschland. Vet. Med. Diss. Hannover.

21. ENGVALL, A. (1985): Survival of Contagious Equine Metritis Organism in different transport media as influenced by storage time, temperature and contamination flora. Zbl. Vet. Med. B, **32**, 454–459.
22. FERNIE, D. S., I. CAYZER & S. R. CHALMERS (1979): A passive haemagglutination test for the detection of antibodies to the contagious equine metritis organism. Vet. Rec. **104**, 260–262.
23. FÖRSTER, D., & M. SCHEER (1976): Infektiöse septikämisch-thrombosierende Meningoenzephalitis in einem Mastbullenbestand. IV. Bakteriologische Untersuchungen: Nachweis von Haemophilus-ähnlichen Bakterienstämmen (Haemophilus somnus). Dtsch. tierärztl. Wschr. **83**, 149–152.
24. GLÄSSER, K. (1912): Die fibrinöse Serosen- und Gelenkentzündung der Ferkel. In: Die Krankheiten des Schweines. S. 122–125. Hannover: M. & H. Schaper.
25. GUNNARSON, A., E. L. BIBERSTEIN & B. HURWELL (1977): Serological studies on porcine strains of Haemophilus parahaemolyticus (pleuropneumoniae): Agglutination reactions. Am. J. Vet. Res. **38**, 1111–1114.
26. HEIDT, M., & R. WEISS (1982): Zum Vorkommen bakterieller Infektionserreger in pathologisch-anatomisch veränderten Lungen von Schweinen unter besonderer Berücksichtigung der Gattung Haemophilus. II. Biochemische Untersuchungen an Haemophilus-Stämmen. Berl. Münch. tierärztl. Wschr. **95**, 453–458.
27. HINZ, K. H. (1975): Der »ansteckende Hühnerschnupfen«. Beitrag zur Differenzierung von Haemophilus-Stämmen aus Hühnern. Habilitationsschrift, Hannover.
28. HINZ, K. H., & CH. KUNJARA (1977): Haemophilus avium, a new species from chickens. Int. J. System. Bact. **27**, 324–329.
29. HOERLEIN, A. B., K. GOTO & S. YOUNG (1973): Haemophilus somnus agglutinins in cattle. J. Am. Vet. Med. Ass. **163**, 1375–1377.
30. HUMPHREY, J. D., & L. R. STEPHENS (1983): Haemophilus somnus: A review. Vet. Bull. **58**, 987–1004.
31. HUMPHREY, J. D., P. B. LITTLE, L. R. STEPHENS, D. A. BARNUM, P. A. DOIG & J. THORSEN (1982): Prevalence and distribution of Haemophilus somnus in the male bovine reproductive tract. Am. J. Vet. Res. **43**, 791–795.
32. HUMPHREY, J. D., P. B. LITTLE, D. A. BARNUM, P. A. DOIG, L. R. STEPHENS & J. THORSEN (1982): Occurrence of Haemophilus somnus in bovine semen and in the prepuce of bulls and steers. Can. J. Comp. Med. **46**, 215–217.
33. KAMADA, M. (1982): Studies on equine infectious metritis. I. Effects of disinfectants against Haemophilus equigenitalis. J. Jap. Vet. Med. Ass. **35**, 90–96.
34. KAMADA, M., T. ODA, H. OHISHI, R. WADA, Y. FUKUNAGA & T. KUMANOMIDO (1983): Studies on contagious equine metritis. II. Evaluation of media for isolation, subculture and storage of Haemophilus equigenitalis. Bull. Equine Res. Inst. **20**, 126–132.
35. KENNEDY, P. C., E. L. BIBERSTEIN, J. A. HOWART, L. M. FRAZIER & D. L. DUNGWORTH (1960): Infectious meningoencephalitis in cattle, caused by a Haemophilus-like organism. Am. J. Vet. Res. **21**, 403–409.
36. KILIAN, M. (1974): A rapid method for the differentiation of Haemophilus strains. The porphyrin test. Acta path. micriobiol. scand. B, **82**, 835–842.
37. KILIAN, M., J. NICOLET & E. L. BIBERSTEIN (1978): Biochemical and serological characterization of Haemophilus pleuropneumoniae (MATTHEWS & PATTISON, 1961) SHOPE, 1964 and proposal of a serotype strain. Int. J. Syst. Bact. **28**, 20–26.
38. KIELSTEIN, P., K. D. FLOSSMANN, B. ROHRMANN & H. BOCKLISCH (1985): Genotypische Untersuchungen an Erregern der hämorrhagisch-nekrotisierenden Pleuropneumonie des Schweines. Zbl. Vet. Med. B, **32**, 93–100.
39. KIRPAL, G., & W. BISPING (1980): Die bakteriologische Untersuchung von Genitaltupfern auf den Erreger der kontagiösen equinen Metritis (CEM). Dtsch. tierärztl. Wschr. **87**, 401–403.
40. KROGH, H. V., K. B. PEDERSEN & E. BLOM (1983): Haemophilus somnus in semen from Danish bulls. Vet. Rec. **112**, 460.
41. LITTLE, T. W. A., D. G. PRITCHARD & J. E. SHREEVE (1980): Isolation of Haemophilus species from the oropharynx of British sheep. Res. Vet. Sci. **29**, 41–44.
42. LINNEWEBER, B., R. WEISS & T. SCHLIESSER (1986): Bakteriologische Untersuchungen über Vorkommen, Biochemie und Antibiotika-Resistenz von Haemophilus somnus (spec. incertae sed.) bei Rindern. Berl. Münch. tierärztl. Wschr. **99**, 221–225.
43. LOW, J. C., & M. M. GRAHAM (1985): Histophilus ovis epididymitis in a ram in the UK. Vet. Rec. **117**, 64–65.
44. LUND, M. E., & D. J. BLAZEVIC (1977): Rapid specification of Haemophilus with the porphyrin production test versus the satellite test for X. J. clin. Microbiol. **5**, 142–144.
45. MACMILLAN, A. D., & S. A. KIDD (1986): Antibodies with Taylorella equigenitalis in equine sera. Vet. Rec. **118**, 562.
46. MATSCHULLAT, G. (1982): Über die Hämophilus-Pleuropneumonie. Prakt. Tierarzt **63**, 1047–1054.
47. MERKT, H., W. BISPING, A. R. GÜNZEL & G. KIRPAL (1980): Die Tupferprobe in der gynäkologischen Untersuchung der Stute. Prakt. Tierarzt **61**, 301–308.
48. MILLER, R. B., D. H. LEIN, K. E. MCENTEE, C. E. HALL & S. SHIN (1983): Haemophilus somnus infection of the reproductive tract of cattle: A review. J. Am. Vet. Med. Ass. **182**, 1390–1392.
49. MITTAL, K. R., R. HIGGINS & S. LARIVIERE (1982): Evaluation of slide agglutination and ring precipitation tests for capsular serotyping of Haemophilus pleuropneumoniae. J. clin. Microbiol. **15**, 1019–1023.
50. MUMME, J., & L. AHLSWEDE (1979): Nachweis von Haemophilus equigenitalis im Zervixtupfer einer Warmblutstute. Dtsch. tierärztl. Wschr. **86**, 257–259.
51. MUSHÖVEL, S. (1981): Vergleichende Prüfung der Eignung von Amies- und Stuart-Transportmedien für die Entnahme und Einsendung von Uterustupferproben zur bakteriologischen Untersuchung. Vet. Med. Diss. Hannover.
52. NAKASHIRO, H., M. NARUSE, C. SUGIMOTO, Y. ISAYAMA & C. KUNIYASU (1981): Isolation of Haemophilus equigenitalis from an aborted equine fetus. Nat. Inst. Anim. Hlth. Quart. **21**, 184–185.
53. NICOLET, J. (1981): Haemophilus. In: H. BLOBEL & T. SCHLIESSER (Hrsg.): Handbuch der bakteriellen Infektionen bei Tieren, Bd. III, S. 495–544. Jena: VEB Gustav Fischer.
54. NICOLET, J. (1971): Sur l'hémophilose du porc. III. Différentiation sérologique de Haemophilus parahaemolyticus. Zbl. Bakt. I. Orig. A, **216**, 487–495.
55. NICOLET, J. (1971): Sur l'hémophilose du porc. IV. L'épreuve de fixation du complément, un test de dépistage des infections à Haemophilus parahaemolyticus. Schweiz. Arch. Tierhk. **113**, 191–200.
56. NICOLET, J., H. KÖNIG & E. SCHOLL (1969): Zur Hämophilus-Pleuropneumonie beim Schwein. II. Eine kontagiöse Krankheit von wirtschaftlicher Bedeutung. Schweiz. Arch. Tierhk. **111**, 166–174.
57. NIELSEN, R. (1979): Haemophilus parahaemolyticus serotypes. Nord. Vet. Med. **31**, 401–406.
58. NIELSEN, R., & V. DANIELSEN (1975): An outbreak of Glässer's disease. Nord. Vet. Med. **27**, 20–25.
59. PLATT, H., J. G. ATHERTON, D. J. SIMPSON, D. F. J. BROWN & T. G. WREGHITT (1977): Genital infection in mares. Vet. Rec. **101**, 20.
60. POHL, S., H. U. BERTSCHINGER, W. FREDERIKSEN & W. MANNHEIM (1983): Transfer of Haemophilus pleuropneumoniae and the Pasteurella haemolytica organism causing porcine necrotic pleuropneumonia to the genus

Actinobacillus on the basis of phenotypic and desoxyribonucleic acid relatedness. Intern. J. System. Bact. 33, 510–514.

61. PRITCHARD, D. G., & N. S. M. MACLEOD (1977): The isolation of Haemophilus somnus following sudden deaths in suckler calves in Scotland. Vet. Rec. 100, 126–127.

62. RAUTH, S. (1985): Bakteriologische Untersuchungen über die Verbreitung von Haemophilus somnus im Genitaltrakt von Rindern. Vet. Med. Diss. Hannover.

63. RICKETTS, S. W., P. D. ROSSDALE, N. H. WINGFIELD-DIGBY, M. M. FALK, R. HOPES, M. D. N. HUNT & C. K. PEACE (1977): Genital infection in mares. Vet. Rec. 101, 65.

64. ROMMEL, F. A., A. H. DARDIRI, S. P. SAHU & R. E. PIERSON (1978): Serological identification of the bacterial agent of contagious equine metritis. Vet. Rec. 103, 564.

65. ROSENDAL, S., & D. A. BOYD (1982): Haemophilus pleuropneumoniae serotyping. J. clin. Microbiol. 16, 840–843.

66. SAHU, S. P., A. H. DARDIRI, F. A. ROMMEL & R. E. PIERSON (1979): Survival of contagious equine metritis bacteria in transport media. Am. J. Vet. Res. 40, 1040–1042.

67. SCHWEIGHARDT, H., P. PECHAN & E. LAUERMANN (1984): Q-Fieber und Haemophilus somnus-Infektion — vergleichsweise seltene Verwerfensursache beim Rind. Tierärztl. Umschau 39, 581–584.

68. SHREEVE, J. E. (1978): Preliminary observations on X-factor growth requirement of the bacterium responsible for CEM. Vet. Rec. 102, 20.

69. SLEE, K. J., & L. R. STEPHENS (1985): Selective medium for isolation of Haemophilus somnus from cattle and sheep. Vet. Rec. 116, 215–217.

70. SONNENSCHEIN, B., & E. KLUG (1979): Erfahrungen mit der kontagiösen equinen Metritis (CEM 77). Dtsch. tierärztl. Wschr. 86, 268–270.

71. STÖBER, M., & D. PITTERMANN (1975): Infektiöse septikämisch-thrombosierende Meningoenzephalitis in einem Mastbullen-Bestand. I. Klinisches Bild. Dtsch. tierärztl. Wschr. 82, 97–102.

72. STEPHENS, L. R., J. D. HUMPHREY, P. B. LITTLE & D. A. BARNUM (1983): Morphological, biochemical, antigenic and cytochemical relationships among Haemophilus somnus, Haemophilus agni, Haemophilus haemoglobinophilus, Histophilus ovis, and Actionobacillus seminis. J. clin. Microbiol. 17, 728–737.

73. SUGIMOTO, C., K. MITANI & M. NAKAZAWA (1983): In vitro susceptibility of Haemophilus somnus to 33 antimicrobial agents. Antimicrob. Ag. Chemoth. 23, 163–165.

74. SWANEY, L. M., & H. M. KISLOW (1981): Desinfection of the causative agent of contagious equine metritis by Nolvasan and Roccal II. Vet. Microbiol. 6, 59–68.

75. TAINTURIER, D. J., C. F. DELMAS & H. J. DABERNAT (1981): Bacteriological and serological studies of Haemophilus equigenitalis, agent of contagious equine metritis. J. clin. Microbiol. 14, 355–360.

76. TAYLOR, C. E. D., R. O. ROSENTHAL, D. F. J. BROWN, S. P. LAPAGE, L. R. HILL & R. M. LEGROS (1978): The causative organism of contagious equine metritis 1977: Proposal for a new species to be known as Haemophilus equigenitalis. Equine vet. J. 10, 136–144.

77. TIMONEY, P. J., J. SHIN & R. H. JACOBSEN (1982): Improved selective medium for isolation of the contagious equine metritis organism. Vet. Rec. 111, 107–108.

78. TIMONEY, P. J., J. WARD & P. KELLY (1977): A contagious genital infection of mares. Vet. Rec. 103, 103.

79. WALDHAM, D. G., R. F. HALL, W. A. MEINERSHAGEN, C. S. CARD & F. W. FRANK (1974): Haemophilus somnus infection in the cow as a possible contributing factor to weak calf syndrome. Am. J. Vet. Res. 35, 1401–1403.

80. WARD, J. M. HOURIGAN, J. MCGIRK & A. GOGARTY (1984): Incubation times for primary isolation of the contagious equine metritis organism. Vet. Rec. 114, 298.

81. WEISS, R., & M. HEIDT (1982): Zum Vorkommen bakterieller Infektionserreger in pathologisch-anatomisch veränderten Lungen von Schweinen unter besonderer Berücksichtigung der Gattung Haemophilus. I. Isolierungsergebnisse aus Lungen von Schlachtschweinen und Sektionsfällen. Berl. Münch. tierärztl. Wschr. 95, 442–446.

82. WHITE, D. C. (1963): Respiratory systems in the hemin-requiring Haemophilus. J. Bact. 85, 842–850.

Brucellae
Brucellen

The species and their biotypes included in the genus *Brucella* are shown in tables 75 and 78 along with their properties.

Die zu der Gattung Brucella gehörenden Arten einschließlich ihrer Biotypen sind mit ihren Eigenschaften in den Tabellen 75 und 78 zusammengestellt.

Table 75: Identification of *Brucella* species and their biotypes

Tabelle 75: Bestimmung der Brucellenarten und ihrer Biotypen

Species	Biotype	CO_2 dependence	H_2S production	Ure	Thionin[1]			Basic fuchsin[1]	
					a	b	c	b	c
Br. melitensis	1	−	−	v	−	+	+	+	+
	2	−	−	v	−	+	+	+	+
	3	−	v	−	−	+	+	+	+
Br. abortus	1	v$^+$	+	1–2 h	−	−	−	+	+
	2[5]	+	+	1–2 h	−	−	−	−	−
	3	v$^+$	+	1–2 h	+	+	+	+	+
	4	v$^+$	+	1–2 h	−	−	−	+	+
	5	−	−	1–2 h	−	+	+	+	+
	6	−	v	1–2 h	−	+	+	+	+
	7	−	v	1–2 h	−	+	+	+	+
	8	+	−	1–2 h	−	+	+	+	+
	9	v	+	1–2 h	−	+	+	+	+
Br. suis	1	−	++	0–30 min	+	+	+	−	−
	2	−	−	0–30 min	−	+	+	−	−
	3	−	−	0–30 min	+	+	+	+	+
	4	−	−	0–30 min	+	+	+	+	+
Br. neotomae	1	−	+	0–30 min	−	−	+	−	−
Br. ovis	1[5]	+	−	−	+	+	+	+	+
Br. canis	1	−	−	0–30 min	+	+	+	−	(+)

1 Brucella (Br.) melitensis, Br. abortus and Br. suis

These classical types of brucella resemble one another very closely in their properties, so that they can be described together.

Incidence and veterinary significance, see table 76.

1.1 Properties, demonstration and identification

■ **Morphology and microscopic examination** (figs. 181 and 182)
The types cannot be differentiated from one another by microscopy. They are Gram-negative, non-motile coccoid rods 0.5–0.7 × 0.6–1.5 µm.

Selective staining: the methods of Köster or Hansen (p. 335) rely on the special affinity of brucellae to basic dyes, which subsequent decolourization removes more slowly than in other bacteria.

1 Brucella (Br.) melitensis, Br. abortus und Br. suis

Diese klassischen Brucellenarten sind sind in ihren Eigenschaften sehr ähnlich, so daß sie zusammen dargestellt werden.

Über ihr Vorkommen und ihre medizinische Bedeutung s. Tab. 76.

1.1 Eigenschaften, Nachweis und Bestimmung

■ **Morphologie und mikroskopische Untersuchung** (Abb. 181 u. 182)
Die einzelnen Arten sind mikroskopisch nicht voneinander zu unterscheiden, es handelt sich um 0,5–0,7 × 0,6–1,5 µm große kokkoide, gramnegative, unbewegliche Kurzstäbchen.

Selektivfärbungen: Die Färbungen nach Köster oder Hansen (S. 335) beruhen auf der besonderen Affinität der Brucellen zu alkalischen Farbstoffen, die sie bei anschließender Entfärbung langsamer abgeben als andere Bakterien.

Table 75: Continued

Species	Agglutination with type-specific sera[2]			Lysis with phage Tb[4]		Principal host
	A	M	R	RTD[3]	10,000 × RTD	
	−	+	−	−	−	sheep, goat
Br. melitensis	+	−	−	−	−	sheep, goat
	+	+	−	−	−	sheep, goat
	+	−	−	+	+	cattle
	+	−	−	+	+	cattle
	+	−	−	+	+	cattle
	−	+	−	+	+	cattle
Br. abortus	−	+	−	+	+	cattle
	+	−	−	+	+	cattle
	+	+	−	+	+	cattle
	−	+	−	+	+	cattle
	−	+	−	+	+	cattle
	+	−	−	−	+	pig
	+	−	−	−	+	pig, hare
Br. suis	+	−	−	−	+	pig
	+	+	−	−	+	reindeer (Rangifer tarandi)
Br. neotomae	+	−	−	−	−	wood rat (USA) (Neotoma lepida)
Br. ovis	−	−	+	−	−	sheep
Br. canis	−	−	+	−	−	dog

[1] Dye concentration: a = 1 : 25,000; b = 1 : 50,000; c = 1 : 100,000; [2] Monospecific sera: A = abortus serum, M = melitensis serum, R = anti-rough serum; [3] routine test dilution; [4] Tbilisi phage; [5] the addition of 5 % serum is necessary for growth

[1] Farbstoffkonzentrationen: a = 1 : 25 000; b = 1 : 50 000; c = 1 : 100 000; [2] monospezifische Seren: A = Abortus-Serum, M = Melitensis-Serum, R = anti-Rauh-Serum; [3] routine test dilution; [4] Tbilisi-Phage; [5] für das Wachstum ist Zusatz von 5 % Serum erforderlich

Staining by the method of Stamp and Stableforth (p. 335) has a certain advantage in that it will demonstrate chlamydiae at the same time, especially in chlamydial abortion of sheep.

■ Culture (figs. 183 and 184)

The examination routine and the required media (6, 35, 70) are shown in the figure 180. Brucellae are aerobic, and only for primary culture of *Br. abortus* is it necessary to have an atmosphere of 10 % CO_2. Small, round, shiny, transparent to blue-green colonies are produced by 2 to 4 days at the earliest. With subsequent passages the brucellae tend to produce R-forms (tab. 77) (49).

■ Biochemical properties

See figure 180, tables 75 and 78.

■ Antigenic structure

The three types of brucella possess the same A-antigen (abortus) and M-antigen (melitensis) but in varying amounts. *Br. abortus* is said to have 20 times as much A- as M-antigen; the reverse applies to *Br. melitensis*. *Br. suis* is similar in its antigenic structure to *Br. abortus*. The latter can be differentiated from *Br. melitensis* by means of agglutination

Table 76: Incidence and clinical manifestations of brucellosis in animals

Brucella	Clinical disease and distribution
abortus	Cause of bovine brucellosis with clinical signs: Abortion (usually 5th–8th months) with retention of after-birth; subclinical granulomatous to interstitial mastitis (29, 48), acute, necrotizing to subacute orchitis with granuloma formation and fibrosis, epididymitis, ampullitis (8), arthritis (particularly tarsal and carpal joints), polyarthritis, tenovaginitis, bursitis (31). Apart from cattle, other warm-blooded domestic and wild animals can be infected. The infection is either latent (positive serological titres) or clinically manifest. The disease is seen mainly in mink (abortion), the horse (20, 23, 36) (arthritis, bursitis, fistulous withers) and in the dog (abortion, bacteraemia) (21, 41, 55). A spread of brucellosis from Europe would involve particularly biotypes 1 and also 2, 3 and 4 (10, 53, 67, 68).
melitensis	Cause of brucellosis of sheep and goats; clinical course is similar to that of bovine brucellosis. Spontaneous infection can occur in other domestic animals; they are usually asymptomatic but antibodies are produced. In cattle abortions and the excretion of organisms through the milk are possible but rare. The infection remains only for a limited time in dogs, but it must be assumed that they continue to excrete the organism (45). The most common is biotype 1; there is no reliable information about the geographical distribution of the various biotypes.
suis	Cause of brucellosis of pigs, characterized by abortion and orchitis. In the course of the infection numerous granulomata can develop in various organs, especially the reproductive organs (e. g. miliary brucellosis of the uterus). The organism has marked pyogenic properties and abscesses may be formed in many organs, the subcutis and long bones (22). Biotype 1 (TRAUM, 1914): world-wide distribution, Biotype 2 (THOMPSON, 1934): Europe, occurs simultaneously in hares, either as latent infection or with the development of granulomatous nodules and abscesses in the testes, liver, spleen, lung, subcutis etc. Slight virulence in man (24, 43, 58, 65, 66), Biotype 3: America, SE Asia.

using monospecific (absorbed) A- and M-sera. It is not possible to separate *Br. abortus* from *Br. suis* serologically (tab. 75 and fig. 180) (51, 52, 59).

■ Animal inoculation

See figure 180.

sis mit der Agglutination bestimmt werden. Eine serologische Trennung von *Br. abortus* und *Br. suis* ist nicht möglich (Tab. 75 u. Abb. 180) (51, 52, 59).

■ Tierversuch

Siehe Abb. 180.

Specimens

Placenta, foetal stomach content, milk, pus from abscess, etc.

Microscopic demonstration of pathogens

For staining methods see p. 335, these are of particular diagnostic value in cases of abortion, because 90 % can be diagnosed by microscopic examination

Demonstration of pathogen by culture

1. Media:
   Brucella agar base from various commercial sources, e. g.
   Meat peptone-casein peptone-dextrose agar,
   Tryptose agar, Columbia agar base;
   Serum (5 %)-dextrose (1 %) agar
2. Selective additives:
   Dyes: 1.4 ml of 0.1 % crystal violet solution per ml;
   Antibiotics: Medium of Kuzdas and Morse (35) contains per ml – 100 mg cycloheximide, 25,000 IU bacitracin, 6000 IU polymyxin B;
   Oxoid supplement: polymyxin B, bacitracin, cycloheximide, nalidixic acid, nystatin, vancomycin;
3. Incubation atmosphere: for primary isolation of *Br. abortus* about 10 % CO_2.
   Incubation temperature: 37 °C, time 4–10 days

Demonstration of pathogen by animal inoculation

Guinea pigs are suitable for this, the homogenized sample (1–2 ml) is injected subcutaneously into the knee fold. In positive cases agglutinins can be detected in the serum after 3–6 weeks and brucella can be cultured from the organs (liver, spleen)

Pure culture

Rapid identification of the genus

1. Microscopic examination: alkali-fast (Köster or Hansen stain), Gram-negative, coccoid, non-motile rods, 0.5–0.7 x 0.6–1.5 µm,
2. Catalase +, Oxidase +, Urease + (quantitative differences tab. 75)
3. Carbohydrate breakdown without acid production
4. Positive slide agglutination test with brucella serum

Rapid identification of species (not all biotypes are identified)

Brucella	CO_2 requirement	H_2S formation	Growth on media with basic fuchsin 1 : 50000	Growth on media with Thionine 1 : 25000	Agglutination with monospecific sera: abortus	Agglutination with monospecific sera: melitensis
abortus	+	+[1]	+	–	+	–
melitensis	–	–	+	+	–	+
suis	–	++[2]	–	+	+	–

[1] On agar slopes positive after 5–8 days; [2] positive after 2–4 days

Fig. 180: Demonstration and identification of brucellae

Abb. 180: Nachweis und Bestimmung von Brucellen

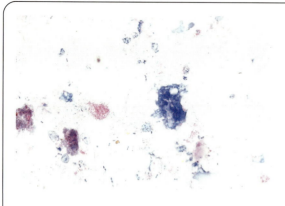
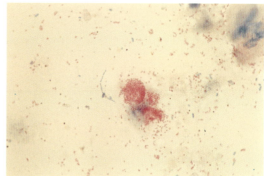
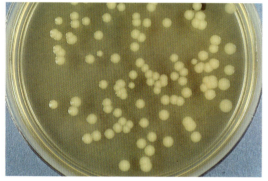
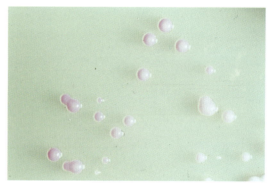

▲ Fig. 181: *Brucella abortus*, smear from placenta, Stableforth stain, groups of brucella stained red. Magnification x 1000

▼ Fig. 183: *Brucella abortus*, cultured from a bovine placenta brucella medium base with selective supplement (polymyxin B, bacitracin, cycloheximide, nalidixic acid, nystatin, vancomycin; Oxoid), 8 d 37°C, incubated in a 10% CO_2 atmosphere. Magnification x 0.4

▲ Fig. 182: *Brucella melitensis*, placental smear of sheep, brucella are red, lying in groups, cannot be differentiated microscopically from other brucellae, Stableforth stain. Magnification x 1000

▼ Fig. 184: *Brucella suis*, pure culture on a crystal violet selective medium, the colonies are coloured because they have taken up the crystal violet, 5 d, 37°C. Magnification x 2.6

▲ Abb. 181: *Brucella abortus*, Nachgeburtsausstrich, Färbung nach Stableforth, rote in Nestern gelagerte Brucellen, Abb.-M. 1000:1

▼ Abb. 183: *Brucella abortus*, kulturelle Isolierung aus der Eihaut eines Rindes, Brucella-Medium-Basis mit Selektivsupplement (Polymyxin B, Bacitracin, Cycloheximid, Nalidixinsäure, Nystatin, Vancomycin; Oxoid), 8 d, 37°C, bebrütet in einer 10%igen CO_2-Atmosphäre, Abb.-M. 1:2,5

▲ Abb. 182: *Brucella melitensis*, Eihautausstrich vom Schaf, rote in Nestern gelagerte Brucellen, mikroskopisch von anderen Brucellen nicht zu unterscheiden, Färbung nach Stableforth, Abb.-M. 1000:1

▼ Abb. 184: *Brucella suis*, Reinkultur auf einem Kristallviolett-Selektivnährboden, die Kolonien haben sich durch Aufnahme von Kristallviolett verfärbt, 5 d, 37°C, Abb.-M. 2,6:1

■ Identification of Brucella species and their biotypes

The identification of brucellae can present difficulty, because there are many strains in which some characters are divergent, so that they form transitions between the classical types. This has led to the establishment of biotypes (tab. 75). A further complicating factor is that many of the characters used to date, such as CO_2 requirement, dye resistance and H_2S production (tab. 75) are variable and only

■ Bestimmung der Brucellenarten einschließlich ihrer Biotypen

Die Bestimmung der Brucellen kann schwierig sein, da es viele Stämme gibt, die aufgrund einzelner abweichender Eigenschaften Übergangsformen zwischen den klassischen Arten bilden. Dies hat zur Aufstellung von Biotypen geführt (Tab. 75). Es kommt erschwerend hinzu, daß viele der bisher benutzten Merkmale (z. B. CO_2-Bedarf, Farbstoffresistenz, H_2S-Bildung; Tab. 75) variabel und nur

quantitative. This is also true of the agglutination with monospecific sera. It is for this reason that lysotyping is being applied today for species identification, along with metabolic studies using the Warburg technique to test the oxygen consumption of brucella strains in the presence of carbohydrates and amino acids (tab. 78) (4, 19, 39, 67). But since these methods are relatively expensive the simplified methods, which rely on the following parameters, have not lost their practical application (tab. 75 and fig. 180).

▷ Growth dependence on a 10% CO_2 atmosphere: The bacterial strain must be tested as soon as possible following its isolation, because CO_2-independent mutants can appear in subsequent passages.

▷ Effect of basic fuchsin and thionine on growth: The test is performed on solid medium and tryptose agar, serum dextrose agar or casein-peptone soyapeptone agar are used as basic media. The dye solutions are produced in strengths of 0.1%, autoclaved and added in the desired amounts to the fluid media (tab. 75 and figs. 191 and 192).

▷ Production of hydrogen sulphide: The production of H_2S is demonstrated on agar slopes (trypsinized meat peptone, with a maximum of 0.1% dextrose) and a strip of lead acetate paper. Results: Br. abortus positive from 5th to 8th day, Br. suis positive from 2nd to 4th day and Br. melitensis negative (tab. 75 and fig. 180) (68).

▷ Production of urease: All brucellae form urease with quantitative variation. This is demonstrated with urea agar of CHRISTENSEN (4), (results in tab. 75) or the urea solution of BAUER (68).

quantitativ sind. Dies trifft auch für die Agglutination mit monospezifischen Seren zu. Deswegen werden nach den derzeitigen Erkenntnissen die Lysotypie sowie Stoffwechseluntersuchungen, die mit der Warburgtechnik den Sauerstoffverbrauch von Brucellenstämmen in Anwesenheit von Kohlenhydraten und Aminosäuren messen (Tab. 78), zur Artbestimmung benutzt (4, 19, 39, 67). Da diese Methoden jedoch relativ aufwendig sind, hat für die Bestimmung typischer Stämme sowie der Biotypen ein vereinfachtes Verfahren seine praktische Bedeutung nicht verloren. Dieses beruht auf der Feststellung folgender Merkmale (Tab. 75 und Abb. 180):

▷ Wachstumsabhängigkeit von einer 10%igen CO_2-Atmosphäre: Der Stamm muß möglichst frühzeitig nach seiner Isolierung geprüft werden, bei nachfolgenden Passagen können CO_2-unabhängige Mutanten auftreten.

▷ Wachstumsbeeinflussung durch basisches Fuchsin und Thionin: Die Prüfung erfolgt auf festen Nährböden, als Basismedium haben sich Tryptose-Agar, Serum-Dextrose-Agar oder Caseinpepton-Sojamehlpepton-Agar bewährt. Die Farbstofflösungen werden 0,1%ig hergestellt, im Dampftopf sterilisiert und in den gewünschten Mengen dem flüssigen Medium zugesetzt (Tab. 75 und Abb. 191 u. 192).

▷ Schwefelwasserstoffbildung: Nachweis auf Schrägagar (tryptisches Fleischpepton, höchstens 0,1% Dextrose) und Bleiacetatstreifen. Ergebnis: Br. abortus positiv ab 5.–8. Tag, Br. suis positiv ab 2.–4. Tag, Br. melitensis negativ (Tab. 75 u. Abb. 180) (68).

▷ Ureasenachweis: Alle Brucellen bilden Urease, jedoch bestehen quantitative Unterschiede. Zum Nachweis sind der Harnstoffagar nach CHRISTENSEN (Ergebnisse s. Tab. 75) (4) sowie die Harnstofflösung nach BAUER (68) geeignet.

Table 77: Dissociation of brucellae

Tabelle 77: Dissoziation der Brucellen

Character	S-form	R-form
Colony form	moist, glistening, smooth border, homogeneous or finely granular	dry, rough, irregular border, coarsely granular
Growth in broth	even turbidity	sediment
Suspension in physiological saline	even and persistent	uneven and unstable
Agglutination with antiserum[1]	+	−
Agglutination with 1 : 1000 acriflavin[2]	−	+
Trypaflavin test	persistent suspension	rapid agglutination and flocculation
Henry's illumination[3]	round, blue to bluish-grey colonies	granular, reddish-yellow to yellow-white colonies

[1] Slide agglutination, interpretation may necessitate microscopy,
[2] Suspension of brucellae in 1 : 2000 trypaflavin solution is kept in the incubator for 6–8 hours,
[3] Light is passed obliquely from below through the culture plate at an angle of 45 °C

[1] Objektträgeragglutination, ev. mikroskopische Kontrolle;
[2] Brucellensuspension in Trypaflavinlösung 1 : 2000, 6–8 h im Brutschrank aufbewahren;
[3] mit einem Winkel von 45 °C schräg von unten in die Plattenkultur eindringendes Licht

Table 78: Classification of brucellae according to lysotypes and by the oxidative metabolic processes established by the Warburg technique

Tabelle 78: Einteilung der Brucellen nach der Lysotypie und nach den mit der Warburg-Technik ermittelten oxidativen Stoffwechselleistungen

Species	Biotype	Lysis with phage						oxidation of												
		Tb	Wb	Fi	Bk2	R/O	R/C	L.alanine	L.asparagine	L.glutamic acid	L.arabinose	D.galactose	D.ribose	D.glucose	DS.xylose	L.arginine	Dl.citrulline	Dl.ornithine	L.lysine	Meso erythritol
Br. melitensis	all	nl	nl	nl	l	nl	nl	+	+	+	−	−	−	+	−	−	−	−	−	+
Br. abortus	all	l	l	l	l	pl	nl	+	+	+	+	+	+	+	v	−	−	−	−	+
Br. suis	1	nl	l	pl	l	nl	nl	v	−	−	+	v	+	+	+	+	+	+	+	+
	2	nl	l	pl	l	nl	nl	−	v	v	+	v	+	+	+	+	+	+	−	+
	3	nl	l	pl	l	nl	nl	v	−	v	−	−	+	+	+	+	+	+	+	+
	4	nl	l	l	l	nl	nl	−	−	v	−	−	+	+	+	+	+	+	+	+
Br. ovis	−	nl	nl	nl	nl	l	l	v	+	+	−	−	−	−	−	−	−	−	−	−
Br. neotomae	−	pl	l	l	l	nl	nl	v	+	+	+	+	v	+	−	−	−	−	−	+
Br. canis	−	nl	nl	nl	nl	nl	l	v	−	+	v	v	+	+	−	+	+	+	+	v

l = lysis; nl = no lysis; pl = partial lysis

l = Lysis, nl = keine Lysis, pl = partielle Lysis

▷ Agglutination with monospecific sera: The sera are produced by absorbing the abortus and melitensis sera respectively with the heterologous strains (4, 52, 68).

▷ Bacteriophages: The known bacteriophages have a preference for certain species of brucella (tab. 75). Phage Tb (Tbilisi) is active only against *Br. abortus* and it is therefore most important for its identification.

▷ Agglutination mit monospezifischen Seren: Die Seren werden durch Absättigung von Abortus- und Melitensisimmunseren mit den heterologen Stämmen hergestellt (4, 52, 68).

▷ Bakteriophagen: Die bekannten Bakteriophagen befallen bevorzugt bestimmte Brucellenarten (Tab. 75). Für die Differenzierung ist vor allem der Phage Tb (Tbilisi) von Bedeutung, der nur gegen *Br. abortus* aktiv ist.

1.2 Serological diagnosis

The serological procedures, together with methodology and interpretation, are laid down in the supplement to the German Government Order of the 26.6.72, for the protection of cattle, pigs, sheep and goats against brucellosis (BGBl. I S. 1046) in the version of 9.4.86 (BGBl. I S. 403). They are also to be found in Appendix C (Brucellosis) of the guidelines issued on 26.6.1964 by the Council of the EEC responsible for decisions on zoonoses in respect of the cattle and pig trade within the Com-

1.2 Serologische Diagnose

Die serologischen Verfahren sind mit ihrer Methode und Auswertung in der Anlage zur Verordnung zum Schutz gegen die Brucellose der Rinder, Schweine, Schafe und Ziegen vom 26.6.1972 (BGBl. I, S. 1046) in der Fassung der Verordnung vom 9.4.1986 (BGBl. I, S. 403) sowie in der Anlage C (Brucellose) der Richtlinien des Rates vom 26.6.1964 zur Regelung viehseuchenrechtlicher Fragen beim innergemeinschaftlichen Handelsverkehr mit Rindern und Schweinen (Amtsblatt der

Table 79: Grading the agglutination at each dilution step

Tabelle 79: Beurteilung des Agglutinationsgrades einer Verdünnungsstufe

++++	Complete agglutination and sedimentation; supernatant fluid is 100 % clear (clumps appear when tube is shaken)
+++	almost complete agglutination and about 75 % clearing of the supernatant fluid (clumps appear when tube is shaken)
++	Still distinct agglutination and about 50 % clearing of the supernatant (small clump are formed when tube is shaken)
+	Traces of agglutination (only the finest precipitate can be seen when the tube is shaken)
−	No visible agglutination, button-like sediment which flows out when the tube is tilted, even turbidity of supernatant fluid

munity (EEC Gazette No. 121, page 1977). This was most recently amended by the guidelines of the 20. 12. 1985 (EEC Gazette No. L 372, page 44).
The following are used:
▷ Blood serum tube agglutination: At least the dilutions 1 : 20, 1 : 40 and 1 : 80 must be examined. One of the three possible methods is shown in figure 185, see table 79 for the interpretation of the degree of agglutination. This assessment must be carried out for every single dilution.
▷ Complement fixation test (CFT): For the method see supplement to above-mentioned Order. The serum is considered to be positive to the CFT, if a 50 % haemolysis inhibition has taken place in the first tube (0.1 ml serum).
▷ Rapid Coombs test: For the method see supplement to the above-mentioned Order.
▷ Abortus ring test: The tests are performed on milk samples from bulk tankers, churns, individual animals or single quarters. 1 ml of fresh milk is placed into tubes of 8–10 mm diameter, a drop of test fluid is added (0.05 ml brucellae stained with haematoxylin, in standardized pipette). Incubation at 37 °C in a waterbath or incubator. After 45 minutes a dark purple ring develops and the milk is discoloured in positive cases.
▷ Milk whey agglutination test: Before the test is set up the cream is removed by centrifugation and casein is precipitated with rennet (30 to 45 minutes at 37 °C). The whey is examined at least in dilutions of 1 : 5 and 1 : 10.

Fig. 185: Procedure for tube agglutination test
Taken from BISPING, W.: Kompendium der veterinärmedizinischen Mikrobiologie, Teil II. Hannover: M. & H. Schaper
Abb. 185: Technik der Blutserumlangsamagglutination Entnommen aus BISPING, W.: Kompendium der veterinärmedizinischen Mikrobiologie, Teil II. Hannover: M. & H. Schaper

Procedure:
1) Making up the dilutions
2) Addition of test fluid
   (Agglutinogen, suspension of bacteria)

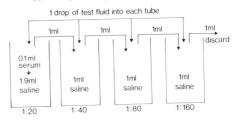

3) Reaction time: 18—24 hours at 37 °C (incubator)
4) Assessment of agglutination
   a) by sediment

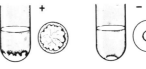

   b) by turbidity or clearing of supernatant fluid and formation of sediment
5) Reading of agglutination titre
   (– the last dilution to give a definite reaction)

Table 80: Evaluation of the serological reactions for the identification of brucellosis (after the supplement to the Order for the protection of cattle, pigs, sheep and goats against brucellosis of 26.5.1972)

Tabelle 80: Beurteilung der serologischen Reaktionen zur Feststellung von Brucellose (nach der Anlage der Verordnung zum Schutz gegen die Brucellose der Rinder, Schweine, Schafe und Ziegen vom 26.5.1972)

Animal species	Test sample	Assessment of agglutination	Supplementary reaction	Presence of brucellosis
A Cattle	I blood serum	negative 1:20 − to 1:20 +	not required	−
		doubtful 1:20 ++ to 1:40 +	CFT: + CFT: −[1]	+ −
		positive 1:40 ++[2] & above	not absolutely necessary	+
	II a milk whey	negative 1:5 −	not required	−
		doubtful 1:5 +	repeat and/or test of blood serum	?
		positive 1:5 ++	not absolutely necessary	+
	II b milk	*Abortus ring test* negative — tanker or churn milk sample	not required	−
		positive	test individual cow milk/blood samples	as in AI or AIIa
	III semen	negative 1:5 −	not required	−
		doubtful 1:5 ++ to 1:10 +	not absolutely necessary	?
		positive 1:10 ++ & above	confirmation by tests as in AI	+
B Pig	blood serum	as in AI	irrespective of results, CFT is done in every case[4]	assessment as in AI[3]
C sheep goat	blood serum[5]	negative as in AI	not required	−
		doubtful as in AI	CFT: + CFT: −	+ −
		positive as in AI	not absolutely necessary	+

[1] The rapid Coombs test can be used in addition, if that is positive too then the animal is to be considered as infected; [2] the diagnostic titre of 1:40 ++ corresponds to 62.5 international agglutination units; [3] if there is doubt concerning the final assessment of an animal, then the serological examination is to be graded doubtful and the test repeated no earlier than after 3 to 4 weeks; [4] in pigs the agglutinins can disappear quickly from the blood and therefore evidence of infection may in certain individuals depend solely on a positive reaction to the complement fixation test; [5] the dilution is to be made with 5% saline

▷ Semen agglutination test: In order to obtain the seminal plasma the semen is centrifuged until the supernatant is clear. The sample is tested in dilutions 1:5, 1:10 and 1:20.

The application of these tests in the various animal species, their combination and interpretation are summarized in table 80. It can be difficult to attempt to follow this routine exactly, because one can encounter not only false positive results but also false negatives.

▷ False negative reactions: They are found particularly in the serum tube agglutination test because the IgG 1 class antibodies, which frequently appear after infections, agglutinate brucellae with difficulty and may even mask the agglutinating properties of the IgM antibodies. The best methods of demonstrating IgG 1 antibodies is with the CFT and the rose Bengal test. The latter is a plate agglutination test using buffered brucella antigen set to pH 3.5 and dyed with rose Bengal. This test is not common in the German Federal Republic but is widely used, especially in the Anglo-Saxon countries.

The blood serum tube agglutination test identifies mainly antibodies of the IgM and IgG 2 classes (tab. 81).

Cows may still give a serologically negative reaction at the time of a brucella abortion (30).

▷ False positive (non-specific) reactions: They can occur in cattle, sheep, goats and pigs without an infection of the herd having taken place and yet it

Table 81: The Ig classes which can be identified in brucellosis by serological means

Serological Methods	Principal Ig class identified	Remarks
Tube agglutination (TA)	IgM, IgG 2, (IgG 1)	the IgG 1 class of antibodies are most numerous after infection, but they are difficult to identify and false negatives are possible
CFT, Rose Bengal test	IgG 1, IgM	The rose-Bengal test is neither proscribed in Germany nor popular, but is especially suitable for the diagnosis of pig brucellosis
Coombs test	IgM, IgG 1, IgG 2	very sensitive test, which identifies »Incomplete« antibodies which do not react in TA
Abortus ring test	IgM, IgG 1, IgA	
Heat inactivation, Rivanol precipitation, mercaptoethanol treatment	IgG	supplementary procedures to differentiate »non-specific« reaction in TA, which are due to IgA which is destroyed by heat, rivanol, mercaptoethanol and other substances

can affect a fair proportion of the tests (26, 27, 33, 54, 64 etc.).

The reason for this is uncertain, it is possible that endotoxins of other Gram-negative bacteria (e.g. pasteurellae, salmonellae, proteus OX 19, *E. coli*), natural antibodies or food additives (26) lead to the development of low, non-specific titres, which are usually the result of IgM antibody interaction. See table 81 for the method of action of the immunoglobulin classes that appear after an infection. Therefore, a limited differentiation is possible if the IgM is destroyed. This can be achieved by:

▷ Agglutination at higher temperature: In this the antigen/antibody mixture is kept not at 37 °C but at 56 °C (5, 7, 26, 28). A similar effect can be obtained by inactivating the serum beforehand at 56 °C or 65 °C for 15 minutes.

▷ Mercaptoethanol treatment: The serum dilutions are made with a mercaptoethanol saline solution (8.5 g NaCl, 7.14 ml mercaptoethanol, distilled water to 1 l). The antigen, without the addition of phenol is added as for the tube agglutination. Instead of mercaptoethanol one can also use dithiothreitol, which is not carcinogenic. The destruction of IgM follows by the breakdown of the disulphide links in the antibody molecules (42, 44).

▷ Rivanol test: Serum is mixed with a 0.4 % solution of rivanol at a ratio of 1 : 3. The interfering proteins are precipitated and can be removed by centrifuging. The remaining serum is then used for the tube agglutination test.

The results of these procedures should always be compared with those of the serum tube agglutination test before an assessment is made. If doubtful titres disappear or weakly positive ones fall into the negative range, then this can be taken as an indication that no infection is present.

■ **Serological cross reactions**

When interpreting the results of the agglutination test one must bear in mind that there is an overlap in antigenic structure between brucellae and certain other bacteria *(Francisella, Campylobacter, Salmonella, Pasteurella)*. Of particular practical importance is the similarity in antigenic pattern between *Br. abortus, Br. suis* and *Yersinia enterocolitica*, especially the serotype 09 (p. 205), which involves the O-antigens. Monospecific *Br. melitensis* serum does not agglutinate *Y. enterocolitica* (2). Such cross reactions are found in the pig, because it is most frequently affected with *Y. enterocolitica*. But the cross reactions also occur in cattle, dogs and other species (1, 3, 11, 66). An infection with *Y. enterocolitica* serotype 09 can not only cause interference with the agglutination test but in rare cases

even the brucella CF test can become positive. There are no sure and easy methods to date for differentiating such cross reactions. No satisfactory results have been obtained with experimental serological procedures such as absorbed sera, the use of ELISA or precipitation tests (60). One can try the parallel test with brucella and *Y. enterocolitica* serotype 09 O- and OH-antigens. The production of OH-antigens (suspensions of yersinia, live or killed with 0.3 % formalin) and of O-antigens (boiled or autoclaved suspensions) must be done at 22–28 °C, since it is only at this temperature that smooth, stable cultures of yersinia are obtained. The agglutination test is read after 8 to 16 hours of incubation in a waterbath at 50–52 °C (32).

If the yersinia titres (O and/or OH titres) are distinctly higher than the brucella titres, then this indicates an infection with *Yersinia enterocolitica* (62). Other methods consist in cross absorption of sera showing a brucella titre with *Brucella* and *Yersinia* respectively. This might be achieved by setting up an agglutination test first with brucellae and after the test has been read, and the brucellae centrifuged off, the test is repeated with yersinia, and vice versa. Brucellosis is indicated if, after absorption with yersinia (09), the brucella titre remains unaltered or has dropped by no more than one dilution.

The serological differentiation is of limited value, particularly in respect of single sera, where it does not always provide a definite answer. For further confirmation of the diagnosis the cultural isolation of *Y. enterocolitica* should be attempted from faecal samples or the tonsils. It can be assumed with certainty that titres to brucella agglutination are probably due to *Y. enterocolitica* if:
▷ no clinical signs of brucella develop,
▷ no brucellae can be isolated in culture,
▷ *Y. enterocolitica* can be isolated and
▷ high titres to *Y. enterocolitica* develop, especially against certain serotypes.

nation auch (seltener) die Brucellen-KBR positiv werden. Zur Zeit gibt es keine einfache und sichere Methode, derartige Agglutinationen zu differenzieren. Versuche mit serologischen Untersuchungsverfahren, wie z. B. Absättigung von Seren oder Anwendung von ELISA- oder Präzipitationstesten, erbrachten keine zufriedenstellenden Ergebnisse (60). Versucht werden kann die vergleichende Untersuchung der Seren mit Brucellen- und *Y. enterocolitica* Serotyp 09 O- und OH-Antigenen. Die Herstellung der OH-Antigene (lebende oder mit 0,3 % Formalin abgetötete Yersiniensuspensionen) und der O-Antigene (gekochte oder autoklavierte Suspensionen) erfolgt bei 22–28 °C, da nur bei dieser Temperatur glatte und stabile Kulturen von Yersinien zu erhalten sind. Die Ablesung der Agglutination erfolgt nach 8–16 h nach einer Inkubation bei 50–52 °C im Wasserbad (32).

Sind die *Yersinia*-Titer (O- und/oder OH-Titer) im Vergleich zu den Brucella-Titern deutlich erhöht, spricht dies für eine Infektion mit *Y. enterocolitica* (62). Andere Methoden bestehen in der kreuzweisen Absättigung der Seren mit einem Brucellentiter mit *Brucella* bzw. *Yersinia*, etwa in der Form, daß ein primärer Agglutinationsansatz mit Brucellen nach der Ablesung und der Abtrennung der Brucellen durch Zentrifugation mit *Yersinia* angesetzt wird und umgekehrt. Wenn nach Absättigung mit *Yersinia* (09) der Brucellosetiter unverändert bleibt oder lediglich um eine Titerstufe absinkt, spricht dies für Brucellose.

Die serologische Differenzierung hat insbesondere in bezug auf Einzelseren eine beschränkte Aussagekraft und führt nicht immer zu einem klaren Ergebnis. Zur weiteren Absicherung der Diagnose empfiehlt es sich, den kulturellen Nachweis von *Y. enterocolitica* aus Kotproben oder aus Tonsillen zu versuchen. Es kann angenommen werden, daß Titer, die bei der Agglutination mit Brucellen auftreten, wahrscheinlich durch *Y. enterocolitica* bedingt sind, wenn
▷ keine klinischen Symptome einer Brucellose auftreten,
▷ Brucellen kulturell nicht nachgewiesen werden,
▷ *Y. enterocolitica* angezüchtet werden kann und
▷ hohe Titer gegen *Y. enterocolitica* auftreten, insbesondere gegen den isolierten Serotyp.

2   Brucella ovis

■ **Incidence and veterinary significance**
Br. ovis was first isolated in New Zealand and Australia (13, 37, 56). In Germany it was first observed in the grey horned »Heidschnucke«, subsequently also in other breeds of sheep (47). HAJDU (25) reports a massive outbreak in Slovakia. The prominent clinical sign is epididymitis, but abortions also

2   Brucella ovis

■ **Vorkommen und medizinische Bedeutung**
Br. ovis ist erstmalig in Neuseeland und Australien isoliert worden (13, 37, 56). In Deutschland wurde das Bakterium zuerst bei der grauen gehörnten Heidschnucke, später auch bei anderen Rassen nachgewiesen (47). Über ein gehäuftes Vorkommen in der Slowakei berichtet HAJDU (25). Klinisch steht

Specimens
Epididymis (especially tail), testis, semen (less well suited, because bacteria are liberated only periodically or may be absent altogether; the medium can be overgrown by contaminants), placenta, foetuses

Demonstration by culture
1. Nutrient media: medium base (eg. brucella agar, Albimi agar, tryptose agar, casein peptone-soya meal-peptone agar etc.) with 10% horse, ox or sheep blood.
2. Selective medium with vancomycin, colistin, nystatin & nitrofurantoin, is only required if the test material is heavily contaminated eg. semen samples (4, 12).
3. Incubation: at 37°C, in 10% CO_2 (no aerobic or anaerobic growth).
4. Appearance of colonies: visible after 2–3 days, 1–2 mm in size and greyish-white after 4–5 days, later yellowish and mucoid (there are no S-forms), they agglutinate in acriflavin.

Serological demonstration of antibodies
1. The Br. abortus and Br. melitensis antigens which are generally used in diagnosis cannot be employed here, because Br. ovis occurs only in the R-form and possesses none of the surface antigen determinants of the S-form.
2. The agglutination test is unsatisfactory because auto-agglutinins occur in the cell suspensions.
3. Complement fixation test is the method of choice, because it is sensitive and specific. Various antigen preparations are used: whole cells, ultrasonic extracts, heat extracts (120°C) (4, 9, 17, 25, 50).
4. Other methods for the demonstration of antibodies, such as agar-gel diffusion, indirect haemagglutination, indirect immunofluorescence, precipitation and the like, are in less common use (38).

Fig. 186: Diagnosis of *Brucella ovis* infection

occur. The organism cannot be transmitted to man. Br. ovis is similar in its properties to the other species of brucella, but it is relatively small (0.7–1.2 × 0.5–0.7 µm).

■ **Cultural and biochemical properties**

See tab. 75, diagnostic demonstration see figs. 186 to 188.

3 Brucella canis

The infection was first reported in the USA in 1966 (14, 15) and in Germany in 1973 (34). It occurs in larger dog breeding concerns and kennels (61). Br. canis causes disturbances of fertility in male dogs (epididymitis and testicular atrophy) and abortion in bitches. Natural infections occur only in dogs and, through contact with dogs or laboratory infections, in man.

Br. canis is similar to other brucellae in its microscopic appearance and its cultural behaviour.

The most important biochemical properties are listed in tab. 75; other characteristics are: Oxy +, Cat +, Nit +, Cit −, Ure +, MR −, VPR −, Ind −, Glu −, Lac − (63). The diagnostic procedure is illustrated in figure 191 and the cultural growth in figures 189 and 190.

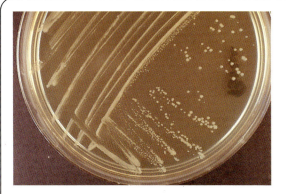
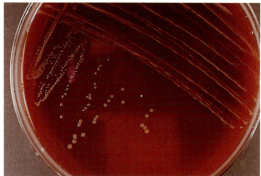
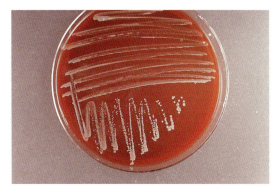
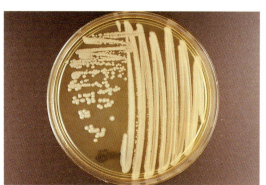

▲ Fig. 187: *Brucella ovis,* pure culture on brucella selective medium (fig. 186), 7 d, incubation in atmosphere of 10 % CO_2. Magnification x 0.33
▼ Fig. 189: *Brucella canis,* pure culture on blood agar, 7 d, aerobic incubation at 37 °C. Magnification x 0.25

▲ Abb. 187: *Brucella ovis,* Reinkultur auf Brucella-Selektivnährboden (Abb. 186), 7 d, bebrütet in 10%iger CO_2-Atmosphäre, Abb.-M. 1 : 3
▼ Abb. 189: *Brucella canis,* Reinkultur auf Blutagar, 7 d, aerob bei 37 °C, bebrütet, Abb.-M. 1 : 4

▲ Fig. 188: *Brucella ovis,* pure culture on blood agar, 7 d, incubation in an atmosphere of 10 % CO_2. Magnification x 0.33
▼ Fig. 190: *Brucella canis,* pure culture on brucella selective medium (fig. 191), 7 d, aerobic incubation. Magnification x 0.25

▲ Abb. 188: *Brucella ovis,* Reinkultur auf Blutagar, 7 d, bebrütet in 10%iger CO_2-Atmosphäre, Abb.-M. 1 : 3
▼ Abb. 190: *Brucella canis,* Reinkultur auf Brucella-Selektivnährboden (Abb. 191) 7 d aerob bebrütet, Abb.-M. 1 : 4

Lact – (63). Der diagnostische Untersuchungsgang ist in der Abb. 191, das kulturelle Wachstum in den Abb. 189 und 190 dargestellt.

Bibliography / Literatur

1. AHVONEN, P., E. JANSSON & K. AHO (1969): Marked cross-agglutination between brucellae and a subtype of Yersinia enterocolitica. Acta path. microbiol. scand. **75**, 291–295.

2. AKKERMANS, J. P. W. M., & W. K. H. HILL (1971): Yersinia enterocolitica serotype 9 infectie als storend element bij de serologische diagnostiek van Brucella-infecties bij het varken. Tschr. Diergeneesk. **24**, 1654–1662.

Specimens
Vaginal discharge, foetuses, milk, urine, semen, spleen, retropharyngeal, bronchial and mesenteric lymph nodes, bone marrow. Cultures of blood are particularly suited for demonstrating the organisms, because of a protracted bacteraemia.

Demonstration by culture
1. Media: medium base (eg. brucella agar, tryptose agar, casein-peptone soya meal peptone agar) with addition of 10 % blood. 2. Selective medium: 25,000 IU bacitracin, 4,500 IU polymyxin B, 100 mg cycloheximidine/l, or addition of crystal violet to tryptose agar (1.4 ml of a 0.1 % solution to 1 l of medium), 3. Incubation: aerobic (increased CO_2 content retards and anaerobic conditions inhibit growth altogether), at 37 °C for 3 days, 4. Blood culture: The blood is cultured either direct or after enrichment in broth (eg. brain heart infusion broth), then plated on solid media. Duration of enrichment 3 weeks. If the agglutination titres are low (1 : 50–1 : 200) the the blood cultures are usually negative, 5. Appearance of colonies: After 3 days on tryptose agar small, slightly opague colonies with a dull sheen appear that have a honey-yellow colour in obliquely transmitted light and a mucoid consistency. Br. canis always grows in the R-form, in both primary and subcultures, the S-form is unknown.

Serological demonstration of antibodies
1. The Br. abortus and Br. melitensis antigens which are generally used in diagnosis cannot be employed here, because Br. canis occurs only in the R-form and possesses none of the surface antigenic determinants of the S-form. 2. Method of choice: tube agglutination test on blood serum. Antigen production has not been standardized to date, and varies from one laboratory to another. The test is carried out at 50 °C or 37 °C and it is assessed 24 to 48 hours later. A titre of 1 : 50 to 1 : 200 is suspect and a titre of 1 : 400 and above is positive. 3. Non-specific titres can occur in the lower serum dilutions, possibly through antigenically related bacteria (bordetella, pasteurella, actinobacillus, moraxella). In such cases it is advisable to repeat the test or to confirm with other methods (complement fixation and mercaptoethanol test).

Fig. 191: Diagnosis of *Brucella canis* infection (4, 34, 40, 46, 61, 63)

Abb. 191: Diagnose der *Brucella-canis*-Infektion (4, 34, 40, 46, 61, 63)

3. AKKERMANS, J. P. W. M., & W. K. H. HILL (1972): Yersinia enterocolitica serotype 9 infections as a factor interfering with the serodiagnosis of Brucella-infections in swine. Netherl. J. Vet. Sci. **5**, 73–80.
4. ALTON, G. G., L. M. JONES & D. E. DIETZ (1975): Laboratory techniques in brucellosis. 2. Aufl., Genf: WHO.
5. ANDERSEN, F. M. (1961): Über die Möglichkeit einer Differenzierung zwischen spezifischen und unspezifischen Brucella-Serumreaktionen beim Rind. Nord. Vet. Med. **13**, 289–332.
6. BAUMGARTNER, H. (1955): Erfahrungen mit der Brucellenzüchtung auf dem Milieu W. Schweiz. Arch. Tierhk. **97**, 357.
7. BEINHAUER, W. (1962): Beitrag zur Differenzierung fraglicher Reaktionen in der Agglutination auf Abortus Bang mittels des sog. Hitzetestes. Mh. Tierhk. **14**, Sonderteil Rindertuberkulose und Brucellose **11**, 86–90.
8. BENDIXEN, H. C. (1950): Brucellose bei Bullen und ihre Bedeutung für die künstliche Besamung. Berl. Münch. tierärztl. Wschr. 253–257.
9. BIBERSTEIN, E. L., & G. MCGOWAN (1958): Epididymitis in rams. Studies on laboratory diagnosis. Cornell Vet. **48**, 31–44.
10. BÖRGER, K. (1958): Ergebnis der Typendifferenzierung von Brucellenstämmen in Schleswig-Holstein. Mh. Tierhk. **10**, Sonderteil »Rindertuberkulose u. Brucellose«, **7**, 53–56.
11. BOCKEMÜHL, J., & J. ROTH (1978): Brucella-Titer bei subklinischen Infektionen mit Yersinia enterocolitica 0 : 9 in einem Schweinezuchtbetrieb. Zbl. Bakt. I. Orig. A **240**, 86–93.
12. BROWN, G. M., C. R. RANGER & D. J. KELLEY (1971): Selective media for the isolation of Brucella ovis. Cornell Vet. **61**, 265–280.
13. BUDDLE, M. B., & B. W. BOYES (1953): A Brucella mutant causing genital disease of sheep in New Zealand. Aust. Vet. J. **29**, 145–153.
14. CARMICHAEL, L. E. (1966): Abortion in 200 beagles. J. Am. Vet. Med. Ass. **149**, 1126.
15. CARMICHAEL, L. E., & R. M. KENNEY (1968): Canine abortion caused by Brucella canis. J. Am. Vet. Med. Ass. **152**, 606–616.
16. CLAPP, K. H. (1961): A comparison of various antigens used in the complement fixation test for ovine brucellosis. Aust. Vet. J. **37**, 188–190.
17. CLAPP, K. H. (1955): A complement fixation test for the diagnosis of ovine brucellosis with special reference to epididymitis. Aust. Vet. J. **31**, 27–28.
18. CLAPP, K. H., L. E. A. SYMONS & J. B. DOOLETTE (1955): The application of a complement fixation test to the diagnosis of ovine brucellosis. Aust. Vet. J. **31**, 29.
19. CORBEL, M. J., & W. J. BRINLEY-MORGAN (1984): Genus Brucella Meyer and Shaw 1920. In: N. R. KRIEG & J. G. HOLT (Hrsg.): Bergey's manual of systematic bacteriology. Vol. 1, S. 377–388. Baltimore, London: Williams & Wilkins.
20. DIETZ, O. (1960): Durch Brucella-Infektionen her-

vorgerufene chirurgische Erkrankungen beim Pferd, Rind, Schwein, Hund und bei der Katze. Mh. Vet. Med. 15, 752–755.
21. EHRLEIN, H. J., I. R. SCHIMMELPFENNIG & W. BISPING (1963): Ein Beitrag zur Brucellose des Hundes. Dtsch. tierärztl. Wschr. 70, 353–357.
22. ENTEL, H. J. (1961): Die Brucellose der Schweine. Mhefte Tierhk. 13, Sonderteil: Rindertuberkulose und Brucellose 10, 131–142, 150–164.
23. FECHNER, J., & W. MEYER (1960): Untersuchungen zur Pferdebrucellose. Arch. exp. Vet. Med. 1327–1339.
24. FENSKE, G. (1963): Untersuchungen über Brucellose bei Hasen. Mh. Vet. Med. 18, 380–390.
25. HAJDU, S. (1962): Ergebnisse der serologischen Untersuchung von Schafen auf Brucelloidose (infektiöse Epididymitis bei Schafböcken, Schafbrucellose) in der Slowakei und die Bekämpfung dieser Krankheit. Arch. exp. Vet. Med. 16, 19–28.
26. HELLMANN, R., & W. HEIN (1960): Untersuchungen an Rinderseren aus brucelloseverseuchten Beständen und Impfbeständen mittels der Serumlangsamagglutination und des Hitzetestes. Dtsch. tierärztl. Wschr. 67, 459–463.
27. HERTER, R. (1955): Phänomene und Probleme bei der serologischen Untersuchung (Agglutination) auf Rinderbrucellose. Dtsch. tierärztl. Wschr. 62, 297–300.
28. HOERLEIN, A. B. (1953): Studies on swine brucellosis. III. The differentiation of specific and nonspecific agglutination titers. Cornell Vet. 43, 28–37.
29. JACOB, KL. (1960): Zur Pathologie des brucelloseausscheidenden Rindereuters. Zbl. Vet. Med. 7, 778–793.
30. KARSTEN, F. (1957): Über den Nachweis von Brucella Ab. Bang in Nachgeburten und in der Milch von Kühen ohne positive serologische Reaktion des Blutes und der Milch. Mhefte Tierhk. 9, 104–105.
31. KELLER, H. (1951): Polyarthritis des Kalbes und Brucellose. Lebensmitteltierarzt 2, 37–39.
32. KNAPP, W., B. PRÖGEL & CH. KNAPP (1981): Immunpathologische Komplikationen bei enteralen Yersiniosen. Dtsch. med. Wschr. 106, 1054–1060.
33. KÖTSCHE, W. (1963): Unspezifische Reaktionen bei der Brucellose-Blutserumlangsamagglutination und ihre Bedeutung für die Diagnostik der Rinderbrucellose. Arch. exp. Vet. Med. 17, 859–875.
34. KRUEDENER, R. v. (1974): Isolierung und Bestimmung von Brucella canis aus einem Beaglebestand. Zbl. Vet. Med. B 21, 307–310.
35. KUZDAS, C. D., & E. V. MORSE (1953): A selective medium for the isolation of brucellae from contaminated materials. J. Bact. 66, 502–504.
36. KRÜGER, A. (1937): Die Brucellose der Pferde. Dtsch. tierärztl. Wschr. 182–186, 198–201.
37. MCFARLANE, D., R. M. SALISBURY, R. M. OSBORNE & J. L. JEBSON (1952): Investigations into sheep abortion in New Zealand during the 1950 lambing season. Aust. Vet. J. 28, 2221–2226.
38. MEYER, M. E. (1982): Brucella ovis. In: H. BLOBEL & T. SCHLIESSER (Hrsg.): Handbuch der bakteriellen Infektion bei Tieren. Bd. 4, S. 309–328. Jena: VEB Gustav Fischer.
39. MEYER, M. E., & H. S. CAMERON (1961): Metabolic characterization of the genus Brucella. J. Bact. 82, 387, 396.
40. MOORE, J. A., B. N. GUPTA & G. H. CONNER (1968): Eradication of Brucella canis infection form a dog colony. J. Am. Vet. Med. Ass. 153, 523–527.
41. MORSE, E. V., M. RISTIC, L. E. WITT & L. WIPF (1953): Canine abortion apparently due to Brucella abortus. Amer. J. Vet. Med. Ass. 122, 18–20.
42. MYLREA, P. J., & G. C. FRASER (1976): The use of supplementary tests in the serological diagnosis of bovine brucellosis. Aust. Vet. J. 52, 261–266.
43. NICOLET, J. H., R. SCHMIDT, H. STUDER & M. DAUWALDER (1979): Ein Ausbruch von Brucella-suis-Biotyp-2-Infektion beim Schwein. Schweiz. Arch. Tierhk. 121, 231–238.
44. NICOLETTI, P. (1969): Further evaluations of serologic test procedures used to diagnose brucellosis. Am. J. Vet. Res. 30, 1811–1816.
45. OSTERTAG, H. G., & H. MAYER (1958): Die Verbreitung der Schafbrucellose bei Herdenhunden. Mhefte Tierhk. 10, Sonderteil: Rindertuberkulose und Brucellose, 7, 57–69.
46. PICKERILL, P. A., & L. E. CARMICHAEL (1972): Canine brucellosis: control programs in commercial kennels and effect on reproduction. J. Am. Vet. Med. Ass. 160, 1607–1615.
47. PÓZVARI, M., & H. BEHRENS (1982): Kultureller Nachweis von Brucella ovis. Prakt. Tierarzt 63, 126–129.
48. RENK, W. (1962): Euterentzündungen bei Brucellose. Zbl. Vet. Med. 9, 487–498.
49. REUSSE, U. (1958): Über die Dissoziation von Brucellen. Mh. Tierhk. 10, Sonderteil: Rindertuberkulose und Brucellose 7, 135–140, 173–180.
50. RIS, D. R. (1974): The complement fixation for the diagnosis of Brucella ovis infection in sheep. N.Z. Vet. J. 22, 143–146.
51. ROOTS, E. (1963): Neuere Untersuchungen über die Antigenstruktur von Brucella melitensis und Brucella abortus. Vet. med. Nachr. 11–15.
52. ROOTS, E., & H. v. SPROCKHOFF (1954): Die Methodik der quantitativen Agglutininabsättigung zur Gewinnung typenspezifischer Brucella-Seren. Zbl. Vet. Med. 1, 660–672.
53. SEELEMANN, M. (1959): L'infection des bovins par Brucella melitensis en Europe. Bull. Off. Int. Epizoot. 52, 337–347.
54. SCHEIBNER, E. (1976): Spezifitätsgrenzen der Brucellose-Langsamagglutination. Berl. Münch. tierärztl. Wschr. 89, 300–302.
55. SCHWARZ, H. (1954): Verwerfen beim Hund infolge Abortus Bang. Mh. Vet. Med. 9, 152–154.
56. SIMMONS, G. C., & W. T. K. HALL (1953): Epididymitis in rams. Preliminary studies on the occurrence and pathogenicity of a Brucella-like organism. Aust. Vet. J. 29, 33–40.
57. STAMP, J. T., A. D. MCEWEN, J. J. A. WATT & D. I. NISBET (1950): Enzootic abortion in ewes. Vet. Rec. 62, 251–254.
58. THOMSON, A. (1959): Das Vorkommen von Brucella-Infektionen bei Schweinen und Hasen mit besonderer Berücksichtigung der Länder Europas. Nord. Vet. Med. 11, 709–718.
59. ULBRICH, F., & E. WEINHOLD (1962): Brucella-Typendifferenzierung mit monospezifischen Seren und Phagen. Zbl. Vet. med. 9, 555–564.
60. WEBER, A. (1982): Zur gegenwärtigen Brucellose-Situation bei Tieren in der Bundesrepublik Deutschland. Tierärztl. Umschau 37, 570–574.
61. WEBER, A. (1976): Untersuchungen über die Verbreitung von Infektionen mit Brucella canis bei Beagle-Hunden in der Bundesrepublik Deutschland. Fortschr. Vet. Med. Heft 25, S. 272–278. Berlin, Hamburg: Paul Parey.
62. WEBER, A., C. LEMBKE, G. BOOS & B. PÜCHNER (1983): Nachweis und Interpretation von Antikörpertitern gegen Brucellen in Serumproben von Hunden. Kleintierpraxis 28, 279–281.
63. WEBER, A., & T. SCHLIESSER (1975): Serologischer und kultureller Nachweis von Brucella canis bei Beagle-Hunden einer Versuchstierhaltung. Zbl. Vet. Med. B 22, 403–410.
64. WOBBEN, J. (1975): Serologische und allergologische Diagnose der Schweinebrucellose — eine Literaturübersicht — und serologische Untersuchungen zum Auftreten der Schweinebrucellose in Nordwestniedersachsen (Emsland). Vet. Med. Diss. Hannover.
65. VALENTINCIC, S. (1964): Beitrag zur Kenntnis der Epizootologie der Brucellose beim Feldhasen. Zschr. Jagdwissensch. 10, 9–19.
66. WILLINGER, H. (1960): Brucellose bei Feldhasen in Österreich. Wiener tierärztl. Mschr. 661–669.

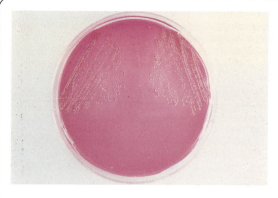
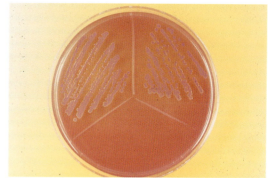
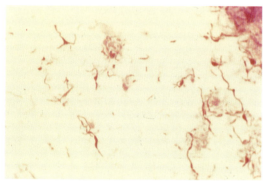
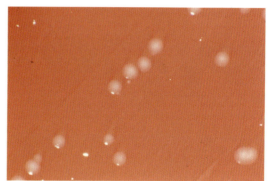

▲ Fig. 192: Differentiation of brucellae by culture on fuchsin (1 : 50,000)-tryptose agar. Lower third: no growth of *Br. suis* (biotype 2), left upper third: *Br. melitensis* and right upper third: *Br. abortus* 6 d, 37 °C. Magnification x 0.25

▼ Fig. 194: *Streptobacillus moniliformis*, culture smear, Gram stain, pleomorphic, Gram-negative rods with spindle-shaped to coccoid swellings. Magnification x 1000

▲ Fig. 193: Differentiaton of brucellae by culture on Thionine (1 : 50,000)-tryptose agar, lower third: no growth of *Br. abortus* (biotype 1), left upper third: growth of *Br. suis* and right upper third: growth of *Br. melitensis*, 6 d, 37 °C. Magnification x 0.25

▼ Fig. 195: *Streptobacillus moniliformis*, pure culture on blood agar, greyish-white, non-haemolytic colonies, anaerobic incubation 3 d, 37 °C. Magnification x 6

▲ Abb. 192: Kulturelle Brucellendifferenzierung auf Fuchsin (1 : 50 000)-Tryptose-Agar, unteres Drittel kein Wachstum von *Br. suis* (Biotyp 2), linkes oberes Drittel Wachstum von *Br. melitensis* und rechtes oberes Drittel von *Br. abortus*, 6 d, 37 °C, Abb.-M. 1 : 4

▼ Abb. 194: *Streptobacillus moniliformis*, Kulturausstrich, Gram-Färbung, polymorphe, gramnegative Stäbchen mit spindelförmigen bis ovoiden Anschwellungen, Abb.-M. 1000 : 1

▲ Abb. 193: Kulturelle Brucellendifferenzierung auf Thionin (1 : 50 000)-Tryptose-Agar, unteres Drittel kein Wachstum von *Br. abortus* (Biotyp 1), linkes oberes Drittel kein Wachstum von *Br. suis* und rechtes oberes Drittel von *Br. melitensis*, 6 d, 37 °C, Abb.-M. 1 : 4

▼ Abb. 195: *Streptobacillus moniliformis*, Reinkultur auf Blutagar, grauweiße, nichthämolysierende Kolonien, anaerobe Bebrütung, 3 d, 37 °C, Abb.-M. 6 : 1

67. WUNDT, W. (1963): Stoffwechseluntersuchungen als experimentelle Grundlage zur Einteilung des Genus Brucella. Zbl. Bakt. I. Orig. **189**, 389–404.
68. WUNDT, W. (1958): Die Typenbestimmung von Brucellen und ihre Bedeutung für die Systematik des Genus Brucella. Z. Hyg. **145**, 235–251.
69. WUNDT, W. (1958): Untersuchungen über die Eignung von Peptonen zur Prüfung der Schwefelwasserstoffbildung von Brucellen. Z. Hyg. **144**, 425–435.
70. WUNDT, W. (1957): Untersuchungen zur Entwicklung leistungsfähiger Brucellennährböden. Zbl. Bakt. I. Orig. **169**, 393–402.

Gram-negative anaerobic rods
Gramnegative, anaerobe Stäbchen

1 Family: Bacteroideaceae

This family groups together rod-shaped, non-spore forming, Gram-negative bacteria, which are obligate anaerobes. 13 genera have been identified to date (30). Among these Gram-negative anaerobic bacteria it is the genera *Bacteroides* and *Fusobacterium* which are of special medical interest.

1.1 Genus: Bacteroides (Ba.)

■ **Incidence and veterinary significance**
Members of the genus *Bacteroides* represent the majority of the resident intestinal flora of man and animals. Furthermore, they also form an important constituent of the oral and skin flora and they inhabit the mucosa of the genital tract. Bacteroides are relatively non-resistant outside the host's body. When they leave their normal habitat, and certain predisposing factors are in play, they can exert a pathogenic action in the body cavities and involve various organ systems. In conjunction with other obligate anaerobes (e.g. Gram-positive cocci, fusobacteria) or facultatively anaerobic species, they produce a purulent necrotizing inflammation and the formation of abscesses (3, 41, 46, 59). In such mixed infections, which are generally of endogenous nature, the synergistic interaction of various pathogenic types plays a potentiating role (4).

These anaerobic infections are most frequently seen in dogs and cats (31, 37) and in cattle (28, 54), but they occur in all other mammalian species as well (46).

All these are non-specific conditions, and most frequently involve members of the *Ba. fragilis* and *Ba. melaninogenicus* group. However, in sheep there is a specific anaerobic infection, known as foot rot which is due to these bacteria. This is a contagious disease of the hoof epidermis the principal

1 Familie: Bacteroideaceae

In dieser Familie werden stäbchenförmige, sporenlose, gramnegative Bakterien, die obligat anaerob wachsen, zusammengefaßt. Man unterscheidet inzwischen 13 verschiedene Gattungen (30). Von diesen gramnegativen Anaerobiern sind insbesondere die Gattungen *Bacteroides* und *Fusobacterium* von medizinischem Interesse

1.1 Gattung: Bacteroides (Ba.)

■ **Vorkommen und medizinische Bedeutung**
Bakterien der Gattung *Bacteroides* repräsentieren den Hauptanteil der residenten Darmflora bei Mensch und Tier, sie sind darüber hinaus wesentlich an der Mundhöhlen- und Hautflora beteiligt und besiedeln auch die Schleimhäute des Urogenitaltraktes. Außerhalb des Wirtsorganismus ist ihre Tenazität relativ gering. Nach Verlassen des natürlichen Standorts können sie unter dem Einfluß prädisponierender Faktoren in verschiedenen Organsystemen und in Körperhöhlen eine pathogene Bedeutung erlangen, indem sie mit anderen obligaten Anaerobiern (z. B. grampositiven Kokken, Fusobakterien) oder fakultativ anaeroben Bakterienarten eitrig-nekrotisierende Entzündungen und Abszeßbildung hervorrufen (3, 41, 46, 59). Bei diesen Mischinfektionen, die meistens endogener Natur sind, spielen synergistische Interaktionen zwischen verschiedenen Erregerarten eine potenzierende Rolle (4).

Besonders häufig wurden diese Anaerobierinfektionen bislang bei Hund und Katze (31, 37) sowie bei Rindern (28, 54) nachgewiesen. Sie kommen aber auch bei allen anderen Säugetierarten vor (46).

Neben diesen als unspezifisch zu bezeichnenden Infektionen, bei denen vornehmlich Vertreter der *Ba. fragilis*- und *Ba. melaninogenicus*-Gruppe beteiligt sind, tritt beim Schaf als spezifische Anaerobier-

agent of which is *Ba. nodosum*, although the synergistic contribution of *Fusobacterium necrophorum* is necessary for the disease to become clinically manifest (11). *Ba. nodosus* also causes a contagious interdigital dermatitis in cattle and healthy individuals harbour the bacterium on the hoofs (33).

■ **Morphology** (figs. 197 and 199)
Gram-negative, pleomorphic rods, 1–10 µm long. Apart from coccoid forms, rods occur with terminal or central enlargements and even vacuoles and filaments are observed. They can be non-motile or

---

```
┌─────────────────────────────────────────┐
│              Specimens                   │
├─────────────────────────────────────────┤
│ Pus, exudate from thoracic or abdominal  │
│ cavities, milk, uterine secretion,       │
│ necrotic tissue etc. Should be worked up │
│ immediately or, if it is to be sent off, │
│ it must be placed into anaerobic         │
│ transport media (e.g. Port-A-Cul medium) │
│ or in special anaerobic shipment         │
│ containers (e.g. Vacutainer anaerobic    │
│ transport)                               │
└─────────────────────────────────────────┘
```

Aerobic culture	Demonstration of Ba. fragilis by means of fluorescence microscopy, gas chromatography can be used for pus and punctates
To show contaminants present	

Microscopic demonstration of pathogens
Gram stain: Gram-negative pleomorphic rods, some with terminal or central enlargements, vacuoles and filaments

Demonstration of organisms by culture

1. Direct culture on pre-reduced solid media with or without additives with selective action (e.g. Schaedler agar)
2. Enrichment in pre-reduced liquid media with and without additives with selective activity (e.g. Schaedler broth). After 48–72 h anaerobic incubation subculture onto solid media
3. Incubation on solid media for 2 to 5 days at 37 °C in special anaerobic systems
4. The colonies of bacteroides are not very characteristic, greyish-white with smooth edges. Members of the Ba. melaninogenicus group can produce black pigment

Identification of bacteroides species in pure culture

1. Provisional identification of genus by its sensitivity (S) or resistance (R) to:
   Kanamycin (1000 µg): R;
   Fosfomycin (10 µg): R;
   Metronidazole (2 µg): S.
2. Provisional group classification
   Ba. fragilis group: grows on bile-aesculin agar, resistant to colistin (10 µg) and vancomycin (5 µg)
   Ba. melaninogenicus group: forms black pigment and colonies fluoresce under ultraviolet light
3. Identification of the species with biochemical methods, conventional biochemical test or the use of miniaturized identification systems (e.g. Minitek, API 20A, table 82)
   For precise species identification the biochemical results should be supplemented with gas chromatographic detection of the fermentation products, see table 82

Fig. 196: Demonstration and identification of *Bacteroides*

motile (peritrichous flagella), and capsule-forming species are encountered (30).

Ba. nodosus is non-motile and 3–6 µm in length. These straight or slightly curved rods often show terminal enlargements, which become less evident in culture specimens (30). The cell surface is covered with numerous fimbriae (45, 55).

■ Culture (figs. 198 and 200)

The specimens for examination must either be dealt with immediately or placed into a semi-solid transport medium for shipment (e.g. swabs into Port-A-Cul medium, Becton and Dickinson) or some other anaerobic transport container (e.g. for tissues Vacutainer-Anaerobic-Transport, Becton and Dickinson). Evacuated tubes, closed with rubber stoppers, may be used for fluid samples (21).

The primary culture is taken on media containing blood and incubation is strictly anaerobic at 37 °C. The cultures should be incubated for at least 2 to 5 days. The appearance of the colonies is not very characteristic for the individual species. Since the generation time of these organisms is 45 to 60 minutes, the colonies only appear after 48 hours incubation. They are greyish-white, round, convex and their size varies between 0.5 and 2 mm. Haemolysis may occasionally be encountered in some strains of various species. After 1 to 2 weeks of incubation the members of the *Ba. melaninogenicus* group produce a black pigment and they fluoresce under UV light (9).

Ba. nodosus differs in that it will grow on solid media without added blood and produce transparent convex colonies, 4–5 mm in diameter in 3 to 7 days. Various colony types occur (11, 50, 55). Eugon agar containing 0.2 % of yeast extract, 10 % of horse blood and 1 µg/ml lincomycin (42), Thorley medium (53) or hoof agar (12) (containing pulverized hoof horn) have been recommended for the primary culture of *Ba. nodosus*.

For the cultural demonstration of all other *Bacteroides* species there are solid media bases such as brucella agar, Columbia agar or BHI agar. They are supplemented with the following: 5 % blood (from horse, sheep or ox), 0.5 % yeast extract, vitamin K1 (Menadion 10 µg/ml), haemin (5 µg/ml) and cysteine hydrochloride (0.5 g/l). Schaedler agar, Wilkins-Chalgren anaerobic agar are complete solid media that are also suitable.

Such solid media may also be selective when kanamycin (0.1 g/l) and vancomycin (7.5 mg/l) have been added. Once made up, the media should be used within 14 days and before inoculation they should be pre-reduced for 6–24 hours in an anaerobic atmosphere (30, 42).

Schaedler and Wilkins-Chalgren anaerobic broths or BHI and thioglycollate broth can be used for the multiplication of *Bacteroides*. It would also be beneficial to add haemin (5 mg/l) and vitamin K

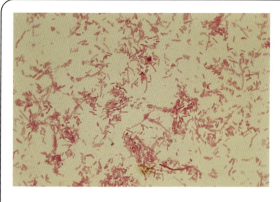
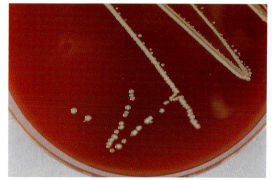
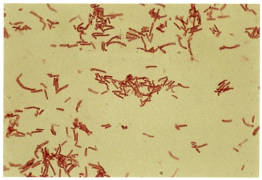
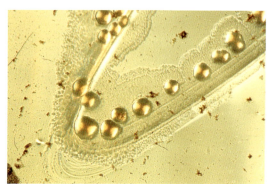

▲ Fig. 197: *Bacteroides fragilis,* culture smear, Gram stain. Magnification x 1000
▼ Fig. 199: *Bacteroides nodosus,* culture smear, Gram stain. Magnification x 1000

▲ Fig. 198: *Bacteroides fragilis,* pure culture on Schaedler agar, greyish-white, shiny colonies, anaerobic incubation 3 d, 37 °C. Magnification x 0.4
▼ Fig. 200: *Bacteroides nodosus,* pure culture on Bacteroides nodosus agar, anaerobic incubation, 3 d, 37 °C. Magnification x 2

▲ Abb. 197: *Bacteroides fragilis,* Kulturausstrich, Gram-Färbung, Abb.-M. 1000 : 1
▼ Abb. 199: *Bacteroides nodosus,* Kulturausstrich, Gram-Färbung, Abb.-M. 1000 : 1

▲ Abb. 198: *Bacteroides fragilis,* Reinkultur auf Schaedler-Agar, grauweiße, glänzende Kolonien, anaerobe Bebrütung, 3 d, 37 °C, Abb.-M. 1 : 2,5
▼ Abb. 200: *Bacteroides nodosus,* Reinkultur auf Bacteroides nodosus-Agar, anaerobe Bebrütung 3 d, 37 °C, Abb.-M. 2 : 1

(1 mg/l). The best reproductive rate is obtained with BHI broth containing 5.0 g/l yeast extract, besides the other additives (13). Improved growth can be obtained by the addition of 5–10 % serum, 0.02 % Tween 80 or 10–30 % of rumen fluid (30).

In order to obtain the necessary environment for the primary culture of these strict anaerobes one need not purchase the relatively expensive anaerobic chamber (glove box technique; 1, 8) because reliable systems are available for the less specialized labora-

anaeroben Milieu vorreduziert werden (30, 42).

Zur Vermehrung von *Bacteroides* in Bouillonkulturen können Schaedler- und Wilkins-Chalgren-Anaerobierbouillon sowie BHI- und Thioglykolatbouillon verwendet werden, günstig wirken sich auch hier Hämin- (5 mg/l) und Vitamin-K-Zusatz (1 mg/l) aus. Die besten Vermehrungsraten wurden in BHI-Bouillon mit 5,0 g/l Hefeextrakt und den anderen Zusätzen erreicht (13). Wachstumsverbesserungen sind auch durch Zugabe von Serum

tory (such as Gaspak system, Becton and Dickinson; anaerobic system, Oxoid). The gas generators liberate hydrogen in the anaerobic flask and with the aid of a palladium catalyst it combines with oxygen to form water. CO_2 is produced at the same time and this is essential for the growth of some species.

A redox indicator checks the anaerobic conditions. In the absence of oxygen it turns from blue (e.g. methylene blue, resazurin) to white. Then the redox potential lies in the range between -100 and -150 mV. The catalysts of this system can be re-used; they are regenerated by heating to 160–170 °C for 2 hours.

The Anaerocult system (Merck) uses no catalyst to produce an oxygen-free CO_2 environment.

■ Biochemical properties

Rapid methods are available for making a provisional identification of the group to which the organisms belongs (fig. 196). Thus, it is possible to separate the *Ba. fragilis* group from the others with the bile aesculin agar, containing 5% sheep blood (35). The identification of fluorescence under UV light and the production of black pigment (haematin) are typical for *Ba. melaninogenicus*. The difference in resistance to antibiotics is also used in making a provisional diagnosis (17). In contrast to the genus *Fusobacterium* all species of *Bacteroides*, with exception of *Ba. ureolyticus*, are resistant to kanamycin. Similarly, the *Ba. fragilis* group is not sensitive to colistin and vancomycin (52).

The further differentiation of the 40 known species is possible with biochemical methods in combination with gas chromatography (tab. 82). The investigative methods are based largely on the comprehensive treatment in "Anaerobe Laboratory Manual" by HOLDEMAN et al. (29). Peptone yeast (PY) and chopped meat medium (CM) are recommended as a basic medium and they are obtainable as PRAS media (pre-reduced anaerobically sterilized).

It is relatively difficult, for routine diagnosis, to make up fluid media and to assess the results. PRESCOTT & CHIRINO-TREJO (42) therefore recommend, that in such instances the medium of DOWELL & HAWKINS (7) is better because, if CHO medium (Difco) is used, it is easier to make up. This medium contains peptone, yeast extract, L-cystine, Na thioglycollate, NaCl, ascorbic acid, brom thymol blue and 0.6% of the carbohydrate to be tested. The tests are read after 1, 2 and 7 days of anaerobic incubation at 37 °C.

The commercially available Minitek system (anaerobic II set, Becton & Dickinson) has been found satisfactory for the biochemical differentiation, and it gave a 97–100% correlation with the conventional methods. Satisfactory results can also be obtained with other miniature systems (e.g. API 20A, bio Merieux) (18, 24, 25).

(5–10%), Tween 80 (0,02%) oder Pansensaft (10–30%) zu erzielen (30).

Zur Erzeugung des anaeroben Milieus für die Anzüchtung strikter Anaerobier stehen neben den relativ teuren Anaerobierkammern (Glove-Box-Technik; 1, 8), für weniger spezialisierte Laboratorien zuverlässige Anaerobiersysteme zur Verfügung (z. B. Gaspak-System, Becton u. Dickinson; Anaerobiersystem, Oxoid). Mit Hilfe von Gasentwicklern wird in den Anaerobiertöpfen Wasserstoff freigesetzt, der im Zusammenwirken mit einem Palladiumkatalysator Sauerstoff unter Bildung von Wasser bindet. Zum anderen entsteht gleichzeitig Kohlendioxyd, das für das Wachstum einiger Arten unbedingt erforderlich ist.

Durch einen Redoxindikator wird das Vorliegen der Anaerobiose kontrolliert. Bei Abwesenheit von Sauerstoff erfolgt ein Umschlag von Blau (z. B. Methylenblau, Resazurin) nach Weiß. Das Redoxpotential liegt dann im Bereich von -100 bis -150 mV. Die Katalysatoren dieses Systems sind wieder verwendbar und können durch 2stündiges Erhitzen auf 160 bis 170 °C regeneriert werden.

Das Anaerocult-System (Merck) arbeitet ohne Katalysator und erzeugt ein sauerstofffreies CO_2-Milieu.

■ Kulturell-biochemische Eigenschaften

Zur vorläufigen Diagnose wird die Möglichkeit der Gruppenzuordnung mit Schnellmethoden genutzt (Abb. 196). So kann durch Verwendung von Galle-Äskulin-Agar mit 5% Schafblut die *Ba. fragilis*-Gruppe von anderen Gruppen abgegrenzt werden (35). Der Nachweis von Fluoreszenz unter UV-Licht und die Bildung von schwarzem Pigment (Hämatin) ist für Kolonien der *Ba. melaninogenicus*-Gruppe charakteristisch. Auch wird das unterschiedliche Resistenzverhalten gegenüber Antibiotika zur vorläufigen Differenzierung herangezogen (17). So sind die *Bacteroides*-Arten mit Ausnahme von *Ba. ureolyticus* im Gegensatz zur Gattung *Fusobacterium* kanamycinresistent. Ebenso ist die *Ba. fragilis*-Gruppe unempfindlich gegenüber Colistin und Vancomycin (52).

Die weitere Differenzierung der 40 bisher bekannten Arten ist mit biochemischen Methoden in Verbindung mit der Gaschromatographie möglich (Tab. 82). Diese Untersuchungsverfahren basieren vornehmlich auf den umfassenden Angaben im »Anaerobe Laboratory Manual« von HOLDEMAN et al. (29). Als Basisnährböden werden danach Pepton-Yeast-(PY) und Chopped-Meat-Medium (CM) als sog. PRAS-Medien (prereduced anaerobically sterilized) empfohlen.

Für die Routinediagnostik ist die Herstellung der präreduzierten flüssigen Medien und auch die Beurteilung des Reaktionsausfalles relativ schwierig, deshalb empfehlen PRESCOTT & CHIRINO-TREJO (42) in diesen Fällen den Einsatz eines Mediums nach DOWELL & HAWKINS (7), das durch Verwen-

According to Holdeman et al. (29) morphological and biochemical methods provide an adequate and reliable differentiation between Gram-negative anaerobic bacteria that were isolated from clinical cases, but they are not sufficient for studies on normal flora.

If an exact species identification is required then the biochemical methods should be supplemented by gas chromatographic investigations to demonstrate volatile and non-volatile end products of carbohydrate metabolism (29, 58, 59).

As example, the Capco Anaerobic Identification System (Gas chromatograph Capco Instruments) has been found satisfactory for this purpose. A detailed description of the gas chromatography procedures for anaerobes is contained in the »Anaerobe Laboratory Manual« by Holdeman et al. (29). The starting materials are cultures on PY or CM media with or without the addition of glucose. Volatile fatty acids (e.g. formic, acetic, propionic, butyric, valeric and capronic acids) are collected by ether extraction and the non-volatile ones (e.g. lactic, pyruvic, succinic) by chloroform extraction after methylation. The results are recorded on the chromatogram. In the interpretation attention is paid not only to the presence or absence of certain metabolites, but also their approximate amounts (tab. 82).

It is now possible to perform a gas chromatographic analysis directly from the pus or a punctate sample, for a rapid provisional diagnosis (10, 40).

dung von CHO-Medium (Difco) einfacher herzustellen ist. Der Nährboden enthält Pepton, Hefeextrakt, L-Cystin, Na-Thioglykolat, NaCl, Askorbinsäure, Bromthymolblau und 0,6 % der zu prüfenden Kohlenhydrate. Die Ergebnisse werden nach 1-, 2- und 7tägiger Bebrütung bei 37 °C im Anaerobiersystem beurteilt.

Für die biochemische Differenzierung hat sich das kommerziell erhältliche Minitek-System (Anaerobier II Set; Becton & Dickinson) bewährt, das eine 97- bis 100%ige Korrelation mit konventionellen Verfahren erbrachte. Ebenso lieferten andere miniaturisierte Systeme (z. B. API 20 A; bio Merieux) brauchbare Resultate (18, 24, 25).

Nach Holdeman et al. (29) erbringen morphologische und biochemische Untersuchungen ausreichende Sicherheit zur Differenzierung gramnegativer Anaerobier aus klinischen Isolaten, nicht jedoch für Studien über die Normalflora.

Wird eine exakte Artdiagnose gewünscht, so sollte die biochemische Differenzierung durch die gaschromatographische Untersuchung zum Nachweis von Stoffwechselendprodukten aus dem Kohlenhydratmetabolismus in Form von flüchtigen und nicht flüchtigen Fermentationsprodukten ergänzt werden (29, 58, 59).

Bewährt hat sich für diese Zwecke z. B. das Capco Anaerobier Identifikationssystem (Gaschromatograph, Capco Instruments). Eine detaillierte Darstellung der Durchführung der Gaschromatogra-

Table 82: Biochemical and gas chromatographic identification of some species of *Bacteroides*

Tabelle 82: Biochemische und gaschromatographische Bestimmung einiger *Bacteroides*-Arten

Group[1]	Bacteroides species	Growth in 20 % bile	Black pigment	Aes	Cat	Ure
Bacteroides fragilis group	fragilis	+	−	+	+	−
	distasonis	+	−	+	v⁻	−
	ovatus	+	−	+	−	−
	uniformis	+	−	+	−	−
	vulgatus	+	−	+	v⁻	−
Bacteroides melaninogenicus group	melaninogenicus	−	+	−	−	−
	intermedius	−	+	−	−	−
	asaccharolyticus	−	+	−	−	−
Bacteroides oralis group	bivius	−	−	−	−	−
	oralis	−	−	+	−	−
	ruminicola	v⁻	−	v⁺	−	−
other species	ureolyticus	−	−	−	−	+
	capillosus	−	−	+	−	−
	nodosus	−	−	−	−	−

[1] group classification after Hamman (23)
A acetate, P propionate, B butyrate, L lactate, F formate, S succinate, iB isobutyrate, iV isovalerate
PYG = peptone yeast glucose medium
Capital letters indicate main product; small letter side products; letters in brackets = variable production

[1] Gruppeneinteilung nach Hamman (23)
A Acetat, P Propionat, B Butyrat, L Lactat, F Formiat, S Succinat, iB Isobutyrat, iV Isovalerianat
PYG = Pepton-Yeast-Glucose-Medium
große Buchstaben: Hauptprodukte; kleine Buchstaben: Nebenprodukte; in Klammern: variable Produktion

phie für Anaerobier wird von HOLDEMAN et al. (29) im »Anaerobe Laboratory Manual« gegeben. Als Ausgangsmaterial werden Kulturen in PY- oder CM-Medien ohne und mit Glucosezusatz verwendet. Flüchtige Fettsäuren (z. B. Ameisen-, Essig-, Propion-, Butter-, Valerian- und Capronsäure) werden über Ätherextrakt, nicht flüchtige erst nach Methylierung (z. B. Lactat, Pyruvat, Succinat) über Chloroformextraktion erfaßt. Das Ergebnis wird im Chromatogramm aufgezeichnet. Zur Interpretation sind An- und Abwesenheit sowie die ungefähren Mengen der gebildeten Stoffwechselprodukte vergleichend zu berücksichtigen (Tab. 82).

Eine gaschromatographische Analyse kann zur Beschleunigung der vorläufigen Diagnose auch schon direkt von Eiter oder Punktaten durchgeführt werden (10, 40).

■ Enzymes and toxins

The endotoxins and neuraminidase are probably the most important virulence factors. Thus, *B. fragilis* the most common pathogen of this group has the greatest neuraminidase activity when compared with the other intestinal species.

Other enzymes have also been demonstrated in various strains, especially those of the *Ba. fragilis* group. These are: hyaluronidase, lecithinase, collagenase, gelatinase, fibrinolysin, heparinase, chondroitin sulphatase (for literature see HENTGES & SMITH, 26).

■ Enzyme und Toxine

Als wichtigste Virulenzfaktoren sind vermutlich das Endotoxin und die Neuraminidase anzusprechen. So zeigte *Ba. fragilis* als häufigster pathogener Vertreter im Gegensatz zu anderen intestinalen Arten die höchste Neuraminidaseaktivität (59).

Bei Stämmen verschiedener Arten, vor allem aus der *Ba. fragilis*-Gruppe, wurden aber auch noch andere Enzyme nachgewiesen: Hyaluronidase, Lezithinase, Kollagenase, Gelatinase, Fibrinolysin, Heparinase und Chondroitinsulfatase (Lit. bei HENTGES & SMITH, 26).

Table 82: Continued   Tabelle 82: Fortsetzung

Ind	Ara	Glu	Lac	Mal	Rha	Sal	Sac	Tre	Xyl	Amy	Gas chromatographic fermentation product from PYG medium
−	−	+	+	+	−	−	+	−	+	+	A, S, p (ib, iv, l, f)
−	−	+	+	+	+	+	+	+	+	+	A, S (ib, iv, p, l)
+	+	+	+	+	+	+	+	+	+	+	A, S, p (ib, iv, f, l)
+	+	+	+	+	−	+	+	−	+	+	A, S, p (ib, iv, f, l)
−	+	+	+	+	+	−	+	−	−	+	A, S, p (ib, iv)
−	−	+	+	+	−	−	+	−	−	+	A, S, p (ib, iv, l, f)
+	−	+	−	+	−	−	+	−	−	+	A, S, ib, iv (l, k)
+	−	−	−	−	−	−	−	−	−	−	A, p, B, ib, iv (l, s)
−	−	+	+	+	−	−	−	−	−	+	A, S, iv (ib, f)
−	−	+	+	+	v	+	+	−	−	+	A, S (F, ib, iv, l)
v+	v+	+	+	+	−	v+	+	−	−	+	A, S, f, p (ib, iv, l)
−	−	−	−	−	−	−	−	−	−	−	a, s (f, p, l)
−	−	+	+	−	−	−	−	−	−	−	a, s (l, f, p)
−	−	−	−	−	−	−	−	−	−	−	a, s, p (ib, iv, b)

Antigenic structure

Besides the O-antigens of the cell wall, polysaccharide antigens have been demonstrated in the capsular material or in the outer layer of the cell wall (59). Although the species-specific cell wall antigen permit the demonstration of *Ba. fragilis* by immunofluorescence (57), further detailed serotyping is not practicable in routine diagnosis, because of the serological complexity. A total of 21 serotypes and several subtypes have been differentiated in the species *Ba. fragilis* (34).

On the other hand, serotyping of *Ba. nodosus* is of practical significance because of the use of specific immune prophylactic procedures. The various fimbrial antigens (K-antigens) which are identical with the immunogens, are utilized in the K-agglutination tests for the separation of 8 different serogroups (A–H) (6, 44, 51). During the examination in Great Britain of sheep suffering from foot rot, all serotypes were identified and groups B and H were found to be the most common (27).

Animal inoculation

It was possible to show in mice, rats and guinea pigs that, following experimental infection of wounds or the abdominal cavity, various *Bacteroides* spp. were able to produce abscesses and sepsis only in syner-

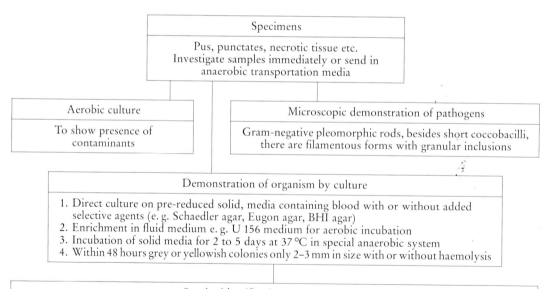

Fig. 201: Demonstration and identification of *Fusobacterium necrophorum*

Family: Bacteroideaceae

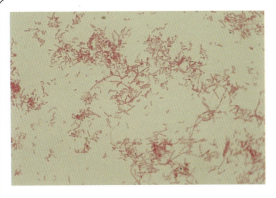
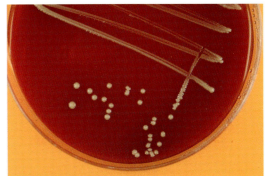

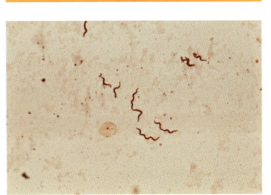

▲ Fig. 202: *Fusobacterium necrophorum*, culture smear, Gram stain. Magnification x 1000
▼ Fig. 204: *Leptospira interrogans* serovar *icterohaemorrhagiae*. Culture smear, silver impregnation, Magnification x 1000

▲ Abb. 202: *Fusobacterium necrophorum*, Kulturausstrich, Gram-Färbung, Abb.-M. 1000 : 1
▼ Abb. 204: *Leptospira interrogans* serovar *icterohaemorrhagiae*. Kulturausstrich, Silberimprägnierung, Abb.-M. 1000 : 1

▲ Fig. 203: *Fusobacterium necrophorum*, pure culture on Schaedler agar, greyish-white, shiny colonies, anaerobic incubation, 3 d, 37 °C. Magnification x 0.4
▼ Fig. 205: *Treponema hyodysenteriae*, culture smear, silver impregnation. Magnification x 1000

▲ Abb. 203: *Fusobacterium necrophorum*, Reinkultur auf Schaedler-Agar, grauweiße, glänzende Kolonien, anaerobe Bebrütung 3 d, 37 °C, Abb.-M. 1 : 2,5
▼ Abb. 205: *Treponema hyodysenteriae*, Kulturausstrich, Silberimprägnierung, Abb.-M. 1000 : 1

gistic interaction with other anaerobic bacteria (4, 32, 60).

1.2 Genus: Fusobacterium (F.)

Fusobacteria are inhabitants of the mouth and intestinal tract of animals and man. However, they are found there less commonly and in smaller numbers

Zusammenwirken mit anderen aeroben oder anaeroben Bakterien Abszeßbildung oder Sepsis hervorrufen (4, 32, 60).

1.2 Gattung: Fusobacterium (F.)

Fusobakterien besiedeln Mundhöhle und Darmkanal von Tier und Mensch. Im Vergleich zu den *Bacteroides*-Arten sind sie dort allerdings seltener

than the *Bacteroides* species. Ten different species comprise the genus (39), and of these *F. necrophorum* is the most common in clinical specimens from animals.

1.2.1 Fusobacterium necrophorum
(Syn.: *Sphaerophorus necrophorus*)

■ **Incidence and veterinary significance**

In many species of animals *F. necrophorum* causes abscesses and necrotizing purulent inflammation after exogenous or endogenous infection and usually in association of other bacterial species (e.g. *Corynebacterium pyogenes*). Not only the internal organs but also the mucous membranes and, after traumatic injury, the skin can be affected. These infections are particularly common in ruminants, which harbour the organism in the rumen. In adult cattle *F. necrophorum* causes interdigital dermatitis and multiple abscesses in the liver, while a necrotizing diphtheritic stomatitis is encountered in calves. *F. necrophorum* is regularly involved in foot rot of sheep together with *Ba. nodosus*. Human infections can occur and the organism is transmitted by animal bites or wound infections from contaminated material. *F. necrophorum* may be found in the vicinity of animals where it can survive in a moist environment for several months (2, 42, 49).

■ **Morphology** (fig. 202)

Gram-negative, non-motile, non-capsulated, pleomorphic bacteria whose form may vary from short coccoid rods (1–3 μm in length) to filaments up to 100 μm long. Their ends may be rounded or pointed. Granular inclusions are often present in the cytoplasm. In culture preparation the morphology depends largely on the age of the culture and the composition of the medium (39).

■ **Culture** (fig. 203)

On solid media which contain blood, *F. necrophorum* grows under strict anaerobic conditions (see genus *Bacteroides*) to produce colonies of 2–3 mm diameter in 48 hours at 37 °C. After prolonged incubation a pattern develops on the surface of the colony which may form lateral processes. Biotypes A, B and AB are differentiated on the basis of colony morphology, haemolysis and the growth in fluid media (20). Type A colonies are flat and grey with an irregular border of distinct haemolysis. In fluid media they form filaments. Type B colonies, on the other hand, are convex with smooth edges, yellowish with a less distinct zone of

1.2.1 Fusobacterium necrophorum
(Syn.: *Sphaerophorus necrophorus*)

■ **Vorkommen und medizinische Bedeutung**

F. necrophorum verursacht nach exogener oder endogener Infektion bei zahlreichen Tierarten, vielfach in Zusammenwirken mit anderen Bakterienarten (insbes. *Corynebacterium pyogenes*), Abszeßbildung und eitrig-nekrotisierende Entzündungen. Neben den inneren Organen können hiervon auch die Schleimhäute bzw. die äußere Haut nach traumatischer Schädigung betroffen sein. Besonders häufig treten diese Infektionen bei Wiederkäuern auf, die den Erreger im Pansen beherbergen. Bei erwachsenen Rindern werden multiple Abszeßbildung in der Leber und interdigitale Dermatitis durch *F. necrophorum* hervorgerufen, bei Kälbern nekrotisierende Stomatitis (Diphtheroid). Außerdem ist der Erreger regelmäßig zusammen mit *Ba. nodosus* an der Entstehung der Moderhinke der Schafe beteiligt. Infektionen beim Menschen kommen vor. Übertragung des Erregers ist durch Tierbisse bzw. durch Wundinfektionen beim Umgang mit infiziertem Material möglich. *F. necrophorum* ist in der Umgebung von Tieren anzutreffen und kann im feuchten Milieu mehrere Monate überleben (2, 42, 49).

■ **Morphologie** (Abb. 202)

Gramnegative, unbewegliche, kapsellose und pleomorphe Bakterien, deren Gestalt von kokkoiden Kurzstäbchen (1–3 μm) bis zu 100 μm langen filamentösen Formen mit runden oder zugespitzten Enden reichen kann. Vielfach sind im Zytoplasma granuläre Einschlüsse zu finden. In Kulturpräparaten ist die Morphologie in hohem Maße abhängig vom Alter der Kulturen und von der Zusammensetzung der Nährmedien (39).

■ **Kultur** (Abb. 203)

F. necrophorum wächst unter strikt anaeroben Bedingungen (s. Gattung *Bacteroides*) auf bluthaltigen festen Nährböden innerhalb von 48 h bei 37 °C in ca. 2–3 mm großen Kolonien, die nach längerer Bebrütung Strukturierung an der Oberfläche und Ausläufer aufweisen können. Aufgrund der unterschiedlichen Kolonienmorphologie, der Hämolyse und dem Wachstum in flüssigen Medien werden die Biotypen A, B und AB unterschieden (20). Typ A-Kolonien sind flach und grau mit unregelmäßiger Randzone und zeigen deutliche Hämolyse; in flüssigem Medium überwiegen filamentöse Formen. Typ B-Kolonien dagegen sind konvex und glattran-

Family: Bacteroideaceae

Table 83: Biochemical and gas chromatographic identification of *Fusobacterium spp.*

Tabelle 83: Biochemische und gaschromatographische Bestimmung von Fusobakterienarten

Fusobacterium spp.	Growth in 20% bile	Lipase	Ind	Aes	Cat	Glu	Lac	Mns
F. necrophorum	–	v⁺	+	–	–	–	–	–
F. nucleatum	–	–	+	–	–	–	–	–
F. varium	+	–	(+)	–	–	+	–	+
F. russii	(–)	–	–	–	–	–	–	–
F. mortiferum	+	–	–	+	–	+	+	+

	Gas chromatography Propionate from		Fermentation products
	Lactate[1]	Threonine[1]	from PYG medium
F. necrophorum	+	+	B, a, p (L, f, s)
F. nucleatum	–	+	B, a, p, s (L, f)
F. varium	–	+	B, A, L (S, p)
F. russii	–	–	B, a (L, f, s)
F. mortiferum	–	–	B, A, p (L, F, iv, s)

[1] Using PY medium with added lactate or threonine (39). For further details see table 82.

[1] Verwendung von PY-Medien unter Zusatz von Lactat bzw. Threonin (39). Weitere Erläuterungen s. Tab. 82

haemolysis. They form a sediment in fluid media, in which short rods predominate. Biotype AB takes up an intermediate position. Eugon agar (5% sheep or ox blood) or Eugon broth with 0.2% yeast extract, are used for the demonstration of these biotypes (15).

One can also employ the media listed for *Bacteroides*. SIMON (47) developed the special medium 156 (Brewer's thioglycollate broth, yeast extract, L-cystine, ascorbic acid), which is suitable for aerobic incubation. The organism will live in this medium for several weeks.

For a selective medium HALLMANN & BURKHARDT (22) recommend the addition of brilliant green (1:3000) and sodium azide (0.3%) and BURGER & HUSSAIN (5) suggests crystal violet (0.005 g/l) and erythromycin (0.04 g/l).

■ **Biochemical properties**

The differentiation of the various types of fusobacteria can be carried out with biochemical tests and gas chromatography (tab. 83). The methods to be used are described in more detail under section 1.1.

The demonstration of lipase production on egg yolk agar is used to identify *F. necrophorum*; especially the haemolytic strains are found to be lipase-positive. Furthermore, an exact species definition can be achieved with the gas chromatographic evidence of propionate production from lactate. A comparative test on ether extracts of cultures on PY medium with and without added lactate will provide the evidence of propionate formation (39).

dig, gelblich gefärbt und besitzen weniger deutlich ausgeprägte Hämolysezonen. Im flüssigen Medium bilden sie einen Bodensatz, in dem Kurzstäbchen überwiegen. Der Biotyp AB nimmt eine Zwischenstellung ein. Zum Nachweis dieser Biotypen wurde Eugon-Agar (5% Schaf- oder Rinderblut) und Eugonbroth mit 0,2% Hefeextrakt verwendet (15).

Ansonsten können auch die für *Bacteroides* aufgeführten Nährböden eingesetzt werden. Von SIMON (47) wurde speziell das Medium 156 (Brewer's Thioglykolbouillon, Hefeextrakt, L-Cystin, Askorbinsäure) entwickelt, das für eine aerobe Inkubation geeignet ist. Der Erreger bleibt in diesem Medium über mehrere Wochen lebensfähig.

Als Zusätze für ein Selektivmedium sind Brillantgrün (1:3000) und Na-acid (0,3%) nach HALLMANN & BURKHARDT (22) oder Kristallviolett (0,005 g/l) und Erythromycin (0,04 g/l) nach BURGER & HUSSAIN (5) geeignet.

■ **Kulturell-biochemische Eigenschaften**

Die Differenzierung der verschiedenen Fusobakterienarten kann mit biochemischen Untersuchungsverfahren und der Gaschromatographie vorgenommen werden (Tab. 83). Die hierbei anzuwendenden Methoden wurden unter 1.1 näher beschrieben.

Zur Abgrenzung von *F. necrophorum* wird der Lipasenachweis auf Eigelbagar empfohlen, wobei sich insbesondere die hämolysierenden Stämme als lipasepositiv erweisen. Außerdem kann gaschromatographisch die Bildung von Propionat aus Lactat zur exakten Bestimmung dieser Art herangezogen werden. Die vergleichende Untersuchung der Ätherextrakte je einer PY-Medium-Kultur mit und ohne Lactatzusatz gestattet eine Aussage über die stattgefundene Propionatbildung (39).

■ Enzymes and toxins

The primary virulence factors are the endotoxin (56) and the exotoxin known as leucocidin (14, 16). But lipase, haemolysin, desoxyribonuclease and haemagglutinin are also of importance. The latter will agglutinate erythrocytes of various species (e.g. sheep, cattle, horse, rabbit, poultry). The haemagglutination inhibition test (HI test) was used by SIMON (48) to obtain a rapid identification of *F. necrophorum*. The virulence difference between biotypes A, B and AB is expressed in the difference in the production of leucocidin and haemolysin (16, 43). Strains of type A, which were isolated from liver abscesses in cattle, were found to be the most virulent.

■ Antigenic structure

Serological investigations based on the various O-antigens and using agglutination, precipitation and complement fixation tests produced evidence of 4 different serogroups (49). This serotyping has not found its way into routine diagnosis, although FALES et al. (19) had described direct immunofluorescence with polyvalent conjugates as a possible rapid identification of *F. necrophorum*.

■ Animal inoculation

Experimental infections with *F. necrophorum* are successful in many animals, but dogs, cats, guinea pigs and poultry appear to be less susceptible than rabbits.

Subcutaneous and intramuscular injections in rabbits will produce local abscesses; intravenous and intraperitoneal administration brings about a generalized spread with miliary necrotic lesions and abscesses (49).

1.2.2 Other types of Fusobacterium

Other types of Fusobacterium, besides *F. necrophorum*, are encountered during the examination of clinical material from various animal species. *F. nucleatum* was frequently isolated from abscess pus and purulent wound secretions of dogs and cats (31, 37) and in such material from cats *F. russii* (38) is also common.

F. nucleatum is morphologically very characteristic. The Gram-negative rods measure between 3 μm and 10 μm in length, their ends are pointed and there is a centrally situated granule. No conclusions as to the species can be drawn from the appearance of the colonies; this requires a biochemical investigation (fig. 201).

■ Enzyme und Toxine

Als Virulenzfaktoren stehen das Endotoxin (56) und das als Leukozidin gekennzeichnete Exotoxin (14, 16) im Vordergrund. Daneben spielen Lipase, Hämolysin, Desoxyribonuklease und Hämagglutinin eine Rolle. Das Hämagglutinin agglutiniert die Erythrozyten verschiedener Tierarten (z. B. Schaf, Rind, Pferd, Kaninchen, Geflügel). Mit Hilfe eines Hämagglutinationshemmungstestes erreichte SIMON (48) eine schnelle Identifizierung von *F. necrophorum*. Die zwischen den Biotypen A, B und AB bestehenden Virulenzunterschiede finden ihren Ausdruck in der unterschiedlichen Produktion von Leukozidin und Hämolysin (16, 43). Virulente Eigenschaften sind bei den Typ A-Stämmen, die überwiegend aus Leberabszessen von Rindern isoliert werden, am ausgeprägtesten.

■ Antigenstruktur

Serologische Untersuchungen (Agglutination, Präzipitation, KBR) erbrachten aufgrund der unterschiedlichen O-Antigene Hinweise auf die Existenz von 4 verschiedenen Serogruppen (49). Für die Diagnostik fand die Serotypisierung bislang keine Verwendung. Von FALES et al. (19) wurde allerdings die direkte Immunfluoreszenz mit polyvalenten Konjugaten als eine Möglichkeit zur schnellen Erfassung von *F. necrophorum* beschrieben.

■ Tierversuch

Experimentelle Infektionen gelingen mit *F. necrophorum* bei zahlreichen Tierarten. Im Vergleich zum Kaninchen scheinen Hunde, Katzen, Meerschweinchen und das Geflügel aber weniger empfänglich zu sein.

Beim Kaninchen kommt es nach subkutaner und intramuskulärer Infektion zu lokaler Abszeßbildung, nach intravenöser und intraperitonealer Verabreichung zur generalisierten Ausbreitung von miliaren Nekroseherden und Abszessen (49).

1.2.2 Weitere Fusobacterium-Arten

Neben *F. necrophorum* kommen in klinischem Untersuchungsmaterial verschiedener Tierarten auch noch andere Fusobakterienspezies vor. So wurde in Abzeßinhalt und eitrigen Wundsekreten von Hund und Katze häufig *F. nucleatum* (31, 37) bzw. bei der Katze auch *F. russii* (38) nachgewiesen.

F. nucleatum zeigt im mikroskopischen Präparat eine recht charakteristische Morphologie. Die 3 bis 10 μm langen gramnegativen Stäbchen besitzen zugespitzte Enden und zentral gelegene Granula. Die Koloniemorphologie läßt bei den Fusobakterienarten keine Rückschlüsse auf die Artzugehörigkeit zu, deshalb muß hierfür die kulturell-biochemische Untersuchung (Abb. 201) herangezogen werden.

Bibliography / Literatur

1. Aranki, A., & R. Freter (1972): Use of anaerobic glove boxes for the cultivation of strictly anaerobic bacteria. Am. J. Clin. Nutr. 25, 1329–1334.
2. Berg, J. N., & C. M. Scanlan (1982): Studies of Fusobacterium necrophorum from bovine hepatic abscesses: Biotypes, quantitation, virulence and antibiotic susceptibility. Am. J. Vet. Rec. 43, 1580–1586.
3. Berkhoff, G. A. (1978): Recovery and identification of anaerobes in veterinary medicine: A 2 year experience. Vet. Microbiol. 2, 237–252.
4. Brook, I., V. Hunter & R. I. Walker (1984): Synergistic effect of Bacteroides, Clostridium, Fusobacterium, anaerobic cocci, and aerobic bacteria on mortality and induction of subcutaneous abscesses in mice. J. Infect. Dis. 149, 924–928.
5. Burger, H., & Z. Hussain (1984): Tabellen und Methoden zur medizinisch-bakteriologischen Laborpraxis. Mainz: Kirchheim.
6. Claxton, P. D., L. A. Ribeiro & J. R. Egerton (1983): Classification of Bacteroides nodosus by agglutination test. Austr. Vet. J. 60, 331–334.
7. Dowell, V. R., & T. M. Hawkins (1977): Laboratory methods in anaerobic bacteriology. CDC Laboratory Manual. Atlanta, Ga.: Center for Disease Control.
8. Drasar, B. S. (1967): Cultivation of anaerobic intestinal bacteria. J. Path. Bact. 94, 417–427.
9. Duerden, B. I., W. P. Holbrook, J. G. Collee & B. Watt (1976): The characterization of clinically important Gram negative anaerobic bacilli by conventional bacteriological test. J. Appl. Bacteriol. 40, 163–188.
10. Egerer, K., & P. Elze (1983): Zur gaschromatographischen Schnelldiagnose anaerober Infektionen. Z. Ges. Inn. Med. 38, 41–44.
11. Egerton, J. R. (1981): Bacteroides nodosus. In: H. Blobel & T. Schliesser (Hrsg.): Handbuch der bakteriellen Infektionen bei Tieren. Bd. III, S. 627–638. Stuttgart: G. Fischer.
12. Egerton, J. R., & E. A. Laing (1979): Characteristics of Bacteroides nodosus isolated from cattle. Vet. Microbiol. 3, 269–279.
13. Eley, A., D. Greenwood & I. O'Grady (1985): Comparative growth of Bacteroides species in various anaerobic culture media. J. Med. Microbiol. 19, 195–201.
14. Emery, D. L., J. H. Dufty & B. L. Clark (1984): Biochemical and functional properties of a leukocidin produced by several strains of Fusobacterium necrophorum. Aust. Vet. J. 61, 382–387.
15. Emery, D. L., J. A. Vaughan, B. L. Clark, J. H. Dufty & D. J. Stewart (1985): Cultural characteristics and virulence of strains of Fusobacterium necrophorum isolated from feet of cattle and sheep. Aust. Vet. J. 62, 43–49.
16. Emery, D. L., R. D. Edwards & J. S. Rothel (1986): Studies on the purification of the leucocidin of Fusobacterium necrophorum and its neutralization by specific antisera. Vet. Microbiol. 11, 357–372.
17. Essers, L. (1982): Simple identification of anaerobic bacteria to genus level using typical antibiotic susceptibility patterns. J. Appl. Bacteriol. 52, 319–323.
18. Essers, L., & E. Haralambic (1977): Erfahrungen mit dem API 20 A-Testsystem bei der Identifizierung von Anaerobiern aus der täglichen Routine. Zbl. Bakt. Hyg. I. Abt. Orig. A 238, 394–401.
19. Fales, W. H., & G. W. Teresa (1972): Fluorescent antibody technique for identifying isolates of Sphaerophorus necrophorus of bovine hepatic abscess origin. Am. J. Vet. Res. 33, 2323–2329.
20. Fievez, L. (1963): Étude comparée des souches des Sphaerophorus isolées chez l'homme et chez l'animal. Bruxelles: Presses Académiques Européennes.
21. Finegold, S. M. (1977): Anaerobic bacteria in human disease. New York, San Francisco, London: Academic Press.
22. Hallmann, L., & F. Burkhardt (1974): Klinische Mikrobiologie. Stuttgart: G. Thieme.
23. Hammann, R. (1986): Das Genus Bacteroides. Forum Mikrobiologie 9, 60–68.
24. Hansen, S. L., & B. J. Stewart (1976): Comparison of API and Minitek to Center for Disease Control methods for the biochemical characterization of anaerobes. J. clin. Microbiol. 4, 227–231.
25. Hanson, C. W., R. Cassorla & W. J. Martin (1979): API and Minitek systems in identification of clinical isolates of anaerobic Gram-negative Bacilli and Clostridium species. J. clin. Microbiol. 10, 14–18.
26. Hentges, D. J., & L. D. Smith (1985): Hydrolytic enzymes as virulence factors of anaerobic bacteria. In: J. A. Holdes (ed.): Bacteriol. enzymes and virulence. Boca Raton, Florida: CRC Press.
27. Hindmarsh, F., & J. Fraser (1985): Serogroups of Bacteroides nodosus isolated from ovine footrot in Britain. Vet. Rec. 116, 187–188.
28. Hoi-Sörensen, G. (1978): Bacteriological examination of summermastitis secretions. The demonstration of Bacteroideaceae. Nord. Vet. Med. 30, 199–204.
29. Holdeman, L. V., E. P. Cato & W. E. C. Moore (1977): Anaerobe Laboratory Manual. 4th ed. Blacksburg, Virginia: Virginia Polytechnic Institute and State University.
30. Holdeman, L. V., R. W. Kelly & W. E. C. Moore (1984): Family I. Bacteroideaceae Pribram 1933. In: N. R. Krieg & J. G. Holt (ed.): Bergey's Manual of Systematic Bacteriology. Vol. 1, S. 602–631. Baltimore, London: Williams & Wilkins.
31. Kanoe, M., M. Kido & M. Toda (1984): Obligate anaerobic bacteria found in canine and feline purulent lesions. Br. Vet. J. 140, 257–262.
32. Kelly, M. J. (1984): A guinea-pig-model demonstrating synergy between Escherichia coli and Bacteroides fragilis in infected surgical wounds. In: M. J. Hill (ed.): Models of anaerobic infection. Dordrecht, Boston, Lancaster: Martimes Nijhoff.
33. Laing, E. A., & J. R. Egerton (1978): The occurrence, prevalence and transmission of Bacteroides nodosus infection in cattle. Res. Vet. Sci. 24, 300–304.
34. Lambe, D. W., & D. A. Moroz (1976): Serogrouping of Bacteroides fragilis subsp. fragilis by the agglutination test. J. clin. Microbiol. 7, 448–453.
35. Livingston, S. J., S. D. Kaminos & R. B. Yee (1978): New medium for selection and presumptive identification of the Bacteroides fragilis group. J. clin. Microbiol. 7, 448–453.
36. Love, D. N., R. F. Jones & M. Bailey (1981): Characterization of Bacteroides sp. isolated from soft tissue infection in cats. J. Appl. Bacteriol. 50, 567–575.
37. Love, D. N., R. F. Jones, M. Bailey & R. S. Johnson (1979): Isolation and characterization of bacteria from abscesses in subcutis of cats. J. Med. Microbiol. 12, 207–211.
38. Love, D. N., R. J. Jones & M. Bailey (1980): Characterization of Fusobacterium species isolated from soft tissue infection in cats. J. Appl. Bacteriol. 48, 325–331.
39. Moore, W. E. C., L. V. Holdeman & R. W. Kelley (1984): Genus II. Fusobacterium. In: N. R. Krieg & J. G. Holt (ed.): Bergey's Manual of Systematic Bacteriology. Vol. 1, S. 631–637. Baltimore, London: Williams & Wilkins.
40. Philipp, I., E. Taylor & S. Eykyn (1980): The rapid laboratory diagnosis of anaerobic infection. Infection 8 (Suppl. 2), 155–158.
41. Prescott, J. F. (1979): Identification of some anaerobic bacteria in nonspecific anaerobic infection in animals. Can. J. Comp. Med. 43, 194–199.
42. Prescott, J. F., & M. Chirino-Trejo (1984): Nonsporeforming anaerobic bacteria. In: G. R. Carter: Diag-

nostic procedures in veterinary bacteriology and mycology. S. 140–160. Springfeld, Illinois: Charles C. Thomas.
43. SCANLAN, C. M., & T. L. HATHCOCK (1983): Bovine rumenitis-liver abscess-complex: A bacteriological review. Cornell. Vet. **73**, 288–297.
44. SCHMITZ, J. A., & J. L. GRADIN (1980): Serotyping and biochemical characterization of Bacteroides nodosus isolates from oregon. Can. J. Comp. Med. **44**, 440–446.
45. SHORT, J. A., C. M. THORLEY & P. D. WALKER (1976): An electron microscope study of Bacteroides nodosus: ultrastructure of organisms from primary isolates and different colony types. J. Appl. Bacteriol. **40**, 311–315.
46. SIERING, H. (1986): Bakteriologische Untersuchungen zum Vorkommen von Infektionen mit Anaerobiern bei Tieren. Vet. Med. Diss., Hannover.
47. SIMON, P. S. (1974): Cultivation and maintenance of Sphaerophorus necrophorus. Part. I: An anaerobic medium for aerobic incubation. Can. J. Comp. Med. **38**, 94–96.
48. SIMON, P. C. (1975): A simple method for rapid identification of Sphaerophorus necrophorus isolates. Can. J. Comp. Med. **39**, 349–353.
49. SIMON, P. C., & M. HARRIS (1981): Fusobacterium necrophorum. In: H. BLOBEL & T. SCHLIESSER (Hrsg.): Handbuch der bakteriellen Infektionen bei Tieren. Bd. III, S. 639–676. Stuttgart: G. Fischer.
50. SHERMAN, T. M., S. K. ERASMUSON & D. EVERY (1981): Differentiation of Bacteroides nodosus biotypes and colony variants in relation to their virulence and immunprotective properties in sheep. Infect. Immun. **32**, 788, 795.
51. STEWART, D. J. (1978): Studies and the antigenic structure of Bacteroides nodosus. Res. Vet. Sci. **24**, 293–299.
52. SUTTER, V. L., D. M. CITION & S. M. FINEGOLD (1980): Wadsworth Anaerobic Bacteriology Manual. 3rd ed. St. Louis: C. V. Mosby.
53. THORLEY, C. M. (1976): A simplified method for the isolation of Bacteroides nodosus from ovine foot-rot and studies on its colony morphology and serology. J. Appl. Bacteriol. **40**, 301–309.
54. TOLLE, A., V. FRANKE & J. REICHMUTH (1982): Zur C. pyogenes-Mastitis. — Bakteriologische Aspekte. Dtsch. tierärztl. Wschr. **90**, 256–260.
55. WALKER, P. D., J. SHORT, R. O. THOMSEN & D. P. ROBERTS (1973): The fine structure of Fusiformis nodosus with special reference to the location of antigens associated with immunogenicity. J. Gen. Microbiol. **77**, 351–361.
56. WARNER, J. F., W. H. FALES, R. C. SUTHERLAND & G. W. TERESA (1975): Endotoxin from Fusobacterium necrophorum of bovine hepatic abscess origin. Am. J. Vet. Res. **36**, 1015–1019.
57. WEINTRAUB, A., A. A. LINDBERG & C. E. NORD (1979): Identification of Bacteroides fragilis by indirect immunofluorescence. Med. Microbiol. Immunol. **167**, 223–230.
58. WERNER, H. (1972): Anaerobierdifferenzierung durch gaschromatographische Stoffwechselanalysen. Zbl. Bakt. Hyg., I. Abt. Orig. A **220**, 446–451.
59. WERNER, H. (1981): Anaerobierinfektionen. Pathogenese, Klinik, Therapie, Stuttgart: G. Thieme.
60. VERWEIJ-VAN VUGHT, A. M. J. J., F. NAMAVAR, M. SPARRIUS, W. A. C. VEL & D. M. MACLAREN (1985): Pathogenic synergy between Escherichia coli and Bacteroides fragilis: studies in an experimental mouse model. J. Med. Microbiol. **19**, 325–331.

Spirochaetes
(Family: Spirochaetaceae)

Spirochäten
(Familie: Spirochaetaceae)

Morphologically the spirochaetes occupy a special position among the bacteria. They are very slim (diameter 0.1 to 0.5 µm), usually very long (up to 30 µm) and spiral shaped. Their motility is dependent not on flagella, but on the presence of contractile fibrils or bundles of fibrils which surround a cylinder of cytoplasm in spiral fashion. The cell is not rigid but motility is achieved by movement, stretching and rotation.

Spirochaetes are Gram-negative and they multiply by binary fission. Their cultural requirements are very variable, their growth can be aerobic to strictly anaerobic.

Spirochaetes occur mainly as saprophytes in the soil and water but some species of the genera *Borrelia*, *Treponema* and *Leptospira* are of veterinary importance (tab. 84).

Die Spirochäten nehmen unter den Bakterien eine morphologische Sonderstellung ein. Es handelt sich um sehr dünne (Durchmesser 0,1–0,5 µm) und meistens sehr lange (bis zu 30 µm), spiralförmige Bakterien. Ihre Beweglichkeit beruht nicht auf Geißeln, sondern auf dem Vorhandensein kontraktiler Fibrillen oder Fibrillenbündel, die einen Cytoplasmazylinder spiralig umschlingen. Die Körperform ist nicht starr, und die Bewegung kommt durch Bewegung, Streckung und Rotation zustande.

Spirochäten sind gramnegativ und vermehren sich durch Querteilung. Ihre Kulturanforderungen sind sehr unterschiedlich, ihr Wachstum kann aerob bis strikt anaerob sein.

Spirochäten kommen überwiegend als Saprophyten im Erdboden und im Wasser vor, von veterinärmedizinischer Bedeutung sind einige Arten der Gattungen *Borrelia*, *Treponema* und *Leptospira* (Tab. 84).

1 Genus: Leptospira (L.)

1 Gattung: Leptospira (L.)

The genus *Leptospira* includes:
▷ *L. biflexa*, a non-pathogenic saprophyte which lives in water or damp soil. It grows in media without serum. Bivalent copper ions in the form of copper sulphate solution up to a dilution of 1 : 100,000 have a bacteriostatic effect on *L. interrogans*, they do not affect *L. biflexa*. Another character which distinguishes *L. biflexa* from *L. interrogans* is that the former will grow at 13 °C and in the presence of 225 µg/ml of azaguanine.
▷ *L. interrogans*: This is a collective group for the pathogenic leptospires. By virtue of the different antigenic structure 19 serogroups and 180 serotypes (serovars) have been identified. The serotypes of importance in Europe are listed in table 85.

Innerhalb der Gattung *Leptospira* werden unterschieden:
▷ *L. biflexa*, apathogen, saprophytär im Wasser oder im feuchten Erdboden lebend. Wächst in Medien ohne Serum. Zweiwertige Kupferionen in Kupfersulfatlösung bis zu einer Verdünnung von 1 : 100 000 wirken (im Gegensatz zu *L. interrogans*) nicht bakteriostatisch. Weitere Unterschiedsmerkmale zu *L. interrogans* sind das Wachstum bei 13 °C sowie bei Anwesenheit von 225 µg/ml Azaguanin.
▷ *L. interrogans*: Sammelgruppe für pathogene Leptospiren. Sie umfaßt aufgrund der unterschiedlichen Antigenstruktur 19 Serogruppen und etwa 180 Serotypen (Serovare). Die für europäische Verhältnisse wichtigsten Serotypen sind in der Tab. 85 zusammengestellt.

■ **Incidence and veterinary significance**
The leptospires are of world-wide distribution with

■ **Vorkommen und medizinische Bedeutung**
Die Leptospiren sind weltweit verbreitet und finden

Table 84: Spirochaetes of clinical importance — Tabelle 84: Medizinisch wichtige Spirochäten

Genus	Species	Appearance	Culture in vitro	Disease	Transmission
Borrelia	B. recurrentis	0.2–0.5 × 3–20 µm in 3–10 lose, often irregular coils	(+)	Epidemic recurrent fever of man	lice
	B. anserina		–	Borreliosis in tropics and subtropics, water fowls, turkeys, fowls	by ticks and blood-sucking insects
	T. pallidum	0.1–0.4 × 3–20 µm mainly regularly wound spirals	–	Syphilis of man and monkeys	venereal
	T. paraluiscuniculi		–	Rabbit "syphilis", latent infections in mice, guinea pigs and others	venereal
	T. hyodysenteriae		+ (anaerobic)	Pig dysentery	contact
	T. innocens		(+ anaerobic)	non-pathogen, occurring in pigs' intestine	contact
Leptospira	L. interrogans with numerous serogroups and serovars	0.1 × 6–12 µm tightly and regularly coiled spirals	+	Leptospirosis of man and animals	Excreted in urine, direct or indirect (water, soil) contact

their biological reservoirs in various animal species, where they produce a latent kidney infection with excretion of the organism. The most important of these reservoirs are:
serotype *icterohaemorrhagiae* rat (dog, fox, pig, ox etc.),
serotype *canicola* dog (fox, ox, pig etc.),
serotype *grippotyphosa* field mouse (horse, ox, pig, sheep, dog, and others),
serotype *hardjo* ox,
serotype *pomona* pig (ox),
serotype *tarassovi* pig.

Man and animals become infected from these reservoirs either directly or indirectly through the agency of water, damp soil, field crops etc.). The

ihr biologisches Reservoir bei verschiedenen Tierarten in Form einer latenten Niereninfektion mit Erregerausscheidung. Die wichtigsten Erregerreservoire sind
Serotyp *icterohaemorrhagiae:* Ratte (Hund, Fuchs, Schwein, Rind u. a.),
Serotyp *canicola:* Hund (Fuchs, Rind, Schwein u. a.),
Serotyp *grippotyphosa:* Feldmaus (Pferd, Rind, Schwein, Schaf, Hund u. a.),
Serotyp *hardjo:* Rind,
Serotyp *pomona:* Schwein (Rind),
Serotyp *tarassovi:* Schwein.

Von diesen Reservoiren kommt es direkt oder indirekt (unter Vermittlung von Wasser, feuchtem

Table 85: The most important serogroups and serovars of *Leptospira interrogans* — Tabelle 85: Die wichtigsten Serogruppen und Serovare von *Leptospira interrogans*

Serogroup	Serovar	Serogroup	Serovar
Australis	australis bratislava	Javanica	javanica
Autumnalis	autumnalis	Pomona	pomona
		Pyrogenes	pyrogenes
Ballum	ballum	Sejroe	hardjo
Bataviae	bataviae		saxkoebing
			sejroe
Canicola	canicola		
Grippotyphosa	grippotyphosa	Tarassovi syn.: hyos	tarassovi
Hebdomadis	hebdomadis		

Genus: Leptospira (L.)

Table 86: Survey of leptospiral infections in the most important domestic animals	Tabelle 86: Zusammenstellung von Leptospireninfektionen bei den wichtigsten Haustieren

Species	Clinical disease
Horse	Mainly latent infections with positive serological titres; periodic ophthalmitis is considered to be caused by leptospira (most often by serovar grippotyphosa), although the aetiology has not been finally solved; acute icterohaemorrhagic and meningoencephalitic forms are extremely rare (9, 50, 59)
Cattle	In Germany the majority of infections are latent; the percentage of positive reactions lies between 5 and 6 % with regional variations; the most common clinical manifestations are abortion or the birth of weak calves, acute, febrile diseases with jaundice, enteritis, haematuria and high mortality are rare in Germany; in Anglo-Saxon countries infections with serovar hardjo have frequently been described in recent years which were associated with abortion and a mastitis-agalactia syndrome. These are of minor importance in Germany. The antibodies found in North Germany are most often against serovar grippotyphosa (85 %), saxkoebing (6 %), australis (5 %), canicola (3 %) and in South Germany predominantly to hardjo and saxkoebing (2, 4, 8, 14, 15, 20, 22, 30, 32, 38, 42, 56).
Pig	Primarily latent infections; in Germany the percentage of positive reactions fluctuates between 1 % and 10 % and in certain areas it is even higher. Clinical manifestations: abortion, piglets weakly from birth, acute general infections with jaundice are rare, the most common serovars are: grippotyphosa, pomona, tarassovi, icterohaemorrhagiae, canicola (2, 21, 23, 25, 26, 32, 35, 40, 41, 46, 52)
Dog and Cat	Acute form: ictero-haemorrhagic, febrile (in first 3 days) generalized disease with central nervous and uraemic (vomiting, diarrhoea) signs. chronic form: lassitude, inappetence, gastro-intestinal signs, cramp latent form: positive titre and excretion of leptospires in the urine Most common serovars: icterohaemorrhagiae (Weil's disease), grippotyphosa and then canicola (Stuttgart disease). Leptospirosis is relatively rare in cats (12, 17, 24, 27, 42, 56).

most important animal diseases are listed in table 86.

Erdboden, Feldfrüchten u. a.) zur Infektion von Mensch und Tier. Die wichtigsten tierischen Infektionsverläufe sind in der Tab. 86 zusammengestellt.

1.1 Properties of leptospires

■ **Morphology** (fig. 204)
Leptospires are protoplasmic spirals that encircle a central thread with about 20 primary coils. They measure $6–20 \times 0.1$ µm. One or both ends may be curved (secondary coils) so as to produce a walking-stick handle- or coat hanger-like shape. Motility is due to rotation about the central axis; there are no flagella.

Microscopically the organisms can be demonstrated under dark ground or phase contrast illumination with a magnification of about $\times 240$ (oil immersion objectives are not necessary). They will not take up the ordinary bacteriological dyes, but can be visualized with Levaditi's silver impregnation.

■ **Culture**
Leptospires are grown aerobically in neutral or slightly alkaline medium at 28–30 °C. Fluid or semisolid media have been found most suitable. In such media the leptospires grow slowly, so that increased

1.1 Eigenschaften der Leptospiren

■ **Morphologie** (Abb. 204)
Leptospiren sind in etwa 20 Primärwindungen um einen Achsenfaden aufgewundene Protoplasmaspiralen. Größe: $6–20 \times 0,1$ µm. Durch Umbiegung einer oder beider Enden (Sekundärwindung) entsteht die Handstock- oder Kleiderbügelform. Die Bewegung geschieht durch Rotation um die Körperachse, Geißeln sind nicht vorhanden.

Ihre mikroskopische Darstellung erfolgt in der Dunkelfeld- (oder Phasenkontrast-)mikroskopie bei einer Vergrößerung bis etwa 240fach (Ölimmersionsobjektive sind nicht erforderlich). Mit den üblichen Bakterienfarbstoffen sind sie nicht anfärbbar, wohl aber mit der Silberimprägnation nach Levaditi.

■ **Kultur**
Die Züchtung der Leptospiren erfolgt aerob, in neutralem oder leichtalkalischem Milieu bei 28–30 °C. Am besten bewähren sich flüssige bis halbfeste Nährböden. Die Leptospiren wachsen in

numbers of organisms can be demonstrated microscopically only after 4–5 days. The maximum bacterial density is not obtained until after 10 to 14 days. In semi-solid media growth is manifest in the form of a ring below the surface. In fluid cultures, and especially in older ones, spherical structures (granules) appear, which are interpreted as evidence of degeneration or signs of breakdown. No new vegetative forms of leptospires can develop from these. For this reason it is impossible to continue to grow cultures where there are only granules and no leptospires of normal appearance.

▷ Maintenance of strains: This is best in Korthof broth or on semi-solid media. They must be subcultured every 4 to 6 weeks and, if granules appear, even earlier.

▷ Media: The media used for the isolation or stock maintenance of leptospires contain rabbit serum or bovine serum albumin as protein supplement. Fluid media are required to perform agglutination tests, semi-solid media (0.2 % agar) are used for the isolation of leptospires and the maintenance of stock strains. Solid media help isolation from contaminated material. Visible colonies of most serotypes require 7 to 14 days to develop on solid media.

The most important media are
▷ supplemented with rabbit serum: Korthof, Stuart, Fletcher media. These are buffered peptone salt solutions (some of which can be obtained commercially) with 10 % rabbit serum added (pooled from several animals on antibiotic-free diet);
▷ supplemented with bovine serum albumin: Medium of ELLINGHAUSEN & MCCULLOUGH (13), modified by JOHNSON & HARRIS (16) which is sold as EMJH medium (Difco) (Tween 80 bovine albumin medium).

These media can be used in the fluid form or, after the addition of agar (see above) in semi-solid or solid form.

The different serotypes of *L. interrogans* have different nutrient requirements. The traditional media (Korthof, Stuart, Fletcher) are adequate for the isolation of the less fastidious serotypes (e. g. *icterohaemorrhagiae, pomona*), Tween 80 bovine albumin (EMJH) is for the more demanding types (e. g. *hardjo*).

■ **Biochemistry, antigenic structure and serological differentiation**

The pathogenic leptospires cannot be identified by their morphological, cultural and biochemical characters. Their enzymatic activity is very low and so far only lipases, haemolysins, oxidases and cata-

lases have been found which are of no consequence in taxonomic classification.

The serotypes are identified by means of agglutination tests. The basis for this is the cross absorption test. Two leptospira strains are compared one with the other. Their identity is proven when in the cross absorption all the antibodies can be removed from the immune sera and the agglutination is negative (47).

1.2 Diagnostic demonstration of causal organism

Although of fundamental importance to diagnosis, it is very difficult to isolate leptospires from specimens of animal origin. This is due to the fact that the microscopic demonstration is complicated; the special cultural demands have already been mentioned. Therefore, the isolation is rarely attempted in routine diagnosis which relies mainly on the demonstration of antibodies.

■ Microscopic demonstration of leptospires

The microscopic demonstration of leptospires in fresh material (blood, urine) under dark ground illumination is prone to a high degree of error because erythrocyte and tissue cell breakdown products (»pseudospirochaetes«) can be confused with leptospires. This method is of little practical importance, therefore.

Blood examination: blood with anticoagulant is centrifuged and the plasma is examined under dark ground illumination. The pseudospirochaetes can be removed by adding streptolysin.

Urine examination: the urine must be centrifuged immediately it is taken. Leptospires can be demonstrated more consistently in kidney homogenate from dead animals (especially in rats and mice) than in urine.

■ Demonstration of leptospires with fluorescent antibodies

Although many authors (10, 38, 40, 45, 46, 55) have found this the most successful method of demonstrating leptospires, it has not been generally accepted in diagnosis. The agreement between this method and culture is variously interpreted, but it allows leptospires to be recognized even in autolyzed material. Cross reactions can occur between the various serotypes. Thus, WHITE & RISTIC (55) also labelled *L. icterohaemorrhagiae, canicola* and *sejroe* with *pomona* serum.

Cultural demonstration

The attempt to culture leptospires in routine diagnosis often fails for the following reasons: there may be insufficient numbers of leptospires in the sample, it may have been taken at an unsuitable stage or it may be impossible to obtain a pure culture. Especially this last point is very important in the isolation of leptospires. When organs are to be examined then the homogenate should be diluted in order to remove growth-inhibiting substances.

The growth of contaminants can be suppressed by the addition of inhibitors to the medium. Fluorouracil has been found effective for this purpose (29). Nalidixic acid (50 mg/l) also produces an inhibitory effect, as do vancomycin (10 mg/l) and polymyxin-B sulphate (500 IU/l) (44).

The method illustrated in figure 206 has proved satisfactory for the demonstration of *L. hardjo* in aborted bovine foetuses.

Kultureller Erregernachweis

Der Versuch, den Erreger kulturell zu isolieren, führt in der praktischen Diagnostik oft nicht zum Erfolg. Die entscheidenden Gründe hierfür sind, daß entweder zu wenige Leptospiren im Untersuchungsmaterial vorhanden sind, daß das Material zu einem ungünstigen Zeitpunkt des Infektionsverlaufes entnommen wurde oder daß es nicht gelingt, Reinkulturen zu bekommen. Insbesondere der letzte Grund spielt bei der Leptospirenisolierung eine wichtige Rolle. Bei der Untersuchung von Organen sollte das homogenisierte Material verdünnt werden, um wachstumshemmende Gewebsfaktoren auszuschließen.

Die Unterdrückung des Wachstums der Begleitbakterien kann durch Zusatz selektiver Substanzen zum Nährmedium versucht werden. Als Zusatzstoff hat sich Fluorurazil bewährt (29). Eine Hemmwirkung kann auch durch Nalidixinsäure (50 mg/l), Vancomycin (10 mg/l) und Polymyxin-B-Sulfat (500 E/l) erzielt werden (44).

Als erfolgreich zum Nachweis von *L. hardjo* aus abortierten Rinderfeten erwies sich das in Abb. 206 dargestellte Verfahren.

Specimens

Blood (in acute leptospirosis), urine, kidney, liver, foetal material (kidneys, eyes) in abortions. Aseptic measures should be taken when organs are to be cultured: they are flamed and sampled from the centre

---

Microscopic demonstration of leptospires

1. Dark ground microscopy fresh material (p. 281)
2. Fluorescence microscopy (p. 281)

Animal inoculation

guinea pigs, golden hamsters followed by cultures

Demonstration of organisms in fluid or semifluid media

1. Uncontaminated or moderately contaminated material (heart blood, urine, possibly organs): direct inoculation of medium (e. g. Korthof broth). Incubation at 29/30 °C for several weeks. Continual microscopic check. Subcultures are set up as soon as structures suggestive of leptospires are found. Even in tubes with no growth it is advisable to carry out blind passages after 3 to 4 weeks.
2. Contaminated material: contaminating flora can be eliminated by diluting the test material and/or adding selective substances to the medium (5-fluorouracil). The following method has proved effective for demonstrating L. hardjo in bovine abortion:
2a. Test material is homogenized and diluted: One part of sample is homogenized in 9 parts of diluting fluid (physiological saline with 1 % bovine serum albumin). From the homogenate a series of dilutions (10^{-2} to 10^{-4}) are made up with the diluting fluid;
2b. Inoculation of the media: 50 µl are taken from each dilution and added to 1 tube EMJH medium (Oxoid; 2.5 ml) with the addition of 1.5 % agar, 1 % inactivated rabbit serum and 100 µg/ml 5-fluorouracil.
2c. Incubation: up to 16 weeks at 29/30 °C.
2d. Assessment of culture: About every second week samples are examined microscopically under dark ground illumination. Very few leptospires are to be expected in positive cases perhaps one in every 20 fields. The search can be facilitated by reducing the viscosity with one drop of fluid medium (without agar) to the semisolid medium. In positive or doubtful cases a new series of dilutions should be set up immediately from which new tubes are inoculated.

Fig. 206: Procedure for demonstrating leptospires (13, 14, 20, 22, 23, 30, 36)

Abb. 206: Untersuchung für den Nachweis von Leptospiren (13, 14, 20, 22, 23, 30 36)

Purification of leptospiral cultures

Contaminated fluid leptospiral cultures can be freed of the unwanted bacteria by the following method:
▷ by animal inoculation — the culture fluid is injected intraperitoneally into guinea pigs and after 15 to 60 minutes blood is withdrawn by heart puncture and inoculated into fresh media;
▷ by filtration — the culture fluid is forced with a syringe through a filter of 0.45 µm pore size (43, 48).

Demonstration by animal inoculation

Animal inoculation is particularly useful when attempting to isolate leptospires from contaminated material. Guinea pigs and golden hamsters can be used. *L. icterohaemorrhagiae* causes a clinical disease in guinea pigs and *L. canicola* in hamsters (5, 7, 39). A generalized febrile disease develops which may or may not be accompanied by jaundice and the leptospires can be found in the blood and the peritoneal fluid. Infection with other types of leptospires usually causes only a brief febrile phase with bacteraemia and subsequent settlement of the bacteria in the kidneys.

For this procedure the material is injected intraperitoneally. From about the 5th to 7th day onwards leptospires can be demonstrated microscopically (even in apparently healthy animals) in the blood and peritoneal fluid (withdrawn with a glass pipette). When the microscopic examination is positive, then blood is withdrawn by heart puncture, placed into culture medium and examined further by cultural means. Sick experimental animals are killed and blood, liver, kidney and urine are cultured. In animals which do not become ill, the experiment is terminated after 20 to 30 days and an attempt is also made to isolate leptospires from blood and organs (liver, kidney).

1.3 Serological diagnosis

The serological diagnosis takes on a special significance in view of the difficulty of demonstrating the organism itself. The most important methods available are the agglutination (-lysis) reaction and the complement fixation test. Other methods such as the indirect haemagglutination, the latex test, ELISA have also been tried (1, 21, 36).
▷ Agglutination: The classical and most frequently tried method is the agglutination-lysis reaction (ALR) with microscopic evaluation. It is usually live leptospires which are mixed with the test serum. If the test is positive an agglutination occurs which is at first in the form of loose clumps that later condense. The reaction is read with the microscope under dark ground illumination at a magnification of about 120 times. This initial reaction is

Table 87: Antigens recommended for serological examination for leptospires

Tabelle 87: Empfehlung der bei serologischen Untersuchungen auf Leptospirose zu benutzenden Antigene

Serovars of L. interrogans	to be used as antigen in					Incidence in animals[2]
	Cattle	Pig	Sheep	Horse	Dog	
copenhageni[1]	+	+	+	+	+	
canicola	+	−	−	+	+	
grippotyphosa	+	+	+	+	+	common
pomona	+	+	+	+	+	
hardjo	+	+	+	+	+	
tarassovi	+	+	+	−	+	
sejroe	−	+	+	+	−	
saxkoebing	+	+	+	+	+	rare
bataviae	+	+	+	+	+	
autumnalis	+	+	+	+	+	
australis	+	+	+	+	+	

[1] serogroup icterohaemorrhagiae; [2] in Germany, but regional variations are possible

followed by »lysis«. Presumably this is only an illusion, because the leptospires are no longer recognizable when they are drawn into the dense agglutination. This process is independent of complement.

There are many variations for the technical procedure of this agglutination. The serum dilutions can be made in tubes or on well plates (slow agglutination at room temperature). After 2 to 4 hours the test is read either by direct microscopy or by taking a loopful from each dilution to be examined under dark ground illumination. The reaction can also be performed on a slide (rapid test). A drop of serum (diluted 1:50) is mixed on a slide with a drop of culture (producing a serum dilution of 1:100). This is kept in a moist chamber at room temperature for 15 minutes, and read by direct examination under dark ground illumination. If agglutination takes place then further dilutions have to be set up until the end point is found. Each slide can be divided into several sectors (8 to 10 is best) by drawing longitudinal and transverse lines with a grease pencil. This permits each slide to be used for testing one serum against antibodies of several types of leptospires (31, 37).

Required serum dilutions: 1:100, 1:200 etc. to the end point. Titres of 1:200 are generally considered doubtful, titres of 1:400 and above as positive.

Required antigen types: the choice of leptospires which are used to test the sera depends on the animal species and the epidemiological situation pertaining in that particular region. The Ministry of Health (Federal German Republic) recommends the serotypes listed in table 87.

The result of the agglutination test is determined by, amongst others, the bacterial density in the culture. The titre rises as the number of leptospires/ml falls. Comparative tests should always be carried

(Dunkelfeld, etwa 120fache Vergrößerung). Im Anschluß daran tritt eine »Lysis« auf, die vermutlich vorgetäuscht wird, indem die Leptospiren in dichte Agglutinate einbezogen werden und dadurch nicht mehr erkennbar sind. Der Prozeß verläuft komplementunabhängig.

In der methodischen Ausführung hat die Agglutination viele Variationen erfahren. Die Serumverdünnungen können in Röhrchen oder Tüpfelplatten angesetzt werden (Langsamagglutination bei Zimmertemperatur). Die Ablesung erfolgt nach 2–4 h entweder durch direkte Mikroskopie oder indem von jeder Verdünnungsstufe eine Öse Material entnommen und im Dunkelfeld untersucht wird. Die Reaktion kann auch auf dem Objektträger (Schnelltest) angesetzt werden. Dabei wird auf dem Objektträger ein Tropfen Serum (Verdünnung 1:50) mit einem Tropfen Kultur vermischt (daraus ergibt sich die Serumverdünnung 1:100). Die Reaktion kann nach etwa 15 min (Aufbewahrung bei Zimmertemperatur in einer feuchten Kammer) durch direkte mikroskopische Untersuchung im Dunkelfeld abgelesen werden. Tritt eine Agglutination ein, muß durch weitere Serumverdünnung der Endtiter bestimmt werden. Der Objektträger kann mit dem Fettstift durch mehrere Quer- und zwei Längsstriche in Felder (am besten 8–10) eingeteilt werden, so daß auf einem Objektträger ein Serum auf Antikörper gegen verschiedene Leptospirentypen untersucht werden kann (31, 37).

Erforderliche Serumverdünnungen: 1:100, 1:200 usw. bis zum Endtiter. Im allgemeinen werden Titer von 1:200 als zweifelhaft, von 1:400 und höher als positiv angesehen.

Erforderliche Antigentypen: Die Auswahl der Leptospiren, mit denen die Seren untersucht werden müssen, richtet sich nach der Tierart und der für eine bestimmte Region gegebenen epidemiologi-

out with constant bacterial concentrations (e. g. 100–200 × 10⁶/ml; 39).

Cross reactions can occur in agglutinations with various serovars because of their antigenic relationship.

Apart from the classical agglutination techniques using live leptospira, methods have been described in which dead leptospira are employed.

▷ Complement fixation test: The CFT has rarely been used for the serological diagnosis of leptospirosis in animals. Killed antigen (heat, formol or phenol) is used. Several serovars (up to 3 or 4) can be used as pooled antigen for the initial survey (6, 8).

schen Situation. Vom Bundesgesundheitsamt sind die in der Tab. 87 zusammengestellten Serotypen empfohlen worden.

Der Ausfall der Agglutination wird u. a. durch die Kulturdichte bestimmt. Mit abnehmender Leptospirenzahl/ml kommt es zu einer Titererhöhung. Bei vergleichenden Untersuchungen sollte deswegen mit konstanten Leptospirenzahlen gearbeitet werden (z. B. 100–200 × 10⁶/ml; 39).

Bei der Agglutination mit verschiedenen Serovaren können aufgrund der antigenen Verwandtschaft Kreuzreaktionen auftreten.

Neben der klassischen Agglutinationsmethode, die lebende Leptospiren benutzt, sind auch Verfahren mit inaktivierten Leptospiren beschrieben worden.

▷ Komplementbindungsreaktion: Die KBR ist zur serologischen Diagnose der Leptospirose bei Tieren selten eingesetzt worden. Es wird mit einem abgetöteten Antigen (Koch-, Formol-, Phenolantigen) gearbeitet. Für orientierende Untersuchungen können mehrere Serovare (3 bis 4) als Antigengemisch benutzt werden (6, 8).

Bibliography / Literatur

1. BABUDIERI, B. (1967): Serologie der Leptospirosen. In: J. KATHE & H. MOCHMANN (Hrsg.): Leptospiren und Leptospirosen. Teil 1, S. 326–350. Jena: VEB Gustav Fischer.
2. BISPING, W., J. DIMITRIADIS, M. POZVARI, H. REDLICH & E. WEILAND (1971): Die Verbreitung der Leptospiren bei Rindern u. Schweinen in Nordwestdeutschland und ihre Bedeutung für die Fleischbeschau. Schlacht- u. Viehhof-Ztg. 71, 173–178, 219–223.
3. BUGNOWSKI, H., U. STRIEN & F. GOTTSCHALK (1981): Erfahrungen bei der Sanierung des Bestandes einer 1040er Sauenanlage von einer Leptospira-tarassovi-Infektion. Mh. Vet. Med. 36, 884–888.
4. BÜRKI, F. (1962): Leptospirenaborte beim Rind. Schweiz. Arch. Tierhk. 104, 650–661.
5. BÜRKI, F. (1960): Zum Nachweis von Leptospiren mittels des Goldhamster-Tierversuches. Zbl. Bakt. I. Orig. 178, 211–222.
6. BÜRKI, F. (1960): Orientierende Untersuchung von Tierseren auf Antikörper gegen Leptospiren mittels Mischantigen in der Komplementbindungsreaktion. II. Mitteilung: Ergebnisse im Vergleich zur Agglutination-Lysis-Reaktion. Zschr. Immunit.-forsch. 119, 333–343.
7. BÜRKI, F. (1952): Der Goldhamster als Versuchstier für Leptospira canicola. Zschr. Hyg. 135, 215–224.
8. BÜRKI, F., & E. WIESMANN (1963): Zur serologischen Diagnostik des Leptospirenaborts beim Rind. Wiener tierärztl. Wschr. 50, 748–761.
9. BÜRKI, F., P. EGLI & E. WIESMANN (1963): Experimentelle Infektion von Pferden mit Leptospira pomona. Berl. Münch. tierärztl. Wschr. 76, 265–269.
10. COFFIN, L., & G. MAESTRONE (1962): Detection of leptospires by fluorescent antibody. Am. J. Vet. Res. 23, 159–164.
11. COX, C. D., & A. D. LARSON (1957): Colonial growth of leptospirae. J. Bact. 73, 587–589.
12. DIETRICH, W. (1962): Leptospireninfektionen beim Hund. Kleintierpraxis 7, 201–209.
13. ELLINGHAUSEN, H. C., & W. G. MCCULLOUGH (1965): Nutrition of Leptospira pomona and growth of 13 other serotypes: fractionation of oleic albumin complex and a medium of bovine albumin and polysorbate 80. Am. J. Vet. Res. 26, 45–51.
14. ELLIS, W. A., J. J. O'BRIEN, S. D. NEILL, H. W. FERGUSON & J. HANNA (1982): Bovine leptospirosis: Microbiological and serological findings in aborted fetuses. Vet. Res. 110, 147–150.
15. ELLIS, W. A., J. J. O'BRIEN & J. CASSELS (1981): Role of cattle in the maintenance of Leptospira interrogans serotype hardjo infection in Northern Ireland. Vet. Rec. 108, 555–557.
16. FAINE, S. (1982): Guideline for the control of leptospirosis. Genf: WHO.
17. FREUDIGER, K. (1969): Leptospireninfektionen bei Katzen. Berl. Münch. tierärztl. Wschr. 82, 390–392.
18. FÜZI, M., & R. CSÓKA (1960): Die Differenzierung der pathogenen und saprophytischen Leptospiren mittels eines Kupfersulfattestes. Zbl. Bakt. I. Orig. 179, 231–237.
19. FUCHS, G. H. P., & H. J. WALTHER (1959): Beiträge zur Leptospirenzüchtung. Zbl. Bakt. I. Orig. 174, 601–615, 175, 570–581.
20. HATHAWAY, S. C., T. W. A. LITTLE & A. S. STEVENS (1982): Isolation of Leptospira interrogans serovar hardjo from aborted bovine fetuses in England. Vet. Rec. 111, 58.
21. HARTWIGK, H., & C. C. MERCK (1964): Canicola-Leptospirose als Ursache eines Verferkelns. Berl. Münch. tierärztl. Wschr. 77, 437–441.
22. HARTWIGK, H., & E. STOEBBE (1963): Zur kulturellen Isolierung von Leptospiren aus Albinoratten. Berl. Münch. tierärztl. Wschr. 76, 3–6.
23. HARTWIGK, H., & E. STOEBBE (1962): Leptospirenfunde im Harn und in den Nieren von Rindern. Berl. Münch. tierärztl. Wschr. 75, 241–245.
24. HORSCH, F., & K. KUTSCHMANN (1974): Die Leptospirosesituation bei Hunden in der DDR. Mh. Vet. Med. 29, 241–243.
25. HORSCH, F., H. U. BRÜSEHABER & A. BÖTTICHER (1973): Zur Sanierung leptospiroseverseuchter Schweinebestände unter Anwendung von Streptomycin. Mh. Vet. Med. 28, 818–824.

26. HORSCH, F., & J. BEER (1968): Zur Epizootiologie der Leptospirose des Schweines in der DDR. Mh. Vet. Med. **23**, 642–648.
27. HÜBNER, D. (1972): Beitrag zum Stand der Leptospiroseverseuchung von Hunden. Fortschr. Vet. Med., Heft 17: 9. Kongreßbericht, S. 87–93. Berlin, Hamburg: Paul Parey.
28. JOHNSON, R. C., & V. G. HARRIS (1967): Differentiation of pathogenic and saprophytic leptospires. I. Growth at low temperatures. J. Bact. **94**, 27–31.
29. JOHNSON, R. C., & P. ROGERS (1974): 5-Fluorouracil as a selective agent for growth of leptospirae. J. Bact. **87**, 422–426.
30. KARASCH, H. (1964): Beitrag zum kulturellen Nachweis von Leptospiren bei Schlachtrindern unter Berücksichtigung der pathologisch-anatomischen Veränderung an den Organen. Arch. Lebensmittelhyg. **15**, 25–28.
31. KRÜGER, A. (1953): Eine einfache Schnellmethode für die Leptospiren-Agglutination. Zschr. Imm.-forsch. exp. Therap. **110**, 17–23.
32. KRÜGER, A. (1952): Vorkommen und Verbreitung der Leptospirosen bei den Haustieren. Berl. Münch. tierärztl. Wschr. **64**, 121–124.
33. LEHNERT, C., & F. MÜLLER (1981): Leptospiroseinfektion bei Besamungsbullen. Mh. Vet. Med. **36**, 756.
34. MENGES, R. W., & M. M. GALTON (1961): Direct cultural methods for the isolation of leptospires from experimentally infected guinea pigs. Amer. J. Vet. Res. **22**, 1085–1092.
35. MICHNA, S. W. (1962): Abortion in the sow due to infection by Leptospira canicola. Vet. Rec. **74**, 917–919.
36. MOCHMANN, H. (1964): Laboratoriumsdiagnose der Leptospirosen und der Leptospiren. Zbl. Bakt. I. Orig. **192**, 385–399.
37. MOCHMANN, H., & S. SCHULZ-PLANETH (1955): Vergleichende Untersuchungen zur serologischen Diagnostik der Leptospirosen mit dem Agglutinations-Lysisversuch im Verfahren der Langsamagglutination und der Objektträgeragglutination. Zschr. Imm.-forsch. exp. Therap. **112**, 482–490.
38. NONNEWITZ, T. (1984): Serologische Untersuchungen zur Leptospirose bei Schweinen und Rindern und ein Verfahren zur Darstellung der Leptospiren mittels indirekter Immunfluoreszenz. Vet. med. Diss., Hannover.
39. POPP, L. (1967): Laboratoriumsdiagnostik der Leptospiren. In: J. KATHE & H. MOCHMANN (Hrsg.): Leptospiren und Leptospirosen, Teil 1, S. 249–287. Jena: VEB Gustav Fischer.
40. PÓZVÁRI, M. (1971): Untersuchungen zur Verbreitung der Schweineleptospirose in Nordwestdeutschland. Vet. med. Diss., Hannover.
41. REDLICH, H. (1970): Verbreitung, Bedeutung und Diagnostik der Schweineleptospirose anhand einer Literaturübersicht sowie eigenen Untersuchungen. Vet. med. Diss., Hannover.
42. RETZLAFF, N., & E. WEISE (1967): Serologische, kulturelle und histologische Untersuchungen an Schlachtrindern auf Leptospirose. Zbl. Vet. Med. B **15**, 581–591.
43. RIEDEMANN, S., C. KORTS & J. ZAMORA (1982): Verfahren zur Entkontamination der Leptospirakulturen. Zbl. Vet. Med. B **29**, 708–714.
44. SCHÖNBERG, A., U. KÄMPE & D. ROHLOFF (1980): Der Einsatz von Hemmstoffen beim kulturellen Nachweis der Leptospiren im Schweinesperma. Berl. Münch. tierärztl. Wschr. **93**, 166–171.
45. SCHRÖDER, H. D. (1965): Zum Nachweis von Leptospiren mit fluoreszierenden Antikörpern. Mh. Vet. Med. **20**, 631.
46. SCHRÖDER, H. D., & W. SENF (1967): Fluoreszenzserologischer Nachweis von Leptospira hyos beim Schwein. Mh. Vet. Med. **22**, 771–773.
47. SCHÜFFNER, W., & H. BOHLANDER (1939): Zur Technik des Absättigungsversuchs mit Leptospiren. Zbl. Bakt. I. Orig. **144**, 434–439.
48. SCHULTZ, J. (1959): Ein Beitrag zur Filtration von bakteriell verunreinigten Leptospirenstämmen. Mh. Vet. Med. **14**, 278–280.
49. SLEIGHT, S. D., & J. A. WILLIAMS (1961): Transmission of bovine leptospirosis by coition and artificial insemination. J. Am. Vet. Med. Ass. **138**, 151–152.
50. SOVA, Z. (1965): Die Beziehung leptospiröser Infektionen bei Pferden zur Iridocyklochorioiditis recidiva. Zbl. Bakt. I. Orig. **197**, 100–110.
51. THIERMANN, A. B. (1981): Use of solid medium for isolation of leptospires of the hebdomadis serogroup from bovine milk and urine. Am. J. Vet. Res. **42**, 2143–2145.
52. WEBER, A., & G. WEBER (1977): Untersuchungen zum Vorkommen von Antikörpern gegen Leptospiren bei Schlachtschweinen des Gießener Schlachthofes. Prakt. Tierarzt **58**, 737–740.
53. WEISE, E. (1967): Serologische und kulturelle Untersuchungen zum Vorkommen von Leptospiren bei Schlachttieren im Hinblick auf die Beurteilung der Leptospirose bei der Fleischuntersuchung. Vet. Med. Diss., Berlin.
54. WHITE, F. H., H. E. STOLIKER & M. M. GALTON (1961): Detection of leptospires in naturally infected dogs using fluorescein-labeled antibody. Am. J. Vet. Res. **22**, 650–654.
55. WHITE, F. H., & M. RISTIC (1959): Detection of Leptospira pomona in guinea pig and bovine urine with fluorescein-labeled antibody. J. infect. Dis. **105**, 118–123.
56. WITTIG, W., F. HORSCH, W. ZIMMERHACKEL & H. HAASE (1967): Leptospira-pomona-Infektion bei Jungrindern. Mh. Vet. Med. **22**, 684–687.
57. WOJTEK, H. L. (1966): Zur Leptospirose der Haus- u. Versuchstiere. Tierärztl. Umschau **21**, 449–455.
58. WORATZ, H. (1952): Ein fester Nährboden für Dauerkulturen pathogener Leptospiren. Z. Hyg. **134**, 78–80.
59. ZAHARIJA, J., M. MAROLT, K. ČERMAK, N. ANDRAŠIĆ & F. SANKOVIĆ (1960): Leptospiren und periodische Augenentzündung beim Pferd. Schweiz. Arch. Tierhk. **102**, 400–408.
60. ZIPPLIES, G. (1958): Zur Züchtung von Leptospiren. Arch. exp. Vet. Med. **12**, 178–192.

2 Genus: Treponema (T.)

2.1 Treponema hyodysenteriae

■ **Incidence and veterinary significance**

T. hyodysenteriae is the causal agent of swine dysentery, an economically important enteric disease of pigs with world-wide distribution. Pigs weighing between 15 and 70 kg are most often affected. Infection is by the oral route. Being an obligate

2 Gattung: Treponema (T.)

2.1 Treponema hyodysenteriae

■ **Vorkommen und medizinische Bedeutung**

T. hyodysenteriae ist der Erreger der Schweinedysenterie, einer weltweit verbreiteten und wirtschaftlich bedeutsamen Darmerkrankung. Schweine im Gewicht von 15 bis 70 kg erkranken am häufigsten. Die Erregeraufnahme erfolgt oral. Als obligater

```
┌─────────────────────────────────────────────────────────────────────┐
│                              Specimens                              │
├─────────────────────────────────────────────────────────────────────┤
│ Faecal samples, diluted 1:10 with phosphate buffered saline         │
│ faecal swab, in transportation medium e. g. Port-a-cul or Amies medium, │
│ abnormal mucosa from caecum or colon as tied off pieces of gut,     │
│ biopsy taken before the start of chemotherapy,                      │
│ cultures should be set up within 24 hours.                          │
└─────────────────────────────────────────────────────────────────────┘
                                  │
┌─────────────────────────────────────────────────────────────────────┐
│                 Microscopic demonstration of pathogen               │
├─────────────────────────────────────────────────────────────────────┤
│ 1. Fresh preparation, examination under dark ground illumination and │
│    phase contrast                                                   │
│ 2. Preparations stained with monochromatic dyes, carbol fuchsin or  │
│    victoria blue R 4,                                               │
│ 3. Immunofluorescence                                               │
│ 4. Silver impregnation.                                             │
│ Methods 1 and 3 are of special diagnostic value.                    │
│ Assessment: test is positive when 3 to 5 treponemes are found per   │
│ microscopic field.                                                  │
└─────────────────────────────────────────────────────────────────────┘
                                  │
┌─────────────────────────────────────────────────────────────────────┐
│                   Demonstration of pathogen by culture              │
├─────────────────────────────────────────────────────────────────────┤
│ 1. Preparation: before taking cultures it is recommended that the intestinal mucosa be rinsed in physio- │
│    logical saline (1:10), centrifuged for 10 minutes and the rinsing fluid is passed through a series of │
│    filters (8, 5, 3, 1.2, 0.8, 0.65 and 0.45 µm pore size). The filtrates which have passed through the three │
│    smallest pore sizes are then inoculated on selective media.      │
│ 2. Solid media: trypticase-soya agar with 5% ox or sheep blood; diagnostic sensitivity test (DST) agar │
│    with added blood,                                                │
│    Selective additives: spectinomycin (400 µg/ml) by itself or with vancomycin and colistin (each │
│    25 µg/ml) (10, 24),                                              │
│    fluid media: trypticase-soya broth with 10% calf (12) or rabbit serum (18) │
│ 3. Incubation: strictly anaerobic in anaerobic jars with catalytic oxidation of $H_2$ (p. 267). Primary │
│    culture can be improved if media are used which have been reduced beforehand for 24 hours under │
│    anaerobic conditions.                                            │
│ 4. Incubation temperature: 37–42 °C, the higher temperature reduces the generation time. │
│ 5. Incubation time: 3–7 d, the search for colonies starts after 2–3 d. │
│ 6. Assessment of cultures: growth in the form of a delicate film which spreads 0.5 to 1 mm beyond the │
│    inoculation streak; there is a strong and sharply defined β-haemolysis. │
└─────────────────────────────────────────────────────────────────────┘
                                  │
           ┌─────────────────────────────────────────────┐
           │           Other tests on pure cultures      │
           ├─────────────────────────────────────────────┤
           │ 1. microscopic confirmation  2. biochemical examination │
           │ 3. serotyping                4. testing resistance      │
           └─────────────────────────────────────────────┘
```

Fig. 207: Demonstration of *Treponema hyodysenteriae*   Abb. 207: Nachweis von *Treponema hyodysenteriae*

anaerobe, *T. hyodysenteriae* finds the large intestine to provide ideal conditions for colonization and multiplication. Synergistic interaction with other bacteria promote the production of disease. Following an incubation period of between 10 and 14 days, diarrhoea of a muco-haemorrhagic nature develops. The disease is an fact, characterized by a muco-haemorrhagic to diphtheritic necrotizing inflammation of the large intestine. Milder forms are also observed with less pronounced clinical symptoms and even latent infections occur which do not become clinically manifest (6). The treponemas are excreted in the faeces and this may persist for more than 7 to 10 weeks after the animals are clinically recovered. A disease outbreak frequently follows on a reduction in resistance and the primary source

Anaerobier findet *T. hyodysenteriae* im Dickdarm optimale anaerobe Bedingungen zur Ansiedlung und Vermehrung. Synergistische Interaktionen mit anderen Darmbakterien begünstigen die Krankheitsentwicklung. Nach einer Inkubationszeit von durchschnittlich 10 bis 14 d kommt es zum Auftreten von schleimigblutigem Durchfall. Die Erkrankung ist gekennzeichnet als mukohämorrhagische bis diphtheroid-nekrotisierende Dickdarmentzündung. Daneben treten milde Verlaufsformen mit weniger ausgeprägten klinischen Symptomen und klinisch nicht erfaßbare latente Infektionen auf (6). Die Erregerausscheidung erfolgt mit dem Kot, sie kann auch nach der klinischen Heilung über 7 bis 10 Wochen fortbestehen. Der Ausbruch der Erkrankung steht häufig im Zusammenhang mit dem Auf-

of infection is carrier pigs, without clinical signs. Rats, mice and liquid manure play a role as infection sources (4, 6).

Treponemas of doubtful pathogenicity, which cannot as yet be classified with certainty in the species *T. hyodysenteriae* or *T. innocens*, have been isolated from the faeces of dogs (19, 22).

A dysentery-like disease was caused by *T. hyodysenteriae* in nutria which were being kept on premises that had previously housed pigs (25).

■ Morphology (figs 205 and 208)

T. hyodysenteriae is a spiral, Gram-negative bacterium, measuring $0.3 \times 6\text{–}9\,\mu m$. The characteristic spiral form has 2 to 4 coils and exhibits motility brought about by fibrillary bundles which project from both poles and cross in the middle part of the cell.

■ Demonstration of organism

The procedure for identification is presented in figure 207. It is generally accepted that the cultural methods are more sensitive than fluorescence microscopy. The combined method is undoubtedly the most reliable.

■ Biochemical properties (fig. 209)

A distinctive character of *T. hyodysenteriae* is the strong β-haemolysis. It is best demonstrated on media containing sheep blood. KINYON et al. (14) recommend the phenomenon of haemolysis intensification. This is achieved in the following way: an agar block with sides of 0.5 cm is cut from a 4-day old plate culture and then the plate is incubated

Table 88: Properties of *T. hyodysenteriae* and *T. innocens*

Properties	T. hyodysenteriae	T. innocens
Size	6–9 µm	6–9 µm
Optimum temperature	42 °C	42 °C
Haemolysis	strong β-haemolysis	weak β-haemolysis
Haemolysis intensification	+	–
Ind	+	–
Glu	+	+
Fru	–	+
other carbohydrates[1]	–	–
Aes	–	–
H$_2$S	–	–
α-galactosidase[2]	–	+
Acetic acid[3]	+	+
N-butyric acid[3]	+	+
Enteropathogenicity[4]	+	–

[1] Ara, Lac, Mal, Man, Sal, Sac, Tre, Xyl; [2] with API-Zym (bio Merieux) after HUNTER & WOOD (9); [3] with gas chromatography after HOLDEMAN et al. (7); [4] in animal experiment by artificial infection of pigs or in the gut ligature test using the same species

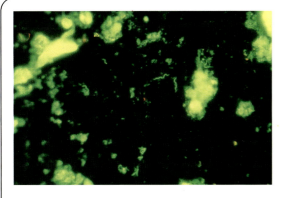
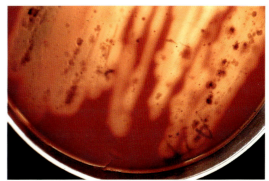
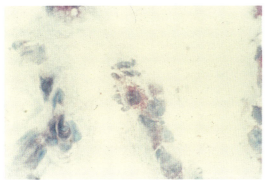
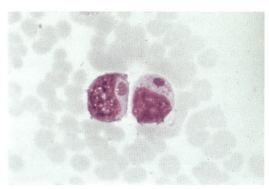

▲ Fig. 208: *Treponema hyodysenteriae*, faecal smear from a pig, microscopic detection by means of fluorescent antibodies. Magnification x 400
▼ Fig. 210: *Coxiella burnetii*, microscopic demonstration of the organism within a disintegrating histiocyte in a cow's udder. Magnification x 1000. (Fig. 210 was supplied by Dr. K. E. Schaal, Leutkirch)

▲ Fig. 209: *Treponema hyodysenteriae*, culture of a pig's faecal sample on selective medium with addition of 5 % bovine blood, anaerobic incubation, severe haemolysis extending beyond the inoculation streak and no clearly defined colonies. Magnification x 0.4
▼ Fig. 211: *Ehrlichia canis,* blood film, Giemsa stain, parasites in mononuclear cells. Magnification x 1000 (Fig. 211 was supplied by Prof. Dr. K. T. Friedhoff, Hannover)

▲ Abb. 208: *Treponema hyodysenteriae*, Kotausstrich vom Schwein, mikroskopischer Nachweis mit fluoreszierenden Antikörpern, Abb.-M. 400 : 1
▼ Abb. 210: *Coxiella burnetii*, mikroskopischer Nachweis des Erregers in einem sich auflösenden Histiozyten im Euter eines Rindes Abb.-M. 1000 : 1 (Abb. von Dr. K. E. Schaal, Leutkirch, zur Verfügung gestellt)

▲ Abb. 209: *Treponema hyodysenteriae*, Kultur einer Schweinekotprobe auf Selektivmedium mit Zusatz von 5 % Rinderblut nach anaerober Bebrütung, kräftige, über den Impfstrich hinausgehende Hämolyse ohne deutlich abgesetzte Kolonien, Abb.-M. 1 : 2,5
▼ Abb. 211: *Ehrlichia canis*, Blutausstrich, Giemsa-Färbung, Parasitenformen in mononukleären Zellen, Abb.-M. 1000 : 1 (Abb. von Prof. Dr. K. T. Friedhoff, Hannover, zur Verfügung gestellt)

anaerobically for a further 4 days. The intensification of haemolysis is recognized by a lighter zone, 1–2 mm broad, along the cut line.

Since *T. hyodysenteriae* is biochemically not very active, the biochemical reactions on their own are really insufficient for the identification of the species, but in combination with serology and cultural methods they make a valuable contribution to this end (tab. 88). Peptone yeast broth is used for

einer 4tägigen Plattenkultur ein Agarblock von 0,5 cm Kantenlänge ausgestanzt. Danach wird die Kultur weitere 4 d anaerob bebrütet. Die Hämolyseverstärkung wird durch eine 1–2 mm breite Aufhellungszone entlang der Ausstanzungslinie sichtbar.

Da *T. hyodysenteriae* biochemisch nicht sehr aktiv ist, kann mit den entsprechenden Reaktionen allein die Artdiagnose kaum gesichert werden. Erst

the carbohydrate breakdown tests and for the gas chromatographic demonstration of volatile fatty acids which are produced during anaerobic metabolism (7). The carbohydrates are added in concentrations of 0.5 to 1%. The reactions are assessed with the pH meter whereby deviations from the control of < 0.25 pH units are considered negative (16).

The presence of α-galactosidase is demonstrated with an API enzyme strip, which indicates another 18 enzyme reactions at the same time. The number-code system of HUNTER & WOOD (9) is recommended for their interpretation.

The essential feature for the identification of *T. innocens* are the strong β-haemolysis, the demonstration of indole, the inability to break down fructose and the formation of α-galactosidase (tab. 88). However, these findings should always be interpreted along with the serological properties (antigenic structure), because of the difficulty of the reliable classification of many haemolytic strains of treponema under one of these two species, even with the aid of biochemical and gas chromatographic tests (1, 17, 20, 22). This is less of a problem in the demonstration of the causal agent in a clinically manifest form of swine dysentery, but it does complicate the interpretation of the findings in the diagnosis of latent infections.

■ Toxins

Lipopolysaccharides have been extracted from *T. hyodysenteriae* as from other Gram-negative bacteria and they have been implicated in possible toxic effects. Haemolysin is viewed as a potential virulence factor; it has been found to be cytotoxic in tissue culture. Haemolysin is produced in smaller amounts by avirulent than by fully virulent strains. It is possible, therefore, that variations in haemolysin production may be the cause of the difference in virulence which is so frequently observed (11).

■ Antigenic structure

Serotypes 1 to 4 have so far been differentiated on the basis of various cell wall antigens (2, 3). They induce a sero-specific immunity in infected animals. The serotypes can be identified with the slide agglutination or growth inhibition tests (16).

im Zusammenhang mit den kulturellen und serologischen Befunden erbringen biochemische Untersuchungsergebnisse wertvolle Hinweise für die endgültige Artdifferenzierung (Tab. 88). Für die Kohlenhydratspaltung, aber auch für den gaschromatographischen Nachweis der im anaeroben Stoffwechsel entstehenden flüchtigen Fettsäuren wird Pepton-Hefe-Bouillon als Basisnährboden verwendet (7). Die Kohlenhydrate werden in Konzentrationen von 0,5 bis 1 % zugesetzt. Der Ausfall der Reaktionen wird mit dem pH-Meter erfaßt, wobei eine pH-Wertabweichung von < 0,25 pH-Einheiten im Vergleich zum Kontrollmedium als negativ zu beurteilen ist (16).

Der Nachweis von α-Galactosidase erfolgt auf API-Enzymstreifen, der gleichzeitig noch weitere 18 Enzymreaktionen berücksichtigt. Für die Beurteilung wird von HUNTER & WOOD (9) die numerische Codierung des Systems empfohlen. Der Indolnachweis ist im flüssigen Anaerobier-TVLS-Nährboden mit Paraffinölüberschichtung unter aeroben Bedingungen möglich (1).

Als wesentliche Merkmale zur Unterscheidung von *T. innocens* werden die kräftige β-Hämolyse, der Indolnachweis sowie die fehlende Fruktosespaltung und α-Galactosidasebildung herausgestellt (Tab. 88). Diese Befunde sollten jedoch stets in Verbindung mit den serologischen Eigenschaften (s. Antigenstruktur) interpretiert werden, da zahlreiche hämolysierende Treponemenstämme von Schweinen und Hunden auch unter Zuhilfenahme von weiteren biochemischen Kriterien und der Gaschromatographie nicht sicher einer der beiden in Frage kommenden Arten zugeordnet werden konnten (1, 17, 20, 22). Diese Problematik berührt weniger den Erregernachweis bei der klinisch manifesten Form der Schweinedysenterie, sondern führt vielmehr in der Diagnostik latenter Infektionen zu Interpretationsschwierigkeiten entsprechender Befunde.

■ Toxine

Wie bei anderen gramnegativen Bakterienarten wurden auch bei *T. hyodysenteriae* Lipopolysaccharide extrahiert und mit möglichen toxischen Effekten in Zusammenhang gebracht. Als potentieller Virulenzfaktor wird bisher das Hämolysin angesehen, es erwies sich in Zellkulturen als zytotoxisch. Das Hämolysin wird von avirulenten Stämmen in geringeren Mengen produziert als von vollvirulenten Isolaten, so daß die unterschiedliche Hämolysinproduktion die Ursache für die häufig zu beobachtenden Virulenzunterschiede sein könnte (11).

■ Antigenstruktur

Aufgrund unterschiedlicher Zellwandantigene ist bislang eine Unterscheidung der Serotypen 1 bis 4 möglich (2, 3), die bei infizierten Tieren eine serotypenspezifische Immunität hervorrufen. Die Bestimmung der Serotypen kann unter Verwendung ab-

The indirect fluorescence antibody technique, which can be employed both for the demonstration of *T. hyodysenteriae* in the test material and for the serological differentiation of isolated treponema species, should also be carried out with absorbed antisera. This is because the common surface antigens of *T. hyodysenteriae* and *T. innocens* can produce false positives.

Various methods have been tried for demonstrating antibodies in the serum. These include, for example, microtitre agglutination, the indirect fluorescent antibody, the passive haemagglutination and the ELISA methods (for literature see HARRIS & GLOCK, 6). Although serological methods are adequate for identifying an outbreak on a farm, they are insufficiently sensitive for pin-pointing latently infected individuals.

■ Animal inoculation

It is best to use pigs for evaluating enteropathogenicity. Acceptable results were obtained with the oral administration in 2-week old SPF piglets.

The colon ligature test on 8–10 week-old pigs was also found suitable. The experimental infection of mice and guinea pigs with *T. hyodysenteriae* produce dysentery-like changes in the large intestine, and this model is therefore recommended for virulence testing. Negative results of the enteropathogenicity test must be interpreted with the greatest circumspection, because passage in pure culture quickly leads to a loss of virulence.

Animal experiments are not essential for routine diagnosis of swine dysentery.

2.2 Treponema innocens

Besides *T. hyodysenteriae* the intestinal tract of pigs also harbours non-pathogenic haemolytic treponemas (8, 9, 14, 26). These were classified by KINYON & HARRIS (12) in their own species *T. innocens* which has since been accepted internationally. *T. innocens* can lead to certain difficulty in the diagnosis of swine dysentery, especially in the case of latent infections with *T. hyodysenteriae*. This is because the two are morphologically identical and the biochemical properties are not always entirely characteristic. Furthermore, serological cross reactions can occur with *T. hyodysenteriae* (1, 17, 20, 23). The most important characters are listed in table 88. Although more extensive serological tests and DNA homology studies support the concept of a separate species *T. innocens*, recent entero-

pathogenicity tests have thrown doubt on the existence of haemolytic non-pathogenic strains of treponema. Thus, BLAHA et al. (4) include the weakly β-haemolytic treponemas in the species *T. hyodysenteriae*, because in animal experiments on pigs using a strain of *T. innocens* they were able to produce symptoms of swine dysentery in 5 passages. Similar observations were made by ANDREWS & HOFFMANN (21). According to the opinions of these authors, the haemolytic treponemas of the pig's gut all belong to a single species which may however encompass strains of different virulence, depending on their adaptation to the large intestine. Therefore, their occurrence invariably represents a risk for the development of swine dysentery. However, the solution to this problem must await the outcome of presently continuing investigations.

schaften wurden in Tab. 88 zusammengestellt. Zwar sprechen weiterführende serologische Untersuchungsergebnisse und DNS-Homologiestudien für das Vorliegen der eigenständigen Art *T. innocens*, in neuerer Zeit werden aber aufgrund von Enteropathogenitätsprüfungen Zweifel an der Existenz einer hämolysierenden, apathogenen Treponemenart geäußert. So rechnen BLAHA et al. (4) die schwach β-hämolysierenden Treponemen zur Art *T. hyodysenteriae*, zumal es ihnen bei Infektionsversuchen an Schweinen in der 5. Tierpassage mit einem *T. innocens*-Stamm gelang, Krankheitserscheinungen der Schweinedysenterie hervorzurufen. Ähnliche Hinweise stammen von ANDREWS & HOFFMANN (zit. nach 21). Nach Ansicht der genannten Autoren gehören die hämolysierenden Treponemen im Darm des Schweines zu einer einzigen pathogenen Art, die allerdings in Abhängigkeit von ihrer Anpassung an den Dickdarm mit unterschiedlich virulenten Stämmen auftreten kann, so daß ihr Vorkommen in jedem Fall eine potentielle Gefahr der Entstehung von Schweinedysenterie darstellt. Eine Klärung dieser Problematik ist sicherlich erst durch weiterführende Untersuchungen zu erwarten.

Bibliography / Literatur

1. AMTSBERG, G., C. MEYER, G. KIRPAL, M. MERKT & W. BISPING (1984): Untersuchungen zum Vorkommen von Treponemen bei Schweinen. 2. Mitteilung: Versuche zur Charakterisierung der Treponemenstämme aufgrund von hämolysierenden und serologischen Eigenschaften sowie der Indolbildung und Virulenzprüfung. Berl. Münch. tierärztl. Wschr. 97, 171–176.
2. BAUM, D. H., & L. A. JOENS (1979): Serotypes of beta-hemolytic Treponema hyodysenteriae. Infect. Immun. 25, 792–796.
3. BAUM, D. H., & L. A. JOENS (1979): Partial purification of a specific antigen of Treponema hyodysenteriae. Infect. Immun. 26, 1211–1223.
4. BLAHA, TH., H. GÜNTHER, K.-D. FLOSSMANN & W. ERLER (1984): Der epizootische Grundvorgang der Schweinedysenterie. Zbl. Vet. Med. B 31, 451–465.
5. COLE, J. R. (1984): Spirochetes. In: CARTER, G. R. (ed.): Diagnostic procedures in veterinary bacteriology and mycology. 4th ed., S. 40–58. Springfield, Illinois: Charles C. Thomas.
6. HARRIS, D. L., & R. D. GLOCK (1981): Swine dysentery. In: DUNNE, H. W., & A. D. LEMAN: Disease of swine. 5th ed. Ames, Iowa: The Iowa State University Press.
7. HOLDEMAN, L. V., E. P. CATO & W. E. C. MOORE (1977): Anaerobe laboratory manual. 4th ed. Blackburg, Virginia: Anaerobe Laboratory Virginia Polytechnic Institute and State University.
8. HUDSON, M. J., T. J. L. ALEXANDER & R. J. LYSONS (1976): Diagnosis of swine dysentery: Spirochaetes which may be confused with Treponema hyodysenteriae. Vet. Rec. 99, 498–500.
9. HUNTER, D., & T. WOOD (1979): An evaluation of the API ZYM system as a means of classifying spirochaetes associated with swine dysentery. Vet. Rec. 104, 383–384.
10. JENKINSON, S. R., & C. R. WINGAR (1981): Selective medium for the isolation of Treponema hyodysenteriae. Vet. Rec. 109, 384–385.
11. KENT, K. A., & R. M. LEMCKE (1984): Purification and cytotoxic activity of a haemolysin produced by Treponema hyodysenteriae. Int. Congr. Pig. Vet. Soc., Ghent, Belgium. S. 185.
12. KINYON, J. M., & D. L. HARRIS (1974): Growth of Treponema hyodysenteriae in liquid medium. Vet. Rec. 95, 219–220.
13. KINYON, J. M., & D. L. HARRIS (1981): Treponema innocens, a new species of intestinal bacteria, and emended description of the type strain of Treponema hyodysenteriae. Int. J. Syst. Bacteriol. 29, 102–109.
14. KINYON, J. M., J. G. SONGER, M. JANC & D. L. HARRIS (1976): Isolation and identification of Treponema hyodysenteriae: Aid to the diagnosis and treatment of swine dysentery. S. 65–74. 19th Ann. Proc. Am. Assoc. Vet. Lab. Diag.
15. KINYON, K. M., D. L. HARRIS & R. D. GLOCK (1977): Enteropathogenicity of varions isolates of Treponema hyodysenteriae. Infect. Immun. 15, 638–646.
16. LEMCKE, R. M., & M. R. BURROWS (1979): A disc growth-inhibition test for differentiating Treponema hyodysenteriae from other intestinal spirochetes. Vet. Rec. 104, 548–551.
17. LEMCKE, R. M., & M. R. BURROWS (1981): A comparative study of spirochaetes from the porcine alimentary tract. J. Hyg. 86, 173–182.
18. LEMCKE, R. M., J. BEW, M. R. BURROWS & R. J. LYSONS (1979): The growth of Treponema hyodysenteriae and other porcine intestinal spirochaetes in a liquid medium. Res. Vet. Sci. 26, 315–319.
19. MEIER, C., B. SRISOPAR & G. AMTSBERG (1982): Untersuchungen zum Vorkommen von Treponemen bei Hunden mit Darmerkrankungen. Berl. Münch. tierärztl. Wschr. 95, 185–188.
20. PICARD, B., S. LARIVIÈRE & S. A. SAHEB (1980): Etude comparative des charactères biochimiques de treponèmes hémolytiques isolés du porc. Can. J. Microbiol. 26, 985–991.
21. POHLENZ, J. F. L., S. C. WHIPP & I. U. ROBINSON (1983): Zur Pathogenese der durch Treponema hyodysenteriae verursachten Dysenterie des Schweines. Dtsch. tierärztl. Wschr. 90, 363–367.

22. Schubert, E. (1983): Kulturell-biochemische und gaschromatographische Untersuchungen an Treponemenstämmen aus dem Darmkanal von Schweinen und Hunden. Vet. Med. Diss., Hannover.

23. Schubert, R. M. (1984): Genus III Treponema Schaudinn 1905. In: Krieg, N. R., & J. G. Holt (ed.): Bergey's Manual of Systematic Bacteriology. Vol. 1, S. 49–57. Baltimore, London: Williams & Wilkins.

24. Songer, J. G., J. M. Kinyon & D. L. Harris (1976): Selective medium for isolation of Treponema hyodysenteriae. J. clin. Microbiol. **4**, 57–60.

25. Sztoikov, V., F. Osztotics & L. Molnár (1982): Durch Treponema hyodysenteriae bedingte Erkrankungen im Tierbestand eines großen Nutriazuchtbetriebes (ungar.) Mag. Allatorv. Lapja **37**, 94–97.

26. Taylor, D. J., & T. J. L. Alexander (1971): The production of dysentery in swine by feeding cultures containing spirochaete. Brit. Vet. J. **127**, 58–61.

27. Whipp, S. C., D. L. Harris, J. M. Kinyon, J. G. Songer & R. D. Glock (1978): Enteropathogenicity testing of Treponema hyodysenteriae in ligated colonic loops of swine. Am. J. Vet. Res. **39**, 1293–1296.

Rickettsiae and Chlamydias
Rickettsien und Chlamydien

This group of bacteria contains obligate cell parasites. They were frequently looked upon as large viruses, but they are true bacteria, because they possess both DNA and RNA, multiply by binary fission, have their own metabolism and are sensitive to antibiotics. In other respects too they exhibit all the structural elements of prokaryotic cells. Their systematic classification is given in table 89, and the most important animal pathogens in table 90.

1   Rickettsiae
1.1   Coxiella (C.) burnetii

■ **Incidence and veterinary significance**
C. burnetii is the causal agent of Q-fever, a zooanthroponosis. The organism occurs in numerous ticks, and in the Federal Republic of Germany its incidence is linked to the distribution of *Dermacentor marginatus,* and is found especially to the south of the Main: Hesse, Baden-Württemberg, Bavaria, North Rhine-Westphalia. Only isolated infections have so far been reported in North-west Germany. Through bites and faeces, the agent is transmitted to wild animals and animals useful to man. The larvae and nymphs of the three-host tick *Dermacentor* transmit the infection to small vertebrates (e. g. field mice, hares, rabbits). The adult form attacks larger animals, especially sheep, goats and cattle, occasionally other mammals and birds.

The disease usually takes a latent form in cattle and sheep but in isolated cases abortions can occur; in sheep these may take on epidemic proportions. Other symptoms, such as weakness, fever and conjunctivitis can occur in exceptional cases.

Affected animals disseminate the organism in large numbers in the milk, the excreta and, at the time of parturition or at abortion, in the placenta or with the amniotic fluid. When dried onto dust particles the agent can survive for long periods (30

Bei dieser Gruppe von Bakterien handelt es sich um obligate Zellparasiten. Sie wurden häufig als große Viren angesprochen, sind aber echte Bakterien, da sie DNS und RNS besitzen, sich durch Querteilung vermehren, einen eigenen Stoffwechsel haben, antibiotikaempfindlich sind und auch sonst alle Strukturelemente einer Prokaryontenzelle besitzen. Ihre systematische Einteilung ist in der Tab. 89 zusammengefaßt. Die wichtigsten tierpathogenen Arten enthält die Tab. 90.

1   Rickettsien
1.1   Coxiella (C.) burnetii

■ **Vorkommen und medizinische Bedeutung**
C. burnetii ist Ursache des Q-Fiebers, einer Zooanthroponose. Der Erreger kommt bei zahlreichen Zecken vor, in der Bundesrepublik ist sein Vorkommen gebunden an die Verbreitung von *Dermacentor marginatus* (insbesondere südlich der Mainlinie, Hessen, Baden-Württemberg, Bayern, Nordrhein-Westfalen). In Nordwestdeutschland kommen bisher nur vereinzelt Infektionen vor. Der Erreger wird durch Biß und Kot auf Wild- und Nutztiere übertragen. Die Larven und Nymphen der dreiwirtigen Zecke *Dermacentor* vermitteln die Infektion besonders auf kleine Wirbeltiere (z. B. Erdmäuse, Hasen, Kaninchen), die adulte Form befällt größere Tiere, insbesondere Schaf, Ziege und Rind, gelegentlich auch andere Säugetiere und Vögel.

Bei Rind und Schaf verläuft die Infektion meistens latent, in Einzelfällen und beim Schaf auch gehäuft kann es zu Aborten kommen. Andere Symptome (Abgeschlagenheit, Fieber, Konjunktivitis) werden nur ausnahmsweise beobachtet.

Von den Tieren wird der Erreger in hohen Zahlen mit Milch, Exkreten und im Zusammenhang mit Geburten oder Aborten mit Eihäuten und Fruchtwasser ausgeschieden und besitzt, angetrocknet an

to 50 days and more). Man is therefore exposed to airborne dust infections (6, 7, 9, 11, 13, 15).

■ Morphology and microscopic demonstration
(fig. 210)

The bacterium is distinctly polymorphic. The most common are rods (0.2–0.4 – 0.4–1.0 µm) which occasionally appear in pairs and spheres (0.3–0.4 µm). The rod forms are distinctly smaller than other rickettsiae. They are Gram-negative and stain with the Stamp, Stableforth, Giemsa and Macchiavello methods.

The demonstration of the causal organism by direct microscopy is only possible if the coxiellae are present in large numbers. This occurs only in placentas after abortion, in smears from the spleen of experimentally infected animals and in the yolk sac of egg cultures. In the placenta the red-stained coxiellae are usually present in groups (for the differential diagnosis of brucellae and chlamydia see figures 181 and 216).

■ Demonstration by culture

This is possible by yolk sac inoculation in embryonated hen's eggs which have been incubated for 6 to 7 days. Penicillin and streptomycin can be added to the test sample to suppress contaminants. Some

■ Morphologie und mikroskopischer Nachweis
(Abb. 210)

Das Bakterium zeigt einen deutlichen Polymorphismus, dabei überwiegen Stäbchen (0,2–0,4 × 0,4–1,0 µm), die gelegentlich paarweise gelagert sind, und Sphärula (0,3–0,4 µm). Die Stäbchenformen sind im Vergleich zu anderen Rickettsien deutlich kleiner. Das Bakterium verhält sich gramnegativ und läßt sich gut nach Stamp, Stableforth, Giemsa oder Macchiavello färben.

Der diagnostische Erregernachweis durch direkte mikroskopische Untersuchung ist nur möglich, wenn im Untersuchungsmaterial mit einem hohen Coxiellengehalt gerechnet werden kann. Dies kann für Plazenten nach Aborten, für Milzausstriche von Versuchstieren nach entsprechender Vermehrung sowie für den Dottersack nach Eikulturen zutreffen. Die Coxiellen sind in den Eihäuten nesterförmig gelagert und rot gefärbt (Differentialdiagnose zu Brucellen und Chlamydien, s. Abb. 181 und 216).

■ Kultureller Erregernachweis

Kultureller Erregernachweis ist über das bebrütete Hühnerei möglich. Es werden 6–7 d bebrütete Eier in den Dottersack beimpft. Dem Untersuchungsmaterial kann Penicillin und Streptomycin zur Un-

Table 89: Taxonomy of Rickettsiales

Tabelle 89: Taxonomische Übersicht zu den Rickettsiales

Order 1: Rickettsiales
Family 1: Rickettsiaceae

Tribus 1: Rickettsieae	Tribus 2: Ehrlichieae	Tribus 3: Wohlbachieae
Genera:	Genera:	Genera:
Rickettsia	Ehrlichia	Wohlbachia
cause of various forms of human epidemic typhus	Cowdria	Ricketsiella (both genera occur mainly in arthropods)
Rochalimaea R. quintala, cause of 5-day fever of man.	Neorickettsia (occurs in canines, USA)	
Coxiella		

Family 2 Bartonellaceae	Family 3: Anaplasmataceae
Genera:	Genera:
Bartonella (human pathogen)	Anaplasma
Grahamella (in hedgehogs and mice in USA)	Paranaplasma
	Aegyptianella
	Haemobartonella
	Eperythrozoon

Order 2: Chlamydiales
Family: Chlamydiaceae
Genus: Chlamydia

Table 90: Rickettsiae of veterinary importance

Tabelle 90: Veterinärmedizinisch wichtige Rickettsien

Family	Genus	Species	Cell parasitism
Rickett-siaceae	Coxiella	burnetii*	in cell vacuoles of the reticulohistiocytic system
	Ehrlichia (Cytoecetes)	equi*	granulocytes
		phagocytophila*	
	Ehrlichia	canis	mononuclear cells
	Cowdria	ruminantium	Cytoplasm of the vascular endothelium
Anaplasma-taceae	Anaplasma	marginale	marginal
		centrale	central — in erythrocytes
		ovis	marginal
	Aegyptianella	pullorum	in erythrocytes
	Haemobartonella	felis*	on erythrocytes (in folds)
	Eperythrozoon	wenyoni*	
		ovis*	on erythrocytes
		suis*	

* This organism has been isolated in Germany

* Der Erreger wurde in Deutschland nachgewiesen

embryos die early (about 6 days after the injection), the remainder are killed after 12 days and examined for the presence of coxiella.

There is no reason why cell culture should not be used, but so far it has not established itself in diagnosis (5, 12).

■ **Demonstration by animal inoculation**
If it is anticipated that the sample to be examined contains but few coxiellae, then animal inoculation is indispensible. The animal of choice is the guinea pig.
▷ Guinea pig experiment with passage: By passaging splenic or testicular material the number of organisms can be increased to such an extent that they can be observed by direct microscopy in impression smears from the spleen. The correct moment for passage can be determined by following the rise in the blood titre in weekly samples of heart blood, or alternatively by the rise in body tempera-

terdrückung der Begleitflora zugegeben werden. Die Embryonen sterben zu einem Teil kurzfristig ab (etwa 6. d p. i.) oder werden am 12. d p. i. getötet und auf Coxiellen untersucht.

Die Zellkultur ist grundsätzlich möglich, hat sich aber bisher in die Diagnostik nicht eingeführt (5, 12).

■ **Erregernachweis durch den Tierversuch**
Wenn in dem Untersuchungsmaterial nur mit wenigen Coxiellen zu rechnen ist, kann auf den Tierversuch nicht verzichtet werden. Versuchstier der Wahl ist das Meerschweinchen.
▷ Meerschweinchenversuch mit Passagen: Dabei kann durch Passageimpfung mit Milz- und Hodenmaterial die Erregermenge so hoch getrieben werden, daß ein direkter mikroskopischer Erregernachweis im Milztupfpräparat möglich wird. Der geeignete Passagezeitpunkt wird durch wöchentliche Kontrolle des Bluttiteranstiegs (Herzpunktion) ermittelt oder durch Temperaturmessung (unspezifi-

Table 90: Continued   Tabelle 90: Fortsetzung

Host	Transmission	Distribution	Disease
sheep, goat, cattle, other mammals, man	ticks, dust, contact	world-wide	Q-fever
horse, dog	unknown, ticks?	USA, Europe	equine ehrlichiosis
sheep, cattle	Ixodes ricinus	Europe	tick-borne fever
canides	Rhipicephalus sanguineus	Asia, Africa, America, Europe	ehrlichiosis in dog tropical canine panleucopenia
cattle, sheep, goat, wild ruminants	various Amblyomma species	Africa	heart water
cattle, zebu, buffalo, sheep, goat	various types of ticks	Africa, Australia, USA	malignant bovine anaplasmosis
cattle		Africa, Asia, America, SE Europe	benign bovine anaplasmosis
sheep, goat			anaplasmosis of sheep and goats
domestic and wild birds	Argas persicus	Africa, Asia SE Europe	aegyptianellosis of poultry
cat	haematophagic arthropods	world-wide	feline infectious anaemia
cattle			anaemia, mild disease
sheep	haematophagic arthropods	world-wide	anaemia, haematoglobinuria
pig			ictero-anaemia

ture. However, it must be borne in mind that nonspecific rises in temperature may occur. It is desirable to carry out the passage during the acute stage of the infectioin, because neutralizing antibodies are produced later. It is also recommended to passage when the complement fixation titre rises. With high infection doses this is the case after 10–14 days. Such a passage procedure presents a high risk of infection to the laboratory personnel (SCHAAL, 8).
▷ Guinea pig experiment without passages: This has been found effective for diagnostic purposes and is without risk to the staff. The method is illustrated in figure 212.

■ **Serological diagnosis**
The serological diagnosis is very important in view of the great difficulty and cost in demonstrating *C. burnetii*. It is also more reliable than animal inoculation and can replace the latter entirely, unless the isolation of the organism is required (REUSCH et al., 4). *C. burnetii* has two surface anti-

sches Fieber möglich) ermittelt. Die Passagierung im akuten Infektionsstadium ist erforderlich, da es später zur Ausbildung neutralisierender Antikörper kommen kann. Es empfiehlt sich, die Weiterverimpfung dann vorzunehmen, wenn die KBR-Titer ansteigen, dies ist bei hohen Infektionsdosen nach 7 bis 9 d, im allgemeinen nach 10 bis 14 d der Fall. Mit dem Passageverfahren ist eine hohe Infektionsgefahr für das Personal verbunden (SCHAAL, 8).
▷ Meerschweinchenversuch ohne Passagen: Hat sich diagnostisch bewährt und ist ohne Gesundheitsrisiko für das Personal möglich. Der Untersuchungsgang ist in der Abb. 212 dargestellt.

■ **Serologische Diagnose**
Angesichts der besonderen Schwierigkeiten und Aufwendungen des Erregernachweises ist die serologische Diagnose besonders wichtig. Da sie zudem eine höhere Sicherheit als der Tierversuch aufweist, kann sie diesen, sofern nicht eine Erregerisolierung erforderlich ist, voll ersetzen (REUSCH et al., 4).

```
┌─────────────────────────────────────────────────┐
│                   Specimens                     │
├─────────────────────────────────────────────────┤
│   Milk, blood, organs etc.; it may be advisable │
│   to chop up or homogenize, filter through gauze,│
│              and centrifuge                     │
└─────────────────────────────────────────────────┘
                        │
┌─────────────────────────────────────────────────┐
│              Animal inoculation                 │
├─────────────────────────────────────────────────┤
│ Guinea pig: about 0.5 ml test sample injected into│
│ both testes until they are tightly filled; additionally│
│   4–5 ml intraperitoneally or subcutaneously    │
└─────────────────────────────────────────────────┘
                        │
┌─────────────────────────────────────────────────┐
│        Interpretation of animal inoculation     │
├─────────────────────────────────────────────────┤
│ 1. Early diagnosis after 10 to14 days: heart puncture and demonstration of antibodies by means of │
│    complement fixation test. At this stage only a positive result is proof. │
│ 2. After 4 weeks: guinea pigs are killed and antibodies are demonstrated in the blood with the complement │
│    fixation test. If the test samples were milk, juices from meat or organ emulsions then coxiellae cannot │
│    be seen at this stage in the guinea pigs organs by microscopy, thus there is little danger of infection of │
│    laboratory staff. │
│    If it is necessary to isolate the organism then the numbers can be increased by passage of splenic or │
│    testicular material through guinea pigs. A direct microscopic observation of the organisms may then be │
│    possible. │
└─────────────────────────────────────────────────┘
```

Fig. 212: Diagnostic inoculation of guinea pigs for the demonstration of coxiellae (after SCHAAL, 8)

Abb. 212: Diagnostischer Meerschweinchenversuch zum Nachweis von Coxiellen (nach SCHAAL, 8)

gens. Strains that occur naturally possess both of these and antigen I overlies and masks the more deeply situated antigen II (phase I strains). Antigen I is lost in egg cultures and such strains then have only antigen II (phase II strains).

The standard method of demonstrating the antibodies is with the complement fixation and agglutination methods. For the CFT antigen II obtained from egg culture is used, but phase I antigen has to be employed for the agglutination test because *C. burnetii* phase II will agglutinate spontaneously.

As a rule the CFT is used with cold fixation in the microtitre system. The antigen is obtainable commercially (e. g. Behringwerke).

The capillary agglutination test of Cuoto requires coxiella stained with haematoxylin (phase I strains from fresh animal material without prolonged egg passage). This method permits cows' milk samples and blood serum from animals and man to be examined (2, 3, 8).

The ELISA test has also proved itself in serological diagnosis (1, 14).

C. burnetii besitzt auf der Zelloberfläche zwei verschiedene Antigene. In der Natur vorkommende virulente Stämme besitzen beide Antigene, wobei das Antigen I das tieferliegende Antigen II überlagert und maskiert (Phase-I-Stämme). Bei Züchtung in der Eikultur geht das Antigen I verloren, so daß solche Stämme nur noch das Antigen II besitzen (Phase-II-Stämme).

Standardmethoden für den Antikörpernachweis sind die KBR und die Agglutination. Als Antigen für die KBR werden in der Eikultur gewonnene Coxiellen mit dem Antigen II benutzt, für die Agglutination müssen Antigene der Phase I verwendet werden, da *C. burnetii* der Phase II spontan agglutiniert.

Die KBR wird im allgemeinen als Kältebindung im Mikrotitersystem durchgeführt. Das Antigen ist käuflich zu erwerben (z. B. Behringwerke).

Die Kapillaragglutination nach Luoto benutzt hämotoxylingefärbte Coxiellen (Phase I-Stämme, gewonnen aus frischem tierischen Material ohne längere Eipassagen). Mit der Methode können Milch vom Rind sowie Blutserum von Tier und Mensch untersucht werden (2, 3, 8).

Für die serologische Diagnose hat sich ferner der ELISA bewährt (1, 14).

Bibliography / Literatur

1. GOUVERNEUR, K., N. SCHMEER & H. KRAUSS (1984): Zur Epidemiologie des Q-Fiebers in Hessen: Untersuchungen mit dem Enzymimmuntest (ELISA) und der Komplementbindungsreaktion (KBR). Berl. Münch. tierärztl. Wschr. **97**, 437–441.

2. LUOTO, L., & D. MASON (1956): An agglutination test for bovine Q-fever performed on milk samples. J. Immunol. **74**, 222–227.

3. LUOTO, L. (1953): Capillar-agglutination at Q-fever of cattle. J. Immunol. **71**, 226–229.

4. REUSCH, C., W. FROST, W. LOHRBACH & G. WACHENDÖRFER (1984): Vergleichsuntersuchungen mit dem Meerschweinchen- und Mäusetest zum Nachweis von Coxiella burnetii — Zugleich eine Studie über die Verbreitung des Q-Fiebers in Süd- und Mittelhessen. Dtsch. tierärztl. Wschr. 91, 47–52.
5. RHODE, M. (1973): Vergleichende Untersuchungen über die Vermehrung von Coxiella burnetii in Zellkulturen unter Berücksichtigung verschiedener mikroskopischer Nachweisverfahren. Vet. Med. Diss., Gießen.
6. SCHAAL, E. H., & J. SCHÄFER (1984): Zur Verbreitung des Q-Fiebers in einheimischen Rinderbeständen. Dtsch. tierärztl. Wschr. 91, 52–56.
7. SCHAAL, E. H. (1982): Zur Euterbesiedlung mit Coxiella burnetii beim Q-Fieber des Rindes. Dtsch. tierärztl. Wschr. 89, 411–414.
8. SCHAAL, E. (1972): Zur Diagnose des Q-Fiebers bei Tieren. Dtsch. tierärztl. Wschr. 79, 25–31.
9. SCHAAL, E. (1969): Coxiella burnetii bei Schlachttieren. Schlacht- u. Viehhof-Ztg. 69, 339–341.
10. SCHAAL, E. (1965): Untersuchungen über das Vorkommen von Rickettsia burnetii in Fleisch und Organen Q-fieberinfizierter Rinder. Fleischwirtschaft 45, 127–130.
11. SCHAAF, J. (1961): Query-Fieber des Rindes. Mhefte Tierhk. 13, 1–18.
12. SCHLIESSER, T., & H. KRAUSS (1982): Bekämpfung des Q-Fiebers. Tierärztl. Prax. 10, 11–22.
13. SCHLIESSER, T. (1969): Das Q-Fieber und seine hygienische Bedeutung. Schlacht- und Viehhof-Ztg. 69, 344–347.
14. SCHMEER, N., H. KRAUSS & B. WILSKE (1984): Untersuchungen zur Serodiagnose des Q-Fiebers beim Menschen — Nachweis von nicht-komplementbindenden IgM-Antikörpern im enzyme-linked-immunosorbent-assay (ELISA). Immun. Infekt. 12, 245–251.
15. WEGENER, K. H. (1957): Das Q-Fieber und seine milchhygienische Bedeutung. Kieler Milchwirtschaftliche Forschungsber. 9, 509–535.

1.2 Ehrlichia (E.)

The most important *Ehrlichia* species are listed in table 90.

Ehrlichia are parasites found in cytoplasmic vacuoles of leucocytes. In that location the small (0.2–0.6 µm) elementary bodies produce first the initial body (2 µm) by continual binary fission, and then colonies (morulae), which are 3–5 µm in size. The genus *Ehrlichia*, which parasitized mononuclear cells, is distinct from the genus *Cytoecetes* which is found in granulocytes.

The diagnosis relies on the microscopic demonstration (fig. 211) of the organism in Giemsa-stained smears (buffy coat [white cell layer] from haematocrit tubes).

Large doses of tetracyclines have proved effective in therapy.

Apart from the species listed in table 90, other Ehrlichia have been described in various animal species (cattle, sheep, goats, rodents etc.), but their classification has not been settled.

1.3 Cowdria, Anaplasma, Aegyptianella

Further information about occurrence, incidence and significance will be found in table 90.

1.4 Haemobartonella (H.)

Haemobartonella are small (0.2–0.4 µm) coccoid rickettsiae, which are found on the depressed cell membrane of erythrocytes. They multiply by binary fission.

H. felis: Haemobartonellosis of the cat is seen only occasionally in Germany and produces the following clinical signs: weakness, apathy, inappe-

tence, emaciation, dehydration and anaemia. There is a rise in body temperature during the acute course.

The diagnosis is made on a Giemsa-stained blood film. The blue-purple coccoid organisms are found to lie singly or in short chains on the surface of the red blood cells (fig. 215). *H. felis* is demonstrable in the blood for only a short period. The blood films should, therefore, be made daily or during an acute episode.

Tetracyclines, chloramphenicol and arsenic preparations have been found effective in treatment (5, 9, 11).

magerung, Exsikkose und Anämie. Bei akutem Verlauf ist die Körpertemperatur erhöht.

Die Diagnose erfolgt im giemsagefärbten Blutausstrich. Der blauviolette, kokkoide Erreger liegt einzeln oder in kurzen Ketten auf der Erythrozytenoberfläche (Abb. 215). *H. felis* ist nur kurzzeitig im Blut nachweisbar, deswegen sollten die Blutausstriche täglich oder während der Fieberschübe angefertigt werden.

In der Therapie haben sich Tetracycline, Chloramphenicol und Arsenpräparate bewährt (5, 9, 11).

1.5 Eperythrozoon (Ep.)

The eperythrozoon are epi-erythrocytic parasites and are seldom found in the blood plasma *(Ep. teganodes)* or on the surface of thrombocytes *(Ep. tuomii)*. They are also observed in Giemsa-stained blood films. The most important species are listed in table 90.

In Germany *Ep. suis* is the most common and is the cause of a spontaneous eperythrozoonosis. This occurs in pigs of all ages, but mainly in weaners and store pigs. The most obvious signs are fever, jaundice and anaemia (1, 6, 7, 8, 10).

Demonstration of the causal agent: in Giemsa-stained blood films taken during the early febrile phase one can see the coccoid to ring-shaped eperythrozoan, which lie on or between the erythrocytes (fig. 214).

The therapeutic agent of choice is oxytetracycline.

1.5 Eperythrozoon (Ep.)

Die Eperythrozoen parasitieren meistens eperythrozytär, seltener im Blutplasma *(Ep. teganodes)* oder auf der Thrombozytenoberfläche *(Ep. tuomii)*. Ihr Nachweis geschieht ebenfalls im giemsagefärbten Blutausstrich. Die wichtigsten Arten sind in der Tab. 90 zusammengestellt.

In Deutschland kommt am häufigsten *Ep. suis* als Ursache einer spontanen Eperythrozoonose vor. Sie tritt bei Schweinen jeden Alters, hauptsächlich jedoch bei Absatzferkeln und Mastläufern auf. Die auffälligsten Krankheitssymptome sind Fieber, Ikterus und Anämie (1, 6, 7, 8, 10).

Erregernachweis: In giemsagefärbten Blutausstrichen aus der frühen Fieberphase sind kokkoide bis ringförmige Eperythrozoen nachweisbar, die auf oder zwischen den Erythrozyten liegen (Abb. 214).

Das Mittel der Wahl zur Behandlung ist Oxytetracyclin.

Bibliography / Literatur

1. BOLLWAHN, W. (1982): Die Eperythrozoonose (Ikteroanämie) der Schweine. Prakt. Tierarzt **63**, 1043–1046.
2. BÜSCHER, G., R. GANDRAS, G. APEL & T. K. FRIEDHOFF (1984): Der erste Fall von Ehrlichiosis beim Pferd in Deutschland. Dtsch. tierärztl. Wschr. **91**, 408–409.
3. FRIEDHOFF, K. T. (1982): Rickettsieninfektionen (Ehrlichia, Eperythrozoon, Haemobartonella) bei Haustieren in Deutschland. Fortschr. der Vet. Med., Heft 35, 204–209. Berlin, Hamburg: Paul Parey.
4. FRIEDHOFF, K., W. DROMMER & M. WOLFHAGEN (1971): Infektionen mit Eperythrozoon ovis bei Schafen in Norddeutschland. Berl. Münch. tierärztl. Wschr. **84**, 361–368.
5. GARBNER, A., & G. SAUERWEIN (1984): Zur Hämobartonellose der Katze. Tierärztl. Umschau **39**, 378–381.
6. HEINRITZI, K., I. WENTZ & W. BOLLWAHN (1984): Hämatologische Befunde bei der akuten Eperythrozoonose der Schweine. Berl. Münch. tierärztl. Wschr. **97**, 401–407.
7. HOFFMANN, H. (1984): Symptomatologie und Diagnostik der Eperythrozoonose in Ferkelerzeugerbetrieben. Tierärztl. Umschau **39**, 474–479.
8. KORN, G., & M. MUSSGAY (1968): Ein Fall von Eperythrozoonose suis mit differentialdiagnostischer Bedeutung bei einem Schweinepestverdacht. Zbl. Vet. Med. B **15**, 617–630.
9. KÜHNERT, R. (1967): Untersuchungen zur Haemobartonellose und Babesiose der Katzen. Vet. Med. Diss., München.
10. MÜLLER, E., & G. NEDDENRIEP (1979): Eperythrozoonose in einem Ferkelerzeugerbetrieb in Norddeutschland. Prakt. Tierarzt **59**, 662–665.
11. SAUERWEIN, G., & A. GRABNER (1982): Zur Behandlung der Haemobartonellose der Katze mit Thiocetarsamid-Natrium (Caparsolate). Kleintierpraxis **27**, 323–328.

2 Chlamydia (Chl.)

The chlamydia (elementary bodies) are coccoid micro-organisms (0.3 µm) which have the following reproductive cycle:
a) Infection of the cell by very dense coccoid elementary bodies, diameter about 0.3 µm, lying in a vacuole within the host cell,
b) grow into a large cell (initial body, reticular body) of 1 µm diameter, non-infectious,
c) division of the initial body, the new initial bodies reduce in size to infectious elementary bodies (condensation),

2 Chlamydia (Chl.)

Die Chlamydien (Elementarkörperchen) sind kokkoide Mikroorganismen (0,3 µm) und durchlaufen bei ihrer Vermehrung folgenden Zyklus:
a) Infektion der Zelle durch kokkoide Elementarkörperchen, Durchmesser etwa 0,3 µm, von sehr dichter Struktur, in einer Vakuole der Wirtszelle gelegen,
b) Heranwachsen zu einer Großzelle (Initialkörperchen, Retikulärkörper), Durchmesser etwa 1 µm, nicht infektiös,
c) Teilung des Initialkörperchen, die neu entstandenen Initialkörperchen verkleinern sich zu infektiösen Elementarkörperchen (Kondensation),

Table 91: Incidence of Chlamydia infections in domestic mammals

Tabelle 91: Vorkommen von Chlamydien-Infektionen bei Haussäugetieren

Species	Clinical signs	Literature
Horse	Pneumonia gastro-intestinal symptoms hepatopathy abortion encephalitis polyarthritis latent infections	11, 19, 20, 23
Cattle	pneumonia enteritis infections of the urinary tract abortion, inflammation of seminal vesicle excretion in semen mastitis encephalitis polyarthritis keratoconjunctivitis (frequently mixed infections with Neisseria catarrhalis, Moraxella bovis, Corynebacterium pyogenes) latent infections	2, 4, 7, 16, 17, 18, 21, 22, 23, 26, 27, 28, 29, 31, 35
sheep goat	pneumonia infections of the digestive tract abortion mastitis polyarthritis keratoconjunctivitis latent infections	3, 5, 13, 14, 20, 23, 24
Pig	pneumonia abortion, orchitis polyarthritis, polyserositis pericarditis latent infections	9, 15, 23, 25, 30
Dog Cat	pneumonia enteritis encephalitis keratoconjunctivitis, keratitis superficialis polyarthritis	6, 10, 20, 32

d) rupture of the host cell and liberation of the elementary bodies; duration of the cycle about 40 hours.

The genus has two species:
▷ *Chl. trachomatis* occurs exclusively in man and is the cause of various illnesses as, for example, trachoma, inclusion conjunctivitis, non-specific genital infections, lymphogranuloma inguinale,
▷ *Chl. psittaci* the cause of various conditions in man and animals (tab. 91).

2.1 Chlamydia psittaci

■ Incidence and veterinary significance

Chl. psittaci is, first and foremost, the cause of psittacosis and ornithosis in birds and of human psittacosis. Besides these, various infections of mammals, which are often latent but may present various clinical signs, are attributed to this organism (tab. 91).

■ Microscopic demonstration of organism

This consists of visualizing the inclusion bodies. The methods of Stamp or Stableforth (modified Ziehl-Neelsen stains) have been found very effective for this. The elementary bodies, lying in groups either intra- or extra-cellularly are stained red (fig. 226). Suitable material for examination in psittacosis are impression smears from air sacs, in abortion from placentas. Other useful methods are the Giemsa stain and the fluorescence microscopic demonstration of the chlamydia.

■ Cultural demonstration

For this purpose the organism is grown in embryonated hen's eggs or in suitable tissue cultures.
▷ Egg culture: The Chlamydia are grown on the wall of the yolk sac of 6-day old chick embryos. The specimen to be examined is homogenized and antibiotics are added to suppress contaminants. This is allowed to stand for 30 minutes by which time the larger particles have settled. 0.25 ml of the supernatant are then injected into the yolk sac. Before inoculation the eggs are placed vertically for two hours, with the blunt end uppermost, so that the yolk sac and the embryo are in the correct position. The shell at the top is then swabbed with iodine solution and pierced with a tuberculin needle, which extends into the air cell. A long hypodermic needle is now passed through the hole in a vertical direction from the top to about the middle of the egg, and the inoculum is injected. The opening is closed with melted paraffin wax and the eggs are replaced horizontally into the incubator. As a rule the embryos die after 5–10 days and the chlamydia can be demonstrated microscopically in the wall of the yolk sac (MITSCHERLICH, 13).
▷ Cell culture: Coverslip culture of Buffalo Green

d) Ruptur der Wirtszelle und Freiwerden der Elementarkörperchen, Dauer des Zyklus etwa 40 h. Die Gattung umfaßt zwei Arten:
▷ *Chl. trachomatis*, kommt ausschließlich beim Menschen vor und ist Ursache unterschiedlicher Erkrankungen wie z.B. des Trachoms, Einschlußkonjunktivitis, unspezifische Genitalinfekte, Lymphogranuloma inguinale,
▷ *Chl. psittaci*, Ursache verschiedenartiger Krankheitsbilder beim Tier und beim Menschen (Tab. 91).

2.1 Chlamydia psittaci

■ Vorkommen und medizinische Bedeutung

Chl. psittaci ist in erster Linie Erreger der Psittakose und Ornithose der Vögel sowie der Psittakose des Menschen. Daneben kommen verbreitet Infektionen bei Säugetieren vor, die oft latent, aber auch unter Ausbildung sehr verschiedener Erkrankungsformen verlaufen (Tab. 91).

■ Mikroskopischer Erregernachweis

Erfolgt durch den Nachweis der Einschlußkörperchen, zu deren Anfärbung sich besonders die Färbungen nach Stamp oder Stableforth bewährt haben (modifizierte Ziehl-Neelsen-Färbungen). Dabei färben sich die intra- oder extrazellulär überwiegend in Nestern gelegenen Elementarkörperchen rot (Abb. 216). Geeignete Untersuchungsmaterialien sind bei der Psittakose Abklatschpräparate von den Luftsäcken, bei Aborten von Eihäuten. Geeignet sind auch die Giemsafärbung sowie die fluoreszenz-serologische Darstellung des Erregers.

■ Kultureller Erregernachweis

Erfolgt durch die Anzüchtung des Erregers im bebrüteten Hühnerei oder über geeignete Zellkulturen.
▷ Eikultur: Die Kultur gelingt in den Dottersackwandungen 6tägiger Hühnerembryonen. Von dem Untersuchungsmaterial wird eine homogene Suspension angefertigt, der zur Ausschaltung der Begleitflora Antibiotika zugesetzt werden können. Nach einer Einwirkungszeit von etwa 30 min und nachdem sich gröbere Gewebsteile abgesetzt haben, werden 0,25 ml in den Dottersack injiziert. Zur Injektion werden die Eier 2 h vor der Beimpfung senkrecht gestellt, damit sich Embryo und Dottersack richtig einstellen. Dann wird die Eischale am obenliegenden stumpfen Pol jodiert und mit einer Tuberkulinnadel, die mit der Spitze nur in die Luftkammer des Eies hineinreicht, durchstoßen. Durch die Stichöffnung wird nunmehr eine lange Injektionsnadel senkrecht von oben bis zur Mitte des Eies geführt und das Injektionsmaterial injiziert. Die Stichöffnung wird mit verflüssigtem Paraffin verschlossen. Die Eier werden in waagerechter Lage weiterbebrütet. Die Embryonen sterben meistens nach 5–10 d ab und in den Dottersackwandungen

Monkey (BGM) cells have been found effective for this. The incubated coverslip cultures are stained by the methods of Gimenez or Stamp, fixed to the slide and examined under the microscope. With both staining methods the chlamydia appear as red intracytoplasmic inclusions on a green background (fig. 217). McCoy cells are also suitable for the demonstration of chlamydia in cell culture.

■ Demonstration by animal inoculation

White mice are preferred as the laboratory animal for the diagnosis of psittacosis/ornithosis. The inoculum is usually administered intraperitoneally, less frequently intranasally or intracerebrally. For the best results the mice are killed on the 6th day after the injection and impression smears from the peritoneum are examined microscopically for the presence of elementary bodies. If the result is negative another 1 or 2 passages are carried out. Antibiotics can be added to the tissue suspension to suppress contaminants (50 mg streptomycin and up to 1000 IU penicillin per ml inoculum).

Mice are much less sensitive to chlamydia strains from mammalian sources than from psittacosis strains. In such cases cell and egg cultures are more suitable methods.

1. Diagnosis during life
1. a) Demonstration of causal organism ▷ Test material: Blood from animals before starting chemotherapy. The blood clot is examined or, if the blood is not clotted, the sedimented erythrocytes are used. Faecal sample: freshly vioded faeces or cloacal rinse. The chlamydia can be demonstrated in this material particularly in the acute, but also in the chronic disease. In latent infections no organisms may be excreted or excretion may be sporadic. ▷ Test methods: Cell culture, which is at least as reliable as the mouse test and usually provides quicker results. Egg culture Mouse test 1. b) Demonstration of antibiodies ▷ Test method: Complement fixation test. Most psittacines procedure antibodies after infection (exceptions: grey parrot and budgerigar, which are erratic in antibody production). A titre of 1:8 is interpreted as positive. Proof of a recent infection is a four fold rise in titre in serum samples taken 10 to 30 days apart.

2. Autopsy diagnosis
2. Plays a more important role in the diagnosis of psittacosis. Pathological changes (enlargement of spleen, hepatopathies with focal necrosis, airsacculitis, pericarditis, enteritis) only add up to a possible diagnosis. Microscopic demonstration of causal organisms: LCM bodies in impression smears from air sacs staining after Stamp, Stableforth, Giemsa, Castaneda or Machiavello) or demonstration by fluorescence microscopy. Isolation of the causal organism: cell culture, egg culture, mouse test.

Fig. 213: Diagnosis of psittacosis/ornithosis (after Wachendörfer, 33)

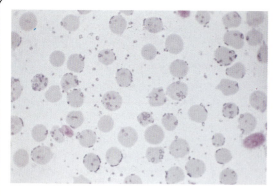 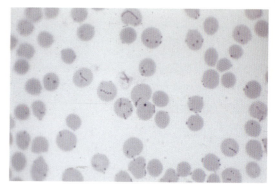

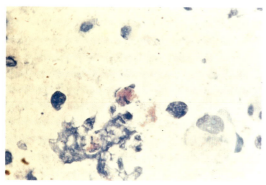 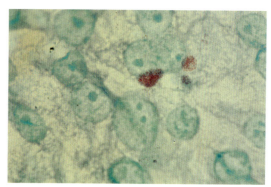

▲ Fig. 214: *Eperythrozoon suis*, blood film, Giemsa stain, coccoid to ring-shaped eperythrozoa on erythrocytes and in the plasma. Magnification × 1000 (This fig. was supplied by Prof. Dr. K. T. Friedhoff, Hannover)

▼ Fig. 216: *Chlamydia psittaci*, smear from the placenta of a ewe after abortion, Stableforth stain, group of red chlamydiae stained red. Magnification × 1000

▲ Abb. 214: *Eperythrozoon suis*, Blutausstrich, Giemsa-Färbung, kokkoide bis ringförmige Eperythrozoen auf Erythrozyten und im Blutplasma, Abb.-M. 1000 : 1 (Die Abbildung wurde von Prof. Dr. K. T. Friedhoff, Hannover, zur Verfügung gestellt)

▼ Abb. 216: *Chlamydia psittaci*, Ausstrich von einer Eihaut eines Schafes nach Abort, Stableforth-Färbung, rote Chlamydiennester, Abb.-M. 1000 : 1

▲ Fig. 215: *Haemobartonella felis*, blood film, Giemsa stain, organisms lying singly or in short chains on the surface of erythrocytes. Magnification × 1000 (This fig. was supplied by Prof. Dr. K. T. Friedhoff, Hannover)

▼ Fig. 217: Demonstration of chlamydia in cell culture (coverslip culture, Buffalo Green Monkey cells) after 6 d incubation, Gimenez stain (fuchsin, malachite green). Magnification × 1000

▲ Abb. 215: *Haemobartonella felis*, Blutausstrich, Giemsa-Färbung, einzeln oder in kurzen Ketten auf der Erythrozytenoberfläche liegende Erreger, Abb.-M. 1000 : 1 (Die Abbildung wurde von Prof. Dr. K. T. Friedhoff, Hannover, zur Verfügung gestellt)

▼ Abb. 217: Nachweis von Chlamydien in der Zellkultur (Deckglaskultur, Buffalo Green Monkey-Zellen) nach 6 d Bebrütung, Färbung nach Giménez (Fuchsin, Malachitgrün), Abb.-M. 1000 : 1

Bibliography / Literatur

1. Arens, M., & W. Weingarten (1981): Vergleichende Untersuchungen an Buffalo Green Monkey (BGM)-Zellen und Mäusen zur Isolierung von Chlamydia psittaci aus Kot- und Organproben von Vögeln. Zbl. Vet. Med. B **28**, 301–309.
2. Danieli, Y., & N. Ayalon (1970): The finding of Bedsonia elementary bodies in uterine discharges as related to post-partum metritis and fertility in a dairy herd. Refuah Vet. **27**, 63–66.
3. Dickinson, L., & B. S. Cooper (1959): Contagious conjunctivo-keratitis of sheep. J. Path. Bact. **78**, 157–266.
4. Dietz, O., J. Wehr, R. Thalmann, A. Popp & W. Buschmann (1983): Neue Untersuchungen zur Ätiologie und Therapie der infektiösen Keratokonjunktivitis. Mh. Vet. Med. **38**, 843–847.
5. Enke, Kh., H. Liebermann & B. Schuckmann (1959): Virusabort und Brucella abortus in einem Schafbestand. Mhefte Tierhk. **14**, 473–475.

6. FRAZER, G., J. NORVAL, A. R. WITHERS & W. E. GREGOR (1969): A case history of psittacosis in the dog. Vet. Rec. **85**, 54–58.
7. JAHN, J., D. AUST & H. ROMER (1972): Genitale Infektionen bei Rindern durch Bedsonien. VIIth Intern. Congr. Animal Prod. Artificial Insemination, München, **1**, 321–325.
8. JOHNSON, F. W. A., M. J. CLARKSON & W. N. SPENCER (1983): Direct isolation of the agent of enzootic abortion of ewes (Chlamydia psittaci) in cell cultures. Vet. Rec. **113**, 413–414.
9. KÖLBL, O., H. BURTSCHER & J. HEBENSTREIT (1970): Polyarthritis bei Schlachtschweinen. Mikrobiol., histol. u. fleischhyg. Untersuchungen und Aspekte. Wien. tierärztl. Mschr. **57**, 355–361.
10. KRAUSS, H. (1982): Die Bedeutung von Rickettsien und Chlamydien bei kleinen Haustieren als Erreger von Zoonosen. Berl. Münch. tierärztl. Wschr. **95**, 470–483.
11. MCCHESNEY, A. D., V. BECERRA & J. J. ENGLAND (1974): Chlamydial polyarthritis in a foal. J. Am. Vet. Med. Ass. **165**, 259–261.
12. MEISSLER, M., & H. KRAUSS (1980): Zur Technik der Isolierung und Züchtung von Chlamydien in der Zellkultur. Fortschr. der Veterinärmed., Heft 30, 13. Kongreßber., 224–230.
13. MITSCHERLICH, E. (1955): Beiträge zum Virusabort des Schafes. 1. Mitt.: Die Ätiologie des Virusabortes des Schafes. Vet. Med. Nachr. Heft 1. 2. Mitt.: Epidemiologie, Seuchenbild und Diagnose des Virusabortes der Schafe. Vet. Med. Nachr. Heft 3.
14. MITSCHERLICH, E. (1954): Der Virusabort des Schafes in Deutschland. Dtsch. tierärztl. Wschr. **61**, 42–45.
15. PLAGEMANN, O. (1981): Chlamydien als Abortursache beim Schwein und als Differentialdiagnose zum Smedi-Komplex. Tierärztl. Umschau **36**, 842–846.
16. ROB, O. (1970): Bewertung der Fertilität und der spermatologischen Befunde bei Bullen mit kulturellem Bedsoniennachweis im Sperma. Veterinari Med. **15**, 369–376.
17. SADOWSKI, M. J., Z. SEMKA & M. FRYMUS (1983): Nachweis von Chlamydien bei Bullen. Mh. Vet. Med. **38**, 724–726.
18. SADOWSKI, J. M., L. JASKOWSKI, L. SZULC & M. TRUSZCZYNSKI (1973): Studies on Bedsonia infection in cattle. II. Occurrence of Bedsonia organism in the semen of suspected bulls. Polskie Arch. Weter. **16**, 491–496.
19. SAITO, (1954): Pneumonie contagieuse de la chèvre. Bull. Off. Int. Epiz. **42**, 676–691.
20. SCHMATZ, H. D., S. SCHMATZ, A. WEBER & J. SAILER (1977): Seroepidemiologische Untersuchungen zum Vorkommen von Chlamydien bei Haus- und Wildtieren. Berl. Münch. tierärztl. Wschr. **90**, 74–76.

21. SCHOOP, G., U. KRÜGER-HANSEN & G. WACHENDÖRFER (1965): Zur Isolierung von Miyagawanellen aus abortierten Rinderfeten. Zbl. Vet. Med. B **12**, 25–32.
22. SCHOOP, G., & E. KAUKER (1956): Infektion eines Rinderbestandes durch ein Virus der Psittakosis-Lymphogranuloma-Gruppe. Gehäufte Aborte im Verlaufe der Erkrankungen. Dtsch. tierärztl. Wschr. **63**, 233–235.
23. SCHOLZ, R. S. (1978): Die Verbreitung, Bedeutung und diagnostische Nachweisbarkeit von Chlamydien-Infektionen bei Tieren (mit Ausnahme der Vögel). Vet. Med. Diss., Hannover.
24. STAUB, H. (1959): Virusabort in einem Ziegenbestand. Dtsch. tierärztl. Wschr. **69**, 98–99.
25. STELLMACHER, H., P. KIELSTEIN, F. HORSCH & J. MARTIN (1983): Zur Bedeutung der Chlamydien-Infektion des Schweines unter besonderer Berücksichtigung der Pneumonien. Mh. Vet. Med. **38**, 601–606.
26. STORZ, I. (1967): Erreger der Psittakose-Gruppe als Ursache von Polyarthritis bei Rindern und Schafen. Vet. med. Nachr. 127–141.
27. STORZ, J., E. J. CARROL, E. H. STEPHENSON, L. BALL & A. K. EUGSTER (1976): Urogenital infection and seminal excretion after inoculation of bulls and rams with Chlamydia. Amer. J. Vet. Res. **37**, 517–520.
28. STORZ, J., E. J. CARROLL, L. BALL & L. C. FAUKNER (1968): Isolation of psittacosis agent (Chlamydia) from semen and epididymis of bulls with seminal vesicultitis syndrome. Am. J. Vet. Res. **29**, 549–555.
29. STORZ, J., A. SMART, M. E. MARIOTT & R. V. DAVIS (1966): Polyarthritis of calves: Isolation of psittacosis agents from affected joints. Am. J. Vet. Res. **27**, 633–641.
30. TOLYBEKOW, A. S., L. A. WISCHNJAKOWA & M. A. DOBIN (1973): Die ätiologische Bedeutung eines Erregers der Bedsoniengruppe für die enzootische Pneumonie der Schweine. Mh. Vet. Med. **18**, 411–414.
31. VEZNIK, Z. (1968): Syndrom der durch Bedsonien verursachten Unfruchtbarkeit des Rindes. Veterinarstvi **18**, 349–352.
32. VOIGT, A., O. DIETZ & V. SCHMIDT (1966): Klinische und experimentelle Untersuchungen zur Ätiologie der Keratitis superficialis chronica. Arch. exp. Vet. Med. **20**, 259–274.
33. WACHENDÖRFER, G. (1971): Zur Diagnostik, Chemoprophylaxe und Therapie der Psittakose bei Sittichen und Papageien. Dtsch. tierärztl. Wschr. **52**, 604–610.
34. WACHENDÖRFER, G., & E. PEHEIM (1962): Zur Züchtung des Schafabortvirus (Miyagawanella ovis) im bebrüteten Hühnerei. Mh. Tierhk. **14**, 220–224.
35. WEHR, J. (1981): Chlamydien als Ursache von Genitalinfektionen beim Bullen. Mh. Vet. Med. **36**, 756.

Mycoplasms
Mykoplasmen

■ **General properties and significance**
■ **Definition and Classification**

Mycoplasms have no cell wall and they are very small. They are the smallest micro-organisms which can multiply independently outside the cell. They can pass through bacterial filters, have a small genome and the guanine and cytosine ratio of their DNA (22–40 mol%) is generally lower than in bacteria (tab. 93).

The classification is based on morphology and biochemical and other properties (tab. 92 and fig. 220). Within the genera the species are identified by their metabolic activity and especially by their surface antigens (growth inhibition and epifluorescence test).

1 Genus: Mycoplasma (M.)

■ **Incidence and veterinary significance**

The mycoplasms of veterinary importance parasitize the mucous membranes. They are found mainly in the respiratory and urogenital tracts, in the udder and joints and they exhibit a relatively strict host specificity. The most important mycoplasms isolated from animals are listed in table 94. The animal pathogenicity of the different species of mycoplasm varies considerably.

Mycoplasms of clinical importance are:
a) for cattle: *Mycoplasma mycoides subsp. mycoides* is the cause of contagious bovine pleuropneumonia, which affects cattle and water buffalo. Strains of this subspecies can be divided into 2 types (21, 75):
▷ SC (small colony) type: Characterized by slow growth (little turbidity in broth) and the formation of small colonies. Included in this type are all the strains of contagious bovine pleuropneumonia and some strains originating from goats which were affected mostly by polyarthritis or pneumonia.

■ **Allgemeine Eigenschaften und Bedeutung**
■ **Definition und Systematik**

Mykoplasmen besitzen keine Zellwand und sind sehr klein (kleinste Mikroorganismen, die sich selbständig und außerhalb von Zellen vermehren können), passieren bakteriendichte Filter, besitzen ein kleineres Genom und einen meist niedrigeren Guanin/Cytosin-Gehalt (22–40 mol%) in ihrer DNA als Bakterien (Tab. 93).

Die Klassifikation erfolgt aufgrund der Morphologie, kulturell-biochemischer und anderer Eigenschaften, s. Tab. 92 und Abb. 220. Innerhalb der Gattungen werden die einzelnen Arten nach ihren Stoffwechselaktivitäten und insbesondere nach der Antigenstruktur ihrer Membranoberfläche bestimmt (Wachstumshemmtest, Epifluoreszenztest).

1 Gattung: Mycoplasma (M.)

■ **Vorkommen und medizinische Bedeutung**

Die medizinisch wichtigen Arten leben als Schleimhautbewohner parasitär. Sie kommen hauptsächlich im Respirations-, Urogenitaltrakt, im Euter und in den Gelenken vor und besitzen eine relativ strenge Wirtsspezifität. Die wichtigsten vom Tier isolierten Mykoplasmen sind in der Tab. 94 zusammengestellt. Bezüglich der Pathogenität für das Tier bestehen für die einzelnen Mykoplasmaarten erhebliche Unterschiede.

Mykoplasmen von besonders großer klinischer Bedeutung sind:
a) für das Rind:
Mycoplasma mycoides subsp. mycoides ist der Erreger der Lungenseuche des Rindes und des Wasserbüffels. Stämme dieser Subspezies lassen sich 2 Typen zuordnen (21, 75):
▷ SC (small colony) Typ: Gekennzeichnet durch langsames Wachstum (geringere Trübung der Bouillon) und Ausbildung kleiner Kolonien, hierzu

Table 92: Classification of Mycoplasms (class Mollicutes, Order Mycoplasmatales)

Tabelle 92: Einteilung der Mykoplasmen (Klasse Mollicutes, Ordnung Mycoplasmatales)

Family	Genus	Properties	Occurrence
Mycoplasmataceae	Mycoplasma ca. 65 species	sterol-dependent digitonin-sensitive	man, animals
	Ureaplasma[1]	sterol-dependent urease-positive digitonin-sensitive	man, animals
Acholeplasmataceae	Acholeplasma 7 species	sterol-independent digitonin-resistant	man, animals
Spiroplasmataceae	Spiroplasma 3 species	spiral form, sterol-dependent digitonin-sensitive	plants and insects

[1] Because of their tiny colonies they were termed »T-mycoplasms«

[1] wurden wegen ihrer oft sehr kleinen Kolonien auch als T-Mykoplasmen bezeichnet (von »tiny«)

Table 93: Property differences of mycoplasms and bacteria

Tabelle 93: Unterschiedliche Eigenschaften von Mykoplasmen und Bakterien

Class	Mollicutes	Schizomycetes
Cell wall	−	+
Filterability (450 nm)	+	−
Size of genome	5×10^8 daltons	2.5×10^9 daltons
G & C ratio (mol%)	22–40	39–90
Membrane contains cholesterol	+[1]	−

[1] Exception Acholeplasms

[1] Ausnahme Acholeplasmen

Sheep strains rarely fall into this group.
▷ LC (large colony) type: Characterized by rapid growth (more pronounced turbidity of broth) and the formation of relatively large colonies. The majority of these strains originate from goats which suffer from pneumonia, conjunctivitis, arthritis, mastitis or abortion. Strains from sheep are less common. These strains do not cause contagious bovine pleuropneumonia.

Other points of difference:
SC types: proteolysis −, caseolysis −, low stability at 45 °C.
LC types: proteolysis +, caseolysis +, greater stability at 45 °C.

It is impossible to differentiate these types by serological means (growth inhibition test) (21).

It appears that under natural conditions cross infections do not occur between these two types, so that in areas free from contagious bovine pleuropneumonia LC types of mycoplasms are isolated from goats (20, 88).

Mycoplasma bovis is not an important species in Germany. Mastitis is the most important condition caused by this species (tab. 94), this is followed in frequency by pneumonia and arthritis of calves and young cattle and by abortion. In cows affected with

zählen alle Lungenseuchestämme des Rindes sowie einige Stämme von Ziegen, die hauptsächlich an Polyarthritis oder Pneumonie erkrankt waren, und seltener von Schafen.
▷ LC (large colony) Typ: Gekennzeichnet durch schnelles Wachstum (stärkere Trübung der Bouillon) und Ausbildung relativ großer Kolonien, die Mehrzahl dieser Stämme stammt von Ziegen, die an Pneumonie, Konjunktivitis, Arthritis, Mastitis, Verlammen erkrankt waren, und seltener vom Schaf. Diese Stämme verursachen keine Lungenseuche beim Rind.

Weitere Unterscheidungsmerkmale:
SC-Typ: Serolyse −, Caseolyse −, geringe Stabilität bei 45 °C,
LC-Typ: Serolyse +, Caseolyse +, größere Stabilität bei 45 °C.

Eine serologische Unterscheidung (Wachstumshemmtest) der Typen ist nicht möglich (21).

Unter natürlichen Verhältnissen bestehen zwischen beiden Typen offenbar keine wechselseitigen Infektionsbeziehungen, so daß es vorkommt, daß in lungenseuchenfreien Ländern von Ziegen Mykoplasmen des LC-Typs isoliert werden (20, 88).

Mycoplasma bovis ist für die BR Deutschland die klinisch wichtigste Mykoplasmenart. Unter den Erkrankungsformen (Tab. 94) steht die Mastitis im

mastitis, intra-uterine spread can infect the foetus where it remains latent to be transferred again during pregnancy to the next generation (79).

b) in the pig: *Mycoplasma hyopneumoniae*

Is the cause of enzootic pneumonia, which takes a relatively benign course if only mycoplasms are involved, but secondary infections (e. g. *Pasteurella multocida*) frequently complicate the picture. This is an interstitial pneumonia with peribronchial and perivascular lymphocyte infiltrations whereby the apical and cardiac lobes are most frequently involved.

c) in poultry: *Mycoplasma gallisepticum*

Cause of a usually chronic inflammation of the respiratory organs of fowls (98).

Mycoplasma synoviae causes not only bursitis and synovitis of fowls but may also affect the respiratory organs (98).

Mycoplasma meleagridis is the cause of mycoplasmosis of turkeys, leading to sinusitis, salpingitis, ovaritis, abnormal feather development and shortening and deformity of the bones, reduced hatchability (98).

Vordergrund, danach folgen Pneumonien und Arthritiden bei Kälbern und Jungrindern sowie Aborte. Die Infektion kann von an Mastitis erkrankten Kühen intrauterin auf die Nachkommenschaft übertragen werden und bei diesen über lange Zeit als oft latente Infektion bestehen und mindestens während der ersten Trächtigkeit erneut auf den Fetus übertragen werden (79).

b) beim Schwein:

Mycoplasma hyopneumoniae als Ursache der enzootischen Pneumonie, die als alleinige Mykoplasmeninfektion relativ gutartig verläuft, aber häufig sekundär durch Bakterien (z. B. Pasteurella multocida) kompliziert wird. Es handelt sich um eine interstitielle Pneumonie mit peribronchialen und perivaskulären Lymphozytenansammlungen und besonderem Befall der Spitzen- und Herzlappen der Lunge.

c) beim Geflügel:

Mycoplasma gallisepticum als Ursache der meistens chronischen Entzündung der Atmungsorgane der Hühner (98).

Mycoplasma synoviae, das neben Bursitis und Synovitis auch Erkrankungen der Atmungsorgane bei Hühnern verursachen kann (98).

Mycoplasma meleagridis als Ursache einer Mykoplasmose bei Puten mit Erscheinungen einer Sinusitis, Salpingitis, Ovariitis, abnorme Entwicklung des Gefieders und Verkürzung und Deformation der Knochen, Brutverlusten u. a. (98).

Table 94: Summary of the most important mycoplasms of animals

Tabelle 94: Zusammenstellung der wichtigsten bei Tieren vorkommenden Mykoplasmen

Animal host	Mycoplasma	Patho-genicity	Clinical signs or organs affected	Literature
Horse	equigenitalium	?	cervical canal, semen	57, 59, 62
horse	equirhinis	?	respiratory tract	4
horse	fastidiosum	?	respiratory tract	66
horse	felis (related-equipharyngis)	?	respiratory tract	4
horse	subdolum	?	cervical canal, aborted foetuses	59, 62, 67
Cattle	alcalescens	+	mastitis, arthritis nasal cavity, prepuce	49, 51
cattle	alvi	−	gut, urogenital tract	
cattle dog	bovigenitalium	+	mastitis, vaginitis, pneumonia, common inhabitant of urogenital tract	2, 12, 15, 22, 43, 80, 81, 85, 96, 99, 109
cattle sheep goat	arginini	?	respiratory tract pneumonia (calves) common in digestive tract of sheep	12, 65

Genus: Mycoplasma (M.)

Table 94: Continued — Tabelle 94: Fortsetzung

Animal host	Mycoplasma	Pathogenicity	Clinical signs or organs affected	Literature
cattle	bovirhinis	−	common resident of respiratory tract, also isolated from pneumonic lungs	11, 12, 35, 44
cattle	bovis	+	greatest clinical importance: mastitis, arthritis, pneumonia, abortion, besides latent infections of respiratory & urogenital tract (especially in young animals) in semen & conjunctiva	5, 10, 12, 14, 29, 32, 49, 79, 80, 83, 92, 93, 111
cattle	bovoculi	+	infectious bovine keratoconjunctivitis	36, 55, 64, 73
cattle	californicum	+	mastitis	50, 51, 54, 69
cattle	canadense	+	mastitis, arthritis, urogenital & respiratory tract	13, 40, 92
cattle	dispar	+	bronchopneumonia (calves)	35, 42
cattle	mycoides subsp. mycoides type SC	+	contagious bovine pleuropneumonia	21, 45, 75
cattle	verecundum	−	conjunctiva, prepuce	42
Sheep, goat	agalactiae	+	mediterranean countries mastitis, arthritis conjunctivitis	52, 53, 90
sheep goat	capricolum	+	acute febrile generalized infection, polyarthritis, mastitis	52, 53, 90
sheep goat	conjunctivae	+	keratoconjunctivitis	52, 74, 90
goat	mycoides subsp. capri	+	contagious caprine pleuropneumonia	52, 53
goat	mycoides subsp. mycoides type LC	+	sporadic diseases, arthritis, mastitis, pneumonia, conjunctivitis	21, 52, 78, 90
sheep	ovipneumoniae	(+)	pneumonia (lambs), often mixed infections with other bacteria	18, 52, 72
goat	putrefaciens	+	mastitis, arthritis	1
Pig	flocculare	(+)	pneumonia, respiratory tract	8, 33
pig	hyopneumoniae	+	enzootic pneumonia; often secondary infection with bacteria	37, 38, 70, 90
pig	hyorhinis	(+)	pneumonia, arthritis, serositis, often latent respiratory infections	19, 46, 91, 101
pig	hyosynoviae	+	polyarthritis, latent infection of tonsils & pharynx widely distributed	91

Table 94: Continued			Tabelle 94: Fortsetzung	
Animal host	Mycoplasma	Patho-genicity	Clinical signs or organs affected	Literature
Dog	cynos	(+)	pneumonia, respiratory, urogenital, digestive tract	19, 48, 87
dog	canis	(+)	pneumonia, respiratory, urogenital, digestive tract	16, 48, 89
dog	edwardii		urogenital, respiratory tract	16, 60, 89
dog cat	feliminutum		respiratory tract	
cat	felis	(+)	conjunctivitis, pneumonia urogenital tract	
dog cat	gateae		urogenital tract	16, 87
dog	maculosum		urogenital, respiratory tract	60, 61, 89
dog	molare		urogenital, respiratory tract	16
dog	opalescens		urogenital tract	16
dog	spumans	(+)	pneumonia, urogenital, respiratory tract	48, 60, 61
Pigeon	columbinum		respiratory tract	98
duck	anatis	?	sinusitis, respiratory tract	98
fowl	gallinarum		respiratory tract	98
fowl, turkey, pigeon, guinea fowl etc.	gallisepticum	+	chronic respiratory disease (CRD)	68, 77, 98
turkey	meleagridis	+	respiratory signs, air sacculitis, sinusitis, arthritis	98
fowl, turkey	synoviae	+	infectious synovitis, bursitis (bursa sternalis & tarsalis subcutanea) diarrhoea can occur	77, 98
Rat, mouse	neurolyticum	+	rolling disease	
rat, mouse	pulmonis	+	pneumonia	
rat, mouse	arthritidis	+	polyarthritis	

2 Genus: Ureaplasma

Ureaplasms are differentiated from mycoplasms by the formation of particularly small, »tiny« colonies (for this reason they were once termed »T-mycoplasms«), and by the breakdown of urea (tab. 92). On solid media they grow within 24 to 48 hours as granular to smooth colonies 5 to 50 µm in size. Ureaplasms are sterol-dependent. Various media have been described for their isolation. One method is described in figure 219.

Ureaplasms occur in cattle as latent infections of the urogenital tract, including the prepuce and semen (104), in the respiratory tract and on the conjunctiva. They have also been associated aetiologically with the following conditions:

Granular vulvitis, endometritis, salpingitis (25, 92, 94, 112), inflammation of the seminal vesicle (11, 105), pneumonia (39), keratoconjunctivitis (86).

They are frequently associated with other bacteria and mycoplasms and their pathogenicity is not yet absolutely determined (94). It appears to differ in the different strains (107). In regions where ureaplasms occur in cattle they have also been isolated from sheep and goats (9), pigs (100, 108) and other species (100, 108), but their pathogenic importance still remains uncertain.

2 Gattung: Ureaplasma

Ureaplasmen unterscheiden sich von den Mykoplasmen durch die Bildung besonders kleiner Kolonien (tiny = winzige Kolonien, deswegen früher auch T-Mykoplasmen genannt) und durch die Spaltung von Harnstoff (Tab. 92). Auf festen Nährböden entstehen innerhalb von 24–48 h 5 bis 50 µm große, granulierte bis glatte Kolonien. Ureaplasmen sind im Wachstum sterolabhängig. Zu ihrer Isolierung sind verschiedene Nährmedien beschrieben worden, eine Möglichkeit ihres Nachweises ist in Abb. 219 dargestellt.

Ureaplasmen des Rindes kommen im Urogenitaltrakt einschließlich Präputium, im Sperma (104), im Respirationstrakt und auf den Konjunktiven in Form von latenten Infektionen vor. Sie sind darüber hinaus mit folgenden Krankheitsbildern in ursächlichen Zusammenhang gebracht worden:

Granuläre Vulvitis, Endometritis, Salpingitis (25, 92, 94, 112), Samenblasenentzündung (11, 105), Pneumonien (39), Keratokonjunktivitis (86):

Sie kommen häufig vergesellschaftet mit anderen Bakterien und Mykoplasmen vor. Ihre Pathogenität läßt sich noch nicht eindeutig beurteilen (94) und scheint für einzelne Stämme unterschiedlich zu sein (107). Ureaplasmen sind ferner aus ähnlichen Lokalisationen wie beim Rind bei Schaf und Ziege (9), Schwein (100, 108) und anderen Tierarten (100, 108) nachgewiesen worden, ihre pathogene Bedeutung ist jedoch offen.

Table 95: The most important Acholeplasma occurring in animals

Tabelle 95: Die wichtigsten beim Tier vorkommenden Acholeplasmen

Animal host	Acholeplasma	Pathogenicity	Clinical signs and organ localization	Literature
Cattle, sheep pig, poultry	axanthum	–	various mucous membranes	12, 53
horse	equifetale	(–)	respiratory and urogenital tract, abortion	56, 58
sheep, goat, pig	granularum	–	various mucous membranes	
all domestic animals	laidlawii	(–)	environment (effluent), on all mucous membranes; especially urogenital and respiratory tract and udder. Mastitis	12, 27, 80, 89, 97
cattle	modicum	–	various mucous membranes	
cattle, sheep, goat, pig	oculi	(+)	keratoconjunctivitis genital tract	55, 106

3 Genus: Acholeplasma (A.)

This is a group of micro-organisms without cell wall which can grow in media without added serum or the cholesterol contained in the serum. Their properties and identification are presented in table 92 and figure 220. The species most important in animals are shown in table 95. They are better able to live outside the animal body (e.g. *A. laidlawii*) than members of the genus *Mycoplasma* and are not very pathogenic to animals.

4 Diagnosis of mycoplasma infections

It is fairly costly to present proof of a mycoplasma infection, because these micro-organisms are very demanding in their cultural requirements. The mere statement that mycoplasms have been demonstrated is of little clinical value, because many species are entirely or largely non-pathogenic, even if they are isolated from a pathological lesion. A further identification is therefore required in order to determine the probable pathogenicity of an isolate. Since this again is very costly and a multiplicity of sera are required for the serological identifications, this work can be performed only to a limited extent in the majority of non-specialist laboratories. It is advisable from the start to direct the diagnostic investigation at certain, clinically relevant mycoplasms as, for example *M. bovis* in figure 218 and to the mycoplasms occurring in the genital organs of cattle (fig. 219).

4.1 Morphology and staining methods

The absence of a cell wall and the enclosure of the cell by a thin, three-layered cytoplasmic cell membrane permit of considerable pleomorphism. The most common basic form is the coccoid (0.3–0.8 µm) but apart from these one encounters disc and filamentous elements, often exhibiting true branching. Mycoplasms have no flagella but they exhibit some form of movement as they glide along the surface of the medium.

Mycoplasms stain very poorly with the ordinary bacteriological stains, the best of these being the Giemsa method. The usual fixation procedures cause considerable distortion of cell form.

Diagnosis of mycoplasma infections

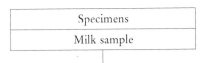

Cultural isolation of *Mycoplasma bovis*

1. Selective media:
    Mycoplasma broth: e. g. 16.8 g Bacto PPLO broth (Difco), 800 ml distilled water, 200 ml horse serum, 10 ml 50% yeast extract, 0.02 g DNA, 200 IU/ml penicillin. Mycoplasma agar: composition similar to broth, but instead of Bacto PPLO broth, 28 g Bacto PPLO agar (Difco), agar concentration 1%.
2. Inoculation of the media:
    Direct culture: one loop of milk is spread onto the mycoplasma agar.
    Culture after enrichment:
    1st tube (mycoplasma broth): addition of 0.2 ml milk (dilution 10^{-1}),
    2nd tube: addition of 0.2 ml of the dilution from the first tube,
    Isolation: After 3 to 10 days a plate is inoculated from each tube.
3. Incubation of cultures:
    Mycoplasma broth: 37 °C aerobic for up to 10 days
    Mycoplasma agar: 37 °C in CO_2 incubator (5% CO_2).
4. Interpretation of culture:
    The mycoplasma plates are examined after 2, 4, 6, 8 and 10 days with a dissecting microscope at a magnification of 40 to 80 times for the appearance of mycoplasma colonies, which take on a typical form (fried egg form)

Diagram of the procedure:

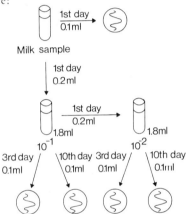

5. prepare pure culture: individual colonies are cut from the medium with a capillary tube and transferred to mycoplasma broth.
6. Differentiation of mycoplasma, see figures 221 and 222.

Fig. 218: Cultural isolation of *Mycoplasma bovis* from milk (110, 111)

Abb. 218: Kulturelle Isolierung von *Mycoplasma bovis* aus Milch (110, 111)

Präparate führt zu erheblichen Veränderungen der Zellform.

4.2 Cultural isolation of mycoplasms

The cultural method is of the greatest significance in the diagnosis of a mycoplasm infection. They require high quality, isotonic media because they are unable to synthesize certain compounds like cholesterol, fatty acids, some amino acids and certain components of their DNA.

High quality basic media to which yeast extract, horse serum, DNA and other substances have been

4.2 Kulturelle Isolierung der Mykoplasmen

Für die Diagnose von Mykoplasmeninfektionen spielt die kulturelle Erregerisolierung die wichtigste Rolle. Mykoplasmen sind auf hochwertige, isotonische Nährmedien angewiesen, da sie wichtige Verbindungen wie Cholesterin, Fettsäuren, einige Aminosäuren sowie einzelne Bausteine ihrer DNA selbst nicht synthetisieren können.

Um diesen Ansprüchen der Mykoplasmen zu

```
┌─────────────────────────┐
│       Specimens         │
├─────────────────────────┤
│     cervical swab       │
└─────────────────────────┘
```

1. Place cervical swab immediately into 2 ml nutrient medium of the following composition (transport medium):
   16.8 g PPLO broth Difco
   800 ml distilled water
   200 ml horse serum
   10 ml 50% yeast extract
   0.02 g DNA (Sigma)
   2000 IU penicillin/ml
   thallium acetate 1 : 100,000
   pH 7.8

2. Isolation of mycoplasma species
   Inoculation of solid media, composition see under (1) above, instead of 16.8 g PPLO broth use 28 g PPLO agar (Difco),
   a) direct inoculation from the cervical swab,
   b) dilution of the transport medium 1 : 10 with more of the same medium diluted and undiluted media are incubated at 37 °C for 4 days, the subcultured onto solid medium,
   incubation at 37 °C in CO_2 incubator (5% CO_2) up to 10 days,
   check with the stereomicroscope for the development of mycoplasma colonies at intervals of 2 to 3 days,
   serological identification of the isolated mycoplasma with the indirect immunofluorescence test, using unfixed mycoplasma colonies on agar blocks with antisera against mycoplasmas which can occur in the bovine genital tract, in particular M. bovis and M. bovigenitalium. The technique is given in figure 221.

3. Demonstration of Ureaplasmas
   Dilute the transport medium 1 : 10 and 1 : 100 with the following medium:
   250 ml Hanks balanced salt solution
   375 ml distilled water
   4.1 g Bacto brain heart infusion (Difco)
   4.35 g Bacto PPLO broth (Difco)
   9 g 1% solution dextran
   15 ml 50% yeast extract
   1.25 ml 1% solution phenol red
   150 ml horse serum
   100,000 IU/ml penicillin
   4 ml 10% solution of urea
   pH 6.5
   Incubation at 37 °C for 10 days,
   If ureaplasmas are present the colour changes to reddish-violet, check with 2 subcultures and discard bacterial growths

Fig. 219: Demonstration of mycoplasmas and ureaplasmas in the bovine genital tract (after WITTKOWSKI et al., 112)

Abb. 219: Nachweis von Mykoplasmen und Ureaplasmen im Genitaltrakt des Rindes (nach WITTKOWKSI et al., 112)

added, must be used in order to satisfy the requirements of the mycoplasms (example in figure 218). Mycoplasms require cholesterol for their growth (contained in the serum); acholeplasms do not (tab. 92).

Penicillin is usually added to the media for selective culture of mycoplasms. These are poured in small Petri dishes of about 6 cm diameter.

The material to be examined is spread onto the surface of the medium. Incubation at 37 °C should last about 10 days. Many mycoplasms will only grow, or grow better under micro-aerophilic conditions. It is advisable as a general principle to incubate primary cultures in an atmosphere with the CO_2 content increased to 5%.

The assessment of the colonies is done under the dissecting microscope with a magnification of 60 to 100 times. Mycoplasm colonies show a more or less dense, darker, granular centre which grows down into the agar and this is surrounded by a thinner lighter veil-like zone (fried egg form) (fig. 223, see

genügen, müssen hochwertige Basismedien benutzt werden, denen meistens Hefeextrakt, Pferdeserum, DNS und andere Substanzen zugesetzt werden (Beispiel s. Abb. 218). Mykoplasmen benötigen zum Wachstum Cholesterin (im Serum enthalten), Acholeplasmen nicht (Tab. 92).

Zur selektiven Züchtung der Mykoplasmen wird den Nährmedien meistens Penicillin zugesetzt. Die Abfüllung erfolgt in kleinen Petrischalen (∅ etwa 6 cm).

Das Untersuchungsmaterial wird auf der Oberfläche der Nährböden ausgestrichen. Die Bebrütung bei 37 °C soll mindestens 10 d dauern, viele Mykoplasmen wachsen besser oder nur unter mikroaerophilen Bedingungen. Allgemein empfiehlt sich bei der Erstkultur eine Erhöhung des CO_2-Gehaltes auf 5%.

Die Auswertung der Kulturen erfolgt unter dem Stereomikroskop (Vergrößerung 60- bis 100fach). Mykoplasmenkolonien weisen ein mehr oder weniger dichtes, dunkleres, granuliertes, in den Agar

page 320). The size of the colony ranges between 0.01 to 0.5 mm.

These colonies can be spotted more easily if they are stained with methylene azur blue after Dienes (2.5 g methylene blue; 1.25 g azur II; 10.0 g maltose; 0.25 g anhydrous sodium carbonate; 0.2 g benzoic acid, distilled water 100 ml; Merck). Agar blocks are excised for this purpose and placed onto a slide with the culture-bearing side uppermost. The staining mixture is poured onto a coverslip and allowed to dry. This is then lightly pressed onto the agar block so that the stain lies next to the colonies. The centre of the colony is deeply stained, the periphery is a lighter blue.

One can assume that mycoplasma colonies are present if: the typical colony picture is seen, there is no growth on serum-free media (acholeplasms are an exception), the colonies adhere to the medium and the blue staining of Dienes persists for at least 1 day.

For enrichment the isolation on solid medium can be preceded with a primary culture in a fluid medium. Examples of the culture procedures for *M. bovis* from milk and suitable media are presented in figure 218. Similarly examples are given in figure 219 for the identification of mycoplasms and ureaplasms occurring on the mucous membranes of the bovine reproductive tract.

4.3 Identification of mycoplasms

A number of different procedures are required in order to identify mycoplasms. The principles of this routine are shown in figure 220. However, abridged methods are used for an identification directed towards certain mycoplasms which are of clinical importance in that particular animal species (example *M. bovis*). Under such circumstances one can forgo the identification of family and genus. The following methods are of practical importance:
▷ Identification of the family: This relies upon the demonstration of the growth inhibiting effect of sodium polyanethol sulphonate or digitonin on *Mycoplasmataceae* (fig. 220); on the demonstration of cholesterol dependence, which is tested in serum-free media containing fatty acids, albumin and cholesterol (31).
▷ Identification of the genus *Ureaplasma*: Urea hydrolysis is positive. It is tested in media containing phenol red and 0.1 % urea, the colour changes within 24 to 48 hours from yellow to red (fig. 220). Ureaplasms grow as very small colonies of about 15 to 60 mm.
▷ Identification of species: A large number of test methods have been described (31), the following are of limited value: biochemical tests (tab. 96) which

include carbohydrate utilization; especially dextrose and mannose.

A suitable medium is mycoplasma broth with phenol red as indicator, additional sugar and horse serum (e.g. Difco supplement), pH 7.8 (29).

The hydrolysis of arginine is demonstrated in the following medium: mycoplasma broth with colour indicator phenol red and 0.2 % L-arginine, pH 7.0–7.3 (29).

Phosphatase activity: some mycoplasms have the ability to hydrolyze phenolphthalein diphosphate added to the medium (29).

Film and spot reaction:
This is tested on media containing horse serum and a yolk suspension and it takes advantage of the ability of mycoplasms to form films (cholesterol

Biochemische Prüfungen (Tab. 96);
Kohlenhydratverwertung: insbesondere von Dextrose und Mannose; Nährmedium: Mykoplasmenbouillon mit Farbindikator Phenolrot, Zuckerzusatz und Pferdeserum (z. B. Difco-Supplement), pH 7,8 (29).

Argininhydrolyse: Mykoplasmenbouillon mit Farbindikator Phenolrot und 0,2 % L-Arginin, pH 7,0–7,3 (29);

Phosphataseaktivität: einige Mykoplasmen sind in der Lage, dem Nährboden zugesetztes Phenolphthaleindiphosphat zu hydrolysieren (29).

Film- und Fleckenbildung (film and spot reaction), beinhaltet die Fähigkeit einiger Mykoplasmen, auf der Oberfläche von Nährböden, die Pferdeserum und Eigelbsuspension enthalten, Filme (Cholesterin

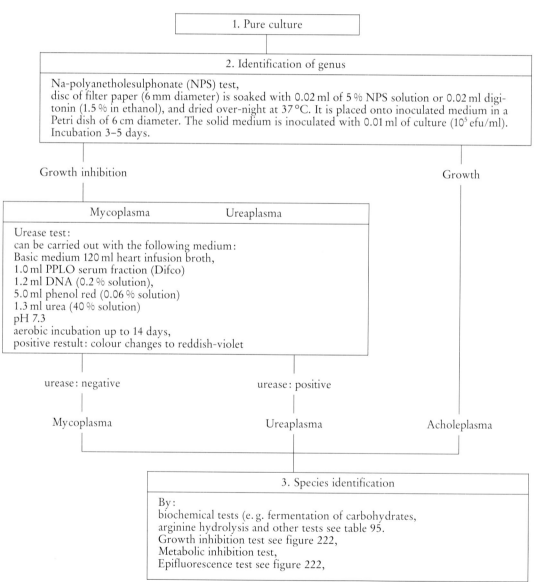

Fig. 220: Differentiation of mycoplasmas   Abb 220: Differenzierung der Mykoplasmen

and phospholipids) and spots (Ca- and Mg-salts of fatty acids) on the surface of the media (28, 29).

Reduction of tetrazolium chloride:
Various mycoplasms are able to reduce 2,3,5-

Table 96: Biochemical behaviour of the most important animal mycoplasms (after FREUNDT & RANZIN, 31)

Main host	Mycoplasma	Glu	Mns	Arg*	Pho*	F & S*	TTC-red* ae[1]	TTC-red* an[1]	Gel	Pro[2]
Horse	equigenitalum	+	+	−	+	+	−	−	−	−
	equirhinis	−		+		+	+	−	−	
	fastidiosum	(+)		−	−	+	−	−		
	subdolum	−	−	+		v	−	−	−	−
Cattle	alcalescens	−		+	+	−	−	−		−
	alvi	+		+	−		−	+		
	arginini	−	−	+	−	−	−	+		−
	bovigenitalium	−	−	−	+	+	−	+	−	−
	bovirhinis	+	−	−	v	−	+	+	−	v
	bovis	−	−	−	+	v	+	+		
	bovoculi	+	v	v	+	−	+	+	−	−
	californicum	−	−	−	+	−	−			
	canadense	−	−	+	(+)	−	−	+		
	dispar	+	+	−	−	−	+	+		
	mycoides subsp. mycoides	+	+	−	−	−	+	+	+	(+)[2]
	verecundum	−	−	−	+	+	−			
Sheep, Goat	agalactiae	−	−	−	+	v	+	+	−	−
	capricolum	+	+	v	+	−	+	+		+
	conjunctivae	+	+	−	−	−	(+)	+		−
	mycoides subsp. capri	+	+	−	−	−	+	+	+	+
	ovipneumoniae	+	−	−	−	−	(+)	+		−
	putrefaciens	+	+	−	+	+	(+)	+		−
Pig	buccale	−	−	+	+	−	−	+	−	−
	flocculare	−	−	−	−	(+)	−	(+)	−	
	hyopneumoniae	−	−	−	−	(+)	−	(+)		
	hyorhinis	+	−	−	+	−	+	+	−	−
	hyosynoviae	−	−	+	−	+	−	−		
	sualvi	+		+	−	−	−	+		
Dog	canis	+	−	−	−	−	−	+	v	
dog	cynos	+	+	−	+	+	(+)	+		
dog	edwardii	+		−	−	+	−	+	−	−
dog, cat	feliminutum			−	−	v	−	+		
cat	felis	+	−	−	+	+	−	+	−	−
dog, cat	gateae	−	−	+	−	−	−	(+)	−	−
dog	maculosum	−	−	+	+	+	−	+	−	−
dog	molare	+	+	−	−	+	+	+		
dog	opalescens	−	−	+	+	+	−	−		
dog	spumans	−	−	+	−	+	−	−		
Pigeon	columbianum	−	−	+	−	+	−	+		
duck	anatis	+	v	−	+	+	−	+		
fowl	gallinarum	−	−	+	−	+	+	+	−	−
fowl, turkey	gallisepticum	+	+	−	−	−	+	+	−	−
turkey	meleagridis	−	−	+	+	−	−	+		
fowl, turkey	synoviae	+	−	−	+	−	(+)			

* Arg = arginine hydrolysis, Pho = phosphatase, F & S = film and spot reaction, TTC-red = reduction of triphenyl tetrazolium chloride
[1] ae = aerobic, an = anaerobic; [2] LC types exhibit a more pronounced proteolysis

triphenyl tetrazolium chloride (29).

Proteolysis: Some mycoplasms can liquify coagulated serum.

Viewed as a whole, the utilization of biochemical characters permits only a rough screening. A more reliable species identification would have to rely on the epifluorescence test (fig. 221) and the growth inhibition test (fig. 222).

Diagnosis of *M. mycoides subsp. mycoides* infections: Pleuropneumonia is diagnosed by the necropsy findings and the cultural isolation of the organism. In the living animals this can be obtained from nasal secretion or blood and in the dead animal from the lung tissue. *M. mycoides subsp. mycoides* is relatively easy to grow aerobically at 37 °C (75). The media consist of high quality basic substrate (bovine heart extract) with the addition of 10–30 % ox or horse serum, yeast extract, preparations of DNA etc. (23, 75). Buffered viande ox serum (BVF-OS) is frequently used. Fluid or solid media will serve equally well. On solid media colonies of 0.2 to 2 mm develop after 3 to 5 days. After 107 hours incubation the colony diameter of is 0.99 mm for the SC type and 2.26 mm for the LC type (21). The colonies resemble a fried egg in shape. The identification can be made with the epifluorescence test.

1. From the mycoplasma culture on solid medium three square agar blocks (side 1 cm) are cut out with a scalpel and placed on a slide with the culture uppermost and glued to a glass slide.
2. M. bovis antiserum (from rabbits, diluted 1 : 50 with phosphate buffered saline is placed onto block 1 with a glass capillary. It is allowed to act for 30 minutes in a moist cabinet at room temperature. The unbound antiserum is washed off in two rinses with PBS and distilled water.
3. Goat anti-rabbit conjugate is placed on blocks 1 and 2 and allowed to react for 30 minutes at room temperature in a moist cabinet. They are then washed as under (2), and covered with a coverslip.
4. Examination under fluorescence microscope M. bovis colonies appear as luminescent spots on a green background. Magnification about 60 times. The specimens can be examined under transmitted UV light or transmitted polychromatic light (epifluorescence).

Diagram of the technique:

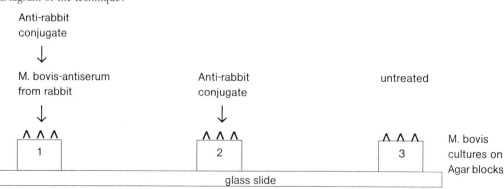

Agar block 1: specific identifiying reaction; agar block 2: control for nonspecific reaction between mycoplasma and conjugate; agar block 3: untreated control, autofluorescence

Fig. 221: Serological differentiation of mycoplasmas by means of indirect immunofluorescence, *Mycoplasma bovis* taken as example (24, 110)

Pure culture as starting material

1. Mycoplasma agar is inoculated with fluid culture in various dilutions
2. Discs of filter paper soaked in mycoplasma antiserum are placed onto the agar plate
3. If the antiserum is specific for that particular strain of mycoplasma, then during incubation the growth is inhibited immediately around the paper disc.
   The assessment is made with the dissecting microscope.

Test procedure in diagrammatic presentation:

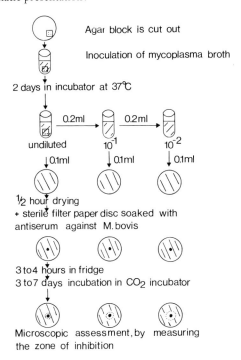

Fig. 222: Serological differentiation of mycoplasmas by the growth inhibition test, presented with the example of *M. bovis* (110)

Abb. 222: Serologische Differenzierung vom Mykoplasmen mit dem Wachstumshemmtest, dargestellt am Beispiel von *Mycoplasma bovis* (110)

Antibodies are demonstrated in infected animals with the complement fixation test.

Diagnosis of *M. hyopneumoniae* infections: Identification of the causal agent is rarely made, because it is difficult to interpret the stained bronchial smears (Giemsa, immunofluorescence) and cultural demonstration is too costly. Clinical and pathological findings are therefore of particular practical importance.

und für den LC-Typ 2,26 mm (21). Die Kolonien sind spiegeleiförmig. Die Identifizierung kann mit dem Epifluoreszenztest erfolgen. Antikörper sind bei infizierten Tieren mittels der KBR nachweisbar.

Diagnose der *M. hyopneumoniae*-Infektion: Der Erregernachweis wird selten durchgeführt, da der färberische Erregernachweis (Giemsa-Färbung, Immunfluoreszenztest) aus einem Bronchialabstrich schwer zu beurteilen und der kulturelle Nachweis sehr aufwendig ist. Deswegen sind klinische und pathologisch-anatomische Befunde von besonderer praktischer Bedeutung.

4.4 Serological diagnosis of mycoplasmosis

Serological methods have been used for the diagnosis of various mycoplasma infections, but these methods are less effective for the identification of infected individuals than for the recognition of the

4.4 Serologische Diagnose von Mykoplasmosen

Bei verschiedenen Mykoplasmeninfektionen sind serologische Methoden zur Diagnose benutzt worden, die Verfahren dienen dabei weniger der Diagnose am Einzeltier als der Bestandsdiagnose. Be-

disease on farms. Special efforts have been put into the following diseases:

▷ Enzootic pneumonia: Various reactions, like the agglutination, complement fixation, indirect haemagglutination and ELISA tests have been used but none have found general acceptance in routine diagnosis (3, 7, 30, 47, 84).

▷ Poultry mycoplasmosis: Tests like slide agglutination and the haemagglutination inhibition are employed especially in infections with *M. gallisepticum* and *M. synoviae* (68, 76, 77).

sondere Bemühungen betreffen folgende Krankheiten.

▷ Enzootische Pneumonie: Angewendet wurden verschiedene Reaktionen wie Agglutination, KBR, indirekte Hämagglutination, ELISA, die jedoch bisher keine allgemeine diagnostische Verbreitung gefunden haben (3, 7, 30, 47, 84).

▷ Geflügelmykoplasmosen, insbesondere die *M. gallisepticum-* und *M. synoviae-*Infektion, angewendet werden verschiedene Reaktionen wie Serumschnellagglutination, Hämagglutinationshemmungstest (68, 76, 77).

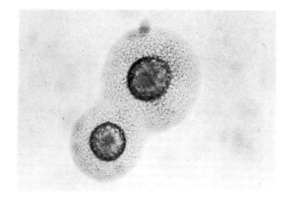

Fig. 223: Morphology of a mycoplasma colony. Magnification × 100. (Fig. 223 was supplied by Prof. Dr. H. Kirchhoff)

Abb. 223: Morphologie einer Mykoplasmenkolonie, Abb. M. 100:1. (Die Abb. wurde von Frau Prof. Dr. H. Kirchhoff zur Verfügung gestellt)

Bibliography / Literatur

1. ADLER, H. E., A. J. DAMASSA & D. L. BROOKS (1980): Caprine mycoplasmosis: Mycoplasma putrefaciens, a new cause of mastitis in goats. Am. J. Vet. Re. 41, 1677–1679.
2. AFSHAR, A. (1967): Granular vulvovaginitis of cattle associated with Mycoplasma bovigenitalium. Vet. Rec. 78, 512–519.
3. AKKERMANS, J. P. W., & W. K. HILL (1972): Complement fixation test in the diagnosis of enzootic pneumonia in pigs. Neth. J. Vet. Sci. 5, 53–59.
4. ALLAM, N. M., & R. M. LEMCKE (1975): Mycoplasma isolated from the respiratory tract of horses. J. Hyg. 74, 385–408.
5. ALLAN, E. M., T. U. OBI, A. WISEMAN, J. C. CORNWALL, I. E. SELMAN, P. M. MSOLLA & H. M. PIRIE (1978): The isolation of Mycoplasma bovis from pneumonic calves in Scotland. Vet. Rec. 103, 139.
6. ARMSTRONG, D. H., M. J. FREEMAN, L. SANDS-FREEMAN, M. LOPEZ-OSUNA, T. YOUNG & L. J. RUNNELS (1983): Comparison of the enzyme-linked immunosorbent assay and the indirect hemagglutination and complement fixation tests for the detecting antibodies to Mycoplasma hyopneumoniae. Can. J. Comp. Med. 47, 464–470.
7. ARMSTRONG, C. H., U. J. FREEMAN, L. L. SAND & D. O. FARRINGTON (1978): The enzyme linked immunosorbent assay (ELISA) for diagnosing mycoplasmal pneumonia of swine. Proc. Am. Ass. Veet. Lab. Diag. 21, 377–389.
8. ARMSTRONG, C. H., & N. F. FRIIS (1981): Isolation of Mycoplasma flocculare from swine in the United States. Am. J. Vet. Res. 42, 1030–1032.
9. BALL, H. J., & W. J. MCCAUGHEY (1982): Experimental production of vulvitis in ewes with a ureaplasma isolate. Vet. Rec. 110, 581.

10. BICKNELL, S. R., R. F. GUNNING, G. JACKSON & C. D. WILSON (1983): Eradication of Mycoplasma bovis infection from a dairy herd in Great Britain. Vet. Rec. 112, 294–297.
11. BITCH, V., N. F. FRIIS & H. V. KROGH (1976): A microbiological study of pneumonic calf lungs. Acta vet. scand. 17, 32–42.
12. BOCKLISCH, H., H. PFÜTZNER, W. ZEPEZAUER, U. KÜHN & H. LUDWIG (1983): Untersuchungen zur Mykoplasmeninfektion des Kalbes. 1. Mitt.: Mykoplasmennachweise bei Pneumonien und Arthritiden von Kälbern. Arch. exp. Vet. med. 37, 435–443.
13. BOUGHTON, E., S. A. HOPPER & P. J. R. GAYFORD (1983): Mycoplasma canadense from bovine fetuses. Vet. Rec. 112, 87.
14. BOUGHTON, E., & C. D. WILSON (1978): Mycoplasma bovis mastitis. Vet. Rec. 103, 70–71.
15. BRANNY, J., S. WIERZBOWSKI, I. ZGORNIAK & K. ROSLANOWSKI (1972): Studies on the occurrence of Mycoplasma in bull semen and experimental infection of heifers. Int. Kongr. tier. Fortpfl. u. Haustierbesam., München, Kongr.ber. 7, 337–341.
16. BRUCHIM, A., I. LUTSKY & S. ROSENDAL (1978): Isolation of mycoplasmas from the canine genital tract: a survey of 108 healthy dogs. Res. Vet. Sci. 25, 243–245.
17. BURCH, D. G. S., & R. F. W. GOODWIN (1984): Use of tiamulin in a herd of pigs seriously affected with Mycoplasma hyosynoviae arthritis. Vet. Rec. 115, 584–595.
18. CARMICHAEL, L. E., T. D. ST. GEORGE, N. D. SULLIVAN & N. HORSFALL (1972): Isolation, propagation and characterization of an ovine mycoplasma responsible for proliferative interstitial pneumonia. Corn. Vet. 62, 654–679.

19. CARTER, G. R. (1954): Observations of pleuropneumonia-like organism recovered from swine with infectious atrophic rhinitis and Glässer's disease. Canad. J. Comp. Med. 17, 413–416.
20. COTTEW, G. S. (1979): Pathogenicity of the subsp. mycoides of Mycoplasma mycoides for cattle, sheep and goats. Zbl. Bakt. I. Orig. A 245, 164–170.
21. COTTEW, G. S., & F. R. YEATS (1978): Subdivision of Mycoplasma mycoides subsp. mycoides from cattle and goats into two types. Aust. Vet. J. 54, 293–296.
22. COUNTER, D. E. (1978): A severe outbreak of bovine mastitis associated with Mycoplasma bovigenitalium and Acholeplasma laidlawii. Vet. Rec. 103, 130–131.
23. DAFAALLA, E. N. (1961): Solid media for the growth of Asterococcus mycoides. J. comp. Path. 71, 259–267.
24. DEL GIUDICE, R. A., F. ROBILLARD & T. R. CARSKI (1967): Immunofluorescence identification of mycoplasma on agar by use of incident illumination. J. Bact. 93, 1205–1209.
25. DOIG, P. A., H. L. RUHNKE & N. C. PALMER (1980): Experimental bovine genital ureaplasmosis. I. Granular vulvitis following vulvar inoculation. II. Granular vulvitis, endometritis and salpingitis following uterine inoculation. Cand. J. comp. Med. 44, 252–258, 259–266.
26. DOIG, P. A., H. L. RUHNKE, I. MACKAY & N. C. PALMER (1979): Bovine granular vulvitis associated with ureaplasma infection. Canad. Vet. J. 20, 89–94.
27. EBERLE, G., & H. KIRCHHOFF (1976): Untersuchungen über das Vorkommen von Mykoplasmen bei neugeborenen und durch Kaiserschnitt entwickelten Hunden. Dtsch. tierärztl. Wschr. 83, 495–497.
28. EDWARDS, D. G. (1950): An investigation of the biological properties of organism of the pleuropneumonia group, with suggestions regarding the identification of strains. J. gen. Microbiol. 4, 311–329.
29. ERNØ, H., & L. STIPKOVITS (1973): Bovine mycoplasmas: Cultural and biochemical studies. Acta. vet. scand. 14, 436–449, 450–463.
30. FREEMAN, M. J., M. LOPEZ-OSUNA, C. H. ARMSTRONG & L. SANDS-FREEMAN (1984): Evaluation of the indirect haemagglutination assay as a practical serodiagnostic test for mycoplasmal pneumonia of swine. Vet. Microbiol. 9, 259–270.
31. FREUNDT, E. A., & S. RAZIN (1984): Genus I Mycoplasma. In: Bergey's manual of systematic bacteriology. Vol. 1, S. 742–770. Baltimore, London: Williams & Wilkins.
32. FREY, M. L., G. B. THOMAS & P. A. HALLE (1973): Recovery and identification of mycoplasma from animals. Ann. New York Acad. Sci. 225, 334–346.
33. FRIIS, N. F. (1974): Mycoplasma suipneumoniae and Mycoplasma flocculare in comparative pathogenicity studies. Acta vet. scand. 15, 507–518.
34. FRIIS, N. F., & E. BLOM (1983): Isolation of Mycoplasma canadense from bull semen. Acta vet. scand. 24, 315–317.
35. FRIIS, N. F., & H. V. KROGH (1983): Isolation of mycoplasma from danish cattle. Nord. Vet. Med. 35, 74–81.
36. FRIIS, N. F., & K. B. PEDERSEN (1979): Isolation of Mycoplasma bovoculi from cases of infectious bovine keratoconjunctivitis. Acta vet. scand. 20, 51–59.
37. GOODWIN, R. F. W., A. P. POMERY & P. WHITTLESTONE (1967): Characterization of Mycoplasma suipneumoniae: A mycoplasma causing pneumonia in pigs. J. Hyg. 65, 85–96.
38. GOODWIN, R. F. W., A. P. POMEROY & P. WHITTLESTONE (1965): Production of enzootic pneumonia in pigs with a mycoplasma. Vet. Rec. 77, 1247–1249.
39. GOURLAY, R. N. (1968): The isolation of T-strains of mycoplasma from pneumonic calf lungs. Res. Vet. Sci. 9, 376–378.
40. GOURLAY, R. M., S. G. WYLD, N. F. S. BURKE & M. J. EDMONDS (1978): Isolation of Mycoplasma canadense from an outbreak of bovine mastitis in England. Vet. Rec. 103, 74–75.
41. GOURLAY, R. N., R. H. LEACH & C. H. HOWARD (1974): Mycoplasma verecundum, a new species isolated from bovine eyes. J. gen. Microbiol. 81, 475–484.
42. GOURLAY, R. N., & R. H. LEACH (1970): A new mycoplasma species isolated from pneumonic lungs of calves (Mycoplasma dispar sp. nov.). J. Med. Microbiol. 3, 111–123.
43. HARBI, M., S. M. EL-HASSAN & M. A. AHMED (1983): Isolation and identification of Mycoplasma bovigenitalium from imported semen of bulls. Vet. Rec. 113, 114–115.
44. HARBOURNE, J. F., D. HUNTER & R. H. LEACH (1965): The isolation of mycoplasma from bovine lungs and nasal swabs. Res. Vet. Sci. 6, 178–188.
45. HEINIKE, W. (1982): Auftreten und Liquidierung eines Herdes von Lungenseuche (Pleuropneumoniae contagiosa bovum) im Herbst 1980 in Frankreich (Ostpyrenäen). Mh. Vet. Med. 37, 818–819.
46. HEITMANN, J., & H. KIRCHHOFF (1978): Weitere Untersuchungen zur Ätiologie der Rhinitis atrophicans des Schweines. Berl. Münch. tierärztl. Wschr. 91, 382–385.
47. HOLMGREN, N. (1974): An indirect haemagglutination test for detection of antibodies against Mycoplasma hyopneumoniae using formalinized tanned swine erythrocytes. Res. Vet. Sci. 16, 341–346.
48. JANG, S. S., G. V. LING, R. YAMAMOTO & M. A. WOLF (1984): Mycoplasma as a cause of canine urinary tract infection. J. Am. Vet. Med. Ass. 185, 45–47.
49. JASPER, D. E. (1977): Mycoplasma and mycoplasma mastitis. J. Am. Vet. Med. Ass. 170, 1167–1172.
50. JASPER, D. E., E. ERNO, J. D. DELLINGER & C. CHRISTIANSEN (1981): Mycoplasma californicum, a new species from cows. Int. J. System. Bact. 31, 339–345.
51. JASPER, D. E., J. D. DELLINGER, M. H. ROLLINS & H. D. HAKANSON (1979): Prevalence of mycoplasmal bovine mastitis in California. Am. J. Vet. Res. 40, 1043–1047.
52. JONES, G. E. (1983): Mycoplasmas of sheep and goats: A synopsis. Vet. Rec. 113, 619–620.
53. JONES, G. E., A. G. RAE, R. G. HOLMES, S. A. LISTER, J. M. JONES, G. S. GRATER & N. RICHARDS (1983): Isolation of exotic mycoplasmas from sheep in England. Vet. Rec. 113, 540.
54. JURMANOVA, K., M. HAJOKOVA & J. VEDOVA (1983): Further evidence of the involvement of Mycoplasma californicum in bovine mastitis in Europe. Vet. Rec. 112, 608.
55. KELLY, J. I., G. E. JONES & A. G. HUNTER (1983): Isolation of Mycoplasma bovoculi and Acholeplasma oculi from outbreaks of infectious bovine keratoconjunctivitis. Vet. Rec. 112, 482.
56. KIRCHHOFF, H. (1979): Bestimmung von Acholeplasmen und Mykoplasmen aus abortierten Feten von Pferden. Berl. Münch. tierärztl. Wschr. 92, 504–506.
57. KIRCHHOFF, H. (1978): Mycoplasma equigenitalium, a new species from the cervix region of mares. Int. J. System. Bact. 28, 496–502.
58. KIRCHHOFF, H. (1978): Acholeplasma equifetale and Acholeplasma hippikon, two new species from aborted horse fetuses. Intern. J. System. Bact. 28, 76–81.
59. KIRCHHOFF, H., J. HEITMANN & W. BISPING (1980): Isolierung von Mykoplasmen aus dem Genitaltrakt von Stuten. Zbl. Bakt. I. Orig. A 246, 228–235.
60. KIRCHHOFF, H., A. BASU & M. LOH (1973): Mykoplasmen bei Hunden. Zbl. Vet. Med. B 20, 466–473, 474–490.
61. KOSHIMIZU, K., & M. OGATA (1974): Characterization and differentiation of mycoplasmas of canine origin. Jap. J. Vet. Sci. 36, 391–406.
62. KRABISCH, P., H. KIRCHHOFF & J. v. LEPEL (1973): Nachweis von Mykoplasmen auf Genitalschleimhäuten von Stuten. Dtsch. tierärztl. Wschr. 80, 493–495.
63. KUNZE, M. (1971): Natrium-Polyanethol-Sulfonat als diagnostisches Hilfsmittel bei der Differenzierung von Mykoplasmen. Zbl. Bakt. I. Orig. 216, 501–505.

64. LANGFORD, E. V., & R. H. LEACH (1973): Characterization of a mycoplasma isolated from bovine keratoconjunctivitis M. bovoculi sp. nov. Can. J. Microbiol. **19**, 1435–1444.
65. LEACH, R. H. (1970): The occurrence of Mycoplasma arginini in several animal hosts. Vet. Rec. **87**, 319–320.
66. LEMCKE, R. M. & J. POLAND (1980): Mycoplasma fastidiosum: a new species from horses. Int. J. System. Bact. **30**, 151–162.
67. LEMCKE, R. M., & H. KIRCHHOFF (1979): Mycoplasma subdolum, a new species isolated from horses. Intern. J. Syst. Bact. **29**, 42–50.
68. LIN, M. Y., & S. H. KLEVEN (1984): Evaluation of the microagglutination test in the diagnosis of Mycoplasma gallisepticum infection in chickens. Av. Dis. **28**, 289–294.
69. MACKIE, D. P., H. J. BALL & E. F. LOGAN (1982): Isolation of Mycoplasma californicum from an outbreak of bovine mastitis and the experimental reproduction of the disease. Vet. Rec. **110**, 578–580.
70. MARÉ, C. J., & W. P. SWITZER (1965): New species: Mycoplasma hyopneumoniae. A. causative agent of virus pig pneumonia. Vet. Med. **60**, 841–846.
71. MÉSZÁROS, J., T. STIPKOVITS, T. ANTAL, I. SZABÓ & P. VESZELY (1985): Eradication of some infectious pig diseases by perinatal tiamulin treatment and early weaning. Vet. Rec. **116**, 8–12.
72. NICOLET, J., A. TONTIS, M. SCHÄLLIBAUM, P. WÜTHRICH-PARVIAINEN, M. KRAWINKLER, P. PAROZ, G. BESTETTI & P. H. BOSS (1979): Beteiligung von Mycoplasma ovipneumoniae bei einer enzootisch auftretenden, proliferativen interstitiellen Pneumonie der Schafe. Schweiz. Arch. Tierhk. **121**, 341–353.
73. NICOLET, J., W. DAUWALDER, P. H. BOSS & J. ANETZHALER (1976): Die (primär) infektiöse Keratokonjunctivitis des Rindes. Mögliche ätiologische Rolle von Mycoplasma bovoculi. Schweiz. Arch. Tierhk. **118**, 141–150.
74. NICOLET, J., & E. A. FREUNDT (1975): Isolation of Mycoplasma conjunctivae from chamios and sheep affected with kerato-conjunctivitis. Zbl. Vet. Med. **22**, 302–307.
75. NITZSCHKE, E. (1985): Mycoplasma mycoides subsp. mycoides. In: H. BLOBEL & T. SCHLIESSER (Hrsg.): Handbuch der bakteriellen Infektionen bei Tieren, Bd. 5, S. 413–446. Jena: VEB Gustav Fischer.
76. NOUGAYREDE, P., D. TOQUIN, B. ANDRAL & M. GUITTET (1984): Depistage serologique des mycoplasmoses aviaires: agglutination rapide sur lame, inhibition de l'hémagglutination, inhibition metabolique, techniques appliquées au serodiagnostic des infections à Mycoplasma gallisepticum. Av. Path. **13**, 753–768.
77. OPITZ, H. M., J. B. DUPLESSIS & M. J. CYR (1983): Indirect micro-enzyme-linked immunosorbent assay for the detection of antibodies to Mycoplasma synoviae and M. gallisepticum. Av. Dis. **27**, 773–786.
78. PERREAU, P. (1979): Mycoplasmose caprine à Mycoplasma mycoides subsp. mycoides en France. Bull. Acad. Vet. France **52**, 575–581.
79. PFÜTZNER, H., & D. SCHIMMEL (1985): Mycoplasma-bovis-Nachweise bei Nachkommen von an M. bovis-Mastitis erkrankten Kühen und ihre epizootiologische Bedeutung. Zbl. Vet. Med. B **32**, 265–279.
80. PFÜTZNER, H., K. ILLING, D. SCHIMMEL, G. TEMPLIN & C. WEHNERT (1983): Untersuchungen zur Mykoplasmenmastitis des Rindes. 10. Mitt.: Prüfung von Mycoplasma bovis, Mycoplasma bovigenitalium und Acholeplasma laidlawii auf Euterpathogenität. Arch. exp. Vet. med. **37**, 361–374.
81. PFÜTZNER, H., D. SCHIMMEL & CH. WEHNERT (1981): Nachweis und Bedeutung von Mykoplasmen beim Bullen. Mh. Vet. Med. **36**, 673–677.
82. PFÜTZNER, H., & D. SCHIMMEL (1981): Nachweis und Bedeutung von Mykoplasmen beim Bullen. Mh. Vet. Med. **36**, 755.
83. PFÜTZNER, H., H. BOCKLISCH & V. ZEPEZAUER (1980): Nachweis von Mycoplasma bovis bei Pneumonien der Kälber. Mh. Vet. Med. **35**, 499–561.
84. PIFFER, I. A., T. F. YOUNG & R. ROSS (1984): Comparison of complement fixation test and enzyme-linked immunosorbent assay for detection of early infection with Mycoplasma hyopneumoniae. Am. J. Vet. Res. **45**, 1122–1126.
85. RAE, A. G. (1982): Isolation of mycoplasma from bovine semen. Vet. Rec. **111**, 462.
86. ROSENBUSCH, R. F., & W. U. KNUDTSON (1980): Bovine mycoplasmal conjunctivitis: experimental reproduction and characterization of the disease. Cornell Vet. **70**, 307–320.
87. ROSENDAL, S. (1978): Canine mycoplasmas: Pathogenicity of mycoplasma associated with distemper pneumonia. J. infect. Dis. **138**, 203–210.
88. ROSENDAL, S., H. ERNØ & D. S. WYAND (1979): Mycoplasma mycoides as a cause of polyarthritis in goats. J. Am. Vet. Med. Ass. **175**, 378–380.
89. ROSENDAL, S., & G. LABER (1973): Identification of 38 mycoplasma strains isolated from the vagina of dogs. Zbl. Bakt. I. Orig. A **225**, 346–349.
90. ROSS, R. F. (1985): Mycoplasma of sheep and goat. In: H. BLOBEL & T. SCHLIESSER (Hrsg.): Handbuch der bakteriellen Infektionen bei Tieren. Bd. 5, S. 345–373. Jena: VEB Gustav Fischer.
91. ROSS, R. F., R. WEISS & H. KIRCHHOFF (1977): Nachweis von M. hyorhinis und M. hyosynoviae in arthritischen Gelenken von Schweinen. Zbl. Vet. Med. B **24**, 741–745.
92. ROTH, B., G. WITTKOWSKI & H. KIRCHHOFF (1985): Nachweis von Mycoplasma canadense im Genitaltrakt einer Kuh in Norddeutschland. Zbl. Vet. Med. B **32**, 169–172.
93. SCHAREN, W., J. NICOLET, J. MARTIG & D. SCHIFFERLI (1983): Ein Ausbruch von Mycoplasma bovis-Mastitiden in der Schweiz. Schweiz. Arch. Tierhk. **125**, 129–136.
94. SCHIFFMANN, M., F. CLOUX, U. KÜPFER & J. NICOLET (1982): Ureaplasmen im Genitaltrakt des Rindes. Schweiz. Arch. Tierhk. **124**, 493–501.
95. SCHULLER, W., R. SWOBODA & W. BAUMGARTNER (1977): Vergleichende Untersuchungen über die Ergebnisse verschiedener nichtklinischer diagnostischer Verfahren zur Diagnose der enzootischen Pneumonie des Schweines. Wien. tierärztl. Wschr. **64**, 236–241.
96. SPECK, J. (1962): Vorkommen und Bedeutung von Mycoplasma laidlawii und Mycoplasma bovigenitalium im Genitaltrakt des Rindes. Mh. Tierhk. **14**, 244–256.
97. STEINER, A. (1982): Darstellung des Verlaufs und der ökonomischen Bedeutung der durch Acholeplasma laidlawii verursachten Mastitiden in einer Milchviehanlage des Bezirkes Magdeburg. Mh. Vet. Med. **37**, 863–864.
98. STIPKOVITS, L. (1985): Mykoplasmose des Geflügels. Mh. Vet. Med. **40**, 167–170.
99. STIPKOVITS, L., J. ROMVÁRY, J. MESZÁROS & J. RÓZSA (1979): Die Bedeutung der Mykoplasmen-Infektionen bei Krankheiten der Geschlechtsorgane des Rindes. Wien. tierärztl. Wschr. **66**, 52–56.
100. STIPKOVITS, L., A. RASHWAN, J. TAKACS & K. LAPIS (1978): Occurrence of ureaplasmas in swine semen. Zbl. Vet. Med. B **25**, 605–608.
101. SWITZER, W. P. (1955): Studies on infectious atrophic rhinitis. Am. J. Vet. Res. **16**, 540–544.
102. SWITZER, W. P. (1972): Mycoplasmal pneumonia of swine. J. Am. Vet. Med. Ass. **160**, 651–653.
103. TAYLOR-ROBINSON, D. (1979): Pathogenicity of ureaplasmas for animals and man. Zbl. Bakt. I. Orig. A **245**, 150–163.
104. TAYLOR-ROBINSON, D., M. THOMAS & P. L. DAWSON (1969): The isolation of T-mycoplasmas from the urogenital tract of bulls. J. Med. Microbiol. **2**, 527–533.
105. TAYLOR-ROBINSON, D., M. H. WILLIAMS & D. A. HAIG (1968): The isolation and comparative biological and physical characteristics of T-mycoplasmas of cattle. J. gen. Microbiol. **54**, 33–46.

106. TIWANA, J. S., & N. SINGH (1982): Isolation of Acholeplasma oculi from genital lesions in sheep. Vet. Rec. 111, 417.
107. TRUSZCZYŃSKI, M., & J. PILAZEK (1984): Differences in the pathogenicity for calves of ureaplasma strains depending on the site of their isolation. Zbl. Vet. Med. B 31, 701–706.
108. WAELCHLI-SUTER, R. O., P. A. DOIG, H. L. RUHNKE, N. C. PALMER & C. A. V. BARKER (1982): Experimental genital ureaplasmosis in the bull. Schweiz. Arch. Tierhk. 124, 273–295.
109. WEHNERT, C., H. KUTZER, W. SCHICK & H. PFÜTZNER (1983): Nachweis von Mycoplasma bovigenitalium bei Mastitiden des Rindes. Arch. exp. Vet. med. 37, 415–419.
110. WIENHUES, M. (1982): Verbreitung von Mycoplasma bovis in Norddeutschland unter besonderer Berücksichtigung seines Vorkommens in Kuhmilch. Vet. med. Diss., Hannover.
111. WIENHUES, M., A. TAOUDI, H. KIRCHHOFF & U. WEIGT (1984): Untersuchungen über das Vorkommen von Mycoplasma bovis in Milchproben von Kühen aus dem norddeutschen Raum. Berl. Münch. tierärztl. Wschr. 97, 311–313.
112. WITTKOWSKI, G., B. ROTH & H. KIRCHHOFF (1984): Nachweis von Mykoplasmen und Ureaplasmen im Genitaltrakt des Rindes. Berl. Münch. tierärztl. Wschr. 97, 189–197.

Appendix
Anhang

1 Abbreviations

Aci	acid
ADH	arginine dihydrolase production
Ado	adonitol fermentation
Aes	aesculin hydrolysis
Alk	alkaline
Amy	amylase production
Ara	arabinose fermentation
C	clotting
Cat	catalase production
Cel	cellobiose fermentation
Cit	citrate utilization
Dul	dulcitol fermentation
F	fermentation
Fru	fructose fermentation
Ga	gas production
Gal	galactose fermentation
Gel	gelatinase production
Glu	glucose fermentation
Gly	glycerol fermentation
Hae	haemolysis
H_2S	hydrogen sulphide production
Hip	hippurate hydrolysis
Ind	indole production
Inu	inulin fermentation
ip	intraperitoneal
iv	intravenous
Lit	litmus milk
Lac	lactose fermentation
Lec	lecithinase production
Lev	laevulose fermentation
LDC	lysine decarboxylase production
Mal	maltose fermentation
Man	mannitol fermentation
Mel	melibiose fermentation

1 Abkürzungen

A	Alkalisierung
Abb. M.	Abbildungsmaßstab
Ado	Adonitabbau
Amy	Stärkeabbau
Ara	Arabinoseabbau
ADH	Arginindihydrolasebildung
Äsk	Äskulinspaltung
Bew	Beweglichkeit
Cel	Cellobioseabbau
Cit	Citratverwertung
Dul	Dulcitabbau
F	fermentativer Abbau
Fru	Fructoseabbau
G	Gerinnung
Ga	Gasbildung
Gal	Galactoseabbau
Gel	Gelatinasebildung
Glu	Glucoseabbau
Gly	Glycerinabbau
Häm	Hämolysebildung
H_2S	Schwefelwasserstoffbildung
Hipp	Hippurathydrolyse
Ind	Indolbildung
Ino	Inositabbau
Inu	Inulinabbau
ip.	intraperitoneal
iv.	intravenös
Kat	Katalasebildung
Lack	Lackmusmilch
Lact	Lactoseabbau
Läv	Lävuloseabbau
LDC	Lysindecarboxylasebildung
Lez	Lezithinasebildung

Mlo	malonate utilization		M	Molkebildung
Mns	mannose fermentation		Mal	Maltoseabbau
Mot	motility		Malo	Malonatabbau
MR	methyl red reaction		Man	Mannitabbau
			Mel	Melibioseabbau
Nit	nitrate reduction		Mns	Mannoseabbau
			MR	Methylrot-Reaktion
O	Oxidation			
OF	oxidation-fermentation test		Nit	Nitratreduktion
ODC	ornithine decarboxylase production			
Oxi	oxidase production		O	oxidativer Abbau
			OF	Oxidations-Fermentationstest
P	peptonization		ODC	Ornithindecarboxylasebildung
PAD	phenyl alanine deaminase test		Oxi	Oxidasebildung
Raf	raffinose fermentation		P	Peptonisierung
Rha	rhamnose fermentation		PAD	Phenylalanindeaminase-Test
Sac	saccharose fermentation		R	Rötung durch Säurebildung
Sal	salicin fermentation		Raf	Raffinoseabbau
Sbs	sorbose fermentation		Rha	Rhamnoseabbau
sc	subcutaneous			
Sel	selenite reduction		Sac	Saccharoseabbau
Sor	sorbitol fermentation		Sal	Salicinabbau
			sbk.	subkutan
Tre	trehalose fermentation		Sbs	Sorboseabbau
			Sel	Selenitreduktion
Ure	urease production		Sor	Sorbitabbau
Vir	viridans reaction		TierSG	Tierseuchengesetz
VPR	Voges-Proskauer reaction		Tre	Trehaloseabbau
W	whey separation		Ure	Ureasebildung
Xyl	xylose fermentation		Vgr	Vergrünung
			VPR	Voges-Proskauer-Reaktion
			Xyl	Xyloseabbau

Evaluation of biochemical reactions

+	90 % or more strains react positively
−	90 % or more strains react negatively
v	variable result
v^+	variable, mostly positive
v^-	variable, mostly negative
(+)	weak and/or late reaction

Abkürzungen für den Ausfall kulturell-biochemischer Reaktionen:

+	90 % und mehr der Stämme reagieren positiv
−	90 % und mehr der Stämme reagieren negativ
v	unterschiedlicher Reaktionsausfall
v^+	unterschiedlicher Reaktionsausfall, meistens positiv
v^-	unterschiedlicher Reaktionsausfall, meistens negativ
(+)	schwach und (oder) verzögert positiver Reaktionsausfall
E	volle Empfindlichkeit
e	geringe Empfindlichkeit
R	Resistenz

2 Taxonomy and nomenclature of bacteria of veterinary importance

2 Systematik und Nomenklatur der veterinärmedizinisch bedeutsamen Bakterien

Source: Bergey's Manual of Systematic Bacteriology, Baltimore, London: Williams & Wilkins. Gram-negative Bacteria: Vol. 1, 1984, Gram-positive Bacteria: Vol. 2, 1986.

Quelle: Bergey's Manual of Systematic Bacteriology, Baltimore, London: William & Wilkins, Gramnegative Bakterien: Vol. 1, 1984, grampositive Bakterien: Vol. 2, 1986.

Family Familie	Genus Gattung	Species Art
	Gram-positive cocci	
I. Micrococcaceae	I. Micrococcus (9 species)	M. luteus M. roseus M. varians
	II. Stomatococcus	Sto. mucilaginosus
	III. Planococcus (motile)	Pl. citreus Pl. halophilus
	IV. Staphylococcus	St. aureus St. epidermidis St. capitis St. warneri St. haemolyticus St. hominis St. saccharolyticus St. auricularis St. saprophyticus St. cohnii St. xylosus St. simulans St. carnosus St. intermedius St. hyicus St. caseolyticus St. sciuri St. gallinarum St. caprae
	Streptococcus (29 species and others of uncertain classification, which are included in the list on the right)	a) pyogenic haemolytic streptococci b) oral streptococci c) enterococci d) lactic acid-forming streptococci e) anaerobic streptococci f) other streptococci
	Peptococcus (anaerobic)	P. niger
	Peptostreptococcus (anaerobic, 9 species)	Psc. anaerobicus Psc. indolicus
	Sarcina	S. ventriculi S. maxima

Family Familie	Genus Gattung	Species Art
	Endogenous spore formers Endogene Sporenbildner	
	Bacillus (aerobic, 34 species)	Bac. anthracis Bac. subtilis Bac. pumilus Bac. cereus Bac. stearothermophilus Bac. alvei Bac. larvae
	Clostridium, (anaerobic, 83 species)	Cl. bifermentans Cl. sordellii Cl. sporogenes Cl. botulinum Cl. histolyticum Cl. novyi Cl. perfringens Cl. chauvoei Cl. septicum Cl. difficile Cl. tetani
	Monomorphic non-sporulating, Gram-positive rods Gleichförmige, sporenlose, grampositive Stäbchen	
	Lactobacillus (44 species)	L. acidophilus
	Listeria	L. monocytogenes L. innocua L. welshimeri L. seeligeri L. ivanovii
	Erysipelothrix	E. rhusiopathiae
	Renibacterium	R. salmoninarum
	Pleomorphic, non-sporulating, Gram-positive rods Ungleichförmige, sporenlose, grampositive Stäbchen	
	Corynebacterium (16 species without plant pathogens)	C. diphtheriae C. pseudotuberculosis C. xerosis C. kutscheri C. renale C. cystitidis C. pilosum C. pyogenes (uncertain taxonomic position, see Actinomyces)
	Eubacterium	E. suis
	Actinomyces (10 species)	A. bovis A. israelii A. odontolyticus A. viscosus A. pyogenes
	Bifidobacterium (24 species)	B. bifidum

Family Familie	Genus Gattung	Species Art
	Mycobacteria Mykobakterien	
Mycobacteriaceae	Mycobacterium	M. tuberculosis M. africanus M. microti (M. muris, vole bacillus) M. bovis M. intracellulare M. avium M. phlei M. fortuitum and other atypical mycobacteria M. paratuberculosis M. leprae
	Nocardioform bacteria Nokardioforme Bakterien	
	Nocardia (9 species)	N. asteroides N. farcinica N. brasiliensis
	Rhodococcus (19 species)	Rh. equi
	Spirochaetes (Order Spirochaetales) Spirochäten (Ordnung Spirochaetales)	
I. Spirochaetaceae	III. Treponema (13 species)	Tr. pallidum Tr. hyodysenteriae Tr. innocens
	IV. Borrelia (19 species)	Bor. anserina Bor. recurrentis
II. Leptospiraceae	I. Leptospira	L. interrogans, parasitic leptospires with 19 serogroups and about 180 serotypes L. biflexa, free-living leptospires with 38 serogroups and more than 60 serotypes
	Aerobic/micro-aerophilic, motile, curved to coiled Gram-negative rods Aerobe/mikroaerophile, bewegliche, gebogene bis gewundene gramnegative Stäbchen	

	Campylobacter	C. fetus
		  subsp. venerealis
		  subsp. fetus (intestinalis)
		C. jejuni
		C. sputorum
		  subsp. bubulus
		  subsp. mucosalis

	Gram-negative aerobic rods and cocci Gramnegative, aerobe Stäbchen und Kokken	
I. Pseudomonadaceae	I. Pseudomonas (27 species)	Ps. aeruginosa Ps. fluorescens Ps. putida Ps. stutzeri Ps. alcaligenes Ps. mallei Ps. pseudomallei Ps. cepacia Ps. maltophilia

Family / Familie	Genus / Gattung	Species / Art
VII. Legionellaceae	I. Legionella	L. pneumophilia
VIII. Neisseriaceae	I. Neisseria	N. gonorrhoeae
		N. meningitidis
		N. canis
	II. Moraxella subgenus Moraxella	M. bovis
	subgenus Branhamella	M. (B.) catarrhalis (N. catarrhalis)
		M. (B.) caviae (N. caviae)
		M. (B.) ovis (N. ovis)
		M. (B.) cuniculi (N. cuniculi)
	III. Acinetobacter	Ac. calcoaceticus
	Flavobacterium (7 species)	F. meningosepticum
	Alcaligenes	Alc. faecalis
		Alc. denitrificans
	Brucella	Br. melitensis
		Br. abortus
		Br. suis
		Br. ovis
		Br. neotomae
		Br. canis
	Bordetella	B. pertussis
		B. parapertussis
		B. bronchiseptica
	Francisella	Fr. tularensis

Facultative anaerobic, Gram-negative rods
Fakultativ anaerobe, gramnegative Stäbchen

Family / Familie	Genus / Gattung	Species / Art
I. Enterobacteriaceae	I. Escherichia	E. coli
	II. Shigella	Sh. dysenteriae
		Sh. flexneri
		Sh. boydii
		Sh. sonnei
	III. Salmonella	S. choleraesuis
		subsp. choleraesuis (subgenus I)
		subsp. salamae (subgenus II)
		subsp. arizonae (subgenus III, monophasic, Arizona)
		subsp. diarizonae (subgenus III, diphasic, Arizona)
		subsp. houtenae (subgenus IV)
		subsp. bongori (subgenus V, Bongor group)
	IV. Citrobacter	Cit. freundii
		Cit. diversus (Cit. koseri)
		Cit. amalonaticus
	V. Klebsiella	K. pneumoniae
		subsp. pneumoniae
		subsp. ozaenae
		subsp. rhinoscleromatis

Family Familie	Genus Gattung	Species Art
		K. oxytoca
	VI. Enterobacter	Ent. cloacae Ent. sakazakii Ent. agglomerans Ent. aerogenes Ent. gergoviae
	VII. Erwinia	15 species
	VIII. Serratia	Ser. marcescens Ser. liquefaciens Ser. rubidaea (6 species)
	IX. Hafnia	Haf. alvei
	X. Edwardsiella	Ed. tarda Ed. hoshinae Ed. ictaluri
	XI. Proteus	Prot. vulgaris Prot. mirabilis
	XII. Providencia	Pr. alcalifaciens Pr. stuartii Pr. rettgeri (Prot. rettgeri)
	XIII. Morganella	Morg. morganii (Prot. morganii)
	XIV. Yersinia	Y. pestis Y. pseudotuberculosis Y. enterocolitica Y. intermedia Y. frederiksenii Y. kristensenii Y. ruckeri
II. Vibrionaceae	I. Vibrio (20 species)	V. cholerae V. metschnikovii V. parahaemolyticus

	III. Aeromonas	A. hydrophila
		A. caviae
		A. sobria
		A. salmonicida
		    subsp. salmonicida
		    subsp. achromogenes
		    subsp. masoucida

	IV. Plesiomonas	Ples. shigelloides
III. Pasteurellaceae	I. Pasteurella	P. multocida P. pneumotropica P. haemolytica P. ureae P. aerogenes P. gallinarum
	II. Haemophilus	H. influenzae H. haemoglobinophilus H. parainfluenzae H. pleuropneumoniae H. paracuniculus

Family Familie	Genus Gattung	Species Art
		H. parasuis H. paragallinarum H. avium
		Species incertae sedis: H. somnus H. agni H. equigenitalis
	III. Actinobacillus	Act. lignieresii Act. suis Act. equuli Act. actinomycetemcomitans
	Streptobacillus	Streptob. moniliformis
	Anaerobic, Gram-negative, straight or curved rods Anaerobe, gramnegative, gerade oder gebogene Stäbchen
I. Bacteroidaceae	I. Bacteroides (39 species)	Bact. fragilis Bact. vulgatus Bact. distasonis Bact. ovatus Bact. thetaiotaomicron Bact. uniformis Bact. melaninogenicus
	II. Fusobacterium (10 species)	F. necrophorum
	Anaerobic, Gram-negative cocci Anaerobe, gramnegative Kokken
I. Veillonellaceae	I. Veillonella (7 species)	V. parvula V. rodentium V. ratti
	Rickettsiae Rickettsien
I. Rickettsiaceae	Tribus I: Rickettsieae I. Rickettsia	R. prowazekii and other human pathogens of typhus
	II. Rochalimaea	R. quintana
	III. Coxiella	C. burnetii
	Tribus II: Ehrlichieae IV. Ehrlichia	Ehrl. canis Ehrl. phagocytophilia Ehrl. equi
	V. Cowdria	C. ruminantium
	VI. Neorickettsia	N. helminthoeca
	Tribus III: Wolbachieae VII. Wolbachia	3 species
	VIII. Ricketsiella	3 species
II. Bartonellaceae	I. Bartonella	Bart. bacilliformis

Family / Familie	Genus / Gattung	Species / Art
	II. Grahamella	Gr. talpae
		Gr. peromysci
III. Anaplasmataceae	I. Anaplasma	A. marginale
		A. centrale
		A. caudatum
		A. ovis
	II. Aegyptianella	Aeg. pullorum
	III. Haemobartonella	H. muris
		H. felis
		H. canis
	IV. Eperythrozoon	Ep. coccoides
		Ep. ovis
		Ep. suis
		Ep. parvum
		Ep. wenyonii

Chlamydias
Chlamydien

Family / Familie	Genus / Gattung	Species / Art
I. Chlamydiaceae	I. Chlamydia	Chl. trachomatis
		Chl. psittaci

Mycoplasms (Class: Mollicutes, Order: Mycoplasmatales)
Mykoplasmen (Klasse: Mollicutes, Ordnung: Mykoplasmatales)

Family / Familie	Genus / Gattung	Species / Art
I. Mycoplasmataceae	I. Mycoplasma (more than 60 species)	M. agalactiae
		M. alvi
		M. arginini
		M. arthritidis
		M. bovigenitalium
		M. bovirhinis
		M. bovis
		M. bovoculi
		M. californicum
		M. canadense
		M. canis
		M. conjunctivae
		M. dispar
		M. equigenitalium
		M. equirhinis
		M. felis
		M. gallinarum
		M. gallisepticum
		M. hyopneumoniae
		M. hyorhinis
		M. hyosynoviae
		M. meleagridis
		M. mycoides
		M. neurolyticum
		M. ovipneumoniae
		M. synoviae
	II. Ureaplasma	U. urealyticum
		U. diversum
II. Acholeplasmataceae	I. Acholeplasma	A. laidlawii
		A. granularum
		A. axanthum

Family Familie	Genus Gattung	Species Art
		A. modicum
		A. oculi
		A. equifetale
		A. hippikon
		A. morum
III. Spiroplasmataceae	I. Spiroplasma	4 species
	Anaeroplasma	2 species
	Thermoplasma	Th. acidophilum

3 Bacteriological stains
3.1 Dyes and staining solutions

The solutions for bacterial stains are seldom purely aqueous or purely alcoholic, but usually a mixture of both.

Aniline dyes

Basic dyes: methylene blue, fuchsin, safranin, malachite green, gentian violet, crystal violet and others.
Acid dyes: Eosin

Staining solutions
are made as dilutions of the stock solutions.
Stock solution: saturated alcoholic solutions
Staining solutions: 1 part stock solution : 9 parts distilled water

Mordants
can be added to the staining solution to increase the dye action (e.g. KOH, phenol).

Making up the stock solution:
10 to 15 parts of the dye in powder form is mixed with 100 parts of 96% alcohol in a brown bottle with well fitting stopper. This is shaken repeatedly to dissolve it quickly. After at least 2 days the saturated dye solution which overlies the undissolved sediment, can be passed through filter paper. It is preferable to allow the solution to stand for a longer time and pour off carefully as required.

3 Bakterienfärbungen
3.1 Farbstoffe und Farbstofflösungen

Zur Färbung von Bakterien werden meistens wässerig-alkoholische (selten rein wässerige oder alkoholische) Lösungen benutzt.

Anilinfarbstoffe

Basische Farbstoffe: Methylenblau, Fuchsin, Safranin, Malachitgrün, Gentianaviolett, Kristallviolett u. a.
Saure Farbstoffe: Eosin.

Farbstofflösungen
werden durch Verdünnung von Stammlösungen hergestellt.
Stammlösung: gesättigte alkoholische Lösung,
Gebrauchslösung: 1 Teil Stammlösung : 9 Teile Aqua dest.

Beizen
können zur Erhöhung der Farbstoffwirkung den Farbstofflösungen zugesetzt werden (z. B. KOH, Phenol).

Herstellung der Stammlösungen
In einer dicht verschließbaren braunen Flasche werden 10 bis 15 Teile des pulverförmigen Farbstoffes mit 100 Teilen 96%igem Alkohol übergossen und anfangs zur beschleunigten Lösung mehrfach geschüttelt. Frühestens nach 2 d kann die über dem Bodensatz befindliche, gesättigte Farbstofflösung durch ein Papierfilter gegossen werden. Besser läßt man die Lösung noch längere Zeit stehen und gießt bei Bedarf vorsichtig ab.

Most important staining solutions:

Fuchsin solution
    fuchsin stock solution   10 ml
    distilled water   90 ml

Carbol fuchsin solution
(for Ziehl-Neelsen stain)
    fuchsin stock solution   10 ml
    phenol (liquefied)   5 ml
    distilled water   100 ml

Carbol gentian violet solution
(for Gram stain)
    gentian violet stock solution   10 ml
    phenol (liquefied)   1 ml
    distilled water   100 ml

Dilute Lugol's solution
(for Gram stain)
    iodine   1 g
    potassium iodide   2 g
    distilled water   300 ml

Aqueous solution of malachite green
(for spore stain of Rakette)
    malachite green   5 g
    distilled water   100 ml

Methylene blue solution
    methylene blue stock solution   10 ml
    distilled water   90 ml

Aqueous solution of methylene blue
(for Köster's brucella stain)
    methylene blue   3 g
    distilled water   100 ml

Loeffler's alkaline methylene blue
    methylene blue stock solution   30 ml
    0.1 % potassium hydroxide   70 ml

Aqueous safranin
(for Olt's capsule and Hansen's brucella stains)
    safranin   3 g
    boiling distilled water   100 ml
    filter when cold

3.2 Staining methods

Only one dye is used in simple monochromatic staining, but in combined double staining methods several dyes act on the preparation either successively or simultaneously.

Rezepte wichtiger Gebrauchslösungen:

Fuchsinlösung
    Fuchsinstammlösung   10 ml
    Aqua dest.   90 ml

Karbolfuchsinlösung
(für Ziehl-Neelsen-Färbung)
    Fuchsin-Stammlösung   10 ml
    Acid. carb. liquef.   5 ml
    Aqua dest.   100 ml

Karbolgentianaviolettlösung
(für Gramfärbung)
    Gentianaviolett-Stammlösung   10 ml
    Acid. carb. liquef.   1 ml
    Aqua dest.   100 ml

Verdünnte Lugolsche Lösung
(für Gramfärbung)
    Jod   1 g
    Kaliumjodid   2 g
    Aqua dest.   300 ml

Wässerige Malachitgrünlösung
(für Sporenfärbung nach Rakette)
    Malachitgrün   5 g
    Aqua dest.   100 ml

Methylenblaulösung
    Methylenblau-Stammlösung   10 ml
    Aqua dest.   90 ml

Wässerige Methylenblaulösung
(für Brucellenfärbung nach Köster)
    Methylenblau   3 g
    Aqua dest.   100 ml

Alkalische Methylenblaulösung nach Loeffler
    Methylenblau-Stammlösung   30 ml
    Kalilauge (0,1 ‰)   70 ml

Wässerige Safraninlösung
(für Kapselfärbung nach Olt und
Brucellenfärbung nach Hansen)
    Safranin   3 g
    Aqua dest. (siedend)   100 ml
    nach Erkalten filtrieren

3.2 Färbemethoden

Einfache (monochromatische) Färbungen bestehen in der Anwendung nur eines Farbstoffes.
Kombinierte (Doppel-)Färbungen benötigen mehrere Farbstoffe, die entweder nacheinander (sukzessiv, sukzedan) oder gleichzeitig (simultan) auf das Präparat einwirken.

Brucella stains

Köster method
1. The heat-fixed preparation is stained with safranin-KOH (5 drops of a 3% aqueous safranin solution are added to 1.5 ml N KOH. This must be freshly prepared every time) for 1 minute.
2. Rinse with water
3. Decolourize 8 seconds in 0.05% H_2SO_4
4. Counterstain 8 seconds with 3% aqueous methylene blue
5. Rinse with water and blot dry.

Hansen method
1. Stain the heat-fixed preparation with Loeffler's methylene blue.
2. Rinse with water.
3. Counterstain 15–20 seconds with 3% aqueous safranin.
4. Rinse with water and blot dry.

In the Köster method the groups of brucellae are stained red, in the Hansen method they are blue.

Stamp method
1. Stain heat-fixed preparation for 5 minutes with carbol fuchsin solution, diluted 1:5.
2. Rinse with water.
3. Decolourize for 30 seconds in 0.5% acetic acid.
4. Rinse with water.
5. Counterstrain for 20 seconds with aqueous methylene blue.
6. Rinse with water and blot dry.

Stableforth method
1. Stain the heat-fixed preparation for 2 minutes with a dilute solution of carbol fuchsin (1 part carbol fuchsin to 2 parts of water).
2. Rinse with water.
3. Decolourize for 30 seconds in 0.5% H_2SO_4.
4. Rinse with water.
5. Counterstain for 10 seconds with 3% aqueous methylene blue.
6. Rinse with water and blot dry.

In the Stamp and Stableforth methods the groups of brucellae are stained red. These stains (modifications of Ziehl-Neelsen) have the advantage that they will also demonstrate chlamydias.

Fuchsin staining
Stain the heat-fixed preparations for 1 to 2 minutes.

Brucellenfärbungen

Färbung nach Köster
1. Hitzefixiertes Präparat mit Safranin-Kalilauge färben (5 Tropfen einer 3%igen wässerigen Safraninlösung zu 1,5 ml N KOH geben, muß für jede Färbung frisch hergestellt werden). Färbedauer 1 min.
2. Abspülen mit Wasser.
3. 8 sek in 0,05%iger H_2SO_4 entfärben.
4. 8 sek nachfärben mit 3%igem wässerigen Methylenblau.
5. Mit Wasser abspülen und im Fließpapierblock abtrocknen.

Färbung nach Hansen
1. Hitzefixiertes Präparat mit Loefflers Methylenblau färben.
2. Abspülen mit Wasser.
3. 15–20 sek mit 3%iger wässeriger Safraninlösung nachfärben.
4. Mit Wasser abspülen und im Fließpapierblock abtrocknen.

Bei der Köster-Färbung erscheinen die Brucellen als rote, bei der Hansen-Färbung als blaue Nester.

Färbung nach Stamp
1. Hitzefixiertes Präparat mit 1:5 verdünnter Karbolfuchsinlösung färben. Färbedauer 5 min.
2. Abspülen mit Wasser.
3. 30 sek in 0,5%iger Essigsäure entfärben.
4. Abspülen mit Wasser.
5. 20 sek mit wässerigem Methylenblau nachfärben.
6. Mit Wasser abspülen und im Fließpapierblock abtrocknen.

Färbung nach Stableforth
1. Hitzefixiertes Präparat mit verdünnter Karbolfuchsinlösung (1 Teil Karbolfuchsin und 2 Teile Wasser) färben. Färbedauer 2 min.
2. Abspülen mit Wasser.
3. 30 sek entfärben in 0,5%iger H_2SO_4.
4. Abspülen mit Wasser.
5. 10 sek nachfärben mit 3%igem wässerigem Methylenblau.
6. Mit Wasser abspülen und im Fließpapierblock abtrocknen.

Bei der Stamp- und Stableforth-Färbung erscheinen die Brucellen in Eihautausstrichen als rote Nester. Die Färbungen (modifizierte Ziehl-Neelsen-Färbungen) weisen den Vorzug auf, daß mit ihr gleichzeitig Chlamydien erfaßt werden können.

Fuchsinfärbung
Hitzefixiertes Präparat 1 bis 2 min färben.

Giemsa method

The stock solution is obtainable ready made up. It consists of azur II-eosin, Azur II, glycerol and methanol. For use the stock solution is diluted 1:1.
1. Fixation with methyl alcohol.
2. Staining for 20 to 30 minutes.

Gram method

1. A thin smear is made on a clean slide, heat fixed and allowed to cool.
2. Flood slide completely with carbol gentian violet, stain for 3 minutes and pour off the stain (do not rinse with water).
3. Counterstain with Lugol's iodine, 2 minutes.
4. Decolourize with alcohol while agitating the slide, until stain will just come off and the smear appears greyish-blue.
5. Counterstain for 15 seconds with dilute fuchsin.
6. Rinse and dry.

Foth capsule stain
(to demonstrate the capsules of *Bacillus anthracis*)
1. Air-dry and flood the unfixed preparation with 2 drops of Giemsa stock solution.
2. After 1 to 2 minutes add about 20 drops (1 ml) of neutral distilled water and mix by lightly tilting the slide back and forth.
3. Allow the stain to act for 2 to 5 minutes.

Olt capsule stain
(to demonstrate the capsules of *Bacillus anthracis*)
1. The heat-fixed preparation is flooded with a 3% aqueous solution of safranin and heated to boiling.
2. Allow the stain to act for 2 minutes.

Methylene blue staining

The heat-fixed preparation is stained for 5 minutes.

Loeffler's alkaline methylene blue method
(specially useful for demonstrating bipolarity)
1. Fixation with methyl alcohol, 3 minutes
2. Staining with Loeffler's methylene blue, 2 to 5 minutes.

Rakette spore stain

1. Fix the air-dried preparation by passing it 6–8 times through a flame.
2. Cover the slide completely with 5% aqueous malachite green, allow to act for 20 seconds, heat and allow to act for a further 30 seconds.
3. Rinse thoroughly.
4. Decolourize for 1 minute with 2.5% aqueous eosin (or dilute fuchsin).
5. Rinse and dry.

Giemsa-Färbung

Die Stammlösung wird fertig aus dem Handel bezogen und besteht aus Azur II-Eosin, Azur II, Glycerin und Methanol. Die Gebrauchslösung wird durch Verdünnung der Stammlösung mit Aqua dest. im Verhältnis 1:1 hergestellt.
1. Fixation des Präparates mit Methylalkohol.
2. Färbedauer 20 bis 30 min.

Gram-Färbung

1. Dünnen Ausstrich auf sauberem Objektträger anfertigen und hitzefixieren, erkalten lassen.
2. Objektträger vollständig bedecken mit Karbolgentianaviolett, 3 min färben, Farbstoff abschütten (keine Wasserspülung).
3. Nachfärben mit Lugolscher Lösung, 2 min.
4. Objektträger in Alkohol schwenkend entfärben, bis sich gerade noch Farbstoff ablöst und der Ausstrich graublau erscheint.
5. Nachfärben mit verdünntem Fuchsin, 15 sek.
6. Abspülen und trocknen.

Kapselfärbung nach Foth
(zum Kapselnachweis bei *Bacillus anthracis*)
1. Lufttrocknen, nicht fixierten Ausstrich mit 2 Tropfen Giemsa-Stammlösung bedecken.
2. Nach 1 bis 2 min etwa 20 Tropfen (1 ml) neutrales Aqua dest. zugeben und durch leichtes Hin- und Herneigen des Objektträgers mischen.
3. 2 bis 5 min färben lassen.

Kapselfärbung nach Olt
(zum Kapselnachweis bei *Bacillus anthracis*)
1. Hitzefixiertes Präparat färben mit 3%iger wässeriger Safraninlösung.
2. Erhitzen bis zum Aufkochen, 2 min einwirken lassen.

Methylenblaufärbung

Hitzefixiertes Präparat 5 min färben.

(Alkalische) Methylenblaufärbung nach Loeffler
(besonders geeignet zum Nachweis der Bipolarität)
1. Fixation mit Methylalkohol, 3 min.
2. Färbung mit Methylenblau nach Loeffler, 2 bis 5 min.

Sporenfärbung nach Rakette

1. Fixieren des lufttrockenen Präparats: 6–8mal durch die Flamme ziehen.
2. Färben: Objektträger vollständig bedecken mit 5%iger wässeriger Malachitgrünlösung. 20 sek. aufkochen, weitere 30 sek einwirken lassen.
3. Kräftig abspülen.
4. Nachfärben 1 min mit 2,5%iger wässeriger Eosinlösung (oder verdünntem Fuchsin).
5. Abspülen, abtrocknen.

Ziehl-Neelsen method
1. Cover slide with carbol fuchsin, heat until bubbles form and allow to act for 2 to 3 minutes.
2. Pour off (without rinsing in water), decolourize in 3 % hydrochloric acid alcohol until the preparation appears to be colourless.
3. Rinse with water.
4. Counterstain for 15 seconds with methylene blue.
5. Rinse and dry.

Assessment:
The background of the preparation must be distinctly light blue. The bacteria may be red or blue, depending on their reaction to acid. The red acid-fast bacteria are clearly differentiated from the blue background only when the colour differences from red to blue are quite distinct, but not if they are transitional, i. e. violet.

Ziehl-Neelsen-Färbung
1. Färbung mit Karbolfuchsin unter Erhitzen bis zur Blasenbildung; 2 bis 3 min einwirken lassen.
2. Abgießen (ohne Wasserspülung), entfärben in 3%igem salzsauren Alkohol, bis das Präparat farblos erscheint.
3. Abspülen mit Wasser.
4. Gegenfärbung mit Methylenblau, 15 sek.
5. Abspülen, abtrocknen.

Beurteilung:
Der Gewebsuntergrund des Präparats muß eindeutig hellblau sein. Die Bakterien können je nach ihrem Verhalten den Säuren gegenüber rot oder blau gefärbt sein. Nur wenn klare Farbunterschiede von blau und rot (nicht dagegen Übergangsfarben wie violett) vorhanden sind, heben sich die roten säurefesten Bakterien von dem blauen Untergrund deutlich ab.

4 Index

Only one integrated index is provided, because most of the headings are identical in German and in English:
■ Scientific names are printed in *italics;* they are the same in both the English and the German versions.
■ All other terms, in normal type, are either in German or English and refer to the corresponding text.

4 Sachverzeichnis

Da eine Vielzahl der Begriffe für den deutschen und den englischen Text identisch ist, sind beide Teile in einem Verzeichnis zusammengefaßt:
■ Die wissenschaftlichen Bezeichnungen der Erreger sind *kursiv* hervorgehoben und verweisen gleichermaßen auf den englischen und den deutschen Text.
■ Von den anderen – nicht kursiven – Stichworten verweisen die deutschen auf den deutschen Teil, die englischen auf den englischen.

Acholeplasma 312
Acinetobacter 209
Actinobacillus 124, 135
– *equuli* 137
– *lignieresii* 137
– *salpingitidis* 136
– *seminis* 136
– *suis* 138
Actinomyces bovis 101
– *israelii* 101
– *naeslundii* 101
– *odontolyticus* 101
– *pyogenes* 45
– *viscosus* 101
Aegyptianella 299
Aeromonas 124, 140
– *caviae* 141
– *hydrophila* 141
– *salmonicida* 143
– *sobria* 141
Alcaligenes 153
Anaplasma 299
Arizona group 177
Arizona-Gruppe 177

Bacillus alvei 77
– *anthracis* 72
– *cereus* 76
– *larvae* 77
– *megaterium* 78
– *mesentericus* 77
– *pumilus* 77
– *stearothermophilus* 78
– *subtilis* 77
Bacteriological stains 333
Bacteroides 263
– *fragilis* 263
– *melaninogenicus* 263
– *nodosum* 264
Bakterienfärbung 333
Bordetella avium 156
– *bronchiseptica* 153
Borrelia 278
Brucella abortus 247
– *canis* 258
– *melitensis* 247
– *ovis* 257
– stains 335
– *suis* 247
Brucellenfärbung 335

Brucellose, serologische Diagnose 252
Brucellosis, serological diagnosis 252

Campylobacter, aerotolerant 223
–, aerotolerante 223
– *coli* 226
– *cryaerophilia* 223
– *fecalis* 228
– *fetus subsp. fetus* 217
– *fetus subsp. venerealis* 217
– *hyointestinalis* 228
– *jejuni* 224
– *laridis* 226
– *sputorum subsp. bubulus* 218
– *sputorum subsp. mucosalis* 228
CEMO 241
Chlamydia 301
– *psittaci* 302
Citrobacter 169
Clostridium bifermentans 82
– *botulinum* 95
– *chauvoei* 82
– *difficile* 93
– *histolyticum* 82
– *novyi Typ A* 82
– *novyi Typ B* 88
– *novyi Typ C* 88
– *novyi Typ D* 88
– *perfringens* 82, 89
– *septicum* 82, 88
– *sordellii* 82, 93
– *spiroforme* 94
– *sporogenes* 82
– *tetani* 94
Corynebacterium 45
– *(Actinomyces) pyogenes* 45
– *bovis* 54
– *cystitidis* 49
– *(Eubacterium) suis* 53
– *kutscheri* 55
– *pilosum* 49
– *pseudotuberculosis* 50
– *renale* 48
– *(Rhodococcus) equi* 51
– *xerosis* 55
Cowdria 299
Coxiella burnetii 294
Coxiellose, serologische Diagnose 297

Coxiellosis, serological diagnosis 297

Dermatophilus congolensis 105

Edwardsiella ictaluri 185
– *tarda* 184
Ehrlichia 299
Enterobacter 189
– *agglomerans* 198
Enterobacteriaceae 160
Enterococci 28, 39
Enterokokken 28, 39
Eperythrozoon 300
– *suis* 300
Erwinia 197
– *herbicola* 198
Erysipelothrix rhusiopathiae 63
Escherichia coli 160
– –, Antigenic structure 161
– –, Antigenstruktur 161
– –, Enterotoxine 164
– –, Enterotoxins 164
– –, Neurotoxine 167
– –, Neurotoxins 167
Eubacterium suis 53

Flavobacterium 152
Foth capsule stain 336
Francisella novicida 213
– *tularensis* 212
Fuchsinfärbung 335
Fuchsin staining 335
Fusobacterium necrophorum 264, 272
– *nucleatum* 274
– *russii* 274

Giemsa-Färbung 336
Giemsa method 336
Gram-Färbung 336
Gram method 336

Haemobartonella 299
– *felis* 299
Haemophilus 232
– *avium* 238
– *haemoglobinophilus* 239
– *paragallinarum* 238
– *parahaemolyticus* 236
– *parasuis* 236
– *pleuropneumoniae* 236

– *somnus* 239
– *suis* 236
– *(Taylorella) equigenitalis* 241
Hafnia 191
Histophilus ovis 242

Kapselfärbung nach Foth 336
– nach Olt 336
Kauffmann-White-Schema 180
Kauffmann-White system 180
Klebsiella oxytoca 188
– *pneumoniae* subsp. *pneumoniae* 187

Lactis streptococci 29
Lactis-Streptokokken 29
Lactobacillis 69
Leptospira 277
– *biflexa* 277
Leptospirae, serogroups 278
Leptospira interrogans 277
Leptospiren, Serogruppen 278
Leptospirose, Agglutination 283
Leptospirosis, agglutination 283
Listeria innocua 58, 60
– *ivanovii* 60
– *monocytogenes* 56
– *seeligeri* 60
– *welshimeri* 60

Methylenblaufärbung 336
Methylene blue staining 336
Micrococcus 26
Moraxella bovis 158
– *(Branhamella) catarrhalis* 160
– – *caviae* 159
– – *cuniculi* 159
– – *ovis* 159
– *equi* 159
Morganella 197
Mycobacteria, atypical 108
Mycobacterium avium 108
– *bovis* 108
– *paratuberculosis* 119
– *tuberculosis* 108
Mycoplasma 306
– *bovis* 307
– *gallisepticum* 308
– *hyopneumoniae* 308
– *meleagridis* 308
– *mycoides* subsp. *mycoides* 306
– *synoviae* 308
Mykobakterien, atypische 108

Neisseria 157
Nocardia asteroides 103
– *brasiliensis* 103
– *caviae* 103

Ödemkrankheit 167
Oedema disease 167
Olt capsule stain 336
Oral streptococci 29
Oralstreptokokken 29

Oxidation-fermentation test 121
Oxidations-Fermentations-Test 121

Pasteurella 123, 124
– *aerogenes* 133
– *anatipestifer* 133
– *gallinarum* 133
– *haemolytica* 130
– *multocida* 126
– *pneumotropica* 133
– *ureae* 133
Planococcus 15
Proteus 195
Providencia 196
Pseudomonas aeruginosa 146
– *cepacia* 149
– *fluorescens* 149
– *mallei* 149
– *maltophilia* 149
– *pseudomallei* 151
– *putida* 149
– *stutzeri* 149

Rakette spore stain 336
Renibacterium salmoninarum 71
Rhodococcus equi 51
Rickettsiae 294
Rickettsien 294
Salmonella 171
Salmonellae, H-antigens 179
–, initial enrichment 175
–, O-antigens 177
–, Phase variation 180
–, selective media 175
Salmonellen, H-Antigene 179
–, O-Antigene 177
–, Phasenwechsel 180
–, Selektivmedien 175
–, Voranreicherung 175
Serratia 192
Shigella 182
Spirillum 215
Spirochaetes 277
Spirochäten 277
Sporenfärbung nach Rakette 336
Staphylococcus aureus 16
– –, Clumping factor 20
– –, Coagulases 19
– –, Enterotoxine 22
– –, Enterotoxins 22
– –, Hämolysine 19
– –, Haemolysins 19
– –, Hyaluronidase 20
– –, Koagulasen 19
– –, Nucleases 20
– –, Nukleasen 20
– –, Protein A 20, 21
– –, Reduction of tellurite 21
– –, Tellurithreduktion 21
– –, Thermonucleases 20
– –, Thermonukleasen 20
Staphylococcus epidermidis 26
– *hyicus* 23
– *hyicus* subsp. *chromogenes* 25

– *hyicus* subsp. *hyicus* 23
– *saprophyticus* 26
– *Streptobacillus moniliformis* 213
Streptococci, Bacitracin test 30
–, Aesculin hydrolysis 31
–, Antigenic structure 31
–, CAMP test 30
–, group E 37
–, group L 37
–, group P 37
–, groups R, S and T 37
–, group U 38
–, group V 38
–, haemolysis 30
–, Hippurate hydrolysis 31
Streptococcus 28
– *agalactiae* 33
– *bovis* 39
– *durans* 39
– *dysgalactiae* 34
– *equi* 35
– *equinus* 39
– *equisimilis* 38
– *faecalis* var. *faecalis* 39
– *faecalis* var. *liquefaciens* 39
– *faecalis* var. *zymogenes* 39
– *faecium* 39
– *pneumoniae* 40
– *uberis* 34
– *zooepidemicus* 35
Streptokokken, Antigenstruktur 31
–, Äskulinspaltung 31
–, Bacitracintest 31
–, CAMP-Test 30
–, Gruppe E 37
–, Gruppe L 37
–, Gruppen R, S und T 37
–, Gruppe P 37
–, Gruppe U 38
–, Gruppe V 38
–, Hämolyse 30
–, Hippurathydrolyse 31

Taylorella equigenitalis 241
Treponema hyodysenteriae 286
– *innocens* 291
Tubercle bacilli 108
Tuberkelbakterien 108

Ureaplasma 311

Vibrio 124, 139
– *anguillarum* 139
– *metschnikovi* 139
– *parahaemolyticus* 140

Yersinia enterocolitica 203, 257
– *frederiksenii* 206
– *intermedia* 206
– *kristensenii* 206
– *pseudotuberculosis* 200
– *ruckeri* 207

Ziehl-Neelsen-Färbung 337
Ziehl-Neelsen method 337

Veterinärmedizinische Parasitologie

Von Prof. Dr. Dr. h. c. J. Boch, München, und Prof. Dr. R. Supperer, Wien. Unter Mitarbeit von Prof. Dr. J. Eckert, Zürich, Prof. Dr. E. Kutzer, Wien, und Prof. Dr. M. Rommel, Hannover. 3., völlig neubearb. Aufl. 1983. 552 S. mit 192 Abb. und 28 Tab. Gebunden DM 98,–
ISBN 3-489-66116-8

Atlas zur Hämatologie von Hund und Katze

Von Dr. P. Keller, Basel, und Prof. Dr. U. Freudiger, Bern. 1983. 160 S. mit 284 Abb. in 665 Einzeldarst., davon 381 farbig, einer schem. Zeichnung und 2 Tab. Gebunden DM 218,–
ISBN 3-489-65516-8

Handbuch der Schutzimpfungen in der Tiermedizin

Ein Lehr- und Handbuch der prophylaktischen Infektionsmedizin, der allgemeinen und speziellen Tierseuchenbekämpfung, der Populationsmedizin sowie der Immunologie und der Impfstoffherstellung.
Von Prof. Dr. Dr. h. c. A. Mayr, München, Prof. Dr. G. Eißner, Tübingen, und Prof. Dr. B. Mayr-Bibrack, München. 1984. 1026 S. mit 160 teilw. farb. Abb., davon 50 auf 8 Farbtaf. Gebunden DM 198,–
ISBN 3-489-66416-7

Lehrbuch der Veterinär-Physiologie

Begründet von A. Scheunert und A. Trautmann. Herausgegeben von Prof. Dr. Günter Wittke, Inst. für Veterinär-Physiologie, -Biochemie, -Pharmakologie und -Toxikologie der Freien Universität Berlin. Unter Mitarbeit von Prof. Dr. E. Bamberg, Wien, Prof. Dr. Dr. h. c. K. Bronsch, Berlin, Prof. Dr. H. Eder, Gießen, Dr. M. Fromm, Berlin, Prof. Dr. J. Gropp, München, Prof. Dr. med. K. H. Hierholzer, Berlin, Prof. Dr. H. Hörnicke, Stuttgart, Prof. Dr. G. Hofecker, Wien, Dr. K. Männer, Berlin, Prof. Dr. E. Pfeffer, Bonn, Prof. Dr. E. Scharrer, Zürich, Prof. Dr. Dr. h. c. H. Spörri, Zürich, Prof. Dr. A. Wels, Gießen, Prof. Dr. G. Wittke, Berlin, Prof. Dr. K. Zerobin, Zürich sowie Prof. Dr. H. Zucker, München.
7., völlig neubearbeitete Auflage. 1987. 739 Seiten mit 418 Abbildungen, davon 2 farbig auf 2 Tafeln sowie 116 Tabellen. Gebunden. DM 198,–
ISBN 3-489-66216-4

Grundlagen der Fischpathologie

Mit einer Einführug in die Anatomie, Physiologie, Pathophysiologie und Immunologie sowie in den aquatischen Lebensraum der Knochenfische.
Hrs. von Prof. Dr. R. J. Roberts, Glasgow. Übers., bearb. und erg. von Fachtierarzt für Fische Dr. H.-J. Schlotfeldt, Hannover. 1985. 425 S. mit 348 Abb., davon 67 farb. auf 9 Taf., und 48 Tab. Gebunden DM 198,–
ISBN 3-489-62516-1

Morphological and Epidemiological Aspects of Simian Herpesvirus Infections

By Dr. M. Brack, Göttingen. 1977. 63 pp. with 1 tab. Soft cover DM 24,–
(Versuchstierkunde, Heft 5)
ISBN 3-489-75518-9

Preise: Stand Juni 1988

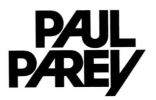 Berlin und Hamburg

Pareys Studientexte

45 Kompendium der veterinärmedizinischen Bakteriologie
Von Prof. Dr. J. Nicolet, Bern. 1985. 280 S. mit 26 Abb. und 71 Tab. Kartoniert DM 38,–
ISBN 3-489-69416-3
In diesem Kompendium werden neben den grundlegenden Kenntnissen die Entwicklungen aus dem Gebiete der veterinärmedizinischen Bakteriologie dargestellt, indem ein übersichtliches Bild der Hauptgruppen der pathogenen Erreger, ihrer Biologie und ihrer Wechselbeziehungen zu Wirt und Umwelt vermittelt wird. Für die Studierenden als Grundlage für die Vorlesung und für praktizierende Tierärzte als Hilfsmittel bei der Beurteilung mikrobiologischer Situationen.

19 Kompendium der allgemeinen medizinischen Bakteriologie
Von Prof. Dr. H. Fey, Bern. 1978. 227 S. mit 77 Abb. und 13 Tab. Kartoniert DM 28,–
ISBN 3-489-61516-6

54 Toxikologisch-hygienische Beurteilung von Lebensmittelinhalts- und -zusatzstoffen sowie bedenklicher Verunreinigungen
Von Prof. Dr. H.-G. Classen, Stuttgart, Prof. Dr. P. S. Elias, Karlsruhe, Prof. Dr. W. P. Hammes, Stuttgart. 1987. 285 S. mit 16 Abb. und 51 Tab. Kartoniert DM 39,80
ISBN 3-489-62514-5
Eine Sammlung von Basisdaten über Wirkungen und Risiken aus dem Verzehr von Lebensmitteln. Die verwendeten biologischen Modelle werden unter hygienischen und toxikologischen Aspekten der Lebensmittelsicherheit ausführlich beschrieben, um Möglichkeiten und Grenzen der Vorhersage und Erfassung gesundheitlicher Risiken zu erkennen. Das abschließende Kapitel enthält eine Übersicht gesetzlich festgelegter Höchstmengen für Kontaminanten und ähnliche Stoffe sowie Richtwerte und Empfehlungen.

20 Kompendium der allgemeinen Immunologie
Von Dr. R. v. Fellenberg, Zürich. 1978. 201 S. mit 64 Abb. und 21 Tab., 2 Anhängen mit 28 Tab. Kartoniert DM 29,–
ISBN 3-489-61416-X

25 Kompendium der medizinischen Mykologie
Von Prof. Dr. B. Gedek, München. 1980. 395 S. mit 195 Abb., davon 8 farbig, und 34 Tab. Kartoniert DM 48,–
ISBN 3-489-62816-0

4 Kompendium der allgemeinen Virologie
Von Prof. Dr. M. C. Horzinek, Utrecht. Unter Mitarbeit von Dr. B. A. M. van d. Zeijst, Utrecht, und Prof. Dr. J. van d. Want, Wageningen. 2., neubearb. Aufl. 1985. 159 S. mit 86 Abb. und 16 Tab. Kartoniert DM 29,–
ISBN 3-489-68116-9
Zugleich mit dem gesicherten Wissensgut der allgemeinen Virologie vermittelt das Buch die Grundlagen für das Verständnis von Viruskrankheiten bei Mensch, Tier und Pflanze. Im Mittelpunkt der Betrachtung steht das Virus als infektiöse Einheit, als Krankheitserreger und als Seuchenursache.

30 Einführung in die veterinärmedizinische Immunologie
Für Tiermediziner, Biologen und Agrarwissenschaftler. Von Prof. I. R. Tizard, Ontario/Canada. Bearb. und übers. von Prof. Dr. H. G. Buschmann, München. 1981. 363 S. mit 161 Abb. und 52 Tab. Kartoniert DM 19,80
ISBN 3-489-62416-5

53 Rückstände in von Tieren stammenden Lebensmitteln
Von Prof. Dr. D. Großklaus, Berlin. In Vorbereitung
ISBN 3-489-62414-9

Journal of Veterinary Medicine
Zentralblatt für Veterinärmedizin

Series B: Infectious Diseases, Immunology, Food Hygiene, Veterinary Public Health.

This journal includes reports on topics in epidemiology, pathogenesis, diagnostic techniques, laboratory methods, application of chemotherapy and vaccines to infectious and parasitic diseases. It is of equal importance to the researcher, teacher, pharmaceutical industry, and governmental institutions. The Journal of Veterinary Medicine Series B is unique in its complete coverage of all aspects of veterinary microbiology and parasitology.

A supplement series "Advances in Veterinary Medicine" is being published in irregular sequence.

Hrsg. Prof. Dr. Dr. h. c. A. Mayr, München; Prof. Dr. E. Scharrer, Zürich; Prof. Dr. Dr. h. c. H. Spörri, Zürich; Prof. Dr. E. G. White, Merseyside.

Erscheinungsweise: Jährlich 10 Hefte, die jeweils einen Band bilden. Jedes Heft umfaßt etwa $5^{1}/_{2}$ Druckbogen à 16 Seiten. Abonnementspreis 1988: DM 998,– zzgl. Versandkosten.

Reihe B: ISSN 0931-1793

Berliner und Münchener Tierärztliche Wochenschrift

Hrsg. Prof. Dr. W. Bisping, Hannover; Prof. Dr. H. Elkmeier, Gießen; Prof. Dr. M. Merkenschlager, München; Prof. Dr. H.-J. Sinell, Berlin; Prof. Dr. H.-J. Wintzer, Berlin.

Erscheinungsweise: monatlich, Umfang je Heft 36 Seiten, zzgl. Umschlag, im Format DIN A 4, Abonnementspreis 1988 DM 338,– zzgl. Versandkosten. Studenten und Praktikanten in nicht vollbezahlter Stellung erhalten gegen entsprechenden Nachweis auf das Jahresabonnement eine Ermäßigung von 20 % auf den Abonnementspreis.
ISSN 0005-9366

Preise: Stand Juni 1988

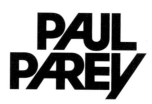

Berlin und Hamburg